Second Edition

Pharmacy Practice Manual:
A Guide to the Clinical Experience

Second Edition

Pharmacy Practice Manual: A Guide to the Clinical Experience

Editor

Larry E. Boh, M.S., R.Ph.

Professor and Chair
University of Wisconsin School of Pharmacy
Madison, Wisconsin

Consulting Editor

Lloyd Y. Young, Pharm.D.

Professor and Chair
Department of Clinical Pharmacy
Thomas A. Oliver Endowed Chair in Clinical Pharmacy
School of Pharmacy
University of California, San Francisco
San Francisco, California

Editor: Daniel Limmer
Managing Editor: Matthew J. Hauber
Marketing Manager: Anne E.P. Smith
Production Editor: Paula C. Williams
Compositor: Maryland Composition, Inc.
Printer: R.R. Donnelley & Sons Company

Printed in the United States of America

Library of Congress Cataloging-in-Publication Data

Pharmacy practice manual : a guide to the clinical experience / editor, Larry E. Boh, consulting editor, Lloyd Y. Young.—2nd ed.
   p. ; cm.
  Rev. ed. of: Clinical clerkship manual / edited by Larry E. Boh, c1993.
  Includes bibliographical references and index.
  ISBN 0-7817-2541-0
    1. Pharmacy—Practice—Handbooks, manuals, etc. 2. Hospital pharmacies—Handbooks, manuals, etc. I. Boh, Larry E. II. Young, Lloyd Y. III. Clinical clerkship manual.
  [DNLM: 1. Pharmacy Services, Hospital—Handbooks. 2. Clinical Clerkship—Handbooks. 3. Pharmacy—Handbooks. QV 735 P5365 2001]
  RS122.5 .P83 2001
  615.1—dc21

                                               00-067322

01 02 03 04 05

1 2 3 4 5 6 7 8 9 10

Preface

Pharmacy practice has evolved rapidly over the past several decades from a practice that primarily focused on the preparation of medication to one that emphasizes rational pharmacotherapeutics in patients. During this time, pharmacy education has moved forward to incorporate these changes and make more coursework available in the clinical pharmacotherapy laboratory and experiential practice setting to improve students' understanding and appreciation of the application of pharmacotherapy in patients.

Development of the first manual (*Clinical Clerkship Manual*) was done primarily through the work of my colleagues at the University of Wisconsin Hospital and Clinics. The goal of this first manual was to provide the novice clinical practitioner with a reference source during the first few weeks of an introductory clerkship experience, which may have occurred either in the pharmacotherapy laboratory or patient care setting. This manual was well received by our students and others throughout the United States, as it helped to alleviate some of the anxiety and uncertainty during this challenging and exciting time in pharmacy education. It also helped to establish a clear code of conduct for our students and stated expectations for their responsibilities to patients primarily in the acute care setting.

It is from a unique perspective as a patient with a recent serious chronic illness that I approached the first revision of this manual. This challenge provided me with an understanding of the difficulty that our patients often encounter in today's constantly changing health care system. As educators and students, we must always remember that each patient has his or her own unique set of needs and concerns. They may not be identical to the expectations that we have for them, but we must constantly look beyond the diagnosis and laboratory value.

With this Second Edition, we introduce a new title, *Pharmacy Practice Manual: A Guide to the Clinical Experience*. This edition expands on the breadth and depth of pharmacy practice to include not only acute care, but also ambulatory, geriatric, and other issues often discussed by clinical instructors and students during a rotation. We are fortunate to be a part of the exciting and challenging times in health care. I trust you will find that this new revision will complement the various types of practices you will encounter during your pharmacy educational career.

Larry E. Boh

Acknowledgment

I am sincerely appreciative to the contributing authors for their outstanding dedication, patience and commitment to the second edition of this manual. The past two and half years have been difficult to move this project from a planning stage to the production stage, often taking longer than any of us could have ever anticipated. Your sacrifices on weekends and evenings to meet the many deadlines has produced a work that is of the highest quality and one that I anticipate will quickly gain widespread application by students.

I would also like to thank Lloyd Young, who served as a consulting editor to keep the process moving during times when it was not possible because of my health related concerns. You are a true friend.

To the publishing staff at Lippincott Williams & Wilkins, especially Dan Limmer and Matt Hauber, thank you for constantly demonstrating a commitment to excellence and maintenance of the rigor which we so often expect in any of the work we undertake in academia. Your leadership, tolerance, and positive attitude have been greatly appreciated.

To all of my friends, students, and colleagues in Madison and beyond, who are too numerous to mention here, thank you for your never-ending letters, cards, and e-mails. You have been a constant source of support and motivation during a difficult three years. Your professionalism and friendship have meant more than words can express.

Finally, to my wife Dawn and daughters Kimberly and Andrea, thank you for your understanding of the importance of this project to me, but mostly for your constant love, support, and encouragement.

Notice To Reader

Drug therapy information is constantly evolving. Our ever-changing knowledge and experience with drugs and the continual development of new drugs necessitates changes in treatment and drug therapy. The editors, authors, and publisher of this work have made every effort to ensure the information provided herein was accurate at the time of publication. *It remains the responsibility of every practitioner to evaluate the appropriateness of a particular opinion or therapy in the context of the actual clinical situation and with due consideration of any new developments in the field.* Although the authors have been careful to recommend dosages that are in agreement with current standards and responsible literature, we recommend the student or practitioner consult several appropriate information sources when dealing with new and unfamiliar drugs.

Contributor

Kenneth R. Baker, R.Ph., J.D.
Vice President, General Counsel
Pharmacists Mutual Insurance Company
Algona, Iowa

Diane Beck, Pharm.D.
Professor and Director, Experiential Education
School of Pharmacy
Auburn University
Auburn, Alabama

Larry E. Boh, M.S., R.Ph.
Professor and Chair
University of Wisconsin School of Pharmacy
Madison, Wisconsin

Robert M. Breslow, R.Ph., BCPS
Clinical Assistant Professor
School of Pharmacy
University of Wisconsin
Madison, Wisconsin

Shelley L. Chambers, Ph.D.
Assistant Professor
Department of Pharmaceutical Sciences
Washington State University
Pullman, Washington

C.Y. Jennifer Chan, Pharm.D.
Clinical Assistant Professor
College of Pharmacy
The University of Texas
Austin, Texas

Mary Beth Elliott, Pharm.D., Ph.D.
Assistant Professor
School of Pharmacy
University of Wisconsin-Madison
Madison, Wisconsin

Marie Gardner, Pharm.D., BCPP, CGP
Clinical Associate Professor
Department of Pharmacy Practice and Science
The University of Arizona College of Pharmacy
Tucson, Arizona

William R. Garnett, Pharm.D.
Professor
School of Pharmacy
Virginia Commonwealth University
Richmond, Virginia

Kathryn L. Grant, Pharm.D., FASHP
Assistant Professor
College of Pharmacy
The University of Arizona
Tucson, Arizona

Stacy L. Haber, Pharm.D.
Clinical Assistant Professor
College of Pharmacy
University of Arizona
Tucson, Arizona

Timothy J. Hoon, Pharm.D.
Clinical Assistant Professor
School of Pharmacy
University of Wisconsin
Madison, Wisconsin

Randolph W. Hurley M.D.
Assistant Professor of Medicine
Regions Hospital
University of Minnesota
St. Paul, Minnesota

Connie Kraus, Pharm.D., BCPS
Clinical Associate Professor
University of Wisconsin School of Pharmacy
Madison, Wisconsin

Y. W. Francis Lam, Pharm.D.
Associate Professor
College of Pharmacy
The University of Texas
Austin, Texas

Michael G. Madalon, R.Ph., BCPS
Senior Clinical Pharmacist
University of Wisconsin Hospital and Clinics
Clinical Instructor
University of Wisconsin School of Pharmacy
Madison, Wisconsin

Beth A. Martin, R.Ph.
Clinical Assistant Professor
Director of Pharmacotherapy Labs
University of Wisconsin-Madison School of Pharmacy
Madison, Wisconsin

Teresa A. O'Sullivan, Pharm.D.
Department of Pharmacy
University of Washington
Seattle, Washington

Paul G. Rosowski, M.S., R.Ph.
Clinical Assistant Professor
School of Pharmacy
University of Wisconsin
Madison, Wisconsin

Ronald L. Sorkness, Ph.D., R.Ph.
Associate Professor (CHS) of Pharmacy, Medicine, and Pediatrics
University of Wisconsin
Madison, Wisconsin

Bernard Sorofman, Ph.D.
Associate Professor
College of Pharmacy
The University of Iowa
Iowa City, Iowa

Avery L. Spunt
College of Pharmacy
University of Illinois at Chicago
Chicago, Illinois

Susan M. Stein, M.S., R.Ph.
Clinical Instructor and Experiential Education
Coordinator
University of Wisconsin-Madison
School of Pharmacy
Madison, Wisconsin

Denise L. Walbrandt Pigarelli, Pharm.D.
Clinical Assistant Professor of Pharmacy
University of Wisconsin-Madison, School of
Pharmacy
Madison, Wisconsin

Joanne Whitney, Ph.D., Pharm.D.
Associate Clinical Professor
Director, Drug Product Services Laboratory
Department of Clinical Pharmacy
University of California, San Francisco
San Francisco, California

Ann K. Wittkowsky, Pharm.D., CACP
Director, Anticoagulation Services
Clinical Pharmacist, Cardiology
Clinical Associate Professor
University of Washington Medical Center
Seattle, Washington

Timothy D. Wolf, Pharm.D.
Senior Clinical Pharmacist and Clinical Assistant
Professor
Department of Pharmacy
School of Pharmacy
University of Wisconsin Children's Hospital
Madison, Wisconsin

David A. Zilz, M.S., R.Ph.
School of Pharmacy
University of Wisconsin
Madison, Wisconsin

Contents

Chapter 1

Overview of the Health Care System

David A. Zilz

For students to understand and appreciate their roles as practitioners, it is important to understand the societal and economic forces driving the rapidly changing health care system in the United States. It is also important to realize the effects of these forces on health care providers (physicians, nurses) and the health care industry entities (hospitals, nursing homes, clinics, agencies) in which they practice.

SETTING THE STAGE

The United States is being transformed from a society that has been a traditional "democracy" to one that is becoming basically a "corpocracy," that is, one dominated by corporations. The 1990s saw a convergence of companies into very large corporate entities that have grown ever larger through mergers and acquisitions. With U.S. corporations' ever-increasing size and financial base of billions of dollars of annual revenues, and their increasing amount of actual net profits to reinvest in the corporate infrastructure, their influence individually and collectively has increased. This influence has affected every sector of society—including political, financial, and production and distribution—as well as the dynamics of individual work and career patterns. This should not necessarily be thought of as a bad evolution because it is so intertwined with our technological revolution.

The technology era, dominated by commercialization of computers and telecommunications, has created the need for and the means of restructuring society. As significant financial resources are required to support and fund these technologies, only mammoth organizations with access to Wall Street finances and other significant venture capital are able to succeed and thrive. It has been suggested that by the year 2000, there will be five national or international corporations that will dominate and influence 80% of every industry in the United States.

However, it is important not to forget the other 20% of revenues—a significant amount of money. Although most individuals will likely work in national corporations, there will be many entrepreneurs in small companies or groups who capitalize on their expertise by combining an understanding of business development with the creation of sound financial enterprises. This population will also generate a significant amount of revenue.

This transformation of society and the key trends mentioned are important for pharmacy students to remember because they are equally true of the health care industry.

HEALTH CARE INDUSTRY AND HEALTH CARE SYSTEMS MIMIC THE REST OF SOCIETY

The health care industry is defined as all sectors that provide, either directly or indirectly, funding, products, or services that relate to improving health or minimizing illness. Health care systems are usually considered that component of the health care industry that provides services directly to patients. More specifically, the pharmacy system can be thought of as a series of systems resulting in the creation, production, and distribution of drugs from the pharmaceutical manufacturer, to the wholesale distributors, to practitioners, and to patients through various payer and payment systems that intertwine throughout.

The health care industry, health care provider systems, and pharmacy systems are evolving similarly to other industries. There has been a continuous convergence of companies that provide the same or similar services, as well as those that have different but synergistic components. As examples, key sectors of pharmaceutical-related industries illustrate the phenomena of "expanding and expansive corporations." Currently, five drug wholesalers are responsible for more than 80% of the wholesale drug distribution activities in the United States, with plans to consolidate to three, pending governmental approval. Likewise, the research-dominated pharmaceutical companies are converging, with potentially similar results. Ten mega-pharmaceutical corporations currently invest more than 85% of the money spent on clinical research and product development. This is a dramatic change from only a few years ago, when no single company was investing more than a few percent of the total dollars in new product development.

Managed care organizations (MCOs), health maintenance organizations (HMOs), and group purchasing organizations (GPOs) are other sectors of the health industry that have consolidated, converged, and coalesced into very large and influential entities of three to five conglomerates, each representing billions of dollars of health care funding annually. Pharmacy benefit management companies (PBMs) are also dominated by five or fewer very large companies that process and manage drug prescription information for millions of prescriptions annually for millions of patients each.

ELEMENTS OF THE HEALTH CARE SYSTEM

The health care provider system is becoming an integrated health care delivery system. There are few independent physicians, physician practice groups, or hospitals without affiliation with, or ownership of, nursing homes, home care companies, independent pharmacies or pharmacists, or other organizations. First, there is usually a consolidation of similar services, such as several hospitals joining together, physician group practices merging, or home care agencies consolidating into a single entity, with a rearrangement of services to meet various care needs. What generally follows is the structure that is more common today: these entities integrating through various organization structures to provide patients with a continuum of care. Part or all of these integrated systems may be organized as either for-profit or non-profit entities.

The same trend of emerging large organizations is also occurring in direct patient care. The financial success of these organizations requires an effective transfer of patients between each sector as the level of care they require changes. The resulting integrated health care delivery network is intended to provide cost-effective services for patients as they move among the different health care environments. Each level has very different costs associated with the provision of that care. For example, in 1997 the average cost of an acute care facility was approximately $1000 per day. The cost of a subacute care unit was $500 per day, a skilled nursing facility $165 per day, an extended care facility $60 per day, and a community-based residential facility $30 per day. Thus, there is tremendous economic pressure for patients to be moved to the lower-cost facility. This linkage is key to coordinating care for bed-ridden patients. During the transfer of these patients, the one component that must be managed for consistency and continuity is drug therapy management. Pharmacies and pharmacists are critical to the successful management of drug therapy as patients move among these different levels of the health care system.

In addition to institutions for bed-ridden patients, other sectors that provide health care to patients include physicians' clinics, ambulatory surgery centers, dialysis centers, home care and home infusion services, as well as many others. Pharmaceuticals and the pharmacy profession have a significant and ongoing role in the medicinal treatment of these patients across the continuum of care and in all the different sites.

STAGES OF MATURATION OF HEALTH CARE SYSTEM IN RESPONSE TO MARKETPLACE CHANGES

In each local geographic area or health care region within a community, the degree of development of an integrated delivery system varies depending on the stage of the health care marketplace of that community. Independent of what stage any health care provider entity (physician, pharmacist, insurance company) is in at the present time, the changes that occur as an area responds to and evolves toward a common market are predictable.

One model describes four stages or steps that occur as a community evolves toward what is considered a mature health care market. The original model, known as the *Market Evolution Model,* was presented in 1993 at a conference titled *Competing in the Maturing Health Care Mar-*

ketplace: Strategies for Academic Medical Centers, held by the University HealthSystems Consortium. In this scheme, a numeric value is designated for each stage. Stage 1 is considered the unstructured marketplace, stage 2 is considered a loosely structured environment, stage 3 is considered a marketplace undergoing consolidation, and stage 4 is considered a managed competition environment (Box1.1). The forces that cause the changes from the unstructured to the mature stages are the number of patients who are enrolled in health maintenance or other managed care organizations, the extent to which there is an excess number of health care providers, the size and number of collaborations of industries in an area that are responsible for the cost of providing coverage to their employees, and other factors. The following is a brief description of a few of the characteristics and components of each of the stages.

Stage 1   Unstructured. The unstructured health care delivery system was the dominant organization in the United States until the late 1980s and early 1990s and is still prevalent in a few areas. This health care environment is primarily characterized by independent practitioners of medicine, pharmacy, and other services, and reimbursement occurs on a fee-for-service basis. Individual hospitals operate in stand-alone mode. Fewer than 10% of patients are enrolled in managed care plans, and there is little coordination between the industries in the community to collectively influence health care costs. Local industries pay for their employees' care almost strictly through health insurance companies. Pharmacists are not directly connected to the other providers and are independent of the system. The care in these environments is often very fragmented as is the concern for costs, because they are so distributed across all sectors.

Stage 2   Loosely Structured. This marketplace is characterized by physicians moving into ever larger group

---

Box 1.1   The Four-Stage Progression of an Integrated Health Care Delivery System

Unstructured → Loosely Structured → Consolidation → Managed Competition practices and hospitals merging with other hospitals or, in some cases, integrating with nursing homes.

Reimbursement for health services is based on discounted rates for physicians. Hospitals receive payment on a per diem or fixed rate per admission. The number of patients enrolled in managed care plans is 10–30% of the population, as employers begin to encourage their employees to use managed care providers. Rather than only individual practitioners and entities providing care, organizations begin to come together. Patient care is coordinated by a series of ambulatory clinics and surgery centers, hospitals, nursing homes, home care companies, and infusion entities as well as pharmacies that are linked together to provide a continuum of care and to begin focusing on individual "wellness" rather than on caring for persons only when they become ill. Pharmacy costs begin to be controlled independently by employers contracting with pharmacy benefit management (PBM) companies that reduce the employers' drug costs through contractual arrangements with pharmacists, provision of mail drug services, and negotiated rebates with drug manufacturers.

Stage 3   Consolidation. Group practices, primarily physicians, begin to merge into larger groups. Hospitals, nursing homes, and home care agencies begin to integrate to provide services. Then, physician group practices and hospitals begin to link together formally. Managed care enrollees account for 30–50% of the population and have their care reimbursed by their plans. The industrial sector begins to organize to reduce costs among the provider organizations. There are a few (usually three to five) large integrated provider organizations (physicians, hospitals—nursing homes—home care agencies—pharmacies) that evolve in the geographic area and become the dominant players. Pharmacies begin to have contracts with the larger organizations, or the organizations create their own pharmacy service programs to support the needs of their patients.

Stage 4   Managed Competition. This stage is defined as the point at which a few large integrated health care delivery systems remain, with the merged hospital networks having their own physician organizations. Reimbursement for care is based on a capitated payment.

Providers are at risk for the cost of providing care. In this scheme, they cannot charge a fee for each individual service they provide to patients. Managed care is responsible for more than 50% of the population, and companies are well organized and begin to deal directly with providers to set expectations for quality and cost of care. Pharmacies and pharmacists at this stage become an integral part of the system to ensure continuous drug care, to manage the costs for the systems by ensuring good prices for their products, to make sure patients are compliant with their prescribed regimens, and to target outcomes.

These parameters are but a few that have been identified. The University Health Care Systems in Oak Brook, Illinois, has published extensive information on this subject. The information provided here is meant to illustrate to students the need to be aware of the more global forces affecting the health care system or organization they may eventually work for, as that organization competes in different stages of market maturity.

WHERE DOES PHARMACY FIT IN THE TRANSFORMATION OF THE HEALTH CARE SYSTEM?

The expectations of pharmacists and pharmacy services vary in each stage of maturation of a health care system. In the early stages, when fees are charged for services, the expectations of pharmacists, their responsibilities, and their roles differ from the latter stages, when the entire organization is at risk for the costs and quality of the drug-related component of care. As the continuum of care becomes integrated, the necessity to optimize drug therapy and manage the associated costs results in the need for pharmacists who understand the value they bring throughout an organization. There is a shift from focusing on a single prescription or drug-order–related transaction and interaction with a single patient, to a much greater emphasis on the totality of all the drugs the patient consumes over a period of time and on monitoring patients and ensuring they comply with all drug therapy. It is equally important to manage the indi-

---

Box 1.2 Three Stages of Cost Reimbursement for Pharmacy Services

---

Cost Per Unit → Cost Per Case →
Cost per Patient Time Frame

---

vidual patient's therapy in the context of multiple patients with similar diseases. The emphasis changes from review of a single transaction to population-based outcomes of drug and related therapies.

There are three stages or different emphases on reimbursement that pharmacists encounter as the organization they work for progresses through the four different stages of evolution (Box 1.2). These are costs for (1) a product through a single prescription transaction, (2) all drugs for an individual case episode, (3) all drugs for an individual for a set time frame, usually 1 year. During the first stage, pharmacists in each sector (ambulatory, acute care hospitals, long-term care, and home care) concentrate primarily on the individual prescription and drug costs and charges and thus may too often think of the therapeutic management similarly. In the second stage, which occurs primarily in hospitals where the provider organization receives reimbursement for the management of the case, the pharmacists and pharmacy departments focus on the total cost per admission to the facility. In the third phase, when the integrated provider network is at risk for all costs of care for the patient. Pharmacists and their management must take into consideration member-per-month costs and related outcomes if they are to be meaningful contributors to patients and the enterprises for which they work.

INTEGRATED SYSTEMS IN MANAGED CARE PROGRAMS AND THE PRACTICING PHARMACIST

Because of the different sites (inpatient, long-term and nursing home, home care, ambulatory clinics) and diverse number of practice functions pharmacists encounter, there are a plethora of opportunities that exist within an integrated delivery network. It is beyond the scope of this chapter to describe all the specialties and areas in which pharmacists currently practice and for which unique expertise and experience are increasingly important. A listing of the pharmacy service sites that a patient can encounter in an integrated delivery system serves to illustrate the need for pharmacists' involvement and the opportunities they have to fulfill that need. These services include ambulatory care clinics, in which many integrated networks have pharmacists accountable for drugs associated with various conditions; mental health clinics, which often require special experience or training; outpatient and clinical pharmacies, where the majority of clinical and product transfer transactions occur and which require a concentrated attention on the patient's continuum of care; the acute care setting, where a major acute care episode may lead to a significant change in therapeutic direction for a patient; long-term care facilities, which are generally a transition from acute care and require tightly managed distribution and information systems; and the residential or home setting, in which there is minimal oversight. The expectations of patients and payers for pharmacy mail services, with sophisticated clinical communication needs via telephone and other electronic means, is another dimension of integrated care provision.

There is a continuous need across all these sectors to support patients in managing their increasingly complicated drug therapy as they move through the continuum of care. This continuum in the management of pharmaceutical care is crucial to maximize the potential benefits and minimize the problems associated with drug therapy.

Numerous opportunities now exist and many more are likely to be available in the future for pharmacists. It is expected that numerous changes will take place in the functional job descriptions for pharmacists and that new sites for pharmacy practice will emerge in integrated networks. These changes will allow—in fact, require—a pharmacist to gain varied experience in many dimensions of pharmacy practice.

WHY PHARMACY STUDENTS NEED TO UNDERSTAND THE TOTAL HEALTH CARE SYSTEM

Students that come to understand the totality of the health care delivery system in which they will practice can better provide the clinical care needed by patients. If as students, one can reach a comfort level with the ever-changing clinical care outcome mandates and economic pressures their future employers face, the advanced practice experiences will take on additional meaning beyond the sole function of clinical care. Furthermore, an understanding that there is continuous change not only in therapies but also in the broader environment in which those therapies are delivered will allow individuals to bring a greater wisdom to their learning efforts and will ultimately lead to greater rewards and influence as practitioners.

APPLICATION TO ADVANCED PRACTICE EXPERIENCE

The clerkship, or advanced practice experience (APE), and subsequent residency training programs are ideal times to conceptualize the significant role drug therapy and pharmacists have in patient care throughout integrated health care organizations. During advanced practice rotations it is likely that students are focusing intently on pharmacotherapy issues. The focus on the patient, because of the site in which the rotation is being held, can easily be too short term and form a limited care perspective. By understanding the total health care environment and the components of the integrated delivery system, students can begin to associate the complexity of the immediate pharmaceutical management with the overall scheme in which the patient and the other practitioners jointly develop an optimum drug therapy plan.

The APE is an ideal time to think about every aspect of therapeutic knowledge being gained and to translate and transfer that knowledge to a patients' needs as they move through the complete cycle of care settings: acute care hospitals, long-term and/or rehabilitation facilities, ambulatory clinics, home care organizations, mail services often associated with pharmacy benefit management companies, and residential and home settings. Such a view of drug therapy will likely be different for a student focusing exclusively on the therapeutic need in a specific care setting at a specific time in the patient's disease course.

THE IMPORTANCE OF LEADERSHIP AMONG FUTURE PHARMACY-TRAINED PRACTITIONERS

There is an ever-increasing need for students to develop a career plan that includes a major leadership role in conceptualizing, organizing, implementing, and managing pharmaceutical service organizations for integrated networks. Without this leadership core, the number of pharmacists who will be able to practice at the levels they strive for will not grow in the current or future health care delivery environment. The increased sophistication and associated costs of drug therapy as part of the totality of health care and its costs will require pharmacists in demanding and influential positions to optimize the utility of their profession. As stated, this career path will be demanding and challenging, but rewarding. Students at any stage in their career planning are encouraged to assume the leadership responsibility that the profession will need in decades to come in our rapidly changing health care system.

Chapter 2

Professional Practice Experiences: Goals, Objectives, and Activities

Larry E. Boh and Diane Beck

BACKGROUND

As the pharmacy profession has moved from the traditional product to patient orientation, curricula within the schools and colleges of pharmacy have evolved to include more experiential course work to foster this patient orientation. This change has been supported by the philosophy of pharmaceutical care that encourages pharmacists to assume a patient **advocacy** role in **optimizing** a patient's drug therapy while **minimizing** the adverse effects of the medication. The role of experiential education is to hasten and enhance the development of the student's ability to provide pharmaceutical care. Hepler and Strand define pharmaceutical care as the "responsible provision of drug therapy for the purpose of achieving definite outcomes that improve the patient's quality of life."[1] Pharmaceutical care begins with establishing a covenantal patient relationship and is successfully accomplished when one of the following outcomes has been achieved: (1) curing a disease, (2) eliminating or reducing a patient's symptoms, (3) arresting or slowing a disease process, or (4) preventing a disease or symptomatology.

Before the contents and components of clerkships are described, a brief explanation of the types of experiential education within pharmacy is warranted because there is considerable confusion among students, preceptors, and colleges or schools of pharmacy. The types are categorized and discussed according to whether they are school sponsored. Historically, internship is an experiential program that is not school sponsored and students do not receive academic credit. Oversight of these experiences is solely provided by each state Board of Pharmacy or Pharmacy Internship Board. Internship hours often begin to accumulate once registered as a pharmacy student. Some states require that a proportion of these hours be completed after graduation. Furthermore, many states allow a portion of school-sponsored experiential programs to count toward the total number of internship hours required for licensure. During an internship program not sponsored by an academic program, students and graduates are paid for their work and complete a set number of hours, as determined by each state.

Pharmacy schools in the United States have changed their experiential curriculum to better prepare students to be pharmaceutical care providers. In the past, pharmacy schools have segregated practice experiences into externships and clerkships. *Externships* provided pharmacy students with experiences in a product-oriented pharmacy environment. In the institutional setting, these experiences involved the student in functions such as unit-dose dispensing, preparation of intravenous medications, and the overall operations of an institutional pharmacy department. Community externships engaged students in the dispensing and patient-education activities in a chain or independent community pharmacy setting. In contrast, *clerkships* provided students with experiences in working with other health professionals and patients for the purpose of ensuring appropriate use of medications.

However, as pharmacy has evolved, the line between distributive and patient-centered functions has faded, and both activities are often supervised by the same pharmacist. Technicians and technology are being increasingly relied on to attend to many of the distributive aspects of pharmacy practice. Therefore, while pharmacists must understand and participate in distributive aspects of pharmacy, their major emphasis and concentration has now shifted to a patient-centered focus.

Consistent with these changes in pharmacy practice, rotations in U.S. pharmacy schools are now referred to as practice experiences. During a practice experience, the student has an opportunity to provide pharmaceutical care in an environment where distributive and patient-focused services are provided in a more integrated manner. Experiential education at pharmacy schools is now a longitudinal program consisting of *introductory practice experiences (IPE)* and *advanced practice experiences (APE)*. Students begin *introductory practice experiences* when they enter pharmacy school and then transition to *advanced practice experiences* as their pharmaceutical care abilities grow in breadth and depth.

Compared with experiential education in the past, a larger number of the practice experiences are now occurring in the ambulatory and community settings. These settings more closely reflect the evolution and status of health care delivery in the United States. In these settings, the student sees more gradual changes in patient response compared with the inpatient setting. For example, a patient with rheumatoid arthritis who begins methotrexate therapy usually requires at least 1–2 months of continued therapy before a response is observed. Thus, students need to be present in that particular setting for a longer duration to observe responses to therapy. Many pharmacy schools are responding to this challenge by offering ambulatory and community rotations that are longer in duration or as longitudinal experiences during the year of advanced practice experience rotations.

Introductory practice experiences are intended to introduce the student to pharmaceutical care. Introductory practice experiences take place during the first three years of a pharmacy curriculum. These early experiences prepare the student for a higher level of experiential learning during the final year of a pharmacy curriculum. Service-learning and shadowing are two types of experiences that accomplish this goal. *Service-learning* allows students to participate in service projects that meet the needs of the community, foster a sense of caring for others, and lead to student learning through communication and professionalism. Therefore, there are reciprocal benefits for both the community and pharmacy students. The development of caring relationships during service-learning prepares students for establishing covenantal patient-caring relationships as characterized in Hepler and Strand's pharmaceutical care statement.[1] *Shadowing*, another type of introductory practice experience, involves the student in observing senior students and practitioners in a variety of pharmacy practice settings including ambulatory, community, and institutional settings.

In the new experiential education models, advanced practice experiences are offered during the final year of pharmacy school. The student's activities and responsibilities are depicted in Hepler and Strand's pharmaceutical care statement. For example, students establish covenantal patient-caring relationships, identify and solve patient-specific medication-related problems, and evaluate the outcomes of patient care.

Due to the rapid changes in information and technology, future practitioners must be able to learn new information without being dependent on a teacher. Therefore, the development of life-long learning abilities is being emphasized in pharmacy education today. One way this can be accomplished is through self-directed learning. Self-directed learning occurs when an individual identifies learning goals, plans learning activities to achieve those goals, and self-assesses whether those goals have been met. The development of life-long learning abilities are emphasized during experiential course work.

This book provides the reader with guidance in providing patient-focused care during both the pharmacotherapy didactic course work and the introductory practice and advanced practice experiences. The following section outlines the common goals and objectives typically found in programs offering these experiences.

OUTCOME FOR PATIENT-FOCUSED CARE EXPERIENCES

By completion of the experiential education components that emphasize patient-focused care, the student should be able to collaborate with physicians, other health care professionals, and patients or their care-givers to formulate a pharmaceutical care plan, including the recommendation of pharmacotherapy specific to patient needs and desired outcome.

GOALS

Through participation in patient-focused care experiences, the student should be able to:

➤ **apply** the concept and philosophy of pharmaceutical care when providing patient care and justify its importance in the U.S. health care system.

➤ **develop** the skills necessary to effectively and efficiently apply and integrate information from the basic pharmaceutical and medical sciences to direct patient care.
➤ **identify** and solve medication-related problems in a prospective manner.
➤ **develop** pharmaceutical care plans for patients and assess patient outcomes.
➤ **communicate** effectively and accurately with patients and health care professionals using a variety of methods (writing, speaking, verbal and nonverbal communication, media, and computers).
➤ **demonstrate** self-learning abilities and habits.

OBJECTIVES FOR INTRODUCTORY PRACTICE EXPERIENCES

On completion of an introductory practice experience, the student should be able to:

➤ **develop** verbal, written, and listening skills as he or she participates in the provision of service or work with a pharmacy practitioner.
➤ **accept** the responsibilities embodied in the principles of pharmaceutical care.
➤ **demonstrate** life-long learning abilities such as reflective thinking skills.

OBJECTIVES FOR CLERKSHIPS AND ADVANCED PRACTICE EXPERIENCES

On completion of an advanced practice experience, the student shall be able to:

➤ **describe** the symptoms, pathophysiology, significant laboratory tests, physical examination findings, diagnosis, and prognosis of a patient with an acute or chronic disease.

➤ **formulate,** on a prospective basis, a pharmaceutical care plan for a patient that includes recommendations of pharmacotherapy specific to the patient's needs and desired outcomes.

➤ **demonstrate** competency and efficiency in monitoring therapy using subjective and objective parameters for efficacy and toxicity.

➤ **recommend** medication doses and dosage schedules based on relevant patient factors such as pharmacodynamic, physiologic, and pharmacokinetic parameters.

➤ **analyze,** evaluate, and synthesize information and make informed, rational, responsible, and ethical decisions.

➤ **utilize** a problem-solving approach effectively and efficiently in the patient care setting.

➤ **provide** basic life support (i.e., CPR).

➤ **evaluate** the chemical properties such as stability, compatibility, and storage requirements of drugs and drug products that are being considered for a patient.

➤ **explain** the mechanism of action of drugs and drug products.

➤ **determine** the appropriate drug delivery system for the patient based on individual patient needs and characteristics.

➤ **monitor** a patient prospectively for adverse reactions, side effects, or contraindications associated with the patient's medications without preceptor intervention.

➤ **identify** prospectively drug-drug, drug-food, and drug-laboratory interactions for drugs and drug products.

➤ **select** the most appropriate product formulation for drugs and drug products included in the patient's pharmacotherapeutic plan.

➤ **provide** drug information to patients and health care professionals in an effective and efficient manner using written and verbal communication skills.

➤ **communicate** therapeutic recommendations to the provider.

➤ **conduct** a patient medication history to identify medication use and allergies.

➤ **provide** patient education.

➤ **prepare** and present educational information to classmates and preceptors.

➤ **use** primary literature and reference sources to answer questions effectively and provide information.
➤ **communicate** effectively with other health care professionals and patients.
➤ **self-assess** and satisfy learning needs on an ongoing basis when providing pharmaceutical care.
➤ **demonstrate** effective interpersonal and intergroup behaviors in the practice environment.

PRACTICE ACTIVITIES— INSTITUTIONAL

To accomplish the practice objectives outlined above, a variety of structured, patient-oriented activities and experiences are often incorporated into the typical institutional or ambulatory-based experiential program. These include the following.

1. Participating in patient care rounds
2. Performing therapeutic drug monitoring
3. Providing pharmacokinetic consultations
4. Performing admission histories
5. Providing patient counseling
6. Answering drug information questions
7. Presenting case studies

PRACTICE ACTIVITIES— AMBULATORY OR OUTPATIENT

To accomplish the practice objectives outlined previously, a variety of structured, patient-oriented activities and experiences are incorporated into the typical ambulatory-based experiential program. These include the following.

1. Participating in the medication use process from prescription intake, processing, review, and preparation to patient delivery and communication
2. Performing therapeutic drug monitoring as it relates to specific disease populations (e.g., patients who have

       hypertension, diabetes, heart disease, arthritis, or osteoporosis) or vaccination programs
3. Providing documentation for pharmaceutical care reimbursement
4. Performing admission medical and drug histories
5. Providing patient counseling on prescription or over-the-counter (OTC) products or devices
6. Answering drug information questions
7. Presenting case studies and related experiences

   The following sections will provide a brief discussion of some of the activities found in typical experiential rotations.

Patient Care Rounds

In a teaching hospital setting, patient care rounds or "work rounds" typically occur early in the morning (7–9 AM) for medical services and even earlier for surgical services. Rounds are used to assess each patient's response to therapy, to assess the results of diagnostic or therapeutic procedure(s), and to establish overall medical status and treatment plans. A variety of health care professionals take part in rounds depending on the hospital and the types of patients receiving care. Participants in work rounds at a teaching hospital generally include an attending physician, a medical resident, a medical intern, a nurse, a pharmacist, and perhaps one or two students from other health care disciplines.

   Work rounds are an excellent opportunity for learning. For a pharmacy student, this is often the first direct, face-to-face contact with hospitalized patients and health professionals. In this environment, students have the opportunity to review a variety of clinical patient data such as laboratory tests, blood pressure readings, intake and output values, and physical examinations for a variety of medical problems common to that particular service. Most importantly, this provides the opportunity to see patients on a daily basis and to evaluate their response to drug therapy both in terms of alleviating their medical problems and perhaps in generating adverse effects. In addition, with so many students and other health professionals participating in rounds, this is an excellent atmosphere for the discussion of disease state, drug therapy, prognosis, and other patient care issues in a multidisciplinary setting.

Specific objectives and activities that should be accomplished during work rounds are described in Appendix 2.1. A self-assessment to evaluate the effectiveness of participation in work rounds is provided in Appendix 2.2.

Therapeutic Drug Monitoring

Clerkship students are generally required to monitor drug therapy on a daily basis for patients on their assigned service. The goal of this activity is aimed at optimizing the benefits while minimizing the risks associated with medication therapy. Each institution has a different format in which this activity is performed, but it is typically a variation of the traditional "SOAP Note." SOAP is an acronym for the terms Subjective, Objective, Assessment, and Plan, which each describe a portion of the progress note (see Chapter 15, "Clinical Drug Monitoring," for a more detailed discussion).

Pharmacokinetic Consults

When using drugs with narrow therapeutic ranges (i.e., aminoglycosides, digoxin, phenytoin, theophylline), patients' blood levels must be monitored closely to guarantee therapeutic efficacy while preventing toxicity. Pharmacists are active participants in pharmacokinetic programs in most teaching hospitals. Involvement, however, varies greatly among hospitals, ranging from pharmacists operating solely as a consultant when the medical team faces a difficult case, to taking responsibility prescribing and administering the dose and drawing the blood for drug level analysis.

Participation in pharmacokinetic monitoring not only allows the clerkship student to practice the calculations learned in school, but also provides an excellent opportunity to combine these skills with their clinical patient assessment abilities. Fluctuating patient parameters (such as changing renal or liver function, or volume of distribution due to diuresis or fluid overload) require anticipation on the part of the person recommending the dose and a plan for subsequent monitoring.

Pharmacokinetics consults are performed as formal consults in some hospitals. With this type of program, the pharmacist is responsible for evaluating the patient, recommending the dosing regimen, and documenting their actions as a formal note in the patient chart. This documentation must be complete and accurate because it is included in the patient's permanent record.

The format for the written note varies considerably among institutions, but the underlying concept remains the same. Several pieces of information, such as the current regimen (including drug, dose, and frequency), are standard portions of the note. Other items included in the note are the day of therapy, infusion time for the anticipated dose, and the times and results of each level drawn. Calculated values such as the extrapolated peak, half-life, and volume of distribution should follow the demographic data. The pharmacist should complete the note with his or her recommendation, the statement "will continue to follow" if therapy is to continue, and his or her signature and title. Fluctuating laboratory values may also be included (particularly serum creatinine, white blood cell counts, and differentials) to emphasize the recommended need for change (see Appendix 2.3 for examples of pharmacokinetic consult notes).

Admission Histories and Discharge Counseling

To obtain an accurate record of a patient's medication history, pharmacists in many hospitals perform admission interviews for either some or all hospitalized patients. This experience often is included in clerkship rotations. During an admission interview, it is important to collect from the patients themselves or from their care-givers a variety of information, including the following:

1. The patient's height and weight
2. A history of drug allergies or adverse reactions (if present, the type of reaction, how long ago it occurred, and whether the patient was rechallenged)
3. All current prescription medications including dose, route, frequency, indication, duration, and number of doses already taken for the day
4. Any significant past medications the patient has taken (and if pertinent, why they were discontinued)

5. OTC or alternative medications the patient takes and approximately how often
6. A history of social drug use, such as consumption of alcohol, cigarettes, or illicit drugs

During the process of gathering this information, it is important to establish the reliability of the patient or caregiver and the patient's compliance with the prescribed regimen. In addition, any specific requirements the patient has which may affect compliance should be noted. An example of this may be an elderly, frail patient with arthritis who is not capable of opening prescription vials with child-proof caps. This information can be used when counseling the patient at the time of discharge, and the pharmacist should ensure that easy-to-open bottles are dispensed.

In many institutions, pharmacists are responsible for first dose teaching and discharge counseling. This activity may be incorporated into the clerkship experience. The challenge of first dose or discharge teaching is to communicate effectively in terminology that a patient will understand. Specific information that should be included in patient teaching for each drug the patient receives includes (1) drug name; (2) purpose and the expected benefits the patient should watch for (i.e., clearing of a rash, decreased pain); (3) dose, frequency, and route; (4) special dosing instructions; (5) duration for which the patient is to take the medication; (6) frequent minor side effects; and (7) adverse effects that, if a patient experiences them, warrant notification of the physician or health care provider. When performing discharge counseling, information on refills and storage should also be described.

Drug Information Questions

Answering drug information questions, whether formal or informal, is a common activity of clerkships. Frequently, other health professionals will ask questions regarding specific drugs, potential side effects, doses, or a recommended therapy. The answers to these inquiries will often not be obvious. It is important that a pharmacist *never* guess if he or she is not sure of the correct answer. Instead, the best response is to say, "I'm really not sure, let me check some references and get back to you." Health care professionals will respect the pharmacist more if he or she takes the time to research an answer rather than just guess—especially if the guess is incorrect!

In addition to informal questions, formal written answers to drug-related questions that may occur while monitoring a patient's medication therapy are often a component of the clerkship. These formal written responses may be provided to a preceptor, physician, nurse, or other health professional. The prepared answer should restate the question, establish an answer, and support the answer with appropriate references. Researching an answer to a question not only helps the student learn about the issue, but familiarizes the student with the various references available. This assists in establishing which references are the most effective and efficient to use for different types of drug information questions (see Chapter 4, "Providing Drug Information," for a more detailed discussion of how to answer drug information questions).

Case Presentations

The case presentation is a teaching method that uses a patient experience to share information on a disease state and its therapeutic management. It also helps the presenters to develop and strengthen their communication skills. Most clerkships require students to prepare and present patient case(s). In general, the cases are 20–30 minutes in length and may be presented to the pharmacists at the clerkship site, to classmates, or to both. The general format for a case presentation is briefly described as follows (see Appendix 2.4 for a more detailed discussion of the case presentation format, Appendix 2.5 for a case presentation example, and Appendix 2.6 for hints for doing a case presentation).

DISCUSSION OF THE DISEASE STATE

This is a general discussion of the disease process. Underlying pathologic and physiologic changes are explained. The cause of the disease, its symptoms, and physical and laboratory findings of a typical case are stated, and diagnosis and prognosis are discussed. These items are compared and contrasted with the particular patient case under discussion. Possible complications of the disease are also stated.

The discussion of the disease state is important. It will be the foundation for discussing drug therapy and monitoring parameters for both efficacy and toxicity. However, the presentation should be kept brief (approximately 5 minutes).

DISCUSSION OF DRUG THERAPY

Discussion of therapeutic approaches for the disease follows discussion of the disease state. The following guidelines are used.

1. State the objective of drug therapy for the disease, including selection of drug, mechanism of action, dosage, route of administration, and duration of therapy.

2. Discuss common and serious side effects for each medication. The relative importance and frequency of these reactions should be stressed, including limits and management of reactions.

3. Outline and describe monitoring parameters to evaluate response to therapy, including therapeutic endpoints.

4. Define potentially clinically significant drug interactions, drug-lab, or drug-nutrient test interactions.

5. Describe factors that will modify the choice of drug, dose, or route of administration (i.e., a comatose patient can receive no oral medication). Methods for modifying dosages when necessary for patients with compromised renal/hepatic function are included.

6. List administration problems likely to be encountered, compliance problems, or patient education requirements.

7. Describe nondrug treatment modalities (i.e., diet instruction, physical therapy, occupational therapy, or respiratory therapy).

8. Support the therapeutic plan and any therapeutic issues with appropriate literature resources.

In addition to discussing the above points, the student should field any questions related to the rationale for any drug therapy discussed. This portion of the presentation should take approximately 10 minutes. Any questions asked can be used to teach concepts to the group.

CONCLUSIONS AND CRITIQUE OF THERAPY

This is a summary of the entire case presentation and focuses on the following questions.

1. How closely does this patient fit the "classic" case? What were the differences or similarities?
2. Did any adverse reactions occur? Could they have been avoided?
3. Do you agree with the therapy used? If not, what would you do differently and why?
4. What medications were given at time of discharge? What would or did you tell the patient? Is compliance a potential problem?

This portion of the presentation should take approximately 5 minutes.

EVALUATION OF STUDENT PERFORMANCE[2–4]

During a rotation, the preceptor will assess the student's performance and provide feedback about strengths and areas for improvement. The preceptor will make these assessments using evaluation forms and performance criteria that are based on the goals and objectives outlined in the rotation syllabus or manual. Therefore, before the rotation begins, the preceptor and student should meet and review the rotation goals and objectives, student performance expectations, and how performance will be measured.

The rotation goals and objectives are statements that communicate the level of performance and activity students are expected to demonstrate. The verbs in these statements describe the level of performance a student is expected to demonstrate, and the remaining part of the statement describes the activity. Typically, rotation goals and objectives communicate that the student is expected to provide patient care successfully in the clinical setting. Figure 2-1 describes four levels of ability that a student must achieve to provide patient care. Although rotation goals and objectives often

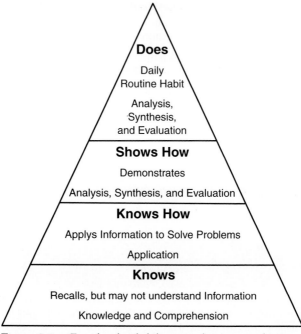

Figure 2-1. Four levels of ability a student must achieve to provide patient care.

include statements depicting each of these levels, most will relate to the highest two levels. The lowest level of this triangle is "*knows*." This tier infers that a student can recall the knowledge gained during classroom courses and the rotation. Goals and objectives describing this level will be statements such as, "The student can *describe* symptoms, pathophysiology, laboratory tests, physical examination, diagnosis, and prognosis of acute and chronic disease." Other verbs that could be used in this statement to describe the lowest tier are *explain, discuss,* and *list.* The second level of Figure 2-1 is "*knows how*." This tier infers that a student knows how to use the knowledge gained during classroom courses and the rotation. However, this tier does not convey that a student can actually provide patient care. An example of an objective describing this tier is, "Use primary literature and reference sources to effectively answer questions and provide information." The third level of Figure 2-1 is "*shows how*." This tier infers the student can actually provide patient care when supervised by a preceptor. The objective, "Demonstrate competency and efficiency in monitoring therapy using subjective and objective parameters for efficacy and toxicity" is representative of this tier. The highest level, "*does*," infers that a student can actually provide patient care and that the correct skills have become habits. At this level, the student performs the task correctly and does not require preceptor intervention. The objective, "Monitor a patient, prospectively, for adverse reactions, side effects, or contraindications associated with the patient's medications without preceptor intervention" is representative of this tier.

The student performance expectations delineate specific activities a student is expected to accomplish during the rotation. These expectations often delineate activities such as attending patient care rounds, providing patient care in the outpatient clinic, providing pharmacokinetic consults, conducting medication histories, providing patient counseling, answering drug information questions, and giving case presentations. These expectations should describe student responsibilities and communicate the frequency in which these activities are to be accomplished. If a student is unsure of performance expectations, he or she should discuss this with the preceptor at the beginning of the rotation.

A description of how performances will be evaluated is often included in a section of the manual or syllabus delineating how grades will be determined. Any forms or instruments used to evaluate student performance will often be included in this section or an appendix. The student should review any forms or instruments with the preceptor at the beginning of the rotation so that the student knows how to use it in self-assessing performance and interpreting the ratings assigned by the preceptor. An example of such a form is provided in Figure 2-2.

Auburn University - School of Pharmacy
Pharmaceutical Care Ability Profile

Student Name: _____   Date: _____   MidPoint☐ Final☐

Directions: Using the scale below, rank the student's performance in each of the outcome areas listed below.

PU	NSD	ND	NR	R
Performance is Unacceptable	**Needs Significant Development**	**Needs Development**	**Needs Refinement**	**Refined**
The student is unable to satisfactorily complete basic and routine tasks despite directed questioning. The preceptor must complete the task. Remediation is necessary.	The student requires guidance/several minutes of directed questioning to complete basic and routine tasks.	The student requires guidance/directed questioning to complete complex tasks; independently completes basic and routine tasks.	The student requires limited prompting to complete complex tasks; independently completes basic and routine tasks.	The student consistently and independently completes complex and basic tasks; confident and automatic application of knowledge and skills demonstrate readiness for developing expertise.

Patient Assessment
- Perform a medication history/patient interview
- Elicit pertinent sociobehavioral information
- Perform physical assessment procedures
- Develop functional patient databases

☐PU ☐NSD ☐ND ☐NR ☐R ☐Not Done
Examples of Patients/Incidents Score is Based On:

Drug Therapy Assessment
- Identify all drug-related problems
- Evaluate status, etiology, and risk factors for each problem
- Prioritize each problem

☐PU ☐NSD ☐ND ☐NR ☐R ☐Not Done
Examples of Patients/Incidents Score is Based On:

Develop, Implement, and Monitor Drug Therapy Plans
- Establish desired therapeutic outcomes
- Consider drug and non-drug therapy alternatives
- Develop comprehensive, logical, and practical drug therapy plans
- Pharmacokinetic/dynamic plan is complete

☐PU ☐NSD ☐ND ☐NR ☐R ☐Not Done
Examples of Patients/Incidents Score is Based On:

• Implements plan promptly, efficiently, and accurately • Monitoring forms are organized, complete, and up-to-date	
Communication Abilities • Communicates effectively with patients and professionals • Defends conclusions/rational regarding drug therapy • Writes effective patient care notes/documents	□PU □NSD □ND □NR □R □Not Done **Examples of Patients/Incidents Score is Based On:**
Thinking Abilities • Critically analyzes and evaluates biomedical literature • Interprets and applies information to patient care appropriately. Uses appropriate patient counseling skills	□PU □NSD □ND □NR □R □Not Done **Examples of Patients/Incidents Score is Based On:**
Pharmacotherapy Decision Making • Identifies and acts upon opportunities proactively	□PU □NSD □ND □NR □R □Not Done **Examples of Patients/Incidents Score is Based On:**
Professional Ethics and Identity • Makes Appropriate Ethical and Legal Decisions • Accepts Responsibility and Provides Patient Centered Care • Maintains Excellence in Personal Practice • Exhibits a Professional Demeanor	□PU □NSD □ND □NR □R □Not Done **Examples of Patients/Incidents Score is Based On:**
Social Interaction, Citizenship, and Leadership • Displays appropriate interpersonal behaviors • Displays appropriate team behaviors	□PU □NSD □ND □NR □R □Not Done **Examples of Patients/Incidents Score is Based On:**
Self-Learning Abilities • Self-assesses, recognizes limitations, develops and implements self-learning plans	□PU □NSD □ND □NR □R □Not Done **Examples of Patients/Incidents Score is Based On:**

Figure 2-2. Pharmaceutical care ability profile.

HINTS ON CLERKSHIP SURVIVAL

The following is a list of suggestions to help the student during the experiential rotation. Of course, each program is unique; the ideas, however, apply to almost all of them.

1. Ask questions of pharmacists, technicians, nurses, physicians, or other health care students. This is a teaching experience, and a part of each professional's job description is education.

2. If you do not know the answer to a question, do not guess or make one up—look up the answer and return with the information promptly.

3. Prepare. This may mean reviewing old class notes or portions of textbooks, especially pharmaco-therapeutics.

4. Prepare for work rounds. This usually requires about 30 minutes depending on the number and complexity of patients on the service. This is the time to review what has happened with each patient since you left the unit and also catch up on new admissions.

5. Participate during rounds. Do not just stand in the back of the group. This is an excellent time to view the manifestations of a disease and also see a patients response to drug therapy.

6. Eat a good breakfast. Not all sights, sounds, and smells are pleasant in various institutions, especially to someone not accustomed to them.

7. Take advantage of any additional opportunities that are available. Examples may include special lectures or conferences. Some hospitals may allow you to observe a variety of tests and procedures or even view surgery. These types of observations are even more beneficial if someone is available to explain what is happening.

8. Dress and act in a professional manner. This will reflect positively on your profession, your school, and most importantly yourself.

9. Maintain patient confidentiality. This is extremely important. Do not discuss patients in public places

or in a loud voice, regardless of whether you are using names or initials. You never know who may be listening.

10. Do not let yourself fall behind. This is an extremely busy time, and if you are stressed to complete work you will not learn from it as well as if you had kept up. In addition, much of what you learn in a clerkship builds on what you learned last week. Therefore, if you never really understood something initially, it will be even more difficult to relate it to a new concept.

11. Remember to "work smart." This translates to completing assignments effectively and efficiently. It does not necessarily require you to work long hours, although this may be necessary if your background is weak in a particular area. A daily calendar will assist you in organizing your day and week to increase your efficiency. Effective time management is an important concept to learn early and apply often.

References

1. Hepler CD, Strand LM. Opportunities and responsibilities in pharmaceutical care. Am J Hosp Pharm. 1990;47:533–543.
2. Beck DE, Boh LE, O'Sullivan PS. Evaluating student performance in the experiential setting with confidence. Am J Pharm Educ. 1995;59(3):236–247.
3. Beck DE, O'Sullivan PS, Boh LE. Increasing the accuracy of observer ratings by enhancing cognitive processing skills. Am J Pharm Educ. 1995;59(3):228–235.
4. Campagna KD et al. Standards and guidelines for pharmacy practice experience program. Am J Pharm Educ. 1994;58:35S–47S.

Appendix 2.1: Work Rounds

The concept and practice of work rounds are used by physicians to evaluate systematically a patient's response to therapeutic intervention and communicate future management plans to the patient and the team. During work rounds, the physician gathers subjective data from patient communication and objective data from physical examination, laboratory test results, and nursing notes. They then analyze the data and further formulate therapeutic or diagnostic plans.

As pharmacists, attendance at work rounds allows direct patient observation and information-gathering. The information gained can be used to monitor a patient's medication therapy, to plan admission and discharge counseling, and to anticipate daily workloads. Work rounds also provide a means for communication between health professionals and serves as a continuing source of educational experiences.

Because of their design, however, work rounds cannot serve as a forum for extensive discussion of any given topic.

The student should be attentive and listen carefully during rounds. Avoid general conversation with other team members unless it relates to patient care.

Objectives

By attending work rounds, the student should be able to:

1. Identify and gather subjective and objective data necessary to monitor medication therapy for efficacy and toxicity.

2. Establish a prospective therapeutic management plan that includes therapeutic endpoints, monitoring parameters, individualization of dosages, and patient counseling.

3. Communicate effectively with other members of the health care team on topics such as therapeutics, drug information, policies and procedures, and patient planning needs.

4. Assess patient medication teaching needs and communicate medication information to the patient, including why drug changes are made and when the patient should expect to note results from the changes.

5. Resolve questionable or unclear medication orders and explain any medication errors such as missed doses, incorrect doses, or incorrect drugs.

6. Prioritize the daily workload.

7. Develop a formal working relationship with the health care team.

8. Assess patient medication needs on discharge, solving problems such as drug and dosage discrepancies, where prescriptions should be filled, and when prescriptions are needed.

Activities

1. Orient new medical housestaff and nursing staff to pharmacy policies and procedures unique to the particular unit.

2. Review patient medication therapy regularly before rounds in terms of indication, dosage, route, duration, efficacy, and toxicity.

3. Obtain information to update and correct the medication profile.

4. Formulate and document a list of problems for new or existing patients seen by the service. The list should focus on disease, drug, or socioeconomic factors.

5. Attend work rounds on a consistent basis and communicate to others on rounds the following information:

   a. Patient's current medication use.

   b. Deviances in patient's therapy—incorrect dosage, missed or refused doses, intravenous (IV) infiltration, and late doses.

   c. Observed subjective or objective signs of efficacy or toxicity.

   d. Drug distribution problems—nonformulary status or medication not ordered for a newly admitted patient.

   e. Prospective therapeutic management plans for patient problems (i.e., change of therapy, discontinuance of medication, change of pain medication, use of prophylactic antibiotics, and identification of therapeutic alternatives).

6. Attend work rounds and gather the following information:

   a. Subjective and objective data for monitoring a patient's medication therapy.

   b. Changes in patient status (condition improved or worsened), discharge date, surgery, diagnostic procedures, and results of procedures.

   c. Changes in nondrug therapy (i.e., dietary changes,

      socioeconomic conditions, physical therapy [PT], respiratory therapy [RT], or occupational therapy [OT]).

  d. Changes in medication therapy—new drug orders, d/c orders, or changes in dose, route, or duration. When chemotherapy is required, what preoperative and IV solutions are needed.

  e. Patient's understanding of medication, name, strength, and expected benefit or toxicities.

  f. Projected discharge needs, including any special teaching requirements such as home antibiotics or total parenteral nutrition (TPN).

7. Communicate developments to the unit pharmacist if he or she is unable to attend all or part of rounds.

Hints for Rounds

1. Introduce yourself to the medical team if not already acquainted.

2. Be prepared to answer and ask questions. Support any information with the necessary literature references.

3. If unable to answer a question, do not hesitate to say so but add that you will attempt to find the answer. Do this in a timely fashion, or if you are unable to do so, communicate the question to the person who receives your report.

4. Obtain the necessary monitoring parameters (such as VS or laboratory tests) before rounds.

5. Before rounds, review the medication record (patient profile), check for the administration of all scheduled or PRN medications, and check for any missed doses.

6. Be assertive and discuss therapeutic management, using a question based approach.

7. Voice disagreements in a calm, courteous manner, stating the rationale for the disagreement.

8. Be consistent; attend daily and for the entire rounds if possible.

9. Anticipate medication orders, especially discharge prescriptions.

10. Carry a clipboard to record information while on rounds.

11. Be attentive and listen to the primary discussion.

Appendix 2.2:
Self-Assessment for Work Rounds

Self-Assessment for Rounds	Yes	No
1. Do you know the names of the members on the service?		
2. Do the members on the service know your name?		
3. Do you actively participate on rounds?		
4. Do members of the service ask you therapeutic questions?		
5. Do you return information accurately and in a timely manner?		
6. Do you communicate in a courteous manner with members of the service?		
7. Do you know the patients' medical problems?		
8. Do you know the rationale for the patients' medications?		
9. Do you ask questions concerning therapeutic rationale that you do not understand?		
10. Do you ask questions about diagnostic or physical exam information as related to drug therapy?		
11. Do you attend all of the rounds?		
12. Do you remind the service to write discharge medication orders, preoperative orders, and to verify chemotherapy on rounds?		

13. What percentage of the time are you asked prospectively (before the medication is ordered) therapeutic questions? (Circle one)

   0% 10% 30% 60% 90% 100%

   If you answer "no" to any of the above questions, you have identified areas of possible improvement, and ones which should be addressed to maximize your learning experience.

Appendix 2.3:
Pharmacokinetic Consults

Example 1: Initial Work-Up

9/26/91   Pharmacokinetic consult
               Day 1 of tobramycin therapy

One-time bolus of 140 mg infused over 60 minutes (0855–0955), followed by 3 postinfusion levels.

Time	Postinfusion Time	Level
1109	1 hour, 14 minutes	3.0 mcg/ml
1303	3 hours, 8 minutes	1.2 mcg/ml
1427	5 hours, 32 minutes	0.6 mcg/ml

Extrapolated peak: 4.4 mcg/ml
Half-life: 1.52 hours
Volume of distribution: 0.25 L/kg

To achieve a peak of 7.0 and a trough of 0.2 mcg/ml, recommended regimen: tobramycin 220 mg every 12 hours. Will continue to follow.

Example 2: Peak and Trough Work-Up

9/27/91   Pharmacokinetic consult
               Day 8 of gentamicin therapy
               Current regimen: 180 mg every 12 hours

Patient afebrile for 3 days
WBC = 9000 cu mm
180 mg gentamicin infused over 60 minutes (0910–1010).

Time	Postinfusion Time	Level
0908	11 hours, 8 minutes (trough)	0.4 mcg/ml
1109	59 minutes (peak)	6.9 mcg/ml

Extrapolated peak: 9.1 mcg/ml
Half-life: 2 hours, 28 minutes
Volume of distribution: 0.33 L/kg

Recommend discontinuing gentamicin therapy.

Appendix 2.4:
Case Presentation Format

The presentation begins with a handout, which should be complete and generally no longer than 1–2 pages. The presentation highlights significant areas of the case. Unnecessary laboratory or physical exam data that is included on the handout only for completeness should be omitted from the presentation. Additional visual aids that assist in clarifying confusing issues are encouraged. References must be in the correct medical journal format.

A. Demographic data (DD) (patient age, sex, race, and weight) and service from which patient receives care.

B. Chief complaint (CC), reason for patient's admission.

C. History, including present illness (HPI), past medical history (PMH), social history (SH), and family history (FH). Briefly, all illnesses, surgical procedures, and previous hospitalizations that have a *direct effect* on the *present illness* should be listed.

D. Medications and allergies—list information that was obtained during medication history; include length of treatment; and identify allergic reaction, how treated, and if patient was rechallenged.

E. *Pertinent* physical examination data (e.g., abnormal examination results in a patient with congestive heart failure may include the presence of 3+ ankle edema, + HJR, + JVP, and presence of rales in both lung fields). Pertinent *negative* results should also be included (e.g., normal rate and rhythm in a patient admitted to rule out myocardial infarct [R/O MI]).

F. *Pertinent* laboratory values (e.g., in a patient with anemia the data may include Hgb 8, HCT 25, MCV 75, MCHC 25, serum iron 30, and TIBC 400). Again, pertinent negative results should also be included. Ranges of normal values should be stated on the handout, as should CrCl and LFT assessment.

G. List of problems.

A list of patient-specific, drug-related problems and rationales for them should be documented.

1. **Failure to receive drugs.** The patient is not receiving

the drug because of pharmaceutical, psychological, sociological, or economic reasons.

2. **Untreated indications.** The patient has a medical problem that requires drug therapy but the patient is not receiving therapy.

3. **Drugs used without indication.** The patient is receiving a drug that is not medically indicated.

4. **Improper drug selection.** The patient is not receiving the right/optimal drug (this includes economic considerations).

5. **Subtherapeutic dosage.** The patient is being treated with too little of the correct drug.

6. **Drug interactions.** The patient has a medical problem or potential problem that is due to a drug-drug, drug-food, or drug-laboratory interaction.

7. **Overdosage.** The patient is receiving too much of the correct drug.

8. **Adverse drug reactions.** The patient has a medical problem that is the result of drug-induced disease.

Time (~ 5 min).

Appendix 2.5:
Case Presentation Example

Gastrointestinal Bleed, Peptic Ulcer Disease

DD: G.Z. is a 48-year-old Asian woman who was admitted to the MICU on 11/25/99. She was transferred to CMS (D6/4) on 11/27/89. GZ weighs 61 kg and is 167.6 cm tall.

CC: Hematemesis.

HPI: GZ presented to UWHC ER on 11/25/99 30 minutes after an episode of hematemesis. She stated she had experienced midepigastric pain with nausea on 11/24, which was relieved by antacids. This morning following breakfast she had one melanotic stool. She is feeling increasingly fatigued and complains of dizziness when standing. She denies abdominal pain, shortness of breath, dysuria, hematuria, or chest pain.

PMH: The patient has no history of liver disease, peptic ulcer disease, gastrointestinal bleeding, hypertension, or diabetes mellitus. She denies previous hematemesis, hematochezia, and melena. She does report several weeks of vague abdominal discomfort. She is status post (s/p) appendectomy.

SH: Negative alcohol and tobacco use.

FH: One brother with peptic ulcer disease.

Medications:

Patient denies use of any medications including aspirin and other nonsteroidal antiinflammatory drugs.

Allergies:

GZ has no known drug allergies (NKDA).

PE: General appearance: Well-nourished Asian female.

Vital Signs:

Lying: pulse = 92 beats/min (normal: 60–80 beats/min); blood pressure = 110/80 mm Hg (normal: 120–140/< 90 mm Hg)

Sitting: 128/80

Temperature = 37.2° C (normal, 35.8–37.3° C)

Review of systems (ROS): noncontributory

Abdomen: soft, negative distention/tenderness; hypoactive bowel sounds

Rectal: melanotic, guaiac-positive stool in vault

Laboratory Test Results:

RBCs 3.4 (3.8–5.0 m/uL)*

Hgb 10.6 (11.8–15.4 g/dL)*

Hct 31 (35–45 ml/dL)*

MCV 92 (82–98 fL/RBC)

MCHC 34 (32–36 g/dL)

Platelets 249 (170–380 K/uL)

Chem:

  Lytes:

    Na 141

      (135–144 mmol/L)

    LFTs: WNL

  K 3.5 (3.6–4.8 mmol/L)*

  Cl 103 (97–106 mmol/L)

  CO_2 25 (22–32 mmol/L)

  Glu 124 (70–110 mg/dL)*

  BUN 24 (7–20 m/dL)*

  Creatinine 0.6

    (0.6–1.3 mg/dL)

  PT 13.6 (11–13 sec)*

  aPTT 25.4 (20–30 sec)

Problem List:

Painless upper gastrointestinal bleeding

Possible hepatitis B

References

1. Grossman MI et al. Gastrointestinal diseases: peptic ulcer. In: Wyngaarden JB, Smith LH, eds. Cecil Textbook of Medicine. 16th ed. Philadelphia: WB Saunders; 1982:635–54.
2. Mitros FA. Atlas of Gastrointestinal Pathology. Philadelphia: JB Lippincott; 1988.
3. Garnett WR. Antacid products. In: American Pharmaceutical Association. Handbook of Nonprescription Drugs. 8th ed. Washington, DC: APhA; 1986:19–51.
4. Berardi RR. Peptic ulcer disease and Zollinger-Ellison syndrome. In: DiPiro JT et al., eds. Pharmacotherapy: A Pathophysiologic Approach. New York: Elsevier; 1989:418–43.

5. Dammann HG et al. The 24-hour acid suppression profile of nizatidine. Scand J Gastroenterol. 1987;22(suppl 136):56–60.

6. Emas S. Medical principles for treatment of peptic ulcer. Scand J Gastroenterol. 1987;22(suppl 137):28–32.

7. Freston JW. H_2-receptor antagonists and duodenal ulcer recurrence: analysis of efficacy and commentary on safety, costs and patient selection. Am J Gastroenterol. 1987;82:1242–9.

8. Lewis JH. Hepatic effects of drugs used in the treatment of peptic ulcer disease. Am J Gastroenterol. 1987;82:987–1003.

9. Ostro MJ. Pharmacodynamics and pharmacokinetics of parenteral histamine (H_2)-receptor antagonists. Am J Med. 1987;83(suppl 6A):15–21.

10. Wolfe MM. Considerations for selection of parenteral histamine (H_2)-receptor antagonists. Am J Med. 1987;83(suppl 6A):82–8.

11. Hollander D. Peptic disease therapy. Am J Med. 1989;86(suppl 6A):152–3.

12. Knodell RG, Garjian PL, Screiber JB. Newer agents available for treatment of stress-related upper gastrointestinal tract mucosa damage. Am J Med. 1987;83(suppl 6A):36–40.

13. Lanza FL, Sibley CM. Role of antacids in the management of disorders of the upper gastrointestinal tract-review of clinical experience 1975–1985. Am J Gastroenterol. 1987;82:1223–41.

Appendix 2.6:
Hints for Case Presentations

1. Think ahead. Be able to answer questions such as, "What if . . . ?" or "If this happens, what would I do?"

2. Remember to be brief; you do not have much time.

3. Define any unusual terminology. Terms may be understood by you but not by your fellow students. When questioned, you should be able to define any medical vocabulary words you have used.

4. Know the proper pronunciation of all terms used. Pronunciation and articulation are important parts of effective communication. If you do not know how to pronounce a term or a drug, find out *before* you present the case. Stumbling over words only serves to decrease your credibility.

5. Remember that you are playing the role of a teacher, and be sure to bring out the important teaching points the patient case illustrates. An important point to remember is that when discussing drug therapy, you should make every attempt to emphasize evidence-based medicine principles during your discussion.

6. Realize that if all questions were answered during the course of your presentation, it would stretch into 2 hours. You should use the outline as a guideline and extract only the most important information under each section to be presented. If all questions in this outline are answered in your mind before the case presentation, you should be able to field any questions offered by your fellow students or the instructor.

7. Be able to answer the following questions if asked.

    a. What was the probability for success with this patient's therapeutic regimen, and how long will it take before success should be achieved? How much time should elapse before a lack of sufficient response during any segment of therapy could be interpreted as therapeutic failure?

    b. What clinically significant interactions or adverse effects of drug therapy could possibly occur?

        1. What would be the nature of this possible interaction, adversity, or side effect, and what would be its significance in this particular patient?

2. What is the probability that an interaction, adversity, or side effect may occur and with what frequency is it encountered in the general population of patients?

3. What parameters will you inspect during treatment as an indication of drug interaction, adversity, or side effect?

c. What is the overall benefit versus risk of therapy? Would long-term treatment modify the overall benefit?

d. What routine alterations in drug therapy can be expected to occur as a matter of course and when should they occur? This might be an alteration of dose, route of administration, or nature of drug. Are there any special procedures to be considered in making these changes (i.e., intramuscular injections being unsuitable for a patient receiving anticoagulants)?

e. What drugs were discontinued during the course of the patient's illness? Why? Was this considered a therapeutic failure?

f. What drugs were added to the therapeutic regimen and why? Was adequate time allowed to determine whether the previous regimen was inadequate?

g. If applicable, how does intravenous therapy affect the overall treatment of the patient?

h. What laboratory tests, symptoms, or other clinical signs were used as criteria to determine the degree of response to therapy?

i. Did any drug-drug or drug-lab interactions occur? If so, what was done? Be sure to include synergism, additive, or antagonistic effects.

j. Did any adverse reactions occur? If so, what was done?

k. If complications arose, how were they treated?

l. If the patient was discharged, were the discharge medications correct? Would you expect any problems with patient compliance or the medications themselves? What directions (by the pharmacist) should be or were given to the patient at the time of discharge regarding their medications?

Chapter 3

Standards of Professional Conduct

Paul G. Rosowski and Avery L. Spunt

Being in the clinical practice environment (clerkship, externship, or internship) provides the student with the opportunity to use the knowledge and skills acquired in the didactic and laboratory course work portions of the academic learning experience. A distinction must be made, however, as this is a new and different environment—an environment that commands the highest academic and professional standards. Soon the student will be interacting with pharmacists, patients, and other members of the health care team. Working to establish a high level of professional integrity from the onset will be important to ensure vitality and success as a pharmacy student and to become an accepted professional.

Developing a professional image requires exhibiting proper behaviors, showing positive attitudes, and maintaining a professional appearance. A good first step in achieving this image is to establish a rapport with coworkers and patients by being respectful, courteous, and willing to listen. Being cheerful and optimistic shows an eagerness to learn. Dressing in an appropriate manner and maintaining a physical appearance that is suitable for the clinical environment complement clinical knowledge and skills. A professional image is something earned and not automatically obtained. The time must be taken to develop a professional image, as this will aid the student in becoming an accepted member of the health care team.

The clinical practice environment is diverse in many ways—from geographic differences to coworkers to patients. As a result, the student must become adept at understanding and accommodating diversities. The language used needs to be tailored to the audience. An effective clinician understands and avoids common communication barriers (e.g., medical jargon, slang, illiteracy, cognitive impairments). Cultural sensitivity is also needed to interpret others' biologic traits, beliefs, and values and to understand their perceptions of disease and health. A failure to understand diversity will only widen the gap between the clinician and others. In turn, this can result in misunderstandings, misinterpretations, and even negative health outcomes.

The clinical practice environment must be a safe environment. Therefore, it should be free of all forms of abuse, discrimination, harassment, and violence. It is the student's responsibility to prevent such instances from occurring and to report any instances that may be harmful to the welfare of others. An environment in which optimum health can be maintained and the risk of adverse health events can be avoided should be promoted. The health policies of the academic institution and clinical practice environment should be read, understood, and followed. Abiding by these practices and policies will help foster an environment that will make learning a success.

The clinical practice experience should be a fruitful and rewarding one. It is a fantastic opportunity to learn and display the wealth of knowledge and skills already attained. New opportunities should be taken advantage of, and the student should work hard to show his or her devotion to the profession. In all, the experience should be enjoyed and valued.

DEVELOPING A PROFESSIONAL IMAGE

Displaying and maintaining a professional image is an essential part of becoming a successful pharmacy practitioner. Professional image can be stated as the interpretation of one's actions, appearance, and attitudes in the clinical practice environment. It should be viewed as a complementary component to the clinical knowledge and skills that must be acquired during the clinical learning experience. Furthermore, professional image is the personification associated with the pharmacy practitioner that is developed over time with a set of norms accepted for the profession.

Learning to display and maintain a professional image should not be a difficult endeavor; however, it should never be presumed. Time must be taken to understand the norms of the clinical practice environment, especially for those who are unfamiliar with it. Time should be set aside early in the clinical learning experience to observe and discuss the norms of the environment with the instructor, other health care team members, and other students. This will help identify the components of how a professional image can be developed and maintained.

Actions

It is important to become acquainted with coworkers. Students should introduce themselves and identify their status (e.g., a fourth-year pharmacy student) to others to establish appropriate expectations. In addition, it is usually required to wear a name badge bearing a professional title (unless restricted in a particular health care setting such as psychiatric unit). Other members of the health care team should always be addressed with their proper titles (e.g., doctor, nurse, laboratory technician). Patients also must be held with the highest regard and should always be referred to by their surnames (i.e., using Mr., Mrs., Ms., Miss), unless they ask to be addressed differently. Practicing in this manner will show respect and sincerity as a member of the health care team.

Proper communication is an essential subcomponent of developing a professional image. The student should be as clear, concise, and accurate as possible. It is best to try to analyze what will be said or written before actually doing it. If a student questions what his or her actions should be, the instructor should be consulted before any actions are taken. Conversations should never be interrupted unless it is absolutely necessary, and careful listening is required when others are voicing opinions. Personal conversations are kept to a minimum, so as not to deter from the focus of the learning experience.

Notes written in patients' charts should refer to patients with the proper titles and should be as clear, concise, and accurate as possible. When making written suggestions or recommendations in a patient's chart based on a consultation, it is customary to thank other health care team members for offering this opportunity. A patient's chart is the official document that health care workers will use to communicate to each other and will be maintained for many years. Any information contained in a patient's chart can enter into legal cases and situations of liability. As a result, considerable attention should be given to written notes because they reflect the clinical practitioner's personal and professional qualities.

Working and taking care of patients should be regarded as a privilege and not a right. Patients entrust members of the health care team to maintain information about their problems and disease states with the strictest confidentiality. To preserve this contract, health care team members must maintain a high legal, ethical, and professional responsibility. A breach of patient confidentiality can not only lead to serious legal action, but also can severely jeopardize the confidence patients place in health care team members. Therefore, it is vital to identify and understand when and where patient confidentiality is at risk.

One common breach of patient confidentiality is referred to as "cafeteria talk." Cafeteria talk can be described as discussing a patient's disease state(s) and/or problem(s) outside the immediate clinical environment. Students may be tempted to discuss the clinical findings of patients with their peers in the lunch room or similar environment, but this puts patient confidentiality at considerable risk. Therefore, such practices should be avoided. It may sometimes be necessary to remind others of their responsibility to refrain from this practice as well.

Another common breach of patient confidentiality is referring to a patient's name in a student presentation (i.e., student case presentation). The instructor's directions or the institution's policies should be followed closely to avoid this practice. One also should never remove (even for a short period) or copy (either manually or mechanically) patient information from the immediate clinical environment that may jeopardize patient confidentiality.

In summary, any patient information or unauthorized use of patients' names (including prescription documents and medication administration records) should be handled very carefully to avoid breaching patient confidentiality.

Appearance

Personal appearance is complementary to professional behavior and attitude in developing and maintaining a professional image. Most people enjoy working with health care team members who are alert, well-groomed, and cheerful. It is wise to recognize that learning in the clinical practice environment will take substantial amounts of energy and brainpower. To look and perform at their best, students should get plenty of sleep and exercise and eat well during the clinical learning experience. Close attention must be paid to personal appearance to promote a positive experience for everyone in the clinical practice environment.

It is essential to dress properly in the clinical practice environment. Clothing styles may change from year to year, but how this affects professional image should not. As a general rule, a conservative approach is best. Many people form opinions of individuals within the first few minutes of meeting them, so clothing should work to establish an immediate good impression.

It is key to know the proper dress code for the clinical practice environment. Clothing should be neat, clean, and pressed at all times. It is unacceptable to wear ripped, stained, or tattered clothing. Men should wear full-length pants (no cut-offs or shorts), buttoned shirts, and ties (tasteful patterns). Women should wear blouses (not overly revealing), dress pants, skirts (not miniskirts), or dresses. All clothing items should match. As for professional attire, a clean, white, pressed laboratory coat should be worn at all times (except in restricted areas such as psychiatric and pediatric units).

Jeans, sweatshirts and sweatpants, t-shirts, athletic outfits, spandex, Lycra (or other body-hugging materials), halter tops or muscle shirts, or other questionable items of clothing should not be worn. Jewelry should be conservative. Metal jewelry can be a potential hazard (especially in resuscitative situations). Sunglasses as well as caps and hats (unless related to religious beliefs) are not suitable for the clinical practice environment. Scrubs and related surgical garb should be worn in restricted areas only. It is, however, important to don proper eye protection, head coverings, bonnets, and gloves in areas where it is required (e.g., sterile products area). Comfortable, cleaned, and shined professional-looking shoes are a must, as the student may be standing for considerable lengths of time. Athletic shoes, high heels, open-toed shoes (e.g., sandals), and work boots are not appropriate. Socks (for men or women) and hosiery (for women) should be worn at all times.

Good grooming habits and good personal hygiene are essential. Hair should be clean, combed, neat, and not excessively long as to interfere with patients or health care team members in the clinical learning environment. One should take note of breath (fresh), nails (clean; for women who wish to polish their nails, a conservative color should be used), and make-up (again, conservatism is best and heavy make-up should be avoided). Bathing regularly is important and proper hand-washing (as stated in an environment's Universal Precautions policy) is essential at all times. It is best to refrain from wearing perfume, cologne, or after-shave lotion, because some individuals may have allergies to it or find it repulsive.

Attitude

Aside from behavior and personal appearance, it is important to maintain a positive attitude in the clinical practice environment. Conveying a positive demeanor and maintaining tact, even when things are not at their best, will enhance the professional image. A clinician's attitude should always be one of empathy, professionalism, responsibility, and understanding.

Personality differences and disagreements will occur between health care team members, patients, instructors, fellow students, and others. However, this should never distract from or compromise patient care. If and when personal disagreements occur, they should first be discussed openly with the instructor. Such discussions should be held outside the immediate clinical practice environment so as not to offend anyone. There are many approaches to providing health care and there is often more than one appropriate method of arriving at an outcome. The student should understand why a certain decision was made and accept any recommendations to avoid future disagreements. It is acceptable to disagree with others (tactfully) but it is always inappropriate to be disrespectful of them.

Many patients the student comes in contact with will be in an unfamiliar environment. Some will be poked, probed, examined, and asked numerous questions repetitively by a variety of health care team members. Some patients may even experience considerable duress on learning of a particular diagnosis or as a result of having undergone a recent surgical procedure. It is, therefore, easy to understand why patients might perceive the clinical practice environment as cold, sterile, and uncomfortable. To help overcome this perception, it is vital to empathize with patients and their families. One effective way to develop empathy skills is to try to see the situation from the patient's point of view. The student must always be courteous, respectful, and willing to listen carefully. It is the patient who ultimately will have to live by the decisions of the health care team. Empathizing with patients and their families will show sincerity and a willingness to understand their decisions.

Finally, responsibility must be acquired and maintained in the clinical learning experience. Responsibility includes being answerable, dutiful, obligated, punctual, reliable, and trusted. The student is responsible to the instructor, other health care team members, other students, and patients. As a member of the team, he or she must ensure positive health outcomes and avoid negative ones. Furthermore, as an advocate of pharmaceutical care, the student must accept the responsibility for all medication-related outcomes.

The student will be expected to maintain a vigilant watch over the medications ordered. It can never simply be assumed that any aspect of medication therapy provided to a patient is correct. All prescription orders are reviewed closely for accuracy and correctness. Any dosing errors, medication interactions, medication omissions, or other problems that might ensue as a result of suboptimal medication therapy must be identified and reported. In addition, the clinician should monitor for positive medication outcomes, because the primary goal of medication therapy should be to improve a patient's quality of life.

It is acceptable to not be able to answer all questions. Nevertheless, these questions should never be dismissed. It is the student's responsibility to follow up on all questions and concerns presented. This also provides an opportunity to develop habits and skills that will foster responsibility.

These efforts will help one mature from a pharmacy student to a professional pharmacist.

USING PROPER LANGUAGE

Language is the primary means of human communication whether it is written, spoken, or transferred via another media. In addition, language involves a process by which an idea that must be interpreted is conveyed by a sender to a receiver. Although it may be regarded as simple, the process inherently has the potential for barriers, misinterpretations, and misunderstandings. Identifying areas in which such problems can occur, and the ways to overcome them, is useful in developing effective language and communications in the clinical learning environment.

The first step in creating effective language is to formulate a well-thought-out idea. Ideas should relate to the problems being solved and be as realistic and concrete as possible. In addition, it is important to prioritize ideas so they are presented logically and rationally. The example of an effective patient consultation can be used to illustrate how to formulate ideas and elaborate further on the communications process.

When formulating ideas to provide a patient consultation, it is important to think carefully beforehand about all the necessary information. This will help to rule out any information or alternatives that might have been overlooked. When consulting with patients, it is important to convey ideas with sufficient detail yet be succinct enough to convey basic medication information.

Once an idea has been formulated, it must be communicated properly to the patient. Ideas must be tailored to the patients who will receive them. Simple terms that the patient can understand should be used. Medical jargon (i.e., medical terminology and medical abbreviations) and difficult words are avoided, because they can cause misunderstandings and cloud the idea being sent. It is essential to speak clearly, at a constant rate, and without great variations in pitch and tone. Patient directions should be explicit (e.g., "Take with 8 ounces of water" should be used instead of, "Take with plenty of water") to help eliminate confusion. Demeaning, derogatory, or perverse language; profanities; and slang terms are unacceptable in the clinical learning environment. Nonverbal mannerisms (e.g., chewing gum, grooming in the immediate clinical environment) that will detract from the idea should be avoided.

Patients come from a variety of knowledge bases and cultures. Correspondingly, assuming that all patients will understand an idea from the onset is improper. To enhance the chances of success, it should first be determined if the patient is receptive to the idea. For example, it is advisable to conduct a patient consultation in an area where the patient is comfortable (e.g., somewhere that is quiet and lacking of distractions). Moreover, it is equally important to determine if the patient's physical, mental, and emotional states are conducive to consultation at that time. Another method to improve comprehension is to solicit feedback by asking patients questions intermittently throughout the consultation. If misunderstandings or misconceptions are revealed, they should be clarified in a courteous and timely manner.

Finally, there are special considerations concerning language and communications that should be borne in mind. Approximately 3–40% of Americans are illiterate, and these individuals are often skilled at hiding their language difficulties. Special care must be taken not to embarrass or demean individuals in any way. Individuals also may have other communication deficits (e.g., those with auditory, cognitive, and visual deficits; those who are terminally ill; or those dealing with emotional situations). In such cases, the clinician should identify individuals (e.g., interpreters) and resources to aid in communication.

IDENTIFYING AND UNDERSTANDING ETHNIC AND CULTURAL DIVERSITY

Patients, health care team members, and health care environments are diverse in many ways and are often shaped by the cultural and ethnic diversities that surround them. According to *The American Heritage Dictionary of the English Language*, culture is the "totality of behavioral patterns, arts, beliefs, institutions, and all other elements of a community or population"; ethnicity is "belonging to a particular ethnic group" (e.g., cultural, national, racial, or religious).

Every individual develops and maintains a unique set of cultural and ethnic beliefs and values. Many beliefs and values stem from personal backgrounds and interactions with certain cultural and ethnic groups. Although beliefs and values are important in identifying individuality, they also can create great problems. Such problems manifest as cultural and ethnic discrimination, misinterpretations, misunderstandings, and prejudices. Most often, such problems are due to a lack of awareness, knowledge, and skills necessary to understand others' cultural and ethnic beliefs and values.

In the clinical practice environment, the student will encounter individuals (patients, health care team members, and others) from a variety of cultural and ethnic backgrounds. It can be easy to draw generalizations, but this should be avoided. Instead, the time should be taken to develop ethnic and cultural sensitivities. Suggestions for developing cultural sensitivity are shown in Box 3.1.

Developing cultural sensitivity comes about through an awareness of how diversity affects the individual and the organization. Knowledge about diversity creates a realistic perspective in which to work with those from different cultures and helps to modify behavior in a multicultural

---

Box 3.1   Ways to Develop Cultural Sensitivity

(1) Recognize that cultural diversity exists

(2) Demonstrate respect for people as unique individuals, with culture as one factor that contributes to uniqueness

(3) Respect the unfamiliar

(4) Identify and examine your own cultural beliefs

(5) Recognize that some cultural groups have definitions of health and illness as well as practices that attempt to promote health and cure illness, which may differ from the health practitioner's own

(6) Be willing to modify health care delivery in keeping with the patient's cultural background

(7) Do not expect all members of one cultural group to behave exactly in the same way

(8) Appreciate that each person's cultural values are ingrained and therefore are very difficult to change

Source: Stule P. Nursing Process and Practice in the Community. St. Louis, MO: Mosby; 1990.

environment. In turn, the benefits gained from an appreciation of ethnic and cultural diversity will improve patient assessment skills and facilitate the use of proper and appropriate language and communication that honors the cultural values and beliefs of others.

Individuals differ in their biologic traits (e.g., skin pigmentation, musculoskeletal systems, and genetic traits). Developing an understanding of the different biologic traits of people from different cultures and backgrounds will augment patient assessment skills. For example, dark-skinned individuals require special expertise to ensure proper assessments of their health and well-being. Disease states such as cyanosis and jaundice may not be as easily apparent in these individuals as they would be in other cultural or ethnic groups. It is especially important to note that the mere presence or absence of certain biologic traits does not imply superiority or inferiority of one ethnic or cultural group over another. Rather, it represents an additional means to understand the biologic features more commonly attributed to a particular group. The ability to understand these differences and to develop the necessary skills to make proper diagnoses and therapeutic recommendations is instrumental in providing good health care to all ethnic and cultural groups.

Cultural values and beliefs also play an important role in the clinical practice environment. In particular, individual values and beliefs can determine how well medical care is accepted, delivered, and followed. Values and beliefs such as familial relationships and kinships; gender dominance roles; parenting roles; self-reliance, self-restraint, and self-control; and social status or social class all must be considered when interacting with individuals. For instance, some cultures regard illness as an extreme self-burden, whereas others do not. Another aspect of cultural values and beliefs involves one's view of health and illness as it relates to diet, nature, health prevention, and religious beliefs. Again, special attention should be given to adapt and modify therapeutic plans and treatments to an individual's cultural values and beliefs.

Cultures and ethnic groups differ in their use and perception of language and communication. This includes cultural and ethnic customs related to the use of a native language (as a primary or secondary language), the types of communication used (written, spoken, or other means), the use of nonverbal gestures, and the manner and willingness to validate information or provide feedback to health care team members. For example, some cultural groups revere illness as a personal issue, whereas others feel obligated to discuss illness more openly with others. The clinician should be aware of language and communications differences and know how to deal with them.

ACADEMIC AND PROFESSIONAL MISCONDUCT

Stated most simply, academic misconduct is cheating. It is an unpleasant and distasteful discovery of dishonesty for all persons involved, including students, instructors, health care team members, and perhaps even patients. Furthermore, it is a breach of one's personal honesty and integrity; it also is absolutely incompatible with a career in the health professions. Although its occurrence may be associated more closely with classroom activities, academic misconduct may prevail in the clinical setting as well.

From the onset of the learning experience, it is crucial that trust be established and maintained with others in the clinical practice environment. Trust means adhering to the rules and policies set forth by the academic institution and/or clinical practice environment. It is, therefore, insightful to become familiar with these rules and policies

Generally, most academic institutions have rules and policies regarding academic misconduct. These can be obtained from the Office of the Dean of Students or other equivalent body. Each professional school is also likely to have a set of rules and policies that apply to academic misconduct that may be more definitive to a particular profession (i.e., pharmacy). Finally, it is important to understand and follow the rules and policies enacted in the clinical learning environment.

Academic misconduct presents itself in many forms. Examples include, but are not limited to, cheating on an examination, collaborating with other students when prohibited by the instructor, falsifying or tampering with data, submitting a paper or assignment that is the work of another individual, knowingly submitting a paper or assignment containing the research of others without providing appropriate acknowledgments, or assisting another student in a paper, assignment, or examination when this is strictly forbidden. Collaboration, plagiarism, and the falsification of data are of special concern in the clinical practice environment.

In some circumstances, it may be acceptable to collaborate on an assignment or a task. For example, an instructor may ask a team of students to present a clinical case on a particular patient or disease state. Conversely, collaboration may be unacceptable if the instructor deems the learning exercise to be one that must be done independently. In any case, the student must understand the instructor's directions before starting any learning exercise.

Another common type of academic misconduct in the clinical setting is plagiarism. Plagiarism is defined by *The American Heritage Dictionary of the English Language* as "using and passing off ideas as one's own" (the ideas or writings of another). At all times, students must give proper credit to words or ideas that are not their own. Plagiarism and the proper rules for citing sources of information must be understood. When there is doubt, the instructor, academic advisor, or a good reference text on writing and systems of citation should be consulted for proper direction.

Falsification of data is another form of academic misconduct that must be avoided. It is never appropriate to "fix" (alter, add, or delete) data in the clinical practice environment. Attempting to provide false or inaccurate data (in patients' charts, assignments, or presentations) is usually the result of poor time management or the inability to draw realistic conclusions from the data at hand. Consequently, the student's goal is to develop accurate data collection techniques and to interpret data as precisely as possible.

Proper professional conduct is equally as important as proper academic conduct. Pharmacy students are expected to maintain a high set of professional and ethical standards as representatives of their academic institutions and profession. These standards are essential for maturation into a good pharmacy professional. Failing to comply with these standards can lead to serious consequences, including course failure or even dismissal from the professional program.

The student should always strive to maintain the highest set of professional and ethical standards. This includes following the Code of Ethics for Pharmacists (Box 3.2). In addition, the standards of the clinical practice environment also must be met (Box 3.3).

Box 3.2   Code of Ethics for Pharmacists

(1) To respect the relationships held between health care providers and patients as conventional ones

(2) To care for patients in a compassionate and confidential manner

(3) To respect the autonomy and dignity of patients

(4) To strive to maintain professional competence

(5) To respect the values of colleagues and other health care team members

(6) To be aware of individual, community, and societal needs

(7) To seek justice in the distribution of health resources

Source: Code of Ethics for Pharmacists. American Pharmaceutical Association; 1994.

Box 3.3   Professional Standards of Conduct in the Clinical Practice Environment

(1) Be honest and cooperative in all professional matters

(2) Refrain from committing threats or acts of violence

(3) Refrain from stealing, defacing, or diverting property

(4) Refrain from possessing, trafficking, or using alcohol, illegal drugs, or other pharmacologically active substances of abuse

(5) Maintain confidentiality in professional matters related to education and training

(6) Avoid impropriety or the appearance of impropriety

Source: University of Wisconsin-Madison School of Pharmacy, 1997–98 Student Handbook and Resource Manual. Madison, WI: University of Wisconsin-Madison School of Pharmacy; 1997.

SEXUAL HARASSMENT

According to *The American Heritage Dictionary of the English Language*, sexual harassment means "unwanted sexual attention from peers, faculty, staff, supervisors, or anyone with whom the victim must interact in order to fulfill job or school duties where the victim's responses are restrained by fear of reprisal." Not only is this behavior unacceptable and intolerable in the clinical practice environment (or anywhere else), it is also against the law. All reports and allegations of sexual harassment should be regarded very seriously.

Sexual harassment can take many forms. Although some persons may regard it as unwelcome sexual advances or requests for sexual favors, other actions can also constitute sexual harassment. For example, sexual harassment can occur as crude or sexually explicit remarks, epithets, or comments (e.g., humor or jokes about bodies); obscene or perverse nonverbal gestures; or the unsolicited distribution of sexually oriented materials. Quite often, sexual harassment comes about in situations in which a power differential exists (where one person has power or authority over another), but it also can occur among peers. Under no circumstances should a position of authority ever be used as a basis for sexual control or enticement.

Examples of sexual harassment in the clinical practice environment include the following: (1) a health care team member talking about and making remarks about a patient's genitalia that are unrelated to a patient's health condition; (2) an instructor who gives a pharmacy student an unsatisfactory grade on a patient case presentation and then offers to give the student a satisfactory mark in exchange for sexual favors; (3) a physician who makes sexually explicit advances toward a pharmacy student; (4) a nurse who shares nude pictures with other health care team members in the workplace and then solicits students to model outside work in exchange for "fun"; (5) a hospital administrator who asks several pharmacy students to go out for drinks at the end of the day and then inquires about their sexual orientations; and (6) a pharmacy student who enters a patient's room to view the patient undressed (permission from the patient or agent of the patient must always be obtained before entering a patient's room).

What should be done if sexual harassment is suspected or occurs? As stated previously, all allegations and reports of sexual harassment are very serious matters and should not be taken lightly. However, this should not preclude one from reporting a suspected sexual harassment incident. If an incident does occur or is suspected, all the facts should be gathered so they can be presented in a confidential, logical, and direct manner. All findings should be reported to, but not be limited to, the instructor (unless directly involved in the case), the director of human resources at the clinical practice site, and the Dean of Students Office. In any case, the polices and procedures at the academic institution and clinical practice site should be referred to for specific guidelines and information relating to sexual harassment. It is common for victims of sexual harassment to feel embarrassed about the situation or feel that they did something to provoke the incident. Despite these feelings, sexual harassment is wrong, and everyone has the right to work and learn in an environment that is free of this type of interference.

Other discriminatory issues and related topics are also important. These include strict prohibition against the discrimination and harassment of others based on their race, color, creed, religion, nationality, disability, ancestry, age, or sexual orientation. It is also improper to discriminate based on an individual's military, marital, parental, or socioeconomic status. Finally, it is important to recognize the concerns and problems surrounding consensual romantic or sexual relationships. Consensual relationships are romantic or sexual relationships in which both parties consent to a relationship but the possibility of a power differential exists (e.g., instructor-student). Because of the high potential for a conflict of interest and abuse in these relationships (e.g., grading of an assignment), they are unwise and are best avoided. Those involved in consensual relationships must take action to eliminate or mitigate the chances that conflict will occur. As with sexual harassment, all discriminatory issues and consensual relationships must be brought to the attention of the proper individuals at the academic institution and clinical learning environment.

STUDENT HEALTH REQUIREMENTS

Through the rigors of the professional program, it is likely that the student will require a few sick days; this is usually of no major consequence. Material presented in a lecture can be obtained from class notes or from the assigned text. However, this can present a host of problems for pharmacy students participating in the clinical practice environment, and a prolonged illness can be devastating. In fact, depending on school policy, too many sick days could result in an automatic failure or withdrawal from the experiential learning course work.

Every effort should be made to avoid being absent from the clinical practice environment. Nevertheless, one should never report to the environment with a communicable disease that could have serious medical complications for patients and other members of the health care team. Therefore, it is incumbent on all pharmacy students to take good care of themselves to avoid illness. Inevitably, some students will be stricken with a communicable illness. If this happens, it is the responsibility of the student to contact a private physician, student health service, or health service of the current assigned clinical practice environment to ascertain the limitations of activities to minimize spreading the disease. Information given to health services is confidential and cannot be used to remove the student from the institution. Prohibiting participation occurs only in the most extreme circumstances when the safety and welfare of patients are at risk.

In addition to preventive measures, colleges of pharmacy and their affiliated clinical practice environments require basic evidence of immunization or natural immunity to disease. Every student should have a good understanding of the school's health policies and the policies of the affiliated clinical practice environments. An example student health policy is shown in Box 3.4. This policy requires students to have documentation of vaccination against mumps, measles, and rubella (or have serologic tests confirming immunity on file) before admission into any clinical practice environment. In addition, a tuberculin skin test is required before beginning experiential learning course work, and

---

Box 3.4   Sample Health Policy for Students Assigned to Patient Care Areas

---

I. PURPOSE

To ensure that students rotating through the hospital and clinics as part of a clinical training program have been:

➤ **Properly** screened for infectious diseases prior to reporting for duty.

➤ **Informed** that if they are susceptible and are exposed to an infectious disease, they must report the exposure to their preceptor/supervisor and will not be allowed in the hospital until it has been determined that they do not pose a risk of transmission.

II. POLICY

It is the responsibility of schools, colleges, and universities sending students to the hospital and clinics for clinical training to ensure that their students have been screened for the infectious diseases listed below.

➤ **Tuberculosis**[*]—A 5TU tuberculin skin test is required within the past 12 months unless it is known that the student or service personnel is already tuberculin positive. Tuberculin-positive (10 mm of induration with standardized 5TU PPD skin test) students or personnel should be able to provide documentation that they have been judged not to be infectious.

➤ **Measles/Mumps/Rubella**[*]—A record of immunization or the results of a serologic (antibody) testing confirming immunity must be on file at the student's school or college. If not contraindicated medically, immunization is required for all students found to be susceptible by serologic testing. The most recent recommendations as promulgated by the Centers for Disease Control (CDC) and the Public Health Service Advisory Committee on Immunization Practices (ACIP) should be used to determine whether additional immunization is necessary.

Box 3.4 *Continued*

➤ **Varicella** (Chicken Pox)—If it cannot be confirmed that the student had chicken pox, an immunofluorescent antibody (IFA) test is strongly recommended. If the history or the antibody test indicates that the student is susceptible, the student must be counseled as to the serious implications of exposing vulnerable hospital patients and staff to chicken pox. It is very strongly recommended that personnel who are found to be susceptible to varicella be immunized through their sponsoring organization before beginning their rotation at the hospital and clinics in order to avoid contracting the disease or spreading it to vulnerable patients.

If a susceptible student/service personnel is exposed to varicella (chicken pox) or herpes zoster (shingles) during the period in which they are working at the hospital and clinics, they must immediately report the exposure to their preceptor (clinical training coordinator) or supervisor, who will contact the Employee Health Service and Infection Control. Employee Health and Infection Control will make a determination on whether the student or service personnel poses a risk of transmission in the current clinical rotation of assignment and whether they will be allowed to continue the rotation or assignment, assigned to another service, or allowed in the hospital until it is determined they no longer pose a risk.

➤ **Other**—In the course of the above assessment, a general health history should be obtained to determine any other conditions that may need to be evaluated medically or for which the student/service personnel may need counseling to protect themselves or patients before reporting to the hospital and clinics. Any questions or concerns in this respect should be directed to the head of the department at the hospital and clinics sponsoring the clinical training or active duty service.

Box 3.4 *Continued*

III. DOCUMENTATION

Schools and colleges sending students to the hospital will be expected to forward documentation confirming that the above screening and education has been done and the results of such screening to the hospital preceptor/supervisor.

Source: University of Wisconsin Hospital and Clinics Administrative Manual - Policies and Procedures. Madison, WI: University of Wisconsin, Madison; 1996.
* *State statute requires testing for rubella and tuberculosis.*

---

yearly tests are required while engaged in experiential experiences. A varicella (chicken pox) antibody test also is now strongly recommended for those who have not had the disease. For those with negative titers, inoculation with the varicella vaccine is advantageous. Unless otherwise contraindicated, students should have their diphtheria, tetanus, pertussis, and polio vaccinations up to date and strongly consider a series of hepatitis B vaccinations, because the possibility of encountering blood or other potentially infectious material is great. Finally, an influenza vaccination should be considered to guard against obtaining and transmitting this disease.

Students with general health conditions (e.g., HIV-positive status) that could preclude them from meeting any health status requirements should contact their instructor and student advisor before entering the clinical practice environment. This policy is meant to reduce the risks and protect the welfare of all individuals from unnecessary medical maladies. As with patients, a student's health status is strictly confidential and will always remain so.

Students must be aware of their responsibility to maintain good medical hygiene practices in the clinical practice environment. In particular, students should familiarize themselves with and follow the Universal Precautions policies advocated in their clinical practice environments. Some examples of Universal Precautions policies related to direct patient care, sterile products preparation, and environmental decontamination are described in Box 3.5. Overall, the

Box 3.5 Sample Universal Precautions for Pharmacy Students Assigned to Patient Care Areas

DIRECT PATIENT CARE

(1) Wash hands thoroughly with liquid soap or antimicrobial skin cleanser after contact with a patient

(2) Do not recap needles

(3) Dispose of syringes and needles in appropriate containers

(4) Care for patients in isolation areas according to the isolation technique specific to that patient's diagnosis

(5) Use clean latex or vinyl gloves for all nonsterile contacts (i.e., if there is a risk of contacting blood or body fluids) requiring a barrier between the patient and the caregiver. Discard gloves between patient contacts

(6) Wash hands routinely after gloves are removed

(7) Wear a gown if there is a risk of splashing blood or body fluids

(8) Wear masks and protective eye wear or face shields during procedures likely to generate splashes or aerosolization of blood or other body fluids

(9) Contact the Employee or Student Health Service to determine the guidelines for patient contact if you have open skin lesions, weeping dermatitis, diarrhea, or rashes of unknown etiology

STERILE PRODUCTS PREPARATION

(1) All personnel involved in sterile compounding must wash their hands with an antimicrobial cleanser before engaging in the preparation of sterile products. If sterile compounding is interrupted, repeat the hand-washing procedure

Box 3.5 *Continued*

(2) All personnel with upper respiratory tract infections who are assigned to compound sterile products must wear a face mask during the compounding

(3) Dispose of sharp objects in appropriate boxes

(4) Clean both the laminar and vertical flow hoods at least once per shift with 70% isopropryl alcohol and wipe with gauze pads

(5) Dispose of needles in the red needle containers that will be removed by the housekeeping staff

(6) Surgical latex gloves and isolation gowns are required for chemotherapy preparation

(7) Prepare all oncology drugs in the Type II vertical flow hood

ENVIRONMENTAL DECONTAMINATION

(1) Dispose of trash items that have been in contact with patients according to institutional isolation techniques

(2) Clean and disinfect blood and body fluid spills with hospital disinfectant detergent (HDD)

Source: Adapted from the University of Wisconsin Hospital and Clinics Department of Pharmacy Policy and Procedure. July 1996.

intent of any of these precautions is to provide adequate direction for health care team members in maintaining proper medical hygiene and decreasing the transmission of communicable diseases.

Acknowledgment

The authors acknowledge Ms. Rosanne Delfosse, Ms. Jennifer Lendbord, and the University of Wisconsin Hospital and Clinics

Pharmacy Department for their assistance and use of materials in the preparation of this chapter.

Suggested Readings

Academic Misconduct Rules and Procedures—Guide for Students. Madison, WI: University of Wisconsin-Madison, Dean of Students Office; 1996;Fall.

Academic Misconduct Rules and Procedures—Guide for Instructors. Madison, WI: University of Wisconsin-Madison, Dean of Students Office; 1997;Spring.

Bourhis RY, Roth S, MacQueen G. Communication in the hospital setting: a survey of medical and everyday language use amongst patients, nurses and doctors. Soc Sci Med. 1989;28(4):339–46.

Furlow TW Jr. Clinical etiquette: a critical primer. JAMA. 1988;260(17):2558–9.

Hepler DC, Strand LM. Opportunities and responsibilities in pharmaceutical care. Am J Hosp Pharm. 1990;47:533–43.

Kilwein JH. Cross-cultural perspectives of health and illness: an elective course. Am J Pharm Educ. 1985;49(Fall):274–6.

Pritchett J. Diversity: where do I go from here. Unpublished instructional handout. Madison, WI: University of Wisconsin-Madison School of Pharmacy; 1997.

Quick Reference to Cultural Assessment. St. Louis, MO: Mosby, 1994.

Gropper RC. Cultural and the Clinical Encounter—An Intercultural Sensitizer for the Health Professions. Yarmouth, ME: Intercultural Press; 1996.

Rantucci MJ. Pharmacists Talking With Patients—A Guide to Patient Counseling. Baltimore, MD: Williams & Wilkins; 1997.

Schneller Hazebrook L. Standard of professional conduct. In: Boh LE, ed. Clinical Clerkship Manual. Vancouver, WA: Applied Therapeutics, 1993:2–1–9.

Social Issues Update—Academic Year 1997–98. Madison, WI: Dean of Students Office and the Equity and Diversity Resource Center, University of Wisconsin-Madison, 1997.

Starr, Gracious C. Guide to good etiquette for the pharmacist. Drug Top. 1993;37(suppl 3):18–9.

Storti Craig. Cross-Cultural Dialogues—74 Brief Encounters with Cultural Difference. Yarmouth, ME: Intercultural Press; 1994.

The American Heritage Dictionary of the English Language. 2nd college ed. Boston, MA: Houghton Mifflin; 1985.

University of Wisconsin Hospital and Clinics Administrative
Manual—Policies and Procedures. Madison, WI: University of
Wisconsin, Madison; 1996.

University of Wisconsin Hospital and Clinics Department of
Pharmacy Policy and Procedure Manual. Madison, WI;
University of Wisconsin, Madison; 1996;July.

University of Wisconsin-Madison School of Pharmacy 1997–98
Student Handbook and Resource Manual. Madison, WI:
University of Wisconsin-Madison School of Pharmacy; 1997.

U.S. Equal Employment Opportunity Commission (EEOC).
Definitions of, and guidelines on, sexual harassment. Fed Reg.
1989:November 10.

Wick JY. Culture, ethnicity and medications. J Am Pharm Assoc
1996;NS36:556–64.

Zinn W. The empathic physician. Arch Intern Med.
1993;153(3):306–12.

Chapter 4

Providing Drug Information

Kathryn L. Grant and Stacy L. Haber

Learning to provide drug information entails efficiently, accurately, and quickly answering drug information questions. This chapter contains questions students frequently ask about providing drug information. Each question reflects an important step in the process of providing quality drug information. As with other clinical skills, the process seems slow and cumbersome at first. Practice and experience help the student to use this process to successfully provide quality drug information. This chapter is not a substitute for a drug literature evaluation course.

WHAT IF I AM ASKED A QUESTION AND I AM UNSURE OF THE ANSWER?

In such cases, the student should always research the answer. The student should never be intimidated into providing an answer when he or she is unsure of its accuracy. A patient's health is not worth the risk.

WHAT TYPES OF QUESTIONS ARE ASKED?

The majority of drug information questions fall into 1 of 10 major categories:

➤ **Adverse** drug reactions
➤ **Alternative** medicines
➤ **Doses**
➤ **Drug** administration
➤ **Drug** identification
➤ **Drug** interactions
➤ **Indications**
➤ **Intravenous** or intramuscular compatibilities

➤ Pharmacokinetics
➤ Teratogenicity

Table 4-1 lists examples in each category. These examples should be reviewed to prepare for the scope of questions

Table 4-1.	Major Drug Information Question Categories
Categories	**Sample Questions**
Adverse drug reactions	What is the incidence of flushing with niacin?
	Can ranitidine cause liver toxicity?
	What are the side effects of nimodipine?
Alternative medicines	Can I take St. John's wort with fluoxetine?
	Will saw palmetto alter prostate serum antigen (PSA) levels?
	What are the adverse effects of high doses (>10 g) vitamin C given intravenously daily for cancer treatment?
Doses	What is the dose of phenytoin for status epilepticus?
	What is the dose of gentamicin in a patient with renal failure?
	What is the dose of acetaminophen in a 6-month-old infant?
Drug administration	Can carbamazepine be given rectally?
	How rapidly can cimetidine be given intravenously?
	Should iron dextran be given as a Z-track injection?
Drug identification	What is a new drug called sirolimus?
	What is the new, approved drug for endometriosis?
	What is the drug's name which is a round, white tablet imprinted MSD 214?

Table 4-1. *Continued*

Categories	Sample Questions
Drug interactions	Can aspirin and wafarin safely be given concurrently? Can tetracycline be taken with milk? Will cephalexin interefere with a serum glucose determination?
Indications	What is epoetin used for? What is the first line drug therapy for endometriosis? How effective is mesalamine for the treatment of ulcerative colitis?
Intravenous or intramuscular compatibilities	Can heparin and nitroprusside be added to the same IV bag/bottle? Can morphine and diphenhydramine be drawn into the same syringe?
Pharmacokinetics	What is the half-life of streptokinase? How much phenytoin should be given to a patient with a steady-state concentration of 5 μg/mL?
Teratogenicity	What would the risk to the fetus be if a woman took aspirin 650 mg twice a day for 2 weeks during her first trimester? Which antibiotics could be used to treat a urinary tract infection in a woman entering her third trimester?

often asked concerning drug therapy or drug delivery. Other drug information categories include requests for information concerning breast-feeding, carcinogenicity/ mutagenicity, chemistry, contraindications, costs, patient information, pharmacology, poisoning/overdose, preparations, stability, and storage.

WHO ASKS DRUG INFORMATION QUESTIONS?

Pharmacists are recognized as drug experts, and pharmacy students are considered "drug experts in training." As a result, patients, nurses, physicians, other pharmacists, students, respiratory therapists, and anyone who needs drug knowledge ask drug information questions. Answers must be tailored to the questioner. A nurse may need a concise, patient-specific answer, whereas a physician may require a more detailed explanation including where the information was found. A patient needs to have information provided in understandable terminology.

HOW CAN I ANSWER DRUG INFORMATION QUESTIONS QUICKLY?

As with any new skill, the student needs to learn a process that—when practiced and used—helps efficiently and accurately locate the necessary information. The key to the process is Step 1 in Box 4.1. A considerable amount of time can be wasted if the question is not thoroughly understood. An inaccurate or incomplete answer can result when insufficient background or patient-specific data are obtained. Table 4-2 provides background and patient-specific data commonly needed to help accurately answer a question.

Box 4.1 Five-Step Process for Providing Drug Information

(1) Define and understand the question
(2) Search for an answer
(3) Evaluate and compile the facts
(4) Formulate an answer
(5) Follow up

Copyright 1993 by Applied Therapeutics, Inc. August 29, 1997.

Table 4-2. Defining Drug Information Questions

Categories	Background or Patient-Specific Information
Adverse drug reactions	Description of reactions
	Medications/duration of therapy
	Known allergies
	Concurrent disease states
	Age, weight, race, sex
Alternative medicines	Determine type:
	Botanical, Chinese herbal, homeopathic flower essences, aromatherapy
	Reputable manufacturer
	Standardized extract, plant part
	Symptoms of adverse effects
	Dose and duration of therapy
Doses	Indication
	Route
	Renal function[a]
	Liver function
	Age, weight, race, sex
	Concurrent medications
	Known allergies
	Concurrent diseases
Drug administration	Route
	Concurrent medications
	If IV:
	Peripheral versus central access
	Infusion fluid
	Other IV medications
	If IM:
	Ability to tolerate pain
	Availability of sites
	Platelet levels
	If oral:
	Bowel sounds present
	Patient absorbing orally
	If rectal:
	Colon disease present
	Diarrhea

Table 4-2. *Continued*

Categories	Background or Patient-Specific Information
Drug identification	Correct spelling
	Imprint code
	Trade versus generic name
	Marketed, investigational, or foreign
	Indication
	Dosage form
	If foreign:
	Country of origin
	Container information
Drug interactions	
Drug-drug	Current medications
	Symptoms of the interaction, if occurring
	Adding a new drug
	Stopping a drug known to be causing an interaction
	Age, weight, race, sex
	Disease state(s)
Drug-food	Current medications
	Dose/schedule
	Timing of meals
	Specific food problem (e.g., milk)
Drug-laboratory	Current medications
	Laboratory test(s)
	Specific test method used
Indications	Disease state (severity, onset, duration)
	Previous drug therapy
	Previous nondrug therapy
	See doses above
Infectious diseases	Microorganism culture and susceptibility results
	Infection site as above
IV or IM compatibilities	Medications/doses/schedules/routes
	Infusion fluid
	IV set-up[b] (number and types of access sites available)

Table 4-2. *Continued*

Categories	Background or Patient-Specific Information
Pharmacokinetics	Medication/dose/schedule
	Age, weight, race, sex
	Previous serum levels
	Drug pharmacokinetic parameters
	Elimination half-life
	Volume of distribution
	Serum peak concentrations
	Serum trough concentrations
	Time to peak concentration
	Compartment model
	Area-under-the-curve (AUC)
Teratogenicity	Medications/doses/schedules/duration
	Trimester
	Medical status
	Drinking/smoking history
	Can therapy be postponed until postpartum

[a] Renal function parameters include serum creatinine, creatinine clearance, dialysis method, and dialysis schedule.

[b] IV set-ups include continuous infusions: two drugs added to the same liter bag/bottle; piggyback or Y site: one drug infused in the IV line of another drug; and injection port: one drug pushed from a syringe into the line of another drug.

HOW LONG CAN I TAKE TO ANSWER A DRUG INFORMATION QUESTION?

The questioner should be asked when he or she needs the answer; it should be remembered that a detailed search for a complicated question takes time. The answer to a patient-related question, however, loses its impact the longer the turnaround time from question to answer. Therefore, a less thorough search may be acceptable if the answer is timely for the patient in question. The student should be prepared to negotiate if the questioner appears to have an unrealistic expectation.

WHERE DO I LOOK FOR INFORMATION?

Hundreds of texts and thousands of journals provide information to answer questions. Knowing which reference to use, along with when and how to use principal references, are the keys to finding pertinent and accurate information quickly. Medical information can be pictured as a pyramid (Fig. 4-1). Medical knowledge relies on reports of clinical experience and clinical trials published in journal articles; these publications are referred to as *primary literature*. The most efficient way to find current, relevant primary literature is to complete a primary literature search using *secondary sources* (guides to primary literature). Performing literature searches for every question, no matter how minor, would be impractical. Health care educators write *textbooks* and *reference books* that, depending on their focus, compile, review, or evaluate the medical information published in primary literature to facilitate access by students and practitioners. An efficient search method is to begin at the top of the pyramid with the compiled information and work down. This approach recognizes that textbooks and reference books, while providing excellent accumulated data, are not as current as more recently published reviews, editorials, and clinical trials.

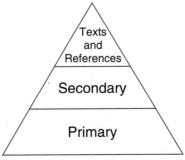

Figure 4-1. Overview of medical information sources.

Table 4-3 lists the most helpful references and is organized by the 10 major categories of drug information inquiries as listed in Table 4-1. Reference entries under each

Table 4-3.	Drug Information Sources: Text and References Organized by Drug Information Categories
Category	**Reference Choices**[a]
Adverse Drug Reactions	AHFS DI[b]/DrugDex[b]/USP DI[b]
	Clinical Pharmacology[b]/Lexicomp[b]/ Physicians GenRx[b]
	Martindale's: The Extra Pharmacopoeia[b]
	Side Effects of Drugs
	Textbook of Adverse Drug Reactions
	Goodman and Gilman's: The Pharmacologic Basis of Therapeutics[b]
Alternative Medicines	Honest Herbal
	Review of Natural Products
	PDR for Herbal Predications
	Natural Medicines Comprehensive Database
	Professional's Handbook of Complementary & Alternative Medicine
	HerbalGram
	Berkley Wellness Letter
Doses	Drug Facts and Comparisons[b]
	AHFS DI[b]/DrugDex[b]/USP DI[b]
	Clinical Pharmacology[b]/Physicians GenRx[b]
	Physicians Desk Reference(s)[b]
	Martindale's: The Extra Pharmacopoeia[b]
Pediatric	Pediatric Drug Handbook
	Pediatric Dosage Handbook
	Harriet Lane Handbook
	Current Pediatric Diagnosis and Treatment

Table 4-3. *Continued*

Category	Reference Choices[a]
Drug Administration	See **Doses**
	If IV/IM see Handbook of Injectable Drugs
Drug Identification	
Marketed	Drug Facts and Comparisons[b]
	PharmIndex
	Identidex[b]
	AHFS DI[b]/DrugDex[b]/USP DI[b]
	Clinical Pharmacology[b]/Lexicomp[b]/ Physicians GenRx[b]
	Physicians Desk Reference(s)[b]
	American Drug Index
	Handbook of Nonprescription Drugs
	Drug Topics Red Book
Investigational	PharmIndex
	Martindale's: The Extra Pharmacopoeia[b]
	DrugDex[b]
	USP Dictionary of USAN and International Drug Names
	Unlisted Drugs
	Merck Index
	FDC Reports: The Pink Sheets
Foreign	Martindale's: The Extra Pharmacopoeia[b]
	Unlisted Drugs
	European Drug Index
	Index Nominum
	Diccionaria de Especialidades Farmaceuticas
	USP Dictionary of USAN and International Drug Names
Drug Interactions	
Drug-drug	Drug Interactions & Updates
	Drug Interactions Facts
	Evaluation of Drug Interactions
	AHFS DI[b]/DrugDex[b]/USP DI[b]

continued

Table 4-3. *Continued*

Category	Reference Choices[a]
	Clinical Pharmacology[b]/Lexicomp[b]/ Physicians GenRx[b]
Side Effects of Drugs	
Drug-food	Drug Interactions & Updates
	USP DI Vol. II: Advice for the Patient
Drug-laboratory	Handbook of Clinical Drug Data
	Clinical Guide to Laboratory Tests
	Interpretation of Diagnostic Tests
	Laboratory Test Handbook
Indications	Pharmacotherapy
	AHFS DI[b]/DrugDex[b]/USP DI[b]
	Clinical Pharmacology[b]/Physicians GenRx[b]
	Applied Therapeutics: The Clinical Use of Drugs
	Drug Information Handbook
	Current Medical Diagnosis and Treatment
	Current Pediatric Diagnosis and Treatment
	Manual of Medical Therapeutics
	Scientific American[b]
	Harrison's: Principles of Internal Medicine
Infectious diseases	Mandell's: Principles and Practice of Infectious Disease
	Medical Letter Handbook of Antimicrobial Therapy
	Sanford's Guide to Antimicrobial Therapy
Intravenous or Intramuscular Compatibilities	Handbook of Injectable Drugs
	King's Guide to Parenteral Admixtures
	Martindale's: The Extra Pharmacopoeia[b]

Table 4-3. *Continued*

Category	Reference Choices[a]
Pharmacokinetics	Applied Pharmacokinetics: Principles of Therapeutic Drug Monitoring Basic Clinical Pharmacokinetics AHFS DI[b]/DrugDex[b]/USP DI[b] Clinical Pharmacology[b]/Lexicomp[b]/ Physicians GenRx[b] Handbook of Clinical Drug Data Goodman and Gilman's: The Pharmacologic Basis of Therapeutics[b] Martindale's: The Exta Pharmacopoeia[b]
Teratogenicity	Physicians Desk Reference[b] Drugs in Pregnancy and Lactation ReproRisk[b] Catalog of Teratogenic Agents[b] AHFS DI[b]/DrugDex[b]/USP DI[b] Clinical Pharmacology[b]/Physicians GenRx[b]

[a] Under each category, the references are listed in roughly the order in which they would most likely provide the answer.
[b] Available on software.

category are listed in descending order from most likely to contain the information to the least likely.

WHEN SHOULD I SEARCH THE PRIMARY LITERATURE?

➤ If the questioner asks for primary literature references.
➤ If the answer is not in text and references.
➤ If the information found in text and references appears to be out of date.

HOW DO I USE SECONDARY SOURCES TO PERFORM A LITERATURE SEARCH?

Medline is one of the most extensive and commonly used secondary sources; however, it is important to recognize that Medline is just one of many secondary sources. Some other secondary sources that may be helpful when searching for answers to drug information questions include the following: International Pharmaceutical Abstracts, Cancer-Lit, PsycINFO, and AIDSLINE. Each of these databases indexes literature that Medline does not. Additionally, there are databases with limited access that are larger in scope than Medline, such as Embase.

Secondary sources are all organized differently. Some secondary sources provide only the citation (defined as the journal article's author[s], article title, journal title, year, volume, issue, and page numbers), whereas others provide the citation along with an abstract. Frequency of publication (e.g., monthly, quarterly), format of publication (e.g., computer access, hard-bound book, section of a journal), and indexing format are additional differences in secondary sources.

Indexing large databases is difficult, and large databases such as Medlars (Table 4-4) standardize medical terms or phrases to facilitate the process. If standardized terms are used, the secondary source publishes a list of synonyms in a thesaurus, and the secondary source's thesaurus must be accessed to use the reference efficiently and accurately. Table 4-4 lists eight commonly used secondary sources including their format(s), how often they are updated, their focus, the type and number of journals reviewed, and whether a published thesaurus is available. Computerized databases can often be searched by the standardized (thesaurus) term and by free text or key words. Key words are any words that appear in the citation or abstract. A detailed explanation of how to use these sources is beyond the scope of this chapter. Students are encouraged to find out which ones are available in the medical or pharmacy libraries or drug information centers accessible to them.

Table 4-4. Drug Information Sources: Secondary References

Secondary References	Format	Updates	Focus	Types of Journals Reviewed	Number of Journals Reviewed	Published Thesaurus
Allied and Complementary Medicine (AMED)	Abstracting service for online searching	Monthly	Complementary medicine palliative care	Medicine, pharmacy, alternative medicine	55,000 records since 1985	No
Clin-Alert. Scheible-Jacobs R, ed. Medford, NJ: Clin-Alert, Inc.	Abstracting service as a newsletter edition	Semi-monthly	Adverse drug reactions	Medicine, pharmacy	600	No
Current Contents: Clinical Practice. Garfield E. Philadelphia, PA: Institute for Scientific Information Inc.	Table of contents indexed by author and key works in either a soft cover edition, floppy-disk, or CD-ROM	Weekly	Clinical practice	Medicine, pharmacy	850	No

continues

Table 4-4. Continued

Secondary References	Format	Updates	Focus	Types of Journals Reviewed	Number of Journals Reviewed	Published Thesaurus
InPharma. Covich K, ed. Langhorne, PA: Australian Drug Information Services	Abstracting service as a newsletter edition or online searching	Weekly	Clinical practice	Medicine, pharmacy	1800	No
International Pharmaceutical Abstracts (IPA). Tousignaut D, ed. Bethesda, MD: American Society of Hospital Pharmacists	Abstracting service as a soft cover edition; CD-ROM and online searching available also	Monthly, quarterly	Pharmacy	Pharmacy practice	800	Yes
Iowa Drug Information Service (IDIS). Seaba H, ed. Iowa City, IA: The University of Iowa	Citation and whole article on microfiche; citation only on CD-ROM	Monthly	Clinical practice	Medicine, pharmacy	170	Yes

Medlars

Index Medicus. Lindberg DAB, ed. Washington, DC: Superintendent of Documents, US Government Printing Office	Citations as a hard cover edition	Monthly	Biomedical research, medicine, pharmacy, nursing	Research, clinical practice	2700	Yes
OVID and other vendors	Abstracting service on CD-ROM	Monthly	As above	As above	3800	Yes
NLM, Grateful Med, Dialog, and other vendors	Abstracting service as online searching	Quarterly	As above	As above	3800	Yes

continued

Table 4-4. Continued

Secondary References	Format	Updates	Focus	Types of Journals Reviewed	Number of Journals Reviewed	Published Thesaurus
Internet Grateful Med, PubMed	Abstracting service on the Internet	Weekly	As above	As above	3800	Yes
PsycINFO	Abstracting service for online searching	Monthly	Psychology, psychiatry	Medicine, pharmacy, nursing, sociology, education, physiology, linguistics	1400	No
Reactions Weekly. Wright T, ed. Langhorne, PA: Australian Drug Information Service	Abstracting service as a newsletter edition	Weekly	Adverse drug reactions	Medicine, pharmacy	1800	No.

HOW DO I CONSTRUCT A SEARCH STRATEGY FOR A COMPUTERIZED LITERATURE SEARCH?

Each computerized secondary source, whether accessed from a personal computer connected to a CD-ROM reader or a modem access to a mainframe, uses different commands and nomenclature. The specific source's user manual should be consulted for detailed instructions. In general, the user types in a search statement (SS). A simple search could be as follows.

> SS
> 1 flumazenil

The secondary source will respond with the number of citations (postings) containing the word/index term "flumazenil."

> postings: 384

Search strategies can be combined to expand or limit the postings. Combinations are made by using the Boolean connecting words "and," "or," and "not." The Boolean operator "and" limits the number of postings retrieved (Fig. 4-2i). The Boolean operator "or" widens retrievals (Fig. 4-2ii). Although the Boolean operator "not" limits retrieval, results can be unpredictable. For now, the use of "not" should be avoided (Fig. 4-2iii). Boolean operators can be combined in series. Figure 4-3i shows the theoretical retrieval if three statements are all combined with an

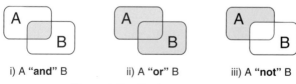

| i) A **"and"** B | ii) A **"or"** B | iii) A **"not"** B |

Figure 4-2. Boolean operators.

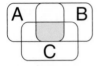 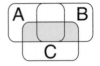

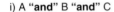

i) A **"and"** B **"and"** C   ii) A **"or"** B **"and"** C

Set A, B and Set C represent theoretical literature citations (e.g., A = Aspirin, B = Arthritis and C = Reviews). The highlighted area represents retrieved citations obtained when the Boolean connectors are combined in series: i) Boolean connector **"and"** combined in series, ii) Boolean connector **"or"** combined with **"and"** in series.

Figure 4-3. Representation of search.

"and": A "and" B "and" C. Figure 4-3ii shows the results when (A "or" B) "and" C are combined.

The following four steps are used to develop a search strategy efficiently:

1. Break the question into component parts (word sets), labeling each set with a heading (A, B, C).
2. Write down all potential thesaurus and key word terms under each word set.
3. Combine each term in the word set with the Boolean operator "or."
4. Combine each word set with the Boolean operator "and."

Be patient. Rarely can a perfect search strategy be constructed the first time.

If too few citations are retrieved, additional terms may need to be used, "and" may have been typed instead of "or" (a common mistake), or not many citations on the topic exist. To come up with more terms, the searcher should type the command to review the thesaurus terms used by the indexer on the citations already retrieved. Perhaps they will provide a clue for other terms to use. Two word sets are usually sufficient for most questions. Using a third word set often limits retrieval to zero postings.

Conversely, if too many citations are retrieved, limiting the search by requesting only English language and human studies may decrease the number of citations. Retrieval can

---

Box 4.2   Example of a Computerized Literature Search

QUESTION

Is flumazenil effective for the treatment of acute alcohol intoxication?

STEP ONE

Break the question into component parts or word sets, labelling each set A, B, etc.
   Is flumazenil effective for the treatment of acute alcohol intoxication?

   A. Flumazenil
   B. Acute alcohol intoxication

Note the concept of efficacy is not searchable.

STEP TWO

Write down all potential thesaurus and key word terms under each heading.

A	B
Flumazenil[a]	Alcoholic intoxication[a]
Flumazepil[b]	Alcohol drinking[a]
Ro 15-1788[b]	Alcohol, ethyl[a]
Mazicon[b]	Ethanol[b]
Romazicon[b]	

---

[a] Thesaurus terms in MEDLINE.
[b] Textword terms in MEDLINE.

continued

---

also be limited, if relevant to the question, by requesting studies by age group, gender, reviews, comparative studies, etc. If only two word sets were used, adding a third word set may limit the number of retrievals.

   Box 4.2 shows an example of a computerized literature search.

Box 4.2   *Continued*

STEP THREE

Combine each term listed together under a heading with the Boolean operator "or".

SS

1. flumazenil or flumazepil or Ro 15-1788 or mazicon or romazicon
2. alcoholic intoxication or alcohol drinking or alcohol, ethyl or ethanol

STEP FOUR

Combine each word set with the Boolean operator "and".

3. #1 and #2.

HOW DO I EVALUATE CLINICAL TRIALS?

Whole college courses are devoted to this topic, and a detailed review of drug literature evaluation is beyond this chapter's objectives. A simplified approach follows.

In general, when evaluating a clinical trial, the reader is trying to determine if biases are apparent in how the study was written, designed, and completed. If biases are evident, the next step is to determine whether these biases are serious enough to invalidate the study's results.

The four basic sections of a written clinical trial other than the abstract are as follows: 1) introduction, 2) methodology, 3) results, and 4) discussion. Each section or subsection is analyzed to answer the evaluative questions.

Introduction

Was a statement of the study's objective(s) clearly provided?

Methods
➤ **What** was the study design? Was the study design explained in sufficient detail to determine how subjects were included or excluded, the number of subjects included, and the subject parameters that might influence the results?
➤ **Were** the data collected retrospectively or prospectively?
➤ **Did** the study use acceptable controls (i.e., placebo, standard drug, historical)?
➤ **Were** subjects randomly assigned to treatment groups?
➤ **If** the study involved a cross-over treatment regimen, was the drug-free interval before cross-over of sufficient duration?
➤ **Did** the design include blinding of the subject or investigator (single blind); the subject and investigator (double blind); or the observer?
➤ **Were** the test methods used to measure results subjective or objective? Were they reliable, sensitive, and specific?

Results
➤ **Were** all pertinent results presented in sufficient detail for adequate analysis?
➤ **Were** the tabular, graphic, and written presentations accurate, distorted, or misleading?
➤ **Was** the statistical method used appropriate for the data collected?
➤ **Did** a statistically significant difference support a clinically significant difference?

Discussion
➤ **Were** the authors' conclusions accurately based on the results presented?
➤ **Were** the authors' conclusions in keeping with the study's stated objectives?

HOW DO I COMPILE THE FACTS TO ANSWER THE QUESTION?

At this point, the student has collected bits and pieces of information from text/references and the primary literature.

The hardest part of providing drug information is summarizing and applying the information to a clinical situation. Students must apply the knowledge from all their didactic courses to put the retrieved information in perspective with their clinical knowledge and to synthesize an answer.

Students usually have difficulties determining how to organize clinical trial information. In general, the following six steps will assist in sorting clinical trial information. Step 1 is to organize by disease state. Step 2 is to organize within the disease state by study design. Then organize by severity of illness (Step 3) and then by doses used (Step 4). Occasionally, further organization by outcomes measured (Step 5) or results (Step 6) would be useful.

This method provides a framework for organizing and summarizing the clinical trial information to more easily see differences and similarities. The following is an example using this method to organize clinical trial information for alteplase.

1. Specific disease state: acute myocardial infarction, pulmonary edema, stroke
2. Study design: case reports, case series, phase I, phase II, phase III, phase IV
3. Severity of illness: mild, moderate, severe
4. Doses used: 100 mg over 3 hours, ≤100 mg
5. Efficacy measurements: mortality, clot lysis
6. Results: results favoring alteplase, results neutral to alteplase, results not favoring alteplase

WHEN SHOULD I USE THE INTERNET?

The answer to this question depends on access to other sources. If there is access to a large number of reputable texts and references, use of the Internet may be minimal; if not, use of the Internet may be substantial. The Internet may be considered a primary, secondary, or tertiary source; it depends on what is being researched. Box 4.3 lists some questions to ask to help determine if an Internet site is reputable, and Box 4.4 lists some common reputable Internet sites.

**Box 4.3   Questions to Ask to Determine the Reliability
            of an Internet Website**

---

(1) Who maintains the website?

(2) Who writes the information?

(3) When was the site last updated?

(4) How is the site funded?

(5) Is there a formal review mechanism for the
    information?

(6) Does the website provide references to support its
    statements?

(7) Is there a disclaimer stating that the information is
    general and not patient-specific?

(8) Can you contact the website's host?

(9) Does the site have a search mechanism?

Box 4.4   Useful Internet Websites

---

(1) Doctor's Guide to the Internet:
    www.docguide.com

(2) Food and Drug Administration: www.fda.gov

(3) National Guideline Clearinghouse:
    www.guideline.gov

(4) Centers for Disease Control and Prevention:
    www.cdc.gov

(5) American Society of Health-System Pharmacists:
    www.ashp.org

(6) American College of Clinical Pharmacy:
    www.accp.com

(7) Institute for Safe Medication Practices:
    www.ismp.org

(8) National Institutes of Health: www.nih.gov

(9) National Library of Medicine: www.nlm.nih.gov

(10) Agency for Healthcare Research and Quality:
     www.ahcpr.gov

HOW DO I FORMULATE AN ANSWER?

Answers to drug information questions must summarize the results of the literature search and be presented with a logical progression of facts to support the answer. Providing the questioner with an unorganized series of facts is unacceptable. For the busy clinician, the summary is begun with one phrase or sentence clearly stating the answer. The reasons supporting the answer follow. Formal or published answers to drug information questions usually start with in-depth background information followed by the summary of clinical data and ending with the answer.

HOW CAN I BE SURE MY ANSWER IS CORRECT?

All sources of drug information contain errors. Therefore, the best way to determine the accuracy of an answer is to validate and verify the information in more than one source. Most of the time, the information provided can be found in more than one source; if not, another practitioner should be consulted about the question.

After information has been provided, the questioner should be contacted and queried if he or she used the information. If the information was not used, the reason why should be discerned. If it was used, the outcome should be stated. This feedback mechanism measures whether the provided information was relevant, timely, and useful.

HOW CAN I KEEP UP WITH NEW INFORMATION ABOUT DRUGS?

Keeping up with new information about drugs after graduation from school or completion of postgraduate training is a difficult but essential task. Basically, there are two ways to do this: routinely scanning biomedical journals for new information, and using the biomedical literature to answer patient-specific clinical questions. If a routine scan of biomedical journals is used, the journals selected will depend on the pharmacist's practice. Box 4.5 lists a selection of reputable journals available in libraries or by subscription for personal use. An increasing number are available on the Internet. *ACP Journal Club*, *Evidence-Based Medicine*, and *Journal Watch* are publications that summarize information from various biomedical journals and may serve as good starting points.

Box 4.5   Leading Medical and Pharmacy Journals

(1) *New England Journal of Medicine* (weekly)
(2) *Journal of the American Medical Association* (weekly)
(3) *Annals of Internal Medicine* (every two weeks)
(4) *Archives of Internal Medicine* (every two weeks)
(5) *The Lancet* (weekly)
(6) *British Medical Journal* (weekly)
(7) *Annals of Pharmacotherapy* (monthly)
(8) *Pharmacotherapy* (monthly)
(9) *American Journal of Health-System Pharmacy* (semi-monthly)

Chapter 5

Physical Examination

Michael G. Madalon and Randolph W. Hurley

This chapter provides an overview of the adult (including geriatric) physical examination. It is not intended to teach the reader how to perform a physical examination.

Subjective and objective information obtained from the history and physical examination is crucial to the assessment of drug efficacy and toxicity. Both positive and negative findings may be noted. A basic understanding of human physiology and gross anatomy are required before the intricacies of a diagnostic examination can be appreciated, and such reference texts should be accessible.

MEDICAL HISTORY

When a patient is admitted to the hospital or undergoes a detailed medical evaluation, the clinician typically obtains a thorough medical history before physically examining the patient. The history describes the events in the life of the patient that are relevant to the patient's mental and physical health. Although this chapter concentrates on physician examination, it should be noted that the history itself contributes the most to understanding a patient's problem or monitoring a drug's effects. The components of the medical history usually follow a standardized format (Table 5-1).

TECHNIQUES IN THE PHYSICAL EXAMINATION

Physical examination uses four main techniques: inspection, palpation, percussion, and auscultation. Inspection is visual observation of the patient with unaided eyes (e.g., examination of the skin), although instruments (otoophthalmoscopic examination) are often used. Palpation is the use of touch to detect normal and abnormal physical findings (e.g., palpating enlarged lymph nodes). Percussion is the

Table 5-1. The Medical History

Section	Contents
Patient profile	Age, race, sex, date of birth, marital status
Chief complaint (CC)	The reason for seeking medical attention
Present illness (PI)	A chronologic account of events and symptoms of the chief complaint; laboratory/diagnostic procedures and negative findings
Past medical history (PMH)	General state of health Childhood illnesses Immunizations Medical illnesses Psychiatric illnesses Surgical procedures Hospitalizations Injuries Medications Allergies
Family history (FH)	Age and health of living relatives Age and cause of death of relatives Occurrence and relation of family members with diabetes mellitus, high blood pressure, cancer, mental illnesses, tuberculosis, and other serious or hereditary illnesses
Social history (SH)	Financial situation, health habits (sleeping, diet, recreation, use of tobacco, alcohol, or other drugs of abuse), education, religion, and family dynamics
Review of systems (ROS)	Common symptoms by body system; the body areas reviewed are: skin, head, eyes, ears, nose, and sinuses, mouth and throat, neck, breasts, chest and lungs, heart, vascular, gastrointestinal, urinary, reproductive, musculoskeletal, neurologic, psychiatric, endocrine, and hematologic

tapping of a body surface with a fingertip to produce sounds that help determine whether underlying structures are air-filled, fluid-filled, or solid (e.g., percussion of the chest). During percussion, the examiner strikes the body surface to sense the vibrations and sounds generated with each tap. Auscultation, with the aid of a stethoscope, is listening for normal and abnormal sounds (e.g., heart tones, breath sounds, blood pressure assessment).

SIGNS AND SYMPTOMS

When interpreting a history and physical examination, clinical signs and symptoms are often described. A sign refers to objective information gathered by the examiner during the physical examination (e.g., heart murmur, ankle edema, rales). A symptom refers to subjective information gathered from the patient while obtaining the history (e.g., nausea, pain). The patient's descriptions of symptoms may be scrutinized further, clarified, and quantified by additional questioning.

ORGANIZATION OF THE PHYSICAL EXAMINATION

Recorded physical examinations are typically arranged in the following order:

➤ **General** appearance
➤ **Vital** signs
➤ **Skin,** hair, and nails
➤ **Lymph** nodes
➤ **HEENT** (head, eyes, ears, nose, throat)
➤ **Neck**
➤ **Back**
➤ **Chest** (general, lung, and breast examination)
➤ **Cardiovascular** system
➤ **Abdomen**
➤ **Genitourinary** and rectal system
➤ **Peripheral** vascular system
➤ **Musculoskeletal** system
➤ **Neurological** system

General Appearance

This portion of the physical examination provides a brief description of the patient's overall appearance. In the geriatric patient, it is an important assessment and may reflect the individual's general health, nutritional status, and general cognitive function. The patient's posture, facial expressions, hygiene, level of distress, and mental status may be noted here as well. Typical observations might include the following:

➤ **This** is a thin, young female in no apparent distress (NAD).
➤ **This** is an 85-year-old black male (85 yo BM) who is alert and appears younger than stated age.
➤ **This** is a pale, tearful, male who is otherwise alert and oriented.
➤ **This** is a crying but easily consolable male infant.

Vital Signs

Just as the name implies, a patient's vital signs are critical in assessing the clinical status of the patient and the acuity of a given problem. Vital signs include body temperature, pulse, blood pressure, and respirations. In addition, height and weight are typically recorded in this section.

BODY TEMPERATURE (T)

Body temperature is measured in the mouth, rectum, or axilla. Identification of the route is essential for interpretation of the result.

Normal adult body temperatures are as follows:

Mouth: 35.8–37.3°C (96.4–99.1°F)
Axillary: 35.3–36.8°C (95.9–99.6°F)
Rectal: 36.3–37.8°C (94.9–99.6°F)

Fever (temperature greater than 37.8°C /100°F) is associated with infection, inflammation (e.g., connective tissue diseases), or cancer (e.g., lymphoma, renal cell carcinoma). The elderly and immunosuppressed patient may not mount a normal febrile response. Fever may also be an adverse drug reaction (e.g., neuroleptic malignant syndrome or drug fever from amphotericin B).

The normal temperature in children ranges by age, with neonates' temperatures being approximately 1°F higher than adolescents in total. There is also a diurnal variation of 1–3°, highest in early evening and lowest close to midnight. Normalization of temperature is a crucial response in monitoring efficacy of antimicrobial therapy.

PULSE (P)

Clinicians typically assess the rate, rhythm, and strength of the pulse. The normal heart rate (HR) is 60 to 100 beats/min (BPM). Deviation from normal, particularly tachycardia (HR greater than 100 BPM), is a sensitive indicator of disease. Bradycardia (HR less than 60 BPM) can be normal in a well-conditioned athlete and can be abnormal in a patient with hypothyroidism. An HR less than 60 BPM can also indicate increased vagal tone, cardiac conduction defects, or the effect of drugs with a negative chronotropic effect (e.g., beta blockers, digoxin). Tachycardia has a broad differential diagnosis encompassing a myriad of conditions including pain, anxiety, volume depletion, tachyarrhythmias, and pulmonary embolism. Tachycardia can also be a side effect of drugs (e.g., sympathomimetic and anticholinergic medications).

Rhythm is difficult to assess accurately without the aid of electrocardiographic monitoring; however, the pulse's regularity or irregularity can be assessed. A pulse characterized as "irregularly irregular" may indicate atrial fibrillation, whereas occasional "regularly irregular" beats may indicate premature atrial or ventricular contraction (PAC or PVC). Assessing an apical pulse by auscultation of the heart is the preferred approach for HR determination, because not all beats in atrial fibrillation may be conducted to the peripheral pulses. The average pulse in the neonate may be about 140. This tapers to an average of 110 at age 1 and about 90 at age 10.

BLOOD PRESSURE (BP)

Blood pressure can vary according to age, race, and gender. It can even vary from minute to minute in any given patient. An appropriate cuff size and careful attention to proper technique are critical to accurate blood pressure assessment (e.g., a small cuff on a large patient's arm could overestimate the true blood pressure).

Adult blood pressure greater than 140/90 mm Hg on more than one occasion is considered abnormal. Hypertension is associated with stroke and renal failure. Systolic hypertension, particularly in the elderly, is also a predictor of vascular risk. Orthostatic blood pressure and pulse are defined as the change in BP and pulse when the patient changes from a sitting to a standing position. A systolic BP drop of greater than 10 mm Hg or a pulse rise of greater than 10 to 20 BPM can reflect intravascular volume depletion, autonomic dysfunction, antihypertensive drug therapy, or a side effect of medications (e.g., anticholinergics and antidepressants). Orthostatic hypotension in an elderly patient may contribute to syncope, falls, and hip fractures.

Pulsus paradoxus originally described the decreased amplitude of the peripheral pulse with inspiration; however, it is now more accurately assessed with a blood pressure cuff and reflects the decrease in systolic BP with inspiration. A normal change is 10 mm Hg, but this value can be accentuated in pericardial tamponade, airway obstruction (such as asthma), or superior vena cava obstruction.

RESPIRATORY RATE (RR)

The rate and pattern of breathing are assessed and can reflect cardiopulmonary or neurologic disease. A normal adult breathes at a rate of 12–18 respirations/min. Tachypnea (RR greater than 20 respirations/min) can be caused by anxiety, pain, cardiopulmonary disease, acidosis, or salicylate toxicity. Bradypnea (RR less than 10 respirations/min) can be a sign of drug-induced respiratory depression such as that associated with opiates.

A number of normal and abnormal patterns of breathing have been described. Cheyne-Stokes breathing is a form of periodic breathing characterized by periods of apnea (absent respirations) alternating with a series of respiratory cycles in which the rate and amplitude increase to a maximum (i.e., hyperpnea or deep rapid breathing). Cheyne-Stokes breathing occurs in patients with brain damage (e.g., trauma or cerebral hemorrhage), patients with congestive heart failure (CHF), and in normal persons at high altitude. Kussmaul's respirations are deep regular respirations that occur independent of the rate. Kussmaul breathing occurs in diabetic ketoacidosis and signals hyperventilatory respiratory compensation for the metabolic acidosis.

Although not a specific physical examination finding, sleep apnea is due to upper airway obstruction occurring

during sleep. It may manifest as snoring and daytime som-
nolence and can be exacerbated by alcohol and central nervous system (CNS) depressants.

HEIGHT AND WEIGHT

Although not classic vital signs, height and weight are typically recorded in this section. Height and weight can be
used together to calculate body surface area (BSA) and lean
body weight (LBW). Day-to-day variation in body weight
reflects changes in total body water (TBW), which is important in assessing the hydration and fluid status of the patient or for assessing response to diuretic therapy. Long-
term weight loss (greater than 10% body weight) may
indicate nutritional deficiency in the elderly or an eating
disorder. It is a poor prognostic feature in patients with human immunodeficiency virus (HIV) or cancer. Height may
diminish with age due to osteoporotic vertebral bone loss
and compression fractures. Osteoporosis may be accentuated by long-term corticosteroid therapy or phenytoin.

Skin, Hair, and Nails

SKIN

The integumentary system is perhaps one of the most as-
sessable organ systems for examination. Skin rashes are a
common form of adverse drug reactions. A notation of the
skin examination in the medical record is typically brief yet
contains a number of descriptive terms and phrases. A more
complete description would include details regarding color
(e.g., brownness, cyanosis, yellowness or jaundice), vascularity (including ecchymoses such as petechiae or purpura),
edema, temperature, texture, mobility and turgor, and the
presence of lesions. Poor skin turgor is a sign of dehydration
but also occurs naturally with aging due to loss of elasticity.

Skin lesions are described in terms of primary and secondary lesions (Fig. 5-1). Primary lesions may arise from
previously normal skin and can be divided into three
categories:

1. Circumscribed, flat, nonpalpable changes in skin color
   (macules and patches).
2. Palpable solid elevations in the skin (nodules, plaques,
   papules, cysts, and wheals).

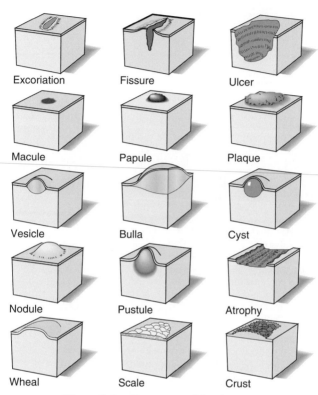

Figure 5-1. Basic types of skin lesions.

3. Circumscribed superficial elevations of the skin formed by free fluid within the skin layers (vesicles, bulla, and pustules).

Secondary lesions result from changes in a primary lesion and include the development of erosions, ulcers, fissures, crusts, and scales.

These descriptive terms can be combined in the record. For example, an erythematous maculopapular eruption (a common manifestation of drug-induced dermatologic toxicity) could be described as circumscribed, flat, red, macules in combination with palpable, solid, raised papules. Table

Table 5-2. Descriptive Dermatologic Terms and Examples

Lesion	Description	Example
Acneiform	Erythematous pustules	Acne
Annular	Ring shaped	Ringworm
Confluent	Lesions run together	Viral exanthems
Discoid	Disc shaped without central clearing	Lupus erythematosus
Eczematoid	An inflammation with a tendency to vesiculate and crust	Eczema
Erythroderma	Diffuse red color	Sunburn
Exfoliative	Sloughing of skin layers	Toxic epidermal necrolysis
Grouped	Clustered lesions	Vesicles of herpes simplex
Iris	"Bulls eye" or target type lesions	Erythema multiform
Keratotic	Thickening	Psoriasis
Linear	In lines	Poison ivy
Papulosquamous	Raised papules or plaques with scaling	Psoriasis
Urticarial	Raised local edema of the skin (wheal)	Hives
Zosteriform	Linear arrangement along a dermatome	Herpes zoster

5-2 and Figure 5-2 provide more information on descriptive dermatologic terms and examples.

Drug-induced cutaneous eruptions occur in many different forms. Common examples include acneiform or pustular (corticosteroids), erythroderma (vancomycin-induced "red man's syndrome"), exfoliation (Stevens-Johnson syndrome from sulfonamides), maculopapular (beta-lactams),

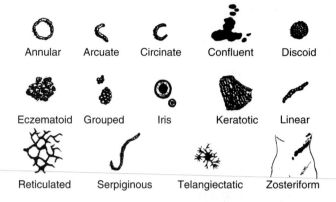

Figure 5-2. Descriptive dermatologic terms.

lupus-like (procainamide, hydralazine), photosensitivity (sulfonamides, fluoroquinolones, methotrexate), urticaria (aspirin sensitivity), and hyperpigmentation (phenothiazines, hydroxychloroquine, amiodarone, oral contraceptives).

HAIR

Hair is considered a skin appendage. It is described according to texture (e.g., dry and coarse as in hypothyroidism) and distribution. Hirsutism (the growth of hair in women in a characteristically male pattern) can be due to androgen excess syndromes, corticosteroids and Cushing's syndrome, oral contraceptives, and androgenic medications. Hypertrichosis (increased hair growth, particularly on the face) is an adverse effect of medications such as minoxidil and cyclosporine. Alopecia, or hair loss, can occur during or after cancer chemotherapy.

NAILS

Nails are also considered a skin appendage. A variety of nail changes have been described, and perhaps the most important is clubbing (Fig. 5-3). Clubbing is the selective bullous enlargement of the distal segment of the digit due to an increase in soft tissue and is associated with flattening of the angle between the nail and nail base from 160° to 180°.

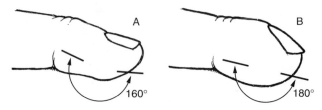

A. Normal angle of the nail.
B. Abnormal angle of the nail seen in late clubbing.

Figure 5-3. Clubbing of the finger.

Clubbing can be hereditary or idiopathic and is associated with a variety of conditions, including cyanotic heart disease and pulmonary disorders (such as chronic obstructive pulmonary disease, cystic fibrosis, tuberculosis, and lung cancer). Pitting and ridging of the nails is another common finding and is characteristic of psoriasis. Beau's lines (horizontal ridge of the nails) can occur during chemotherapy.

Lymph Nodes

Lymph nodes are not usually palpable, unless enlarged (Fig. 5-4 shows the location of lymph node groups.) Enlargement can be due to a variety of disorders including infections, neoplasia (lymphomas and metastatic malignancies), immunologic disorders (rheumatoid arthritis, systemic lupus erythematous), and other illnesses. Rarely, phenytoin produces a pseudolymphomatous enlargement of the lymph nodes.

Lymph nodes are described according to their size, location, firmness, mobility, and tenderness. Tender nodes suggest infection, whereas firm, nontender, immobile nodes suggest malignancy. Shotty nodes are small nodes that feel "like buckshot" underneath the skin and are not necessarily pathologic.

Head, Eyes, Ears, Nose, Throat (HEENT)

HEAD

When the head is described, its shape is noted using the terms normocephalic (occasionally abbreviated NC), hy-

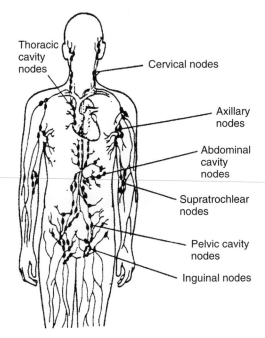

Figure 5-4. Location of lymph nodes in the body.

drocephalic, or microcephalic. Evidence of trauma is discovered by inspection and palpation. Absence of trauma (atraumatic) is occasionally abbreviated AT.

Several disorders have characteristic facial features, including the moon facies of Cushing's syndrome (or corticosteroid use), exophthalmos of Grave's disease, and the masked facies of scleroderma or Parkinsonism. Several skin disorders and rashes affect the face, including acne vulgaris, acne rosacea, the purplish heliotrope rash surrounding the eyelids in dermatomyositis, the butterfly-pattern malar rash over the cheeks in systemic lupus erythematosus (SLE), and the zosteriform rash of herpes zoster.

EYES

The anatomy of the external and internal eye is depicted in Figures 5-5 and 5-6. Routine bedside examination of the

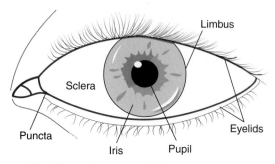

Figure 5-5. External anatomy of the eye. Note how the upper lid normally covers the upper rim of the iris and limbus. Reprinted with permission from Longe RL, Calvert, JC. In: Young LYY, ed. Physical Assessment: A Guide for Evaluating Drug Therapy. Vancouver, WA: Applied Therapeutics, Inc.; 1994.

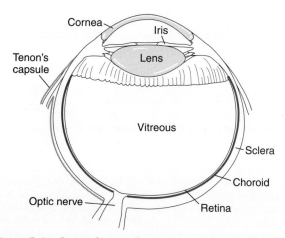

Figure 5-6. Internal eye and optic nerve. Diagram of the internal eye with its three layers (the retina, choroid, and sclera) and the optic nerve, with its posterior chamber filled with vitreous fluid and anterior chamber containing the lens and retina. Reprinted with permission from Longe RL, Calvert, JC. In: Young LYY, ed. Physical Assessment: A Guide for Evaluating Drug Therapy. Vancouver, WA: Applied Therapeutics, Inc.; 1994.

eyes includes observations of visual acuity (VA), visual fields (VF), the external eye, the extraocular muscles (EOM), and pupillary responses as well as a funduscopic examination. If an ophthalmologic problem is suspected, visual acuity is always checked first with a hand-held Snellen chart. Decreased visual acuity with aging is a common geriatric problem and may compromise activities of daily living. Visual fields can only be grossly tested at the bedside. The conjunctiva of the external eye (a thin translucent vascular membrane covering the sclera and inner eyelid surface) is examined for inflammation (conjunctival infection or conjunctivitis), mattering, and exudate. The presence of conjunctival pallor may indicate anemia. A stye (hordeolum) is a painful tender nodule. Scleral icterus (a yellowish pigmentation of the sclera) signifies jaundice in a patient with a bilirubin serum concentration greater than 2–3 mg/dL.

The function of the extraocular muscles (cranial nerves 3, 4, and 6) is described as intact (EOMI) if the patient can follow the examiner's finger through the normal directions of gaze. Thus, a muscle palsy or cranial nerve problem could be detected if the patient is unable to follow the examiner's finger when directed up-down or left-right. Strabismus is the lack of parallelism of the eyes' visual axes. Nystagmus is an abnormal rapid rhythmic spontaneous movement of the eyes (i.e., under conditions of fixation, the eyes drift slowly vertically or horizontally and are corrected by a quick movement to the original position). Nystagmus can indicate inner ear and brain disease and is also part of the triad of findings for Wernicke's encephalopathy. Nystagmus can also be a sign of drug toxicity (e.g., phenytoin, lithium, phencyclidine [PCP]).

In examining the pupillary response, the clinician tests the afferent function of the optic nerve along with the efferent pupillary response of the third cranial nerve. Normally, if a light is shone in one eye, both pupils will constrict (both a direct and consensual response). PERRLA (pupils equal, round, reactive to light and accommodation) is a typical mnemonic description in the medical record. A number of processes, both normal and abnormal, can produce anisocoria (a difference in the size of the pupils). Likewise, a number of drugs can classically affect pupillary size (e.g., barbiturates produce mydriasis or pupillary dilatation; opiates produce miosis or pinpoint pupils).

An ophthalmoscope is used in the funduscopic examination to view the lens, retina, choroid, retinal vessels, and optic disc (termination of the optic nerve). Opacities (e.g., floaters) can sometimes be observed in the vitreous. Cataracts, opacities in the lens, can occur with age or in patients receiving long-term corticosteroid therapy. The retinal vessels are some of the few small-sized vessels that can be seen readily in detail. Characteristic changes in the vessels are observed in a number of diseases (see Chapter 7, "Diagnostic Procedures"). Hypertension produces graded changes based on the severity and duration of the elevated blood pressure (e.g., Keith-Wagener-Barker classifications—normal, I–IV). Arteriovenous narrowing is one of the early changes in hypertension. Hemorrhages, exudates, and papilledema signify more extensive hypertensive retinopathy. Papilledema, edema of optic disc margins, may also be a sign of increased intracranial pressure. Diabetic retinopathy is characterized by early microaneurysm and exudates that can progress to proliferation of blood vessels, retinal detachment, and vitreal hemorrhage. Ophthalmoscopic evaluation can detect cytomegalovirus (CMV) retinopathy and guide assessment of therapy.

Ophthalmologists use several additional instruments in the evaluation of eye complaints. These instruments include planimetry to detect glaucoma, slit lamp examination (which can identify a number of lesions including corneal opacities due to drug toxicity), and visual field testing (which is important to monitor for hydroxychloroquine toxicity).

EARS

The normal anatomy of the external and middle ear is depicted in Figures 5-7 and 5-8. The inner ear contains specialized structures to transmit sound via the auditory branch of the eighth cranial nerve and balance via the vestibular branch of the eight cranial nerve. Damage to this apparatus (from aminoglycosides, furosemide, or cisplatin) can manifest as hearing loss or vestibular dysfunction. Presbycusis, sensorineural hearing loss with age, contributes to communication difficulties. Bedside examination of the ear includes inspection of the external ear and tympanic membrane (TM) with the aid of an otoscope and gross tests of hearing with or without the aid of a tuning fork. Otitis ex-

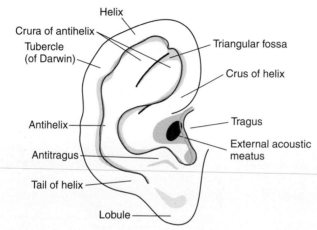

Figure 5-7. External ear (auricle or pinna). The helix, lobule, tragus, and external acoustic meatus (opening into the external auditory canal) are frequently used during physical examination to evaluate deeper structures. Reprinted with permission from Longe RL, Calvert, JC. In: Young LYY, ed. Physical Assessment: A Guide for Evaluating Drug Therapy. Vancouver, WA: Applied Therapeutics, Inc.; 1994.

terna (swimmer's ear) is typified by an inflamed external ear canal (external acoustic meatus) that is tender to the touch. Otitis media (middle ear infection) occurs behind the TM and is common in children. The ear drum can be retracted if eustachian tube dysfunction is present. Bulging of the drum suggests fluid or pus in the middle ear. Pus in the external ear canal might suggest tympanic membrane perforation, whereas blood could suggest basilar skull fracture in a patient with head trauma.

A conical-shaped light reflex is observed on the normal TM due to the reflection of light from the otoscope. Distortion of the reflection's shape is another clinical clue seen in otitis media. In addition, a device is available to insufflate air into the external ear canal through the otoscope. By insufflating air, the TM's ease of mobility can be assessed. Decreased mobility is seen in otitis media and eustachian tube dysfunction.

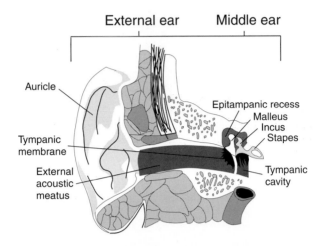

Figure 5-8. Three compartments of the ear. The three compartments of the ear include the external ear (auricle to tympanic membrane), middle ear (tympanic membrane to the round window of inner ear), and inner ear. Reprinted with permission from Longe RL, Calvert, JC. In: Young LYY, ed. Physical Assessment: A Guide for Evaluating Drug Therapy. Vancouver, WA: Applied Therapeutics, Inc.; 1994.

NOSE

The nose is examined for deformities, swelling, septal defects, and discharge. Epistaxis, a nose bleed, may represent an adverse effect of anticoagulant therapy. Nasal polyps are associated with asthma in patients with aspirin hypersensitivity. Rhinitis medicamentosus, a side effect of prolonged nasal vasoconstrictor therapy, may manifest as mucosal swelling and edema.

MOUTH AND OROPHARYNX

Visual examination of the mouth and oropharynx can identify a number of diseases and adverse drug manifestations. Cyanosis of the lips might indicate hypoxemia. Gingival hyperplasia can be caused by phenytoin. Stomatitis (mouth sores) is a common complication of cytotoxic drugs or gold.

Xerostomia (dry mouth) is observed as a lack of saliva and can be caused by a variety of connective tissue diseases (e.g., SLE, rheumatoid arthritis, Sjögren's syndrome) and medications (e.g., anticholinergics). Infectious disease manifestations include pharyngitis, erythema (with or without exudates), oral thrush/candidiasis (e.g., in immunocompromised patients or infants), and herpetic lesions. Aphthous stomatitis is a common nonspecific painful ulceration of the buccal mucosa. Hairy leukoplakia, a common manifestation of acquired immune deficiency syndrome (AIDS), appears as a white, raised lesion on the lateral margins of the tongue.

Neck

Structures examined in the neck include the trachea, carotid arteries, jugular veins, and thyroid gland. The presence of masses or lymphadenopathy is noted. Diffuse thyroid enlargement (goiter) and the presence of thyroid nodules may be detected. If appropriate, the neck's resistance to passive motion (e.g., in a patient with cervical arthritis [motion limited] or meningitis [neck stiffness]) is noted. Additional maneuvers that classically suggest meningeal irritation include Kernig's sign (resistance to extension of the knee after passive flexion at the hip) and Brudzinski's sign (flexion of the hips after passive flexion of the neck).

Jugular venous distention (JVD) reflects central venous pressure as shown in Figure 5-9; the height of distention is measured in centimeters. JVD will be decreased in patients who are hypovolemic. JVD will be increased in patients with conditions such as CHF, right ventricular dysfunction, cardiac tamponade, and cor pulmonale. By applying pressure over the liver, the hepatojugular reflex (HJR) test (i.e., application of pressure over the liver and observation of subsequent neck vein distention) assesses liver congestion and right ventricular function.

The carotid artery pulse is examined for duration and amplitude. A delayed upstroke is characteristic of aortic stenosis. A bounding pulse is characteristic of high-stroke volume states such as aortic regurgitation (waterhammer pulse). Auscultation of the carotid arteries can detect bruits (a blowing or turbulent sound caused by blood flowing past an obstruction such as an atherosclerotic narrowing).

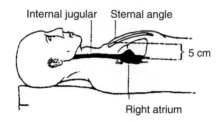

Jugular venous pressure cannot be
measured (in supine patient)

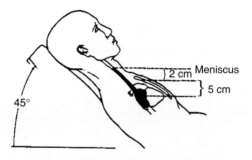

Jugular venous pressure is 7 cm of water

Figure 5-9. Hepatojugular reflex: measuring the jugular venous pressure. The sternal angle (angle of Louis) is a bony ridge
palpable between the manubrium and the body of the sternum
at the level of the second intercostal space. It is always 5 cm vertically above the midright atrium. In any position, therefore,
one may measure the distance from the sternal angle to the
meniscus of the internal jugular vein and add 5 cm to obtain the
jugular venous pressure. Reprinted with permission from Judge
AC et al. Clinical Diagnosis. Little Brown and Co.

Back

Examination of the back discloses any spinal deformities
(e.g., scoliosis, kyphosis) or tenderness. Conditions of
endogenous or exogenous corticosteroid excess can produce a "buffalo hump" over the upper back. Costovertebral

angle (CVA) tenderness in the posterior flank is a classic sign of pyelonephritis. Kyphosis in the elderly can occur due to osteoporosis.

Chest

GENERAL

The lower respiratory tract is composed of the trachea, lungs, and thoracic cage (ribs, sternum or breast bone, intercostal muscles, and diaphragm). Structures in the mediastinum include the heart, great vessels, and esophagus (Fig. 5-10). Examination of the chest includes inspection, palpation, percussion, and auscultation. The chest is inspected for sternal deformities (e.g., pectus excavatum,

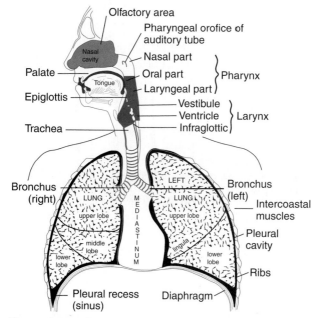

Figure 5-10. Components of the respiratory system from the nose to the alveolus. Reprinted with permission from Longe RL, Calvert, JC. In: Young LYY, ed. Physical Assessment: A Guide for Evaluating Drug Therapy. Vancouver, WA: Applied Therapeutics, Inc.; 1994.

pectus carinatum) (Fig. 5-11). An increased anteroposterior (AP) diameter (i.e., barrel chest) is seen in chronic obstructive airways disease (COAD). Vigorous use of the accessory muscles of respiration (sternocleidomastoid muscle, intercostal muscles) or retraction between the rib spaces on inspiration is a sign of severe airway obstruction.

Palpation of the chest detects masses, tenderness, and fremitus. Fremitus is the normal vibration that can be felt on the thoracic wall during phonation. The patient is asked to repeat a word or phrase ("ninety-nine") while the chest wall is examined with the fingertips. Characteristic changes are noted with consolidation of the lung, pleural effusion, or bronchial obstruction.

Percussion of the chest produces hyperresonant, high-pitched sounds over the air-filled lungs. Lower-pitched

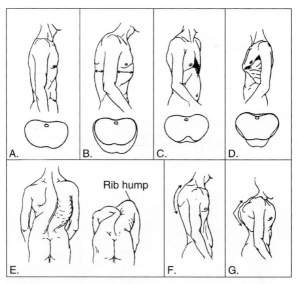

Chest wall contours. A. Normal. B. Barrel chest (emphysema). C. Pectus excavatum (funnel chest). D. Pectus carinatum (Pigeon breast). E. Scoliosis. F. Kyphosis. G. Gibbus (extreme kyphosis).

Figure 5-11. Chest wall contours. Reprinted with permission from Judge AC et al. Clinical Diagnosis. Little Brown and Co.

notes are heard over fluid or solid structures such as the heart or liver. High-pitched hyperresonant, tympanic sounds are observed in emphysema or pneumothorax. Dull, low-pitched sounds are characteristic of pleural fluid or consolidation that might occur with CHF and pneumonia.

LUNG

A stethoscope is used to auscultate the anterior and posterior lung fields. Normal breath sounds are classified according to intensity, pitch, and duration of inspiration/expiration. They include tracheal, bronchovesicular, and vesicular breath sounds. Abnormal sounds include rales, rhonchi, wheezes, rubs, and bronchial breath sounds (Fig. 5-12). Rales are fine crackles emitted from the small airways and alveoli in conditions such as CHF, interstitial pulmonary disease, or pneumonia. Rhonchi are much more coarse and suggest secretions in the larger airways. Wheezes are caused by air movement through narrowed airways as in asthma or COAD. Rubs are "creaking" type noises often caused by inflamed pleura (pleurisy).

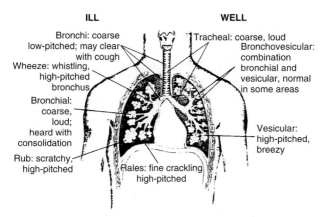

Schema of breath sounds in the well and ill patient.

Figure 5-12. Schema of breath sounds. Reprinted with permission from Seidel HM et al. Mosby's Guide to Physical Examination. St. Louis, MO: CV Mosby; 1987.

Voice sounds discerned with the aid of a stethoscope include bronchophony, whispered pectoriloquy, and egophony. Bronchophony is an increase in the clarity of spoken voice sounds. Whispered pectoriloquy is an increase in clarity of whispered voice sounds. Egophony is a nasal bleating sound detected when the spoken letter "E" sounds more like "A." These voice alterations can occur when a lung is consolidated by pneumonia or compressed by pleural effusion. Improvements in chest findings may occur in response to drug therapy. Thus, signs of airflow obstruction (intercostal muscle retraction, wheezing) may improve with asthma therapy (e.g., sympathomimetics, corticosteroids). Signs of fluid consolidation (dullness to percussion, bronchial breath sounds, and egophony) improve with antibiotic therapy for pneumonia.

BREASTS

Breast cancer occurs in one of nine women but may also occur in men. Breast self-examination should be encouraged in all women. Breast examination is an important component of the physical examination. Inspection might disclose changes in skin texture or coloration or alterations in the contour of the breast. The nipple might become retracted or a discharge may be present. Palpation discloses the presence of breast and axillary masses or tenderness. Galactorrhea, an abnormal milky discharge, can occur in either sex as a result of complex neurohumoral regulation. Dopaminergic antagonists, phenothiazines, and butyrophenones can also cause galactorrhea. Gynecomastia sometimes occurs in alcoholic men (due to testicular atrophy and hyperestrogenemia) and as a side effect of numerous medications (e.g., cimetidine, spironolactone, estrogens).

Cardiovascular (CV) System

The anatomy of the heart is depicted in Figure 5-13. Ventricular relaxation allows opening of the tricuspid and mitral valves, resulting in right and left ventricular filling, respectively. During early systole, the rise in intraventricular pressure due to ventricular contraction causes closure of the tricuspid and mitral valves leading to the first heart sound (S1). Simultaneously, during systole, ventricular contraction opens the pulmonic valve (allowing ejection of blood

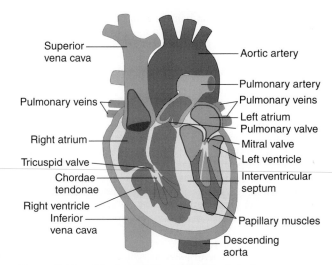

Figure 5-13. The heart. The right side of the heart receives venous blood and pumps it to the lungs to be oxygenated. Oxygenated blood returns to the left side of the heart and is pumped to the systemic circulation through the aorta. Heart valves that do not open or close properly or holes in walls between the chambers (e.g., a defect in the interventricular septum) can result in abnormal function of the heart and heart failure.

from the right ventricle into the pulmonary artery) and aortic valve (allowing ejection of blood from the left ventricle into the aorta). As ventricular contraction ceases in late systole, the aortic and pulmonic valves close, resulting in the second heart sound (S2). Cardiac examination includes inspection, palpation, auscultation, and less commonly percussion. For reference, the apex of the heart is the tip of the left ventricle; the base corresponds to the connections with the great vessels.

Inspection and palpation of the chest wall detects the point of maximal impulse (PMI) corresponding to systole at the apex of the heart. The PMI typically lies in the fifth intercostal space medial to the midclavicular line (a line drawn down the body perpendicular to the middle of the clavicle). A diffuse or laterally displaced PMI is associated with left ventricular enlargement as in CHF. "Heaves," sustained precordial impulses noted by palpation, reflect ventricular hypertrophy. "Thrills" are palpable vibrations due to turbulent flow across an abnormal heart valve. A heart murmur with an associated thrill suggests more severe valve disease.

Auscultation with a stethoscope detects normal physiologic heart tones (S1, S2) and the presence of gallops (S3, S4), murmurs, or rubs. The S3, an abnormal diastolic filling sound created early in diastole after opening of the atrioventricular valves, is associated with CHF. S4, an abnormal gallop occurring in diastole just before systole (presystolic), originates in the ventricle during the latter half of diastole when the atria contract to complete ventricular filling. It suggests poor compliance of the ventricular wall as in left ventricular hypertrophy from hypertension or aortic stenosis and can be a normal finding in otherwise healthy young adults. Murmurs are sounds made by turbulent blood flow, often across a structurally abnormal valve. Either narrowing (stenosis) or insufficiency (regurgitant flow back across a valve that should be closed) can occur. Murmurs are graded by severity from 1 to 6 (Table 5-3).

Pericardial friction rubs are grating sounds caused by the rubbing together of inflamed pericardial surfaces (pericarditis). The rate and rhythm of the heart tones (regular rate and rhythm [RRR], normal sinus rhythm [NSR], or "irregularly irregular" in atrial fibrillation) are noted. A relatively normal heart examination is often abbreviated S1 S2, no M/G/R (i.e., normal S1 and S2 and the absence of any murmurs, gallops, or rubs). Drug therapy can pro-

Table 5-3. Grading of Heart Murmurs

Grade	Description of Heart Murmur
I/VI	Heard only after special maneuvers
II/VI	Very faint, but can be observed
III/VI	Loud, without a thrill
IV/VI	Associated with a thrill; stethoscope must be on chest wall
VI/VI	Heard without a stethoscope; palpable thrill

foundly affect cardiac function and physical examination findings. Antiarrhythmics can slow the heart rate and normalize rhythm disturbances. The stigmata of CHF (increased JVD, HJR, rales, S3 gallop) and lower extremity edema may improve with appropriate drug therapy (e.g., preload reducers like diuretics or afterload reducers like angiotensin-converting enzyme [ACE] inhibitors).

Abdomen

The abdomen is inspected for contour (distended, scaphoid), skin rashes, abnormal venous pattern, and masses. Auscultation is performed to detect bruits and listen to bowel sounds. Midabdominal or flank bruits suggest atherosclerotic disease in the abdominal aorta or renal arteries, respectively. Bowel sounds are diminished in advanced stages of bowel obstruction, ileus due to a variety of reasons (e.g., postoperative, opioid drugs), or peritonitis. Hyperactive bowel sounds are noted in early stages of bowel obstruction and in diarrheal-type illnesses. High pitched "tinkles" and "rushes" suggest small bowel obstruction.

Percussion is performed to elicit tenderness and to detect organ size, masses, and abdominal distention. Gaseous abdominal distention produces a higher-pitched tympanic percussion note, whereas a fluid-filled abdomen (e.g., in ascites) elicits a dull percussion note. Additionally, a fluid wave or succussion splash (i.e., a splashing sound) can be noted by tapping one side of the abdomen and palpating the transmitted vibration on the opposite abdominal wall. Percussion can detect fluid "dullness" that shifts when the patient is rolled from the supine position onto his or her side (e.g., "shifting dullness" of ascites). Liver and spleen enlargement can be detected by both percussion and palpation. Percussion also detects a distended bladder as in bladder outlet obstruction or neurogenic bladder dysfunction.

Palpation determines organ size, the presence of masses, and the degree of abdominal tenderness. The right upper quadrant is palpated for liver size, texture, and tenderness. Hepatomegaly is occasionally quantitated by the degree of distention (in centimeters) below the right costal margin (RCM). A normal-sized liver generally does not distend more than 1–2 cm below the right costal margin. Percussion is an additional method used to measure the liver size, with a span of 4–8 cm being normal. An enlarged liver can be associated with hepatitis, right-sided heart failure, infiltrating diseases, and cancer. The liver is enlarged early in cirrhosis but becomes smaller at later stages when fibrosis occurs. The spleen is normally not palpable, unless it is enlarged. Splenomegaly can be due to portal hypertension, leukemias and lymphomas, hemolytic anemia, and infections. The kidneys are also difficult to palpate unless they are enlarged (e.g., polycystic kidney disease). An enlarged pulsating mass suggests an aortic aneurysm. The gallbladder is not palpable unless enlarged. A tender gallbladder suggests cholecystitis, whereas a nontender gallbladder suggests bile duct obstruction from cancer. Abdominal tenderness in specific locations suggests involvement of the various organs as outlined in Figure 5-14. Rebound tenderness and guarding (involuntary spasm of the abdominal wall muscles) are considered "peritoneal signs" that indicate peritoneal inflammation due to conditions such as appendicitis, diverticulitis, pancreatitis, or cholecystitis.

Murphy's sign and McBurney's point are two eponyms pertinent to the abdominal examination that may be seen in the medical record. Murphy's sign is positive in cholecysti-

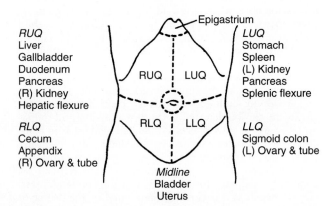

Figure 5-14. Superficial topography of the abdomen: a four-quadrant system. Reprinted with permission from Judge AC et al. Clinical Diagnosis. Little Brown and Co.

tis: during right upper quadrant (RUQ) palpation, as the patient inspires, the inflamed gallbladder descends due to the downward motion of the diaphragm and thus comes in contact with the examiner's fingers. The patient experiences pain and abruptly halts inspiration. Rebound tenderness over McBurney's point (a point on the abdominal wall lying between the umbilicus and the anterior superior iliac spine) suggests acute appendicitis. Numerous drugs target abdominal organ dysfunction. Medications improve symptoms and occasionally abdominal examination findings. Anti-ulcer therapy can improve symptoms of peptic ulcer disease and may improve signs (epigastric and left upper quadrant [LUQ] tenderness). Antibiotics may improve left lower quadrant (LLQ) pain and tenderness of sigmoid diverticulitis, a common problem in the elderly.

Genitourinary (GU) and Rectal System

MALE

The male GU examination is performed with the patient in the upright position. The penis is examined for skin lesions (e.g., syphilitic ulcers, chancroid, herpetic lesions, condyloma) and urethral discharge (suggesting a sexually transmitted disease). Phimosis is the inability to retract the foreskin. The inguinal area is examined for skin rashes (e.g., tinea cruris, candida). Hernias present as inguinal or scrotal masses. An incarcerated hernia cannot be "reduced" by pushing the contents back through the defect in the abdominal wall musculature. Other scrotal masses include varicoceles (dilated scrotal veins) and hydroceles (fluid collections that are translucent on transillumination with a bright light). Testicular size and masses are noted. Testicular self-examination is important for early diagnosis of cancer. Testicular atrophy can accompany alcoholism. Testicular tenderness is noted in testicular torsion (an acute genitourinary emergency) or orchitis. Epididymal tenderness is present in epididymitis.

FEMALE

The female pelvic examination is typically performed in the "dorsal lithotomy" (supine with legs in stirrups) position on a specialized examination table. The examination consists of an examination of the external genitalia, a speculum examination, and a bimanual examination of the pelvic organs. The speculum examination allows direct visualization of the vagina and cervix. Appropriate specimens are obtained to evaluate vaginitis or sexually transmitted diseases. The Papanicolaou (Pap) smear is taken to detect cervical cancer. The bimanual examination is so-named because both hands are used to examine the pelvic organs (one internally and the other externally, on the abdominal wall). The cervix is examined for cervical motion tenderness (CMT), suggesting pelvic inflammatory disease. The uterus and ovaries (adnexa) are examined for size, tenderness, and the presence of masses.

RECTAL EXAMINATION

The rectal examination includes an examination of the prostate gland in men to screen for malignancy or enlargement. The prostate is examined for nodules (suggesting cancer) and tenderness (suggesting prostatitis). Rectal masses can be palpated, and the stool can be tested for occult blood (as a screen for malignancy or occult gastrointestinal bleeding). Hemorrhoids, both internal and external, are also noted. Altered anal sphincter tone is a clue to neurologic dysfunction.

Peripheral Vascular System (PVS)

The location of the peripheral pulses is depicted in Figure 5-15. The peripheral arterial pulses are evaluated by palpation and auscultation to determine occlusion and flow. Typically, a description of the carotid pulse and presence of bruits is found in the neck or cardiovascular section. Similarly, description of the abdominal aorta (if palpable) and abdominal bruits is noted in the abdomen section. Several different grading systems are used to characterize the other peripheral pulses. One such system describes a gradation of pulse intensity from 0 to 4+, with 0 being the absence of a pulse, 3+ being normal, and 4+ denoting a bounding pulse. Acute arterial occlusion due to embolus or thrombosis produces an acutely painful, pale, cool, pulseless extremity and may be treated with thrombolytics. Chronic arterial occlusion from atherosclerotic disease produces symptoms of claudication (exertional extremity pain) and signs of diminished pulses, bruits, and ischemic leg ulcers (see Table 5-4 for an example).

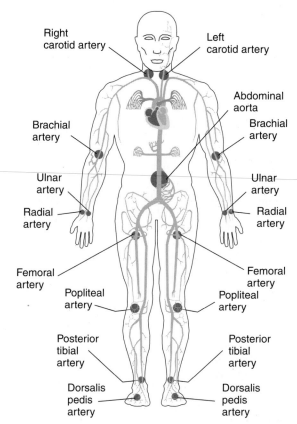

Figure 5-15. Locations of peripheral pulses. Reprinted with permission from Longe RL, Calvert, JC. Physical Assessment: A Guide for Evaluating Drug Therapy. In: Young LYY, ed. Vancouver, WA: Applied Therapeutics, Inc.; 1994.

EXTREMITIES

If not specifically recorded in other sections, examination of the extremities might include notation of skin, nail, hair, and joint abnormalities. The presence of venous disease including varicosities, venous insufficiency, and evidence of

Table 5-4. Sample Recording System for Peripheral Pulses

Pulse	R	L
Carotid	2/4	2/4
Brachial	2+	2+
Radial	3+	3+
Femoral	3+	3+
Popliteal	2+	2+
Dorsalis pedis (DP)	1+	0
Post tibial (PT)	1+	1+

thrombophlebitis is noted. Calf swelling and tenderness may indicate a deep venous thrombosis (DVT). Homans' sign (calf pain produced on passive dorsiflexion of the foot) is a relatively insensitive indicator of DVT. These signs of venous thrombotic disease may improve with anticoagulant therapy.

Edema can have many causes, such as CHF, hypoalbuminemia, and cor pulmonale. "Dependent edema" can occur in the pretibial area in an ambulatory patient. In a bedridden patient, the sacral area is the most dependent portion of the body; thus, early edema might initially manifest in this location. Edema may be pitting or nonpitting. Pitting refers to a noticeable, transient indentation in the tissue subsequent to firm pressure with the fingertips over a bony surface and reflects displacement of the excess interstitial fluid. Pitting is arbitrarily graded depending on severity from trace to 4+. Edema can be a side effect of nifedipine, nonsteroidal anti-inflammatory drugs, and corticosteroids. Diuretics can enhance the resolution of edema.

Musculoskeletal (MSK) System

The musculoskeletal system comprises the supporting structures of the body such as bones, joints, tendons, ligaments, and musculature. Joints are examined for the presence of deformities, swelling, effusions, warmth, redness, and tenderness. Two common types of arthritis, osteoarthritis (OA) and rheumatoid arthritis (RA), have differing patterns of joint involvement. Osteoarthritis often affects the large weight-bearing joints: the knees, hips, and spine with bony proliferation causing swelling and bony proliferation. In the hands, osteoarthritis affects the proximal and distal interphalangeal (PIP and DIP) joints due to nodules known as Bouchard's and Heberden's nodes, respectively. Although RA can also affect weight-bearing joints, it classically causes symmetrical small joint arthritis, particularly of the hands, wrists, elbows, and feet. In contrast to OA, RA affects the metacarpophalangeal joints (MCP) and PIP joints of the hands by causing joint inflammation, swelling, warmth, and pain and spares the DIP joints. A joint's range of motion can become limited by a number of diseases that affect the joint. Improvements in symptoms and examination findings can occur with disease-modifying agents for certain arthritic diseases.

The musculature or motor system is examined for bulk, strength, tone, tenderness, and the presence of abnormal spontaneous movements (e.g., fasciculations). Examination of the motor system is part of the neurologic examination and is discussed in that section.

Neurological System

Examination of the nervous system includes evaluation of the mental status, cranial nerves, motor and sensory function, coordination, deep tendon reflexes (DTRs), and gait. The medical record contains various levels of detail regarding the neurological examination depending on the clinical situation.

MENTAL STATUS

A detailed neurological assessment is an important component of a geriatric physical examination. Impairment of cognitive and motor/sensory function in this population may severely affect quality of life issues and level of function. The mini-mental status examination (Appendix 5.1) is formally used to evaluate a patient's cognitive function.

CRANIAL NERVES

The function of the 12 cranial nerves (CN I to XII) is described in Table 5-5. A common mnemonic uses the first letter of each word in the following sentence: "*On Old Olympus' Towering Tops, A Finn And German Viewed Some Hops*" to identify the 12 cranial nerves (olfactory, optic,

Table 5-5. Cranial Nerves and Their Functions

Cranial Nerves	Function
Olfactory (I)	*Sensory:* smell reception and interpretation
Optic (II)	*Sensory:* visual acuity and visual fields
Oculomotor (III)	*Motor:* raise eyelids, most extraocular movements, changes of lens shape and pupillary constriction
Trochlear (IV)	*Motor:* inward and downward eye movement
Trigeminal (V)	*Motor:* chewing, mastication, jaw opening and clenching
	Sensory: sensation to facial skin, ear, tongue, nasal and mouth mucosa, cornea, iris, lacrimal glands, conjunctiva, eyelids, forehead, and nose
Abducens (VI)	*Motor:* lateral eye movement
Facial (VII)	*Motor:* movement of facial expression muscles except jaw, close eyes, labial speech sounds (M, b, W and round vowels)
	Sensory: tase, anterior two thirds of tongue, sensation to pharynx
	Parasympathetic: secretion of tears and saliva
Acoustic (VIII)	*Sensory:* hearing and balance of equilibrium
Glossopharyngeal (IX)	*Motor:* voluntary muscles for phonation or swallowing
	Sensory: sensation of nasopharynx, gag reflex, taste posterior one third of tongue
	Parasympathetic: secretion of salivary glands, carotid reflex
Vagus (X)	*Motor:* voluntary muscles of phonation (guttural speech sounds) and swallowing

Table 5-5. *Continued*

Cranial Nerves	Function
	Sensory: sensation behind ear and part of external ear canal
	Parasympathetic: secretion of digestive enzymes, peristalsis, carotid reflex, involuntary action of heart, lungs, and digestive tract
Spinal accessory (XI)	*Motor:* turn head, shrug shoulders, some actions for phonation and swallowing
Hypoglossal (XII)	*Motor:* tongue movement for speech sound articulation (l, t, n) and swallowing

oculomotor, trochlear, trigeminal, abducens, facial, acoustic, glossopharyngeal, vagus, spinal accessory, and hypoglossal).

MOTOR EXAMINATION

The motor examination includes evaluation of bulk, strength, tone, tenderness, and the presence of abnormal movements. Both primary muscle diseases and diseases of nerves innervating muscles can cause weakness and atrophy. Muscle strength is graded on a scale of 0 (no movement) to 5 (normal strength) (Table 5-6).

Table 5-6. Muscle Strength Grading

Grade	Muscle Strength
0	No muscle contraction
1	Flicker or trace of contraction
2	Movement possible, but not against gravity
3	Moves against gravity, but not against resistance
4	Can move against resistance
5	Normal strength

Muscle tone can be decreased (flaccid) or increased (spasticity). The phenothiazines and butyrophenones can cause dystonias that are characterized by sustained increased muscle tone and contraction, particularly in the head and neck. The extrapyramidal tract is a system consisting of the basal ganglia and nigrostriatal pathways in the brain. It is involved with initiation of movements, and diseases of these areas cause movement disorders such as Parkinson's disease and Huntington's chorea. The phenothiazines and butyrophenones can have extrapyramidal side effects including dystonias, tremors, and cogwheel rigidity (passive range of motion of an affected muscle group elicits a sensation as if one was pulling on a ratchet or cogwheel).

A number of abnormal movements can be seen in muscles. Fasciculations are miniscule uncoordinated contractions of muscle fibers often due to denervation of the muscle. Tremors are more obvious. A number of drugs can cause tremors (e.g., antipsychotics, lithium, cyclosporine).

SENSORY

Conventionally, the primary sensations include pain, touch, vibration, joint position sense (JPS), and thermal sensation. Pain sensation is conveyed by small unmyelinated fibers and is tested with a pinprick (PP). Light touch (LT) is mediated by a combination of small and larger nerve fibers; this is tested with a wisp of cotton. Vibration and JPS (also called proprioception) are mediated by large myelinated fibers. Vibration sensation is tested with a tuning fork. Neuropathy is a manifestation of diseases such as diabetes as well as an association with drugs such as vinca alkaloids, isoniazid, and didanosine. Peripheral neuropathies often begin distally, affecting the longest nerve fibers first. This gives rise to the term "stocking and glove" distribution to denote abnormalities in the hands and feet. As peripheral nerves convey information back to the spinal cord (and ultimately the brain), the nerve fibers segregate and the dorsal roots enter the dorsal horn of the spinal cord. This allows for a topographically coherent pattern of information entering the spinal cord: each dorsal root receives information from a particular topographic region of the body called a dermatome. In evaluating a sensory abnormality, the clinician tests whether a deficit fits a dermatomal distribution, indicating dorsal root involvement (Fig. 5-16), or the

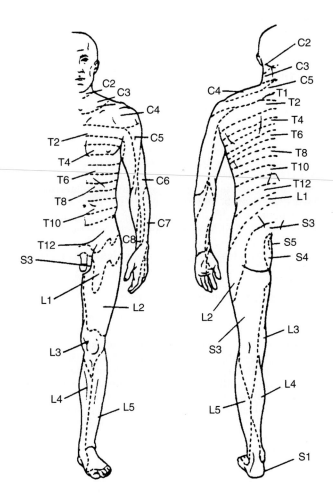

Figure 5-16. Sensory dermatomes. Reprinted with permission from Judge AC et al. Clinical Diagnosis. Little Brown and Co.

distribution of a collection of spinal segments, constituting a peripheral nerve (peripheral neuropathy).

COORDINATION AND VESTIBULOCEREBELLAR TESTING

Coordination of movement is a complex process involving both sensory afferent information regarding proprioception and muscle efferent stimuli. Muscle efferent stimuli cause contraction in certain muscle groups and inhibit muscle contraction in the opposing muscle groups. The Romberg test (testing balance with the patient standing, feet together, eyes closed) evaluates proprioception and cerebellar function. Ataxia (the inability to coordinate voluntary muscle movements) can be tested by asking the patient to alternately point from his nose to the clinician's finger (finger-to-nose test [FTN]). Coordination in the lower extremities is evaluated with the heel-to-shin (HTS) test. The ability to perform rapid alternating movements (RAM) can also be impaired.

DEEP TENDON REFLEXES (DTRS)

Evaluation of DTRs examines the spinal reflex arc. When an already partially stretched tendon is tapped briskly with a reflex hammer, stretch receptors in the tendon send an impulse to the spinal cord that elicits a contraction of the corresponding muscle. The spinal reflex arc is modified by control from the brain via descending corticospinal tracts. Typically, this often has an inhibitory influence. With damage to those higher centers, as in stroke or descending nerve tracts (i.e., the upper motor neurons), the spinal reflex arc is uninhibited and the DTRs are hyperactive. With damage to the peripheral nerve or particular dorsal roots (i.e., low motor neurons), the reflex arc is interrupted and the DTRs are diminished. Reflexes are graded on a scale from 0 to 4. A stick figure typically appears in the chart to designate the elicited reflexes (Fig. 5-17).

The plantar reflexes refer to the reflex motion of the great toe after a noxious stimuli is applied to the bottom of the foot. An up-going toe, Babinski's Sign, is suggestive of an upper motor neuron lesion (but can be normal in infants). A down-going toe is normal.

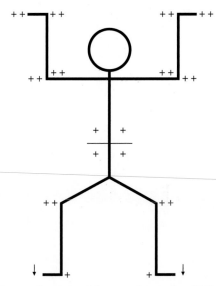

Figure 5-17. Example of deep tendons reflex (DTR) recording. Grading scale: 0 = no response; + = diminished; ++ = normal; +++ = hyperactive; ++++ = hyperactive, often with clonus.

Appendix 5-1. Mini-Mental Status Examination

Maximum Score	Patient Score	Assessment	Questions
			Orientation
5	_____	What is the (year)? (season)? (date)? (day)? (month)?	Ask for the date. Then ask specifically for parts omitted (e.g., "Can you also tell me what season it is?"). One point for each correct answer.
5	_____	Where are we: (state)? (country)? (town)? (hospital)? (floor)?	Ask in turn: "Can you tell me the name of this hospital?" One point for each correct answer.
			Registration
3	_____	Name 3 objects (1 second to say each). Then ask the patient to name all 3 after you have said them.	Ask the patient if you may test his memory. Then say the names of 3 unrelated objects, clearly and slowly, about one second for each.

#Trials		
_____	Give 1 point for each correct answer. Then repeat them until he learns all 3. Count trials and record.	After you have said 3, ask him to repeat them. This first repetition determines his score (0 to 3) but keep saying them until he can repeat all 3, up to 6 trials. **Note:** If he does not eventually learn all 3, recall cannot be meaningfully tested.

Attention and Calculation

5	Serial 7's. (1 point for each correct). Stop after 5 answers.	Ask the patient to begin with 100 and count backwards by 7. Stop after 5 subtractions (93, 86, 79, 72, 65). Score the total number of correct answers.
5	Alternatively spell "world" backwards.	If the patient cannot or will not perform this task, ask him to spell the word "world" backwards. The score is the number of letters in correct order, e.g., dlrow = 5, dlorw = 3.

Recall

3	Ask the patient if he can recall the 3 words you previously asked him to remember. Score 0 to 3.	Ask for the 3 objects repeated above. Give 1 point for each correct.

continued

Appendix 5-1. *Continued*

Maximum Score	Patient Score	Assessment	Questions
			Language
2	————	Name a pencil and a watch (2 points)	*Naming:* Show the patient a wrist watch and ask him what it is. Repeat for pencil. Score 0 to 2.
1	————	Repeat the following: "No ifs, ands, or buts." (1 point)	*Repetition:* Ask the patient to repeat the sentence after you. Allow only one trial. Score 0 to 1.
3	————	Following a 3-stage command: "Take a paper in your right hand, fold it in half, and put it on the floor" (3 points)	*3-State Command:* Give the patient a piece of plain blank paper and repeat the command. Score 1 point for each part correctly executed.
1	————	Read and obey the following: Close your eyes. (1 point)	*Reading:* On a blank piece of paper print the sentence "close your eyes" in letters large enough for the patient to see clearly. Ask him to read it and do what it says. Score 1 point only if he actually closes his eyes.

1	Write a sentence (1 point)	*Writing:* Give the patient a blank piece of paper and ask him to write a sentence for you. Do not dictate a sentence, it is to be written spontaneously. It must contain a subject and verb and be sensible. Correct grammar and punctuation are not necessary.
1	Copy a design (1 point)	*Copying:* On a clean piece of paper, draw intersecting pentagons, each side about 1 inch, and ask him to copy it exactly as it is. All 10 angles must be present and 2 must intersect to score 1 point. Tremor and rotation are ignored.

TOTAL SCORE:	**A score of 27 to 30 is generally considered acceptable.**
_____	*ASSESS level of consciousness along the following continuum: Alert, Drowsy, Stupor, Coma. Estimate the patient's level of sensorium, from alert to coma.*

Chapter 6

Interpretation of Clinical Laboratory Test Results

Mary Beth Elliott

Chapter Roadmap

NORMAL VALUES

LABORATORY ERROR

SENSITIVITY/SPECIFICITY

COMMON LABORATORY ORDERS

LABORATORY TESTS

ROUTINE HEMATOLOGY
  Hematocrit (Hct)
  Hemoglobin (Hgb)
  Red Blood Cell (RBC or Erythrocyte) Count
  Red Cell Indices
    Mean Corpuscular Volume (MCV)
    Mean Corpuscular Hemoglobin (MCH)
    Mean Corpuscular Hemoglobin Concentration (MCHC)
    Red Blood Cell Distribution Width (RDW)
  Reticulocytes
  White Blood Cell, Leukocyte (WBC)
  WBC Differential (Diff)
    Neutrophils (PMNs, Polys, Segs)
    Eosinophils (EOS)
    Basophils
    Monocytes (Monomorphonuclear Monocytes)
    Lymphocytes (Monomorphonuclear Lymphocytes)
    Platelets (PLT)

ELECTROLYTES AND CHEMISTRY SURVEY
  Sodium (Na^+)
  Potassium (K^+)
  Chloride (Cl^-)
  Carbon Dioxide (CO_2) Content
  Glucose (Fasting Blood Sugar [FBS])
  Blood Urea Nitrogen (BUN)

Creatinine
Calcium
Ionized Calcium
Phosphorus, Inorganic (PO_4)
Uric Acid
Magnesium (Mg^{++})
Cholesterol
Total Serum Protein (TSP)
Arterial Blood Gases (ABG)
  Oxygen Saturation (SaO_2)
  Partial Pressure of Oxygen (PaO_2)
  Partial Pressure of Carbon Dioxide ($PaCO_2$)
  pH
Anion Gap (AG)
Bicarbonate Buffer System

URINALYSIS (UA)

LABORATORY TESTS BY ORGAN SYSTEM

CARDIAC DIAGNOSTIC TESTS
  Cardiac Isoenzymes
    Creatine Kinase (CK)
  Troponin I
  Lipoprotein Panel
    Cholesterol
    Low-Density Lipoprotein (LDL) Cholesterol
    High-Density Lipoprotein (HDL) Cholesterol
    Triglycerides

RENAL DIAGNOSTIC TESTS
  Creatinine, Urine
  Na^+/K^+ Ratio, Urine
  Urine Sodium (Na^+)
  Urine Chloride (Cl^-)
  Urine Potassium (K^+)
  Creatinine Clearance, Calculated (ClCr)

GASTROINTESTINAL/HEPATIC DIAGNOSTIC TESTS
  Amylase, Serum
  Lipase
  Alanine Aminotransferase (ALT)
  Alkaline Phosphatase (Alk Phos)
  Ammonia (NH_3)

Aspartate Aminotransferase (AST)
Bilirubin (Bili, T. Bili)
Gamma Glutamyl Transferase (GGT)
Hemoccult (Guaiac or Benzidine Method)
Lactate Dehydrogenase (LD)

ENDOCRINE DIAGNOSTIC TESTS
  Thyroid Function Tests
    Thyroid Stimulating Hormone (TSH)
    Thyroxine, Total, Determination by Radioimmunoassay
      (T_4-RIA)
    Free Thyroxine (Free T_4)
    Triiodothyronine Uptake Ratio (T_3UR)
    Triiodothyronine (T_3)
  Adrenal Gland
    Plasma Cortisol
    Hemoglobin AIC (Hgb A_1C)

HEMATOLOGIC DIAGNOSTIC TESTS
  Anemias
    Iron (Fe)
    Ferritin
    Transferrin
    Total Iron Binding Capacity (TIBC)
    Glucose-6-Phosphate Dehydrogenase (G6PD) in
      Erythrocytes
  Coagulation Tests
    Activated Partial Thromboplastin Time (aPTT) and
      Prothrombin Time (PT)
      International Normalized Ratio (INR)
    Fibrin Degradation Products (Fibrin Split Products, FDP,
      FSP, D dimer)
    Thrombin Time (TT)
    Factor V
    Factor VIII
    Antithrombin III (ATIII)

INFECTIOUS DISEASE/IMMUNOLOGIC/
RHEUMATOLOGIC DIAGNOSTIC TESTS
  Human Immunodeficiency (HIV) Tests
    Enzyme-linked Immunosorbent Assay (ELISA) or Enzyme
      Immunoassay (EIA)
    Western Blot

HIV Antigen Test
HIV RNA by Polymerase Chain Reaction (PCR)
CD4+ T-Cell Counts

OTHER DIAGNOSTIC TESTS RELATED TO
IMMUNOLOGIC/RHEUMATOLOGIC DISEASE AND
INFECTIOUS DISEASE
   Erythrocyte Sedimentation Rate (ESR, Sed Rate)
   $Beta_2$-Microglobulin (B_2M)
   Hepatitis Panel
   Infectious Mononucleosis (IM) Monospot
   Venereal Disease Research Laboratory (VDRL)

NUTRITIONAL DIAGNOSTIC TESTS
   Albumin
   Zinc, Serum

BODY FLUID ANALYSIS
   Cerebrospinal Fluid (CSF) Examination
   Glucose (in CSF)

A clinical laboratory test can provide a useful diagnostic clue, assist with a therapeutic assessment, or have programmatic implications. This chapter contains many commonly encountered laboratory tests used in clinical medicine. The chapter is designed to provide the user with (1) normal values in the traditional and Systeme Internationale (SI) units, (2) descriptions of specific tests, and (3) descriptions of the clinical implications of abnormal findings.

   If specific tests are not included or if more detailed information is desired, the reader is advised to consult the most recent edition of F.K. Widmann's "Clinical Interpretation of Laboratory Tests" published by F.A. Davis Company (Philadelphia, Pennsylvania) or John B. Henry's "Clinical Diagnosis and Management by Laboratory Methods" published by W.B. Saunders (Philadelphia, Pennsylvania). Before using the information in this chapter, it is important to review the following general principles regarding laboratory tests.

NORMAL VALUES

In determining normal values or, more correctly, reference ranges, a variety of factors and the interrelationships of these factors must be considered. Normal values will vary as a function of the patient's age, gender, weight, and height. Changes from normal will also occur when certain medications are used that may either falsely elevate or lower the results of a specific test. Other factors that affect normal values include the timing of the sample, relationship to a meal, the method of analysis, and the disease state itself. Similarly, abnormal values are not always significant, and occasionally normal values can be viewed as abnormal in some diseases. Therefore, it is important to refer to published normal data or reference standards used by the clinical laboratory performing the test and to consider potential interferences with the test in question. The normal values in this chapter refer primarily to adults unless otherwise indicated and may vary slightly among laboratories.

LABORATORY ERROR

Laboratory error is generally an uncommon occurrence. When it does occur, there may be serious implications for patient care. A laboratory error should be suspected when a particularly low or high value occurs or when an unexpected value based on the patient's clinical status is reported. Examples of potential causes of laboratory errors include the following:

➤ A spoiled specimen (e.g., contaminated, wrong container, exposed to improper temperature or light conditions)
➤ **Specimen** taken at the wrong time
➤ **Incomplete** specimen
➤ **Faulty** reagents
➤ **Technical** error
➤ **Medications** (e.g., due to interference with the assay) that can falsely lower or elevate the result

➤ **Diet** (e.g., elevated blood sugar that was obtained soon after eating)
➤ **Specimen** from wrong patient
➤ **Diagnostic** or therapeutic procedures (e.g., digital stimulation of the prostate or a prostate biopsy may increase the prostate-specific antigen [PSA] level)
➤ **Hemolyzed** blood samples

SENSITIVITY/SPECIFICITY

The accuracy and reliability of laboratory tests are based on the sensitivity and specificity of each test. The sensitivity of a test is the likelihood of a positive test result in a person with a disease. Specificity refers to the likelihood of a negative test result in a person without a disease. Therefore, the clinical implications of these two factors are that test performance can change as the test is more widely used. Further, the selection bias of individuals may affect the measurement of a test's sensitivity and specificity. For example, selecting all healthy volunteers may overestimate the specificity of a test, whereas selecting individuals with extensive disease may overestimate the sensitivity of the method. In any case, it is important to remember the following points when evaluating laboratory values:

➤ **Test** values represent probability values (probability that a disease or abnormality is in fact present).
➤ **Many** laboratory values are expressed as continuous variables and provide only an indication that normality or abnormality is present.
➤ **Regardless** of the sensitivity and specificity of a given test, the predictive power of the test will be influenced by the prevalence of the disease in the population from which the patient is drawn.

COMMON LABORATORY ORDERS

Laboratory tests are frequently ordered in groups or as panels of tests to simplify the task. The cost of these panels is often less expensive than the cost of each test ordered individually. The following are descriptions of some of the more commonly used laboratory test panels and associated abbreviations:

➤ *Chemistry Survey (Chem Survey).* Glucose, blood urea nitrogen (BUN), creatinine, calcium, phosphate (PO_4^-), uric acid, magnesium (Mg^{++}), cholesterol, and total serum protein (TSP).

➤ *SMA-6.* Sodium (Na^+), potassium (K^+), chloride (Cl^-), carbon dioxide (CO_2), BUN, and glucose.

➤ *SMA-12.* SMA-6 plus albumin (Alb), TSP, bilirubin (T. Bil), alkaline phosphatase (Alk Phos), calcium, and creatinine.

➤ *Electrolytes (Lytes).* Na^+, K^+, Cl^-, CO_2.

➤ *Complete Blood Count (CBC) with Differential (diff).* White blood cell (WBC) count and differential (segmented neutrophils, bands, eosinophils, basophils, lymphocytes, atypical lymphocytes, and monocytes).

➤ *Arterial Blood Gases (ABG).* pH, PCO_2, PO_2, and base excess and bicarbonate (HCO_3).

➤ *Hematology Panel (Heme Panel).* WBC, red blood cells (RBCs), hemoglobin (Hgb), hematocrit (Hct), RBC indices, and red cell distribution width (RDW).

➤ *Enzymes.* Alanine aminotransferase (ALT), aspartate aminotransferase (AST), amylase, lipase, gamma glutamyltransferase (GGT), lactic acid dehydrogenase (LD), and creatine kinase (CK).

➤ *Isoenzymes.* CK (MM, MB, BB bands) and LD (LD_1, LD_2).

➤ *Urine Electrolytes.* Na^+ and K^+.

Included with most of the tests are examples of conditions that may increase or decrease the values obtained. These examples may not be all-inclusive. In addition to use of abbreviations, test results are frequently recorded in a patient's chart using a variety of formats. It is usually easy to identify particular laboratory tests just by knowing the normal values.

LABORATORY TESTS

ROUTINE HEMATOLOGY

Hematocrit (Hct)

Normal Values
Male: 40–52% SI units = 0.40–0.52
Female: 34–46% SI units = 0.34–0.46

Description
The hematocrit (percent of packed cell volume) describes the space occupied by packed RBCs. It is expressed as a percentage of red cells in volume of whole blood and represents a calculated value.

Clinical Implications
➤ **Decreased** values are seen in anemia (various causes), hemolytic reactions, leukemia, cirrhosis, massive blood loss, and hyperthyroidism.
➤ **Increased** values are seen in erythrocytosis, dehydration, chronic obstructive pulmonary disease (COPD), polycythemia, and shock.
➤ The Hct lacks clinical validity immediately after moderate blood loss or transfusion. It may appear normal after acute hemorrhage.
➤ The Hct usually parallels the RBC count when erythrocytes are of a normal size.
➤ If the patient has iron-deficiency anemia with small RBCs, the Hct decreases because microcytic cells pack into a smaller volume. However, the RBC count may appear normal.
➤ The Hct value is approximately three times the Hgb value.
➤ One unit of blood will increase the Hct value by 2–4%.

Hemoglobin (Hgb)

Normal Values
Male: 13.6–17.2 g/dL   SI units = 8.5–10.7 mmol/L
Female: 11.6–15.6 g/dL   SI units = 7.2–9.7 mmol/L

Description

Hemoglobin is contained in RBCs and transports oxygen (O_2) and carbon dioxide (CO_2). It consists of globin, a protein with two alpha and two beta subunits, surrounding a heme core with an iron atom and a porphyrin ring. The heme structure accounts for hemoglobin's red color. The iron pigment of hemoglobin combines with oxygen. When hemoglobin carries oxygen, blood is scarlet (arterial); when it loses oxygen, the blood becomes dark red (venous). One gram of hemoglobin carries 1.34 mL of oxygen. This oxygen-carrying capacity correlates with the amount of Hgb present, not the number of RBCs. Hgb also serves as a buffer by shifting chloride in and out of RBCs according to the level of O_2 in plasma (for each chloride entering the RBC, one anion of HCO_3 is released).

A decrease in the normal Hgb protein types A_1, A_2, and F (fetal), and the appearance of type S hemoglobin is associated with sickle cell anemia.

The definition of anemia based on a specific hemoglobin value varies because of varying body adaptations (e.g., to high altitudes, pulmonary disease, and exercise); however, a hemoglobin value of ≤ 12 g/dL generally suggests an anemic condition. The total amount of circulating hemoglobin is more important than the number of erythrocytes in determining anemia.

Clinical Implications

➤ The Hgb concentration is decreased in anemia (especially iron-deficiency anemia), hyperthyroidism, cirrhosis, hemorrhage, hemolytic reactions, increased fluid intake, and pregnancy.

➤ The Hgb concentration is increased in hemoconcentration (polycythemia, burns), COPD, congestive heart failure (CHF), and in those living at high altitudes.

➤ Hgb concentration fluctuates in patients with hemorrhages and burns because of fluid replacement and blood transfusions.

➤ The Hgb concentration can be used to assess the severity of anemia, response of anemia to treatment, or progression of disease(s) associated with anemia.

Red Blood Cell (RBC or Erythrocyte) Count

Normal Values

Male: $4.4–5.8 \times 10^6$ cells/mm^3
          SI units = $4.4–5.8 \times 10^{12}$ cells/L

Female: $3.8–5.2 \times 10^6$ cells/mm^3
               SI units = $3.8–5.2 \times 10^{12}$ cells/L

Description

The main function of the RBC is to carry oxygen from the lungs to body tissue and to transfer CO_2 from tissues to the lungs by hemoglobin. RBCs, by virtue of their biconcave disk shape, have a larger surface area than if they were flat. This allows them to combine with more oxygen and also to bend more easily when passing through small capillaries. Erythrocyte production is stimulated by the hormone erythropoietin in response to decreased oxygen.

RBCs have a life span of 120 days and are generally released into the circulation as mature cells. If the demand for erythrocytes is high, immature cells will be released into the circulation. At the end of their life span, older erythrocytes are removed from circulation by phagocytes in the spleen, liver, and bone marrow (reticuloendothelial system or RES).

ERYTHROPOIESIS

In bone marrow, the erythrocyte develops in the following sequence: (1) hemocytoblast (precursor of all blood cells), (2) prorubricyte (synthesis of Hgb), (3) rubricyte (nucleus shrinks, Hgb synthesis increases), (4) metarubricyte (nucleus disintegrates, Hgb synthesis increases), (5) reticulocyte (nucleus absorbed), and (6) erythrocyte (mature red cell without nucleus/reticulum).

Clinical Implications

➤ **Generally,** the Hgb or Hct is used to monitor the associated quantitative changes of the RBCs.
➤ **The** RBC count is decreased in anemias and systemic lupus erythematosus (SLE).
➤ **RBCs** are increased in polycythemia vera, secondary polycythemia (hormone secreting tumors), diarrhea/dehydration, vigorous exercise, burns, and high altitudes.

Red Cell Indices

MEAN CORPUSCULAR VOLUME (MCV)

Calculation

$$MCV = \frac{Hct\ \% \times 10}{RBC\ (10^{12}/L)}$$

Normal Values

$$82\text{--}97 \text{ fL} \qquad SI = 82\text{--}97 \text{ fL}$$
$$(1 \text{ fL} = 10^{-15} \text{ L})$$

Description

The MCV is an index for classifying anemia based on examination of erythrocytes. It expresses the volume (or size) of a single red cell as being normocytic (normal size), microcytic (small size, <75 fL), or macrocytic (large size, >105 fL).

Clinical Implications

➤ **Decreased** values are seen in iron-deficiency anemia, pernicious anemia, and thalassemia. Therefore, these anemias are "microcytic anemias."

➤ **Increased** values are seen in liver disease, alcoholism, antimetabolite therapy, folate/B_{12} deficiency, and valproate therapy. These anemias are "macrocytic anemias."

➤ **In** sickle cell anemia, the MCV is of questionable value, because the Hct is unreliable due to the abnormal erythrocyte shape.

➤ **MCV** is a calculated value; therefore, it is possible to have a wide variation in macrocytes/microcytes and still have a normal MCV.

MEAN CORPUSCULAR HEMOGLOBIN (MCH)

Calculation

$$MCH = \frac{Hgb \text{ (g/dL)} \times 10}{RBC \text{ } (10^{12}/L)}$$

Normal Values

$$28\text{--}33 \text{ pg/cell} \qquad SI = 28\text{--}33 \text{ pg/cell}$$

Description

The MCH index is a calculated value that indicates the average mass of Hgb—and hence the amount of color (i.e., normochromic, hypochromic, hyperchromic)—in the RBC. It is useful in the diagnosis of anemia.

Clinical Implications

➤ **An** increase in MCH indicates macrocytic anemia.
➤ **A** decrease in MCH indicates microcytic anemia.

MEAN CORPUSCULAR HEMOGLOBIN CONCENTRATION (MCHC)

Calculation

$$MCHC = \frac{Hgb\ (g/dL) \times 100}{}$$

Normal Values

32–36 g/dL   SI = 320–360 g/L

Description

The MCHC index measures the average concentration of Hgb in the RBC. For a given MCH, the smaller the cell, the higher the concentration. This index relies on the Hgb and Hct for calculation of MCHC and is a better index of red cell hemoglobin, because cell size affects MCH in contrast to the MCHC.

Clinical Implications

➤ **MCHC** is decreased in iron deficiency, microcytic anemia, pyridoxine-responsive anemia, thalassemia, and hypochromic anemia.
➤ **MCHC** is increased in spherocytosis but not in pernicious anemia.

RED BLOOD CELL DISTRIBUTION WIDTH (RDW)

Normal Values

10.5–15%

Description

Coefficient of variation (CV) of the RBC size.

Clinical Implications

➤ **Normal** RDW with low MCV is seen in thalassemia and in anemia of inflammatory disease.
➤ **Increased** RDW occurs with low MCV seen in iron deficiency.
➤ **Normal** RDW with normal MCV is seen in normal persons but also in anemia of inflammatory disease.
➤ **Increased** RDW with normal MCV occurs in early iron deficiency, B_{12}, or folate deficiency.
➤ **Increased** RDW with high MCV is seen in B_{12} or folate deficiency and in hemolytic anemia.

Reticulocytes

Normal Values

0.5–2.20% red cells   SI = 0.005–0.022 red cells

Description

Reticulocytes are young, nonnucleated cells of the erythrocyte series formed in the bone marrow. An increase in the reticulocyte count indicates that RBC production is accelerated. A decrease in the number indicates that bone marrow red cell production is reduced.

Clinical Implications

➤ **The** reticulocyte count differentiates anemias due to bone marrow failure from those due to hemorrhage or hemolysis (red cell destruction), because hemorrhage or hemolysis should stimulate reticulocytosis in patients with competent bone marrow function.
➤ **The** reticulocyte count should be increased in hemolytic anemias and sickle cell disease.
➤ **If** the reticulocyte count is not increased when the patient is anemic, it implies that the bone marrow is not producing enough erythrocytes (e.g., iron-deficiency anemia, aplastic anemia, untreated pernicious anemia, chronic infection, radiation therapy).
➤ **Following** treatment of anemias, an increase in "retics" reflects the effectiveness of treatment. After adequate doses of iron in iron-deficient anemia, the reticulocyte count increases by approximately 20%; it increases pro-

portionally when pernicious anemia is treated by transfusion. A maximum increase may be expected to occur 7–14 days after appropriate treatment (i.e., iron supplementation).

White Blood Cell, Leukocyte (WBC)

Normal Values

3800–10,500 cells/mm^3 SI = 3.8–10.5 × 10^{9}cells/L

Description

The main functions of the WBC are to fight infection, defend the body by phagocytosis of foreign organisms, and produce or transport/distribute antibodies. There are two major types of white blood cells:

1. Granulocytes: neutrophils, eosinophils, and basophils.
2. Agranulocytes: lymphocytes and monocytes.

Leukocytes are formed in the bone marrow (myelogenous), stored in lymphatic tissue (spleen, thymus, tonsils), and transported via blood to organs or tissues. The average life span of a leukocyte is 13–20 days. Vitamins, folic acid, and amino acids are needed for leukocyte formation. The endocrine system regulates the production, storage, and release of leukocytes.

Granulocyte development begins with myeloblasts (immature cells in the bone marrow) that mature progressively to become promyelocytes, myelocytes (found in the bone marrow), metamyelocytes, bands (neutrophils in early stages of maturity), and ultimately, polymorphonuclear segmented neutrophils (also called "polys" or "segs"). Lymphocyte development begins with lymphoblasts (immature) that mature to prolymphoblasts and finally to lymphocytes (mature cell). Monocyte development begins with monoblasts (immature) that mature to become promonocytes and then to monocytes (mature cell).

Clinical Implications

➤ *Leukocytosis.* 10,500–20,000 (slight); 30,000 (moderate); 50,000 (high).

 • **Usually** due to an increase of only one cell type (e.g., neutrophilia).

- **Absence** of anemia helps to distinguish infection from leukemia.
- **Hemorrhage**, trauma, drugs (e.g., mercury, epinephrine, corticosteroids), necrosis, toxins (eclampsia), and leukemia are other causes.
- **Food**, exercise, emotion, menstruation, stress, seizures, and cold baths can also increase the WBC count.

➤ *Leukopenia* is a decrease to <4000. Causes of leukopenia include:

- **Viral** infections, hypersplenism, and leukemia.
- **Drugs** (antimetabolites, antibiotics, anticonvulsants, chemotherapy).
- **Pernicious/aplastic** anemia.

➤ *Staining* Procedures.

- **Neutral** reaction for neutrophils.
- **Acid** stain for eosinophils.
- **Basic** stain for basophils.

➤ *Concentration.* Concentration of leukocytes follows an hourly rhythm, with low levels in early morning and peak levels in the late afternoon.

➤ *Age.* The normal concentration of leukocytes in newborns and infants is 10,000–20,000 and decreases until age 21.

WBC Differential (Diff)

Normal Values

White Blood Cell, Leukocyte (WBC):	3800–10,500 cells/mm^3	SI units = 3.8–10.5 $\times 10^9$/L
Neutrophils(PMNs; polys; segs): 45–74%	1700–7500 cells/mm^3	SI units = 1.7–7.5 $\times 10^9$/L
Bands: 0–4%	0–400 cells/mm^3	SI units = 0–0.04
Eosinophils: 0–7%	0–500 cells/mm^3	SI units = 0–0.07
Lymphocytes: 16–45%	1000–3500 cells/mm^3	SI units = 0.16–0.45
Mono:4–10%	200–900 cells/mm^3	SI units = 0.04–0.10

Description

➤ **Neutrophils** combat bacterial infection and inflammatory disorders.
➤ **Eosinophils** combat allergic disorders and parasitic infections.
➤ **Basophils** combat blood dyscrasias and myeloproliferative disease.
➤ **Lymphocytes** combat viral infections and bacterial infections.
➤ **Monocytes** combat severe infections

NEUTROPHILS (PMNS, POLYS, SEGS)

Normal Values

Neutrophils: 1700–7500 cells/mm^3 SI units = 1.7–7.5
  45–74% $\times 10^9$/L
Bands: 0–4% 0–400 cells/mm^3 SI units = 0–0.04

Description

The neutrophil is the most abundant leukocyte. Neutrophils primarily defend against microbial invasion by phagocytosis. These cells also play a major role in the tissue damage associated with noninfectious diseases such as rheumatoid arthritis, asthma, and inflammatory bowel disease. Most laboratories report neutrophils by combining segs and bands and reporting as an absolute number (cells/mm^3).

Clinical Implications

➤ **Neutrophilia** is an increased percentage of circulating neutrophils. Its causes include bacterial or parasitic infections, metabolic disturbances, hemorrhage, or myeloproliferative disorders. Stress, excitement, and exercise can temporarily cause increased neutrophils.
➤ **Neutropenia** is a decreased percentage of circulating neutrophils. Its causes include decreased neutrophil production, increased cell disappearance, viral infection, blood diseases, hormonal disorders, toxic agents, and a massive infection.
➤ **"Shift to left"** or an increase in bands (immature cells) occurs when immature neutrophils are released into the circulation. This left shift can be caused by infection, chemotherapeutic agents, a cell production disorder (leukemia), or hemorrhage.

➤ **"Shift to right"** or an increase in "segs" (mature cells) occurs in liver disease, megaloblastic anemia due to B_{12} or folic acid deficiency, hemolysis, tissue breakdown, surgery, and certain drugs (e.g., corticosteroids).

➤ If the neutrophil count is increased to a notably greater extent than the total WBC count, it often indicates the presence of a severe infection.

➤ The degree of neutrophilia is proportionate to the amount of tissue involved in inflammation. Neutrophils will leave the blood to migrate to areas of inflammation; however, marrow storage release usually overcompensates, resulting in neutrophilia.

➤ In cases of tissue necrosis or destruction (e.g., crush injuries, burns, myocardial infarction [MI], surgeries), neutrophilia may occur via a neutrophilic promoting substance and other poorly understood mechanisms.

➤ **Absolute** neutrophil count (ANC) = WBC × (% segs + % bands)

EOSINOPHILS (EOS)

Normal Values

0–7%   0–500 cells/mm³   SI units: 0–0.07

Description

Eosinophils are capable of phagocytosis. They are active in the later stages of inflammation, when they ingest antigen-antibody complexes. These cells are also active in allergic reactions and parasitic infections; thus, an increase in eosinophils serves as a useful diagnostic or monitoring tool in these conditions.

Clinical Implications

➤ **Eosinophilia** represents an increase in the number of eosinophils of more than 7% or an absolute count of more than 500. Causes include the body's response to *n*eoplasm, *A*ddison's disease, *a*llergic reactions, *co*llagen vascular disease, or *p*arasitic infections. The mnemonic "NAACP" is helpful to remember these causes.

➤ **Eosinopenia** is a decrease in the number of circulating eosinophils. Eosinopenia can be encountered with glucocorticoid excess. This can occur when glucocorticoids are produced in response to bodily stress (e.g., infectious mononucleosis), in Cushing's disease, or when administered exogenously.

➤ **Eosinophils** disappear early in pyogenic infections.
➤ **The** eosinophil count is lowest in the morning and increases from noon to midnight.
➤ **Eosinophilia** can be masked by steroid use and can be increased substantially by L-tryptophan (i.e., eosinophilic-myalgia syndrome).

BASOPHILS

Normal Values
0–2%   0–200 cells/mm^3 SI units: 0–0.02

Description
The function of basophils is not clearly understood. Basophils are phagocytic cells that contain heparin, histamine, and serotonin. A high basophil count is often noted when the serum concentration of histamine is high. Tissue basophils are also called mast cells.

Clinical Implications
➤ **Basophilia** (increased basophils) is associated most commonly with granulocytic and basophilic leukemia, myeloid metaplasia, and allergic reactions.
➤ **Basopenia** (decreased basophils) is associated with acute infections, stress reactions, and after prolonged steroid therapy.

MONOCYTES (MONOMORPHONUCLEAR MONOCYTES)

Normal Values
4–10%   200–900 cells/mm^3 SI units: 0.04–0.10

Description
Monocytes are the largest cells in the blood and serve as the body's second line of defense. The histiocyte, a fixed tissue

macrophage, is capable of phagocytosis and performs scavenger functions. Monocytes also produce interferon.

Clinical Implications

➤ **Monocytosis** is associated with certain viral, bacterial, and parasitic infections and collagen, vascular, and hematologic disorders.
➤ **Monocytopenia** or a decreased number of monocytes is not usually identified with a disease but is secondary to stress, glucocorticoids, or myelotoxic or immunosuppressive drugs.

LYMPHOCYTES (MONOMORPHONUCLEAR LYMPHOCYTES)

Normal Values

16–45%   SI units: 0.16–0.45

or 1000–3500 cells/mm^3

Description

Lymphocytes are the second most common white cell. They are small, motile cells that migrate to sites of inflammation during both early and late stages of inflammation. Lymphocytes elaborate immunoglobulins and are also important in the body's cellular immune response. Most lymphocytes are located in the spleen, lymphatic tissue, and lymph nodes. Only approximately 5% of total lymphocytes are present in the circulation.

Clinical Implications

➤ **Lymphocytosis** is associated with viral diseases (e.g., mumps, mononucleosis, upper respiratory infections), bacterial diseases, and hormonal disorders.
➤ **Lymphopenia** is associated with Hodgkin's disease, SLE, burns, and trauma.
➤ **Virocytes** (stress lymphocytes, Downy type cells, atypical lymphocytes) are atypical cells than can also appear in viral, fungoid, and parasitic infections; after transfusions; and as a response to stress.
➤ **Transformed** lymphocytes are used as a measure of histocompatibility.

PLATELETS (PLT)

Normal Values

$160–370 \times 10^3/mm^3$ $SI = 160–370 \times 10^9/L$

Description

Platelets (thrombocytes), the smallest of the formed elements in the blood, are necessary for clot formation. Platelets are activated after contact with nonendothelial surfaces and subsequently adhere to subendothelial components (e.g., collagen). During the adhesion/aggregation phase, coagulation is triggered and thrombin is formed. Platelets then become interspersed with RBCs and WBCs to form a clot. Formation of platelets occurs primarily in the bone marrow. The life span of a platelet is approximately 7.5 days. Two-thirds of all platelets are circulating in the blood, whereas one-third are located in the spleen.

Clinical Implications

➤ **Increased** platelets (thrombocythemia/thrombocytosis) are associated with cancer, polycythemia vera, splenectomy, trauma, cirrhosis, myelogenous/granulocytic leukemia, stress, and active rheumatoid arthritis.

➤ **Decreased** platelets (thrombocytopenia) are associated with idiopathic thrombocytopenia purpura (ITP); pernicious, aplastic, and hemolytic anemia; allergic reactions; and bone marrow lesions.

➤ **Many** drugs (e.g., amrinone, antineoplastic agents, sulfonamides, heparin, quinidine, penicillins, H_2 receptor antagonists, gold salts, and penicillamine) can cause thrombocytopenia.

➤ **Decreases** below 20,000 may be associated with spontaneous bleeding, prolonged bleeding time, petechiae, or ecchymosis.

➤ **The** precise number of platelets necessary for hemostasis is not firmly established. Patients with platelet deficits require observation for signs/symptoms of gastrointestinal (GI) bleeding, petechiae, hematuria, and episodes of spontaneous bleeding.

➤ **Valproic** acid decreases platelet counts in a dose-dependent fashion in some patients. It may also decrease platelet adhesiveness, resulting in increased bleeding time.

➤ **Aspirin** and nonsteroidal antiinflammatory drugs (NSAIDs) (except celecoxib and rofecoxib) primarily affect platelet function rather than platelet number.

ELECTROLYTES AND CHEMISTRY SURVEY

Sodium (Na$^+$)

Normal Values

135–144 mEq/L   SI = 135–144 mmol/L

Description

Sodium is the most abundant cation in extracellular fluid. It maintains oncotic pressure and acid-base balance and aids in the sequence of transmission of nerve impulses. Serum sodium concentrations are regulated by the kidneys, the central nervous system (CNS), and the endocrine system (see Chapter 10, "Fluid and Electrolyte Therapy," for a more detailed discussion of daily requirements).

Clinical Implications

➤ *Hyponatremia.* Hyponatremia generally reflects excess body water rather than low total body sodium. Predisposing factors include burns, diarrhea/vomiting, psychoses associated with excessive water intake, and excessive use of fluids that do not contain electrolytes. Addison's disease, nephritis, and diabetic acidosis can also lead to hyponatremia.

➤ *Syndrome of Inappropriate Antidiuretic Hormone (SIADH).* This is characterized by hyponatremia, inappropriately concentrated urine, and increased urinary sodium concentration in a euvolemic patient with normal renal, adrenal, and thyroid function. SIADH may be caused by certain tumors and some drugs (e.g., thiazide diuretics, chlorpropamide, carbamazepine, clofibrate, cyclophosphamide) and may be associated with some pulmonary disorders (e.g., tuberculosis, pneumonias).

➤ *Cystic Fibrosis.* Patients with cystic fibrosis may become hyponatremic due to increased loss of sodium in sweat.

➤ *Acute Sodium Depletion.* Clinical signs of acute sodium depletion include nausea, fatigue, cramps, psychosis, seizures, and coma.

➤ *Hypernatremia.* Predisposing factors include dehydration, aldosteronism, diabetes insipidus, and the use of osmotic diuretics. Generally, hypernatremia is an uncommon manifestation because thirst is a powerful defense against hypertonicity. Therefore, hypernatremia primarily occurs in patients who are unable to ingest adequate fluids (e.g., comatose patients, infants).

➤ *Intravenous (IV) Therapy Considerations.* A patient receiving >400 mEq/day of sodium (e.g., 3 L/day of normal saline containing 155 mEq/L of sodium) usually will have difficulty with fluid balance and should be checked for signs of edema or elevated blood pressure. Healthy subjects can accommodate large increases in sodium intake as long as thirst mechanisms and renal function are intact.

➤ *Drugs.* Numerous drugs affect sodium concentrations directly (sodium content) or indirectly by affecting urinary excretion of sodium.

➤ *Water Deficit.* Total body water deficit = approximately 1 liter for each 3 mmol/L of Na^+ greater than normal.

Potassium (K^+)

Normal Values

0–17 years of age:	3.5–5.2 mEq/L	SI = 3.5–5.2 mmol/L
18+ years of age:	3.5–4.8 mEq/L	SI = 3.5–4.8 mmol/L

Description

Potassium is the principle intracellular fluid cation, which (with bicarbonate) serves as the primary buffer within the cell. Approximately 80–90% of potassium is excreted in the urine by the kidneys. The mineralocorticoid aldosterone also regulates potassium concentration. Only about 10% of the total body concentration of potassium is extracellular, and about 50 mmol are in extracellular fluid. Therefore, the serum concentration of potassium is a poor measure of total body potassium. Nevertheless, the serum potassium concentration correlates well with its physiologic effects on nerve conduction, muscle function, acid-base balance, and heart muscle contraction.

Clinical Implications

➤ **Predisposing** factors for hyperkalemia are reduced excretion of potassium seen in some types of renal failure, cell damage (e.g., burns, surgery), acidosis, Addison's disease, uncontrolled diabetes, and RBC transfusion.

➤ **A** serum potassium concentration of less than 3.5 mEq/L is usually defined as hypokalemia. As with many laboratory tests, a falling trend (e.g., 0.1–0.2 mEq/liter/day) is more worrisome than just one low laboratory result. Predisposing factors include vomiting/diarrhea, severe burns, primary aldosteronism, chronic stress, liver disease with ascites, renal tubular acidosis, therapy with certain diuretics, steroids, cisplatin, ticarcillin, and amphotericin therapy.

➤ **Potassium** values do not vary with circulatory volume. Potassium is an intracellular ion, and its serum concentration should not be affected by circulatory volume.

➤ **The** chloride salt of potassium (KCl) is preferred for the treatment of hypokalemia. The optimal replacement dose of KCl depends on the degree of hypokalemia and whether electrocardiogram (ECG) changes are present. Adults usually ingest 60–120 mEq/day of potassium, and hospitalized patients not receiving food by mouth often receive 10–30 mEq K^+/L of IV fluids (see Chapter 10, "Fluid and Electrolyte Therapy" for more detailed potassium administration guidelines).

➤ **Hypokalemia** enhances the effects of digitalis preparations and may result in digitalis toxicity.

➤ **As** a very rough guideline, potassium blood levels rise approximately 0.6 mEq/L for every 0.1 decrease in blood pH from normal (pH 7.4).

➤ **Specific** ECG changes are associated with changes in serum potassium levels.

➤ **Hypokalemia** may be difficult to correct with KCl supplementation if the patient is also hypomagnesemic.

➤ **Neuromuscular** function is affected in both hyperkalemia and hypokalemia.

➤ **Glucose** tolerance testing or large ingestions of glucose can decrease potassium blood levels by shifting potassium intracellularly.

➤ **If** the WBC is greater than 50,000/mm^3, the laboratory report of the serum potassium concentration can be spuriously decreased due to an intracellular shift of potassium into the leukocytes if the serum sample remains in the laboratory test tube for a long period.

➤ **Calculation** of total body potassium is not well-defined. Each mmol/L decrement in the serum potassium represents a total 200–400 mmol potassium deficit. If the serum level is <2 mmol/L, this may reflect a total deficit of >1000 mEq.

➤ **Laboratory** measurement of serum potassium values can be elevated up to 50% above normal with moderate hemolysis.

➤ **Protein** synthesis is decreased with potassium deficiency.

Chloride (Cl⁻)

Normal Values

> 97–106 mEq/L   SI = 97–106 mmol/L

Description

The chloride anion resides predominantly in the extracellular space. It participates in the maintenance of acid-base and water balance through its influence on osmotic pressure. Although an alteration in the serum concentration of chloride is seldom a clinical problem, the chloride concentration is monitored because it is helpful in the diagnosis of acid-base disorders.

Clinical Implications

➤ **Decreased** serum chloride concentrations can be caused by vomiting, gastric suctioning, aggressive diuresis, burns, heat exhaustion, diabetic acidosis, and acute infection. A decreased chloride concentration is frequently associated with metabolic alkalosis.

➤ **Increased** serum chloride concentrations can result from dehydration, hyperventilation, metabolic acidosis, and kidney disorders.

➤ **Chloride** values are useful in assessing acid-base disturbances accompanying renal dysfunction. The plasma concentration of chloride, however, can be maintained near normal even in the presence of renal failure.

Carbon Dioxide (CO_2) Content

Normal Values

22–32 mEq/L   SI = 22–32 mmol/L

Description

In normal plasma, 95% of total CO_2 is present as bicarbonate (HCO_3) ions and the other 5% is dissolved CO_2 gas and carbonic acid (H_2CO_3).

There is often confusion by use of the term CO_2. The plasma CO_2 content is mainly bicarbonate, a base that is in solution and regulated by the kidneys. Dissolved CO_2 gas is mainly acid and is regulated by the lungs. Therefore, laboratory values of plasma CO_2 reflect bicarbonate concentrations.

Clinical Implications

➤ **Elevated** CO_2 is associated with severe vomiting, emphysema, and aldosteronism.
➤ **Decreased** CO_2 is associated with acute renal failure, diabetic acidosis, hyperventilation, and salicylate toxicity.

Glucose (Fasting Blood Sugar [FBS])

Normal Values

12 months to
    6 years of age: 60–100 mg/dL   SI = 3.33–5.55
                                                            mmol/L
    7+ years of age: 70–100 mg/dL   SI = 3.89–5.55
                                                            mmol/L

Description

Glucose is formed from the digestion of carbohydrates and by conversion of glycogen in the liver. Testing of the blood for glucose is primarily a screening procedure that indicates the inability of the islet cells of the pancreas to produce insulin, the inability of the intestines to absorb glucose, the inability of cells to utilize glucose efficiently, or the inability of the liver to accumulate and break down glycogen.

Clinical Implications

➤ **Elevated** blood sugar (hyperglycemia) or glucose intolerance (fasting values >120 mg/dL) can accompany Cushing's disease, acute distress, pheochromocytoma, chronic liver disease, potassium deficiency, chronic illness, and bacterial sepsis.

➤ **Glucocorticoids** can increase the blood sugar concentration to greater than 200 mg/dL. Other drugs (estrogen, epinephrine, alcohol, phenytoin, thiazides) can also increase blood glucose.

➤ **Other** interfering factors include diuretics, pregnancy, surgical procedures and anesthesia, obesity, and parenteral glucose administration.

➤ **When** the serum glucose concentration is repeatedly >126 mg/dL, diabetes mellitus must be considered.

➤ **Lowered** blood sugar concentration (hypoglycemia) can result from insulin overdose, Addison's disease, malnutrition, and liver damage (alcoholism).

Blood Urea Nitrogen (BUN)

Normal Values

Adult:	7–20 mg/dL	SI = 2.5–7.4 mmol/L
Child:	5–18 mg/dL	SI = 1.8–6.4 mmol/L

Description

Urea is a nonprotein, nitrogenous end-product of protein catabolism. It is formed in the liver, carried by the blood to the kidneys, and excreted in urine. The BUN, therefore, provides an index of glomerular filtration. The BUN concentration can be affected by tissue necrosis, protein catabolism, and the state of hydration. It is not as sensitive an indicator of renal function as creatinine or creatinine clearance.

Clinical Implications

➤ **Increased** BUN is most commonly caused by inadequate excretion secondary to kidney disease/urinary obstruction. Decreased renal function caused by shock, dehydration, infection, or diabetes mellitus can increase BUN. Major GI bleeding, with subsequent catabolism of blood to nitrogen, or an increased protein intake also could increase BUN.

➤ **BUN** is decreased with end-stage liver failure because the liver is unable to convert ammonia to urea. It is decreased by overhydration because of a dilutional effect, and by impaired absorption disorders because of an inability to absorb nitrogen subsequent to the digestion of protein.

➤ **Elderly** patients may have an increased BUN because of renal impairment.

➤ **Nephrotoxic** drugs (e.g., aminoglycosides, amphotericin B) can increase BUN.

➤ A BUN/Cr ratio of >20 indicates prerenal azotemia. A ratio ≤20 when BUN is elevated is associated with intrinsic renal disease and azotemia.

Creatinine

Normal Values

Child (1 year):	0.0–0.6 mg/dL	SI = 0–53 μmol/L
Child (2–3 years):	0.0–0.7 mg/dL	SI = 0–62 μmol/L
Child (3–7 years):	0.0–0.8 mg/dL	SI = 0–71 μmol/L
Child (7–10 years):	0.0–0.9 mg/dL	SI = 0–80 μmol/L
Child (10–12 years):	0.0–1.0 mg/dL	SI = 0–88 μmol/L
Child (12–17 years):	0.6–1.2 mg/dL	SI = 62–106 μmol/L
Adult (18+ years):	0.6–1.3 mg/dL	SI = 62–115 μmol/L

Description

Creatinine is a breakdown by-product of muscle creatine and phosphocreatine and is excreted renally. Creatinine production is constant as long as muscle mass remains constant. A reduction in kidney function reduces excretion of creatinine.

Clinical Implications

➤ **The** serum creatinine concentration is increased with impaired renal function regardless of whether the renal dysfunction is caused by nephritis, urinary tract obstruction, muscle disease, or severe dehydration.

➤ **The** serum creatinine concentration can be decreased as the result of muscular dystrophy, atrophy (e.g., spinal cord injury), malnutrition, or decreased muscle mass of aging.

➤ **Drugs** such as ascorbic acid, cimetidine (Tagamet), levodopa (Larodopa), and methyldopa (Aldomet) can interfere with the laboratory test measurement of creatinine independent of their effects on renal function.

➤ **Creatinine** values may be normal despite impaired renal function in elderly and malnourished patients due to decreased muscle mass.

➤ **Creatinine** has a serum half-life of approximately 1 day. Therefore, significant improvement in renal function requires several days before a new steady-state level of creatinine is truly reflective of renal function.

➤ A serum creatinine of 2 and 3 mg/dL corresponds to renal function of about 50% and 30% of normal, respectively.

➤ **Creatinine** of 10 mg/dL equals essentially no renal function, and the patient requires dialysis.

➤ **Creatinine** serum concentrations also are dependent on the patient's weight, age, and muscle mass.

➤ **Calculated** creatinine clearance is a better reflection of renal function and takes into account the age and weight of the patient.

➤ **Measured** creatinine clearance is better still, but requires measurement of creatinine in a timed urine collection and measurement of serum creatinine.

Calcium

Normal Values

8.5–10.2 mg/dL   SI = 2.1–2.55 mmol/L

Description

Calcium plays an essential role in muscle contraction, cardiac function, transmission of nerve impulses, and blood clotting. Approximately 98–99% of the body's calcium is stored in the skeleton and teeth. Of the calcium in the blood, 50% is ionized (free) and the remainder is protein-bound. Ionized calcium is the active form. A decrease in the serum albumin concentration of 1 g/dL will decrease the total calcium serum concentration by approximately 0.8 mg/dL (see Chapter 13, "Common Calculations in Pharmacy Practice").

Clinical Implications

➤ **Hypercalcemia** is most commonly the result of hyperparathyroidism or neoplasms. Other causes include parathyroid adenoma or hyperplasia (associated with hypophosphatemia), Hodgkin's disease, multiple myeloma, leukemia, Addison's disease, Paget's disease, respiratory acidosis, bone metastasis, immobilization, and therapy with thiazide diuretics.

➤ **Hypocalcemia** can result from hyperphosphatemia, alkalosis, osteomalacia, hypermagnesemia, inadequate calcium replacement, laxative use, and furosemide and calcitonin administration. It can also be exacerbated by bisphosphonates if the person is not receiving adequate calcium and vitamin D. Pseudohypocalcemia is sometimes encountered when the serum albumin concentration is low because of the association of calcium with albumin as described above.

➤ The following factors influence calcium levels:

- **Parathyroid** hormone is released when serum calcium drops. PTH stimulates bone resorption, which in turn releases calcium and phosphorus into the blood and enhances renal calcium reabsorption. PTH also increases renal conversion of vitamin D to the active form.
- **The** active form of vitamin D (1,25-diOH vitamin D) stimulates intestinal calcium absorption.
- **Estrogen** slows bone resorption and stabilizes bone density and may decrease calcium excretion.
- **Glucocorticoids** and excessive thyroid hormone can lead to hypocalcemia and osteoporosis.
- **When** requesting ionized calcium levels, blood pH should be measured concurrently.

Ionized Calcium

Normal Values

4.60–5.20 mg/dL   SI = 1.15–1.30 mmol/L

Description

Approximately half of calcium is bound to serum proteins, mainly albumin. The above test reports only the unbound or free (ionized) form, which is the active form.

Clinical Implications

➤ See above for effects of elevated or depressed calcium.
➤ The free form of calcium is the biologically active form. It is necessary to either correct for any differences in

binding from normal or to measure the free calcium. For example, in the case of a person who is hypoalbuminemic, he or she may have a low total serum calcium, but because less is bound, the level of free calcium may be appropriate (see above under Calcium).

➤ **Alternatively**, the ionized (free) calcium level can be measured by the clinical laboratory.

Phosphorus, Inorganic (PO$_4$)

Normal Values
Children:

0–6 years	3.9–6.9 mg/dL	SI = 1.26–2.22 mmol/L
6–14 years	3.9–5.7 mg/dL	SI = 1.26–1.84 mmol/L
14–17 years	3.1–5.5 mg/dL	SI = 1.00–1.78 mmol/L
17–20 years	2.9–4.9 mg/dL	SI = 0.93–1.58 mmol/L
20+ years	2.5–4.5 mg/dL	SI = 0.87–1.45 mmol/L

Description
Phosphate, an anion, is required for generation of bony tissue, metabolism of glucose and lipids, maintenance of acid-base balance, and storage and transfer of energy within the body. Approximately 85% of the body's total phosphorus is combined with calcium. When evaluating phosphate levels, the serum calcium values also must be checked.

Clinical Implications
➤ **Hyperphosphatemia** is associated with kidney dysfunction, uremia, excessive phosphate intake, hypoparathyroidism, hypocalcemia, excessive vitamin D intake, bone tumors, respiratory acidosis, lactic acidosis, and bisphosphonate therapy.
➤ **Hypophosphatemia** can be associated with hyperparathyroidism, rickets, diabetic coma, hyperinsulinism, continuous IV glucose administration in a nondiabetic person, antacids, diuretic phase of severe burns, and respiratory alkalosis.

Uric Acid

Normal Values

Men:	3.5–8.0 mg/dL	SI = 208–476 μmol/L
Women:	2.5–6.0 mg/dL	SI = 149–357 μmol/L

Description

Uric acid is formed from the breakdown of nucleic acids. Serum concentrations of urate increase when there is excessive production/destruction of cells (e.g., psoriasis, leukemia) or an inability to excrete urate renally.

Clinical Implications

➤ **Hyperuricemia** is associated with leukemia, lymphomas, shock, chemotherapy, metabolic acidosis, and significant renal dysfunction because of either increased production or decreased excretion.

➤ **Values** below normal are not significant.

➤ **Drugs** that increase urate blood levels include thiazides, salicylates (<2 g/day), ethambutol, niacin, and cyclosporine.

➤ **Drugs** that decrease blood levels include allopurinol (Zyloprim), sulfinpyrazone (Anturane), and salicylates (>3 g/day).

➤ **Serum** uric acid is useful for monitoring gout therapy with allopurinol.

Magnesium (Mg^{++})

Normal Values

1.70–2.3 mg/dL   SI = 0.7–0.95 mmol/L

Description

Magnesium is required for the utilization of adenosine triphosphate (ATP) as an energy source. It also has a role in carbohydrate metabolism, protein synthesis, nucleic acid synthesis, and muscle contraction. Magnesium deficiency in a normal diet is rare; however, high phosphate diets suppress magnesium absorption. Magnesium also regulates neuromuscular irritability, the clotting mechanism, and calcium absorption.

Clinical Implications

➤ **Hypermagnesemia** is associated with renal dysfunction, diabetic acidosis, large doses of magnesium antacids in the presence of renal insufficiency, hypothyroidism, and dehydration.

➤ **Hypomagnesemia** can be associated with diarrhea,

hemodialysis, malabsorption syndromes, drugs (e.g., thiazides, amphotericin B, cisplatin), lactation, acute pancreatitis, and chronic alcoholism.
- ➤ **Magnesium** deficiency may cause apparently unexplained hypocalcemia and hypokalemia resulting in severe neuromuscular irritability.
- ➤ **Increased** magnesium can act as a sedative and can depress cardiac and neuromuscular activity.
- ➤ **Hypomagnesia** may cause ventricular arrhythmias.

Cholesterol

Normal Values

Desirable:	0–199 mg/dL	SI = 0–5.20 mmol/L
Borderline:	200–239 mg/dL	SI = 5.20–6.18 mmol/L
High Risk:	240 mg/dL	SI = 6.21 mmol/L

Description

Cholesterol exists in tissues throughout the body. It is used by the body to form steroid hormones, bile acids, and cell membranes. Elevated cholesterol concentrations are associated with atherosclerosis and an increased risk of coronary artery disease.

Clinical Implications

- ➤ **Increased** levels of >200 mg/dL are considered to be high and require a triglyceride evaluation. Associated conditions include cardiovascular disease, atherosclerosis, Type II familial hypercholesterolemia, and obstructive jaundice.
- ➤ **Decreased** levels are associated with malabsorption, liver disease, sepsis, and pernicious anemia.
- ➤ **A** patient must fast for 12 hours before blood is obtained to measure the serum concentration of cholesterol and should maintain his or her customary diet for 3 days before blood is taken. Alcohol should not be consumed 24 hours before testing.

Total Serum Protein (TSP)

Normal Values

0–3 years of age:	4.5–7.5 g/dL	SI = 45–75 g/L
≥3 years of age:	6.0–8.0 g/dL	SI = 60–80 g/L

Description

The three major protein categories are as follows: (1) tissue or organ proteins, (2) plasma proteins, and (3) hemoglobin. The plasma proteins (albumin and globulins) reflect nutritional status and also serve as buffers in the maintenance of acid-base balance.

Clinical Implications

➤ Hyperproteinemia may be due to hemoconcentration secondary to dehydration. In this case, both albumin and globulin increase. If TSP increases but the albumin serum concentration is unchanged, the albumin/globulin (A/G) ratio falls. Collagen diseases, SLE, acute liver disease, and multiple myeloma are associated with hyperproteinemia.

➤ Hypoproteinemia (decreased total protein) is usually associated with a low albumin level and a small change in globulin yielding a low A/G ratio. It is normally associated with increased loss of albumin in the urine, decreased formation in the liver, insufficient protein intake, or severe burns.

Arterial Blood Gases (ABG)

Description

Arterial blood gas concentrations are analyzed to evaluate the exchange of oxygen and carbon dioxide to assess acid-base status. Arterial blood can be obtained by either an arterial puncture or from an indwelling arterial line to assess pH, pCO_2, pO_2, and SaO_2.

Common indications for the use of arterial gases include:

➤ *Gas Exchange Abnormalities.*

- **Acute** and chronic pulmonary disease
- **Acute** respiratory failure
- **Cardiac** disease
- **Rest** and exercise pulmonary testing
- **Monitoring** O_2 therapy
- **Sleep** disorder studies

➤ *Acid-Base Disturbances.*

- **Metabolic** acidosis
- **Metabolic** alkalosis

OXYGEN SATURATION (SaO$_2$)

Normal Values

$$95\text{–}99\% \text{ oxygen (O}_2)$$

Description

The oxygen saturation (SaO$_2$) describes the amount of oxygen carried by hemoglobin. It is expressed as a total percentage of the total capacity of oxygen to combine with hemoglobin.

Clinical Implications

➤ SaO$_2$ is used with pO$_2$ to evaluate the extent of oxygenation of hemoglobin and the adequacy of tissue oxygenation.

➤ The partial pressure of O$_2$ dissolved in plasma determines the amount of oxygen bound to hemoglobin. The large pool of oxygen carrying hemoglobin allows blood to transport 65 times the amount of oxygen dissolved in plasma. This relationship is determined by pH, temperature, the concentration of 2,3 DPG (diphosphoglycerate), and the molecular species of hemoglobin.

PARTIAL PRESSURE OF OXYGEN (PaO$_2$)

Normal Values (Room Air, Age-Dependent)

$$80\text{–}90 \text{ mm Hg} \qquad SI = 10.6\text{–}12.0 \text{ kPa}$$

Description

PaO$_2$ is a measure of the partial pressure exerted by the amount of O$_2$ dissolved in the plasma. It provides an estimate of the lung's ability to oxygenate blood.

Clinical Implications

➤ Decreased PaO$_2$ values are associated with chronic obstructive airway disease (COAD), restrictive airway disease, anemia, hypoventilation due to physical or neuromuscular impairment, and compromised cardiac function. PaO$_2$ values <40 mm Hg are a major concern.

➤ Increased values are associated with increased O$_2$

delivery by arterial means (e.g., nasal prongs, mechanical ventilation), hyperventilation by the patient, and polycythemia (increase in RBC mass and oxygen-carrying capacity).

PARTIAL PRESSURE OF CARBON DIOXIDE (PaCO₂)

Normal Values

34–46 mm Hg   SI = 4.5–6.1 kPa

Description

$PaCO_2$ reflects the pressure exerted by the CO_2 dissolved in the plasma. It can be used to evaluate the effectiveness of alveolar ventilation and to determine the acid-base status of the blood.

Clinical Implications

➤ **Decreased** $PaCO_2$ is usually associated with hypoxia, anxiety/nervousness, and pulmonary embolism. Values <20 mm Hg are a major concern.
➤ **Increased** $PaCO_2$ is usually associated with obstructive lung disease or reduced function of the respiratory center. $PaCO_2$ values >60 mm Hg are a major concern.
➤ **In** general, a rise in $PaCO_2$ is associated with hypoventilation, whereas a decrease reflects hyperventilation.
➤ **Typically,** for each mEq decrease in HCO_3, the $PaCO_2$ will decrease 1.3 mm Hg

PH

Normal Values

7.36–7.44

Panic Values

<7.25 or >7.65

Description

The serum pH reflects the chemical balance of acids and bases within the body. Hydrogen ion sources within the body include volatile acids and fixed acids (i.e., lactic acid, ketoacids).

Clinical Implications

➤ **pH** is generally decreased in acidemia (due to increased formation of acids).
➤ **pH** is generally increased in alkalemia (due to acid loss).
➤ **When** evaluating a pH value, pCO_2 and HCO_3 should also be obtained to estimate the respiratory or metabolic component contributing to the patient's acid-base status.

Anion Gap (AG)

Normal Values

8–16 mEq/L if potassium is included in the calculation
12–20 mEq/L if potassium is not included in the calculation

Description

The anion gap is used clinically in the diagnosis of metabolic acidosis. Calculations using available electrolyte information assist in quantification of unmeasured cations and anions. The unmeasured cations include Ca^{++} and Mg^{++}; unmeasured anions include protein, phosphate, sulfate, and organic acids. The anion gap can be calculated using two different approaches:

$$Na^+ - (Cl^- + HCO_3^-) \text{ or } (Na + K)$$
$$- (Cl + HCO_3) = AG$$

See Chapter 13, "Common Calculations in Pharmacy Practice," and Chapter 10, "Fluid and Electrolyte Therapy," for further discussions.

Clinical Implications

➤ **A** high anion gap (with a high pH) may indicate extracellular volume contraction or administration of penicillins in large doses.
➤ **A** high anion gap (with a low pH) is demonstrated with the mnemonic "MULEPAK" (*m*ethanol ingestion, *u*remia, *l*actic acidosis, *e*thylene glycol ingestions, *p*araldehyde ingestion, *a*spirin intoxication, and *k*etoacidosis).

➤ A low anion gap is associated with hypoalbuminemia, multiple myeloma, hyponatremia caused by viscous serum, marked hypercalcemia, and lithium toxicity.
➤ A normal anion gap can occur with metabolic acidosis as the result of diarrhea, renal tubular acidosis, potassium-sparing diuretics, and carbonic anhydrase inhibitors.

Bicarbonate Buffer System

Normal Values

$$22\text{--}26 \text{ mEq/L}$$

Description

The bicarbonate buffer system consists of carbonic acid (H_2CO_3) and bicarbonate (HCO_3). Quantitatively, it is the major buffer system in the extracellular body fluid. It reflects the following relationship:

$$\text{Total } CO_2 \text{ content} = \text{carbonic acid} + \text{bicarbonate}$$

Clinical Implications

➤ **Increased** bicarbonate may indicate respiratory acidosis due to decreased ventilation.
➤ **Decreased** bicarbonate may indicate respiratory alkalosis due to increased alveolar ventilation and removal of CO_2 and water, metabolic acidosis due to accumulation of body acids, or a loss of bicarbonate from the extracellular fluid.

URINALYSIS (UA)

Normal Values
See Table 6-1.

Description
UA provides valuable information in the evaluation of patients with renal disease.

Clinical Implications
➤ *Specific Gravity.* A specific gravity >1.025 in the morning indicates good concentrating ability; 1.010–1.012

Table 6-1.   Normal Values for Urinalysis

Parameter	Normal Value
Specific gravity	1.001–1.030
Appearance	Straw-colored, yellow
pH	5.0–7.5
Protein	0-trace (Tr)
Glucose	Negative
Ketones	Negative
Blood	Negative
Sediment analysis	Cell count for RBC, WBC (see Table 6.2)
Gram's stain	Negative

indicates the urine is isotonic with plasma (285–295 mOsm). Glucosuria, iodinated contrast media, and massive proteinuria (>2 g/24 hr) also can increase the specific gravity of urine.

➤ *Alkaline pH.* Urea splitting organisms (such as Proteus, Klebsiella, or *Escherichia coli*) or renal tubular acidosis caused by amphotericin therapy can alkalinize urine.

➤ *Protein.* A trace amount can be noted when a patient stands for prolonged periods. A 24-hour urine specimen is collected to quantitate the urinary protein.

➤ *Proteinuria.* Proteinuria (with dipstick method) may produce a false-positive result in patients with alkaline urine. The urinary protein may be (1) normal, indicating increased glomerular permeability or a renal tubular disorder; or (2) abnormal because of multiple myeloma and Bence-Jones proteins.

➤ *Glucose.* The correlation of urine glucose with serum glucose can be helpful in monitoring and adjusting hypoglycemic medications.

➤ *Ketones.* Starvation, poorly controlled diabetes mellitus, and alcoholism can result in the appearance of ketones in the urine.

➤ *Sediment.* No particular type of urine cast is pathognomonic for a specific renal disorder. However, the presence of red cell casts or white cell casts often signals a serious problem (Table 6-2).

Table 6-2. Cell Types in the Urine Sediment

Cell Type	Normal	Clinical Considerations
RBC	0–2/hpf	Cystitis is the most frequent cause of hematuria, although slight hematuria often occurs secondary to exertion, trauma, or febrile illness Yeast cells may be confused with RBCs; to distinguish between the two, acetic acid addition will result in a lysis of the RBC, but not yeast cells
Epithelial	0–2/hpf	Epithelial cells increase with tubular damage or heavy proteinuria Should be squamous epithelial cells only
Bacteria		Presence of bacteria on Gram's stain of unspun specimen correlates well with culture growth of 10^5 organisms (i.e., indicates presence of urinary tract infection) A culture and sensitivity (C & S) is useful to confirm the presence of bacteria
WBC	0–5/hpf	Polymorphonuclear leukocytes are the most common form of WBCs observed; if seen, and two routine cultures are negative, the culture should be tested for tubercle bacilli

Table 6-2. *Continued*

Cell Type	Normal	Clinical Considerations
Casts	0–occasional per low-power field	Red cell casts usually signify active glomerular disease
		Fatty and waxy casts may be seen with inflammatory or degenerative renal disease
		Leukocyte casts are usually associated by pyelonephritis
		Hyaline or granular casts may also be present normally, up to 0–1 per hpf

hpf, high-power field

LABORATORY TESTS BY ORGAN SYSTEM

CARDIAC DIAGNOSTIC TESTS

Cardiac Isoenzymes

CREATINE KINASE (CK)

Normal Values

Male:	<250 U/L	SI = <4.16 μkat/L
Female:	<175 U/L	SI = <2.91 μkat/L
CK isoenzymes:		
BB or CK1:	0%	
MB or CK2:	0–4% or ≤9ng/mL	
MM or CK3:	96–100%	

Description

Creatine kinase (formerly known as creatine phosphokinase) is an enzyme found in high concentrations in heart and skeletal muscle. It is used as a specific test for the diagnosis of MI and as a reliable measure of skeletal muscle diseases (e.g., muscular dystrophy, polymyositis).

CK can be divided into three isoenzymes: MM or CK3, BB or CK1, and MB or CK2. Skeletal muscle contains primarily MM; cardiac muscle contains primarily MM and MB. Brain tissue contains primarily BB. Normal CK is virtually 100% MM.

Clinical Implications

➤ In MI, the CK begins to rise 3–4 hours after myocardial injury, peaking within 15–24 hours and returning to normal within 3–4 days. If CK-MB is negative throughout 48 hours following onset of chest pain, the patient is unlikely to have suffered an MI.

➤ Other diseases than cause increased CK levels include cerebrovascular disease, muscular dystrophy, polymyositis, dermatomyositis, delirium tremens (DTs), chronic alcoholism, subarachnoid hemorrhage, and CNS trauma.

➤ Elevated MM enzymes occur in muscle trauma, intramuscular (IM) injections, shock, and MI as well as after surgery.

➤ Elevation of the MM level is an indication of skeletal muscle injury; elevation of MB provides a more definitive indication of myocardial injury.

➤ Elevated MB enzymes occur in MI, myocardial ischemia, and muscular dystrophy.

➤ Elevated BB enzymes occur in biliary atresia, brain trauma, and certain other brain injuries or tumors.

Troponin I

Normal Values

In normal cardiac health, troponin I < 0.0–0.4 ng/mL

Description

Troponins are globular proteins found in cardiac and skeletal muscle. Troponins play a key role in triggering muscle contraction in response to increased cytosolic calcium (ex-

citation-contraction coupling). There are three cardiac troponins: troponin I (cTnI), T (cTnT), and C (cTnC). cTnC is
not specific for the heart. cTnI and cTnT are found specifically in the heart. However, cTnT can also be expressed in
noncardiac tissue upon injury, and so cTnI appears to have
the highest selectivity as a marker of cardiac damage.

Levels of cTnI and cTnT can be used to evaluate patients
with suspected MI (6 hours–1 week after the incident).

Clinical Implications

➤ **Cardiac** Troponin I is usually increased within 6 hours
  of myocardial injury. It remains elevated for 7–10 days.
➤ If the level is <0.4 ng/mL, this indicates no myocardial
  injury within the previous several days.
➤ If the level is between 0.4 and 2.0 ng/mL, this is border-
  line and suggests possible MI. Repeat testing is recommended
➤ If Troponin I is >1.6 ng/mL, current myocardial injury
  is suggested.

Lipoprotein Panel

This includes cholesterol, low-density lipoprotein (LDL)
cholesterol, triglycerides, and high-density lipoprotein
(HDL) cholesterol

CHOLESTEROL

See Electrolytes and Chemistry Survey, Cholesterol.

LOW-DENSITY LIPOPROTEIN (LDL) CHOLESTEROL

Normal Values

Desirable:	<130 mg/dL	SI = <3.36 mmol/L
Borderline:	130–159 mg/dL	SI = 3.36–4.11 mmol/L
High Risk:	160 mg/dL	SI = >4.13 mmol/L

Description

LDLs contain cholesterol esters, protein (apoprotein),
triglycerides, and phospholipids. LDL plays a key role in
transporting cholesterol to a variety of tissues where it is
needed for membrane synthesis and other functions.

Clinical Implications
➤ **High** LDL values are associated with coronary vascular disease or familial hyperlipidemia. Levels may also be elevated in samples taken from subjects who have not fasted. Levels may also be elevated in types IIa and IIb hyperliproteinemia, diabetes mellitus, hypothyroidism, obstructive jaundice, nephrotic syndrome, and familial and idiopathic hyperlipidemia.
➤ **Decreased** LDL levels may occur in patients with hypoproteinemia, abetalipoproteinemia, and severe illness as well as in those undergoing estrogen treatment.

HIGH-DENSITY LIPOPROTEIN (HDL) CHOLESTEROL

Normal Values

Desirable:	>60 mg/dL	SI = >1.55 mmol/L
Borderline:	35–60 mg/dL	SI = 0.9–1.55 mmol/L
High Risk:	<35 mg/dL	SI = <0.9 mmol/L

Description
HDLs are the products of liver and intestinal synthesis and triglyceride catabolism.

Clinical Implications
➤ **There** is an inverse relationship between HDL cholesterol levels and the incidence of coronary artery disease.
➤ **Increased** HDL levels are seen in chronic alcoholism and primary biliary cirrhosis. Increased levels are also seen subsequent to exposure to industrial toxins or polychlorinated hydrocarbons. Patients taking estrogens or oral contraceptives, nicotinic acid, or phenytoin may have increased HDL levels.
➤ **Decreased** HDL can occur in patients with cystic fibrosis, severe hepatic cirrhosis, diabetes mellitus, Hodgkin's disease, nephrotic syndrome, malaria, and some acute infections. Patients receiving β-adrenergic blockers may have decreased HDL levels.

TRIGLYCERIDES

Normal Values

10–190 mg/dL   SI = 0.11–2.15 mmol/L

Description

Triglycerides are found in plasma lipids as chylomicrons and very-low-density lipoproteins (VLDLs).

Clinical Implications

➤ **Triglycerides** are increased in patients with alcoholic cirrhosis, alcoholism, anorexia nervosa, biliary cirrhosis, biliary obstruction, cerebral thrombosis, chronic renal failure, diabetes mellitus, Down's syndrome, hypertension, idiopathic hypercalcemia, hyperlipoproteinemia (types I, IIb, III, IV, and V), glycogen storage diseases (types I, III, and VI), gout, ischemic heart disease, hypothyroidism, pregnancy, acute intermittent porphyria, respiratory distress syndrome, thalassemia major, viral hepatitis, and Werner's syndrome.

➤ **Cholestyramine**, corticosteroids, estrogens, ethanol, high carbohydrate diets, oral contraceptives, and spironolactone can increase triglycerides.

➤ **Decreased** triglycerides may be seen with chronic obstructive lung disease, hyperparathyroidism, hyperthyroidism, hypolipoproteinemia, intestinal lymphangiectasia, severe parenchymal liver disease, malabsorption, and malnutrition.

RENAL DIAGNOSTIC TESTS

Creatinine, Urine

Normal Values

Men:	20–26 mg/kg/d	SI = 177–230 μmol/kg/d
Women:	14–22 mg/kg/d	SI = 124–195 μmol/kg/d

Description

Creatinine is a product of creatine metabolism and functions solely as a waste product of creatine. Since creatinine is freely filtered by renal glomeruli and is not appreciably reabsorbed in the tubules under normal conditions, serum creatinine and creatinine clearance reflect glomerular filtration rate.

Clinical Implications

➤ **Creatinine** production decreases with advanced age as muscle mass diminishes.

➤ To calculate creatine clearance, values for serum creatinine and for the total amount of creatinine excreted in urine over a fixed time (usually 24 hours) are required (see Chapter 13, "Common Calculations in Pharmacy Practice").

➤ The utility of measuring the quantity of creatinine excreted over time is to check on the adequacy of the urine collection process. If the value is lower than expected (see above values), then it is likely that the urine collection was not complete and will not allow accurate assessment of creatinine clearance.

Na^+/K^+ Ratio, Urine

Normal Value

0.9–3.88

Description

The Na^+/Ka^+ ratio in urine is useful in evaluating kidney function, fluid and electrolyte balance, acid-base balance, and extent of aldosterone effects on electrolyte composition of the urine.

Clinical Implications

➤ Diurnal variation occurs.

➤ Timed collection is required for an accurate measurement. A single collection may be used to assess responses to spironolactone therapy. The urine Na^+/Ka^+ ratio is >1 with effective spironolactone therapy.

Urine Sodium (Na^+)

Normal Values

40–220 mEq/24 hr   SI = 40–220 mmol/24 hr

Description

The urine sodium concentration is useful in assessing fluid balance, aldosterone effects, and renal concentrating ability. The wide range of normal values reflects dietary variations.

Clinical Implications

➤ Decreased urinary sodium levels may indicate dehydra-

tion, congestive heart failure, liver disease, or nephrotic syndrome.
➤ **Increased** urinary sodium levels may indicate diuretic use, Addison's disease, SIADH, or renal tubular acidosis.
➤ **Urine** sodium >30 mmol/L and oliguria suggest renal tubular necrosis.
➤ **The** wide range for normal values reflects diet, posture, stress, and endocrine effects.

Urine Chloride (Cl⁻)

Normal Values
110–250 mEq/24 hr   SI = 110–250 mmol/24 hr

Description
Used in workup of acid-base status to determine whether metabolic alkalosis is chloride-responsive. Normal values are dependent on diet and perspiration.

Clinical Implications
The chloride value only has meaning if Na^+/K^+ intake and output are also known. It can serve as a guide in monitoring individuals eating salt-restricted diets.

Urine Potassium (K⁺)

Normal Values
25–125 mEq/24 hr   SI = 25–125 mmol/24 hr

Description
Concentration is dependent on diet. It is used in workup of aldosteronism, renal tubular acidosis, and alkalosis.

Clinical Implications
➤ **Elevated** levels of urinary potassium are seen in patients with chronic renal failure, diabetes mellitus, renal tubular acidosis, dehydration, primary aldosteronism, and Cushing's disease.
➤ **Decreased** levels of urinary potassium are seen in acute renal failure and in malabsorption/diarrhea syndromes.
➤ **Urine** pH is decreased in patients who have decreased

potassium levels (hydrogen secreted in exchange for potassium) because less potassium is available for exchange.

Creatinine Clearance, Calculated (ClCr)

Normal Values

See Creatinine Clearance, Measured (Chapter 13).

Description

Creatinine clearance is the rate at which creatinine is cleared from the body by the kidney, essentially a measure of the glomerular filtration rate (GFR).

Clinical Implications

The measured creatinine clearance can provide a more accurate assessment of renal function than the calculated creatinine clearance. (see Chapter 13, "Common Calculations in Pharmacy Practice," and Creatinine, Urine in this chapter.)

GASTROINTESTINAL/HEPATIC DIAGNOSTIC TESTS

Amylase, Serum

Normal Values

20–100 U/L   SI = 0.33–1.66 μkat/L

Description

Amylase is an enzyme that converts starch to sugar. It is produced in the salivary glands, pancreas, liver, and fallopian tubes. More of the enzyme enters the blood if there is inflammation of the pancreas or salivary glands.

Clinical Implications

➤ **Increased** levels are associated with acute pancreatitis; carcinoma of the lung, esophagus, or ovaries; acute exacerbation of chronic pancreatitis; partial gastrectomy; obstruction of pancreatic duct; perforated peptic ulcer; mumps; obstruction or inflammation of salivary duct or

gland; acute cholecystitis; cerebral trauma; burns; traumatic shock; diabetic ketoacidosis; and dissecting aortic aneurysm.
➤ **Decreased** levels are associated with acute pancreatitis subsidence, hepatitis, cirrhosis of the liver, or toxemia of pregnancy.

Lipase

Normal Values

115–285 units/L   SI = 1.92–4.75μkat/L (values vary with methodology)

Description

Lipase converts triglycerides to fatty acids and monoglyceride. The major source of lipase is the pancreas; therefore, lipase appears in the bloodstream following damage to the pancreas.

Clinical Implications

➤ **Increased** levels are associated with pancreatitis, obstruction of the pancreatic duct, pancreatic carcinoma, acute cholecystitis, cirrhosis, severe renal disease, and inflammatory bowel disease.
➤ **Serum** lipase rises when secretions from the pancreas are blocked. Elevation may not occur until 24–36 hours after onset of illness.
➤ **Lipase** may be high when amylase levels are normal.
➤ **Lipase** persists longer in the serum than amylase in patients with pancreatitis.

Alanine Aminotransferase (ALT) (Formerly Serum Glutamic Pyruvic Transaminase [SGPT])

Normal Values

0–65 U/L   SI = 0–1.08 μkat/L

Description

High concentrations of the ALT enzyme are present in the liver. It is also found in the heart, muscle, and kidney. ALT is relatively more abundant in hepatic versus cardiac tissue and is more liver-specific than AST. ALT is used in the diagnosis of liver disease and to monitor the course of treatment for hepatitis, postnecrotic cirrhosis, and hepatotoxic effects of drugs.

Clinical Implications
➤ **Increased** levels are found in hepatocellular disease, active cirrhosis, obstructive jaundice/biliary obstruction, and hepatitis.
➤ **Many** drugs can increase levels.
➤ **A** two-fold increase is significant.

Alkaline Phosphatase (Alk Phos)

Normal Values

Female		Male	
Age (years)	U/L	Age (years)	U/L
1–10	75–375	0–9	75–375
11	150–425	10	150–350
12	159–375	11–13	150–450
13	50–325	14	150–400
14	50–250	15–16	50–300
15	50–175	17	50–225
16–17	50–150	18	50–175
18+	35–130	19+	35–130

Description
This enzyme originates mainly in the bone, liver, and placenta, with different isoenzymes from different tissues. High concentrations can be found in the biliary canaliculi with some located in the kidney and intestines. In liver disease, the alkaline phosphatase blood level rises when its excretion is impaired as a result of biliary tract obstruction. Bone alkaline phosphatase is a marker of bone formation, and there is usually a measurable amount released into the circulation during the process of normal bone turnover (bone resorption coupled with bone formation). Increased alkaline phosphatase is released into the blood in Paget's disease, a disease characterized by excessively high bone turnover, and the enzyme may be increased modestly in patients who have osteoporosis. In most clinical instances, the routine laboratory test used does not distinguish the isoen-

zymes, but for research purposes and for those patients who may have both liver disease and bone disease, it is possible to measure the isoenzymes separately to distinguish the source.

Clinical Implications

➤ **Elevated** levels are associated with obstructive jaundice, liver lesions, hepatocellular cirrhosis, Paget's disease, metastatic bone disease, osteomalacia, hyperparathyroidism, total parenteral nutrition, and hyperphosphatemia.

➤ **Reduced** levels are associated with hypophosphatemia, malnutrition, and hypothyroidism.

➤ **After** IV administration of albumin, there is often a moderate increase of alkaline phosphatase than can last for several days.

➤ **If** a patient exhibits increased serum alkaline phosphatase and the source is unknown, a measurement of GGT can help. If GGT is elevated, then the increased alkaline phosphatase is likely to be hepatic in origin.

Ammonia (NH_3)

Normal Values

0–40 μmol/L   SI = 0–40 μmol/L

Description

Ammonia is formed by bacterial metabolism of proteins in the intestine. Ammonia is normally removed from the blood by the liver and converted to urea. Urea is then excreted by the kidney. Generally, ammonia levels vary with protein intake. Exercise can increase ammonia levels.

Clinical Implications

➤ **Increased** levels are associated with liver disease, pericarditis, severe heart failure, acute bronchitis, pulmonary emphysema, urinary tract obstruction, hepatic coma, azotemia, and Reye's syndrome.

➤ **Measurements** of blood ammonia levels are used to evaluate metabolism as well as the progress of severe liver disease and response to treatment.

➤ **In** Reye's syndrome, elevated ammonia levels and encephalopathy may occur.

Aspartate Aminotransferase (AST) [Formerly Serum Glutamic Oxaloacetic Transaminase (SGOT)]

Normal Values

Male: 0–50 U/L   SI = 0–0.83 μkat/L
Female: 0–40 U/L   SI = 0–0.67 μkat/L

Description

AST, an enzyme of high metabolic activity, is found in heart, liver, skeletal muscle, kidney, brain, spleen, pancreas, and lung. Any disease that causes change in these highly metabolic tissues, or any injury or death of these cells, will release the enzyme into circulation.

Clinical Implications

➤ **Increased** levels occur in MI, liver disease, acute pancreatitis, trauma, acute hemolytic anemia, acute renal disease, severe burns, and with the use of various drugs.
➤ **Decreased** levels occur in the acidotic patient with diabetes mellitus.
➤ **Normal** serum concentrations (0–80 U/L) can be slightly higher in infants 1–60 days of age.

Bilirubin (Bili, T. Bili)

Normal Values

Total: 0–1.4 mg/dL   SI = <23.9 μmol/L
Direct: 0–0.30 mg/dL   SI = <5.1 μmol/L

Description

Bilirubin is a break-down of hemoglobin and a by-product of hemolysis. It is primarily removed by the liver and excreted into the bile, with a small amount found in the serum. A rise in the bilirubin occurs if there is excessive RBC destruction or if the liver is unable to excrete the amount produced.

There are two forms of bilirubin: (1) indirect or unconjugated (which is protein bound), and (2) direct or conjugated that circulates freely in the serum. An increase in conjugated bilirubin is more frequently associated with increased destruction of RBCs, whereas an increase in unconjugated bilirubin is more likely in dysfunction or blockage of the liver.

Bilirubin is important in evaluating liver function, hemolytic anemias, and hyperbilirubinemia (in newborns).

Clinical Implications

➤ **Bilirubin** elevations accompanied by jaundice may be due to hepatocellular injury, disease of parenchymal cells, bile duct obstruction, or red cell hemolysis.

➤ **Elevations** of unconjugated bilirubin levels occur in hemolytic anemia, trauma with evidence of a large hematoma, and pulmonary infarcts.

➤ **Elevations** of conjugated bilirubin levels occur in pancreatic cancer and cholelithiasis.

➤ **Both** levels increase in hepatic metastasis, hepatitis, cirrhosis, and cholestasis secondary to drugs.

➤ **Hemolyzed** blood falsely elevates bilirubin.

Gamma Glutamyl Transferase (GGT)

Normal Values

Men: 0–85 U/L	SI = 0–1.42 μkat/L
Women: 0–40 U/L	SI = 0–0.67 μkat/L

Description

GGT is present mainly in the liver, kidney, prostate, and spleen. The liver is considered the source of normal serum activity, even though the kidney has the highest level of the enzyme. The enzyme is believed to function in the transport of amino acids and peptides. Men have higher levels due to the concentrations found in the prostate.

Monitoring GGT values may be beneficial in detecting acute or chronic alcohol consumption, obstructive jaundice, cholangitis, and cholecystitis.

Clinical Implications

Increased GGT levels are associated with cholecystitis, cholelithiasis, cirrhosis, biliary obstruction, barbiturate use, and hepatotoxic drug use (especially those that induce the cytochrome P450 system). GGT is very sensitive but not specific. Elevations of just GGT (not AST, ALT) do not necessarily indicate liver damage.

Hemoccult (Guaiac or Benzidine Method)

Normal Values
Negative

Description
Commonly used to measure the presence of blood in stools, nasogastric output, and other bodily secretions.

Clinical Implications
➤ **Presence** of blood in stools requires further investigation.
➤ **False-positive** results are observed with large doses of iron, iodides, phenazopyridine, or red meat within 3 days of the test.
➤ **False-negative** results are observed with high doses of ascorbic acid.

Lactate Dehydrogenase (LD) (Formerly LDH)

Normal Values
Reported values vary considerably. The clinician should check with the laboratory.

Adult: 90–200 U/L   SI = 1.50–3.33 μkat/L

Description
An intracellular enzyme, LD is widely distributed in the tissues, particularly in the liver, kidney, heart, lungs, and skeletal muscle. This glycolytic enzyme catalyzes the interconversion of lactate and pyruvate. LD levels are nonspecific but aid in confirmation of myocardial or pulmonary infarction in combination with other findings. The LD may also be helpful in diagnosing muscular dystrophy and pernicious anemia. More specifics can be determined if LD is broken down into isoenzymes. Therefore, specific isoenzymes can be requested (i.e., LD_1:LD_2 for MI).

Clinical Implications
➤ In an acute MI, the LD increases and the LD_1:LD_2 ratio

usually "flips" to >1. Levels increase within 12–24 hours of infarction and usually peak 3–4 days after an MI.

➤ **With** pulmonary infarction, the LD is usually increased within 24 hours after onset of pain.

➤ **Elevated** levels are associated with acute MI, acute leukemia, skeletal muscle necrosis, pulmonary infarct, skin disorders, shock, megaloblastic anemia, and lymphomas. Various drugs and disease states also increase levels.

➤ **Decreased** levels reflect a good response to cancer therapy.

ENDOCRINE DIAGNOSTIC TESTS

Thyroid Function Tests

THYROID STIMULATING HORMONE (TSH)

Normal Values
0.5–4.7 μU/mL   SI = 0.5–4.7 mU/L

Description
TSH, a peptide hormone secreted from the anterior pituitary, stimulates thyroid hormone (T_3 and T_4) release from the thyroid gland. TSH secretion is under negative feedback control from thyroid hormone. It can differentiate primary hypothyroidism from pituitary/hypothalamic hypothyroidism.

Clinical Implications
➤ **TSH** is the best screen for hypothyroidism and hyperthyroidism and is also used for monitoring thyroid replacement therapy.

➤ **In** primary hypothyroidism, pituitary release of TSH is increased in response to low circulating free thyroid hormone. If TSH is elevated, free T_4 should be measured to confirm the diagnosis of hypothyroidism.

➤ **If** clinical evidence for hypothyroidism is present, and thyroid hormone concentrations are low but TSH is not elevated, the implication of possible hypopituitarism exists.

➤ **Decreased** levels of TSH are associated with hyperthyroidism.

THYROXINE, TOTAL, DETERMINATION BY RADIOIMMUNOASSAY (T₄-RIA)

Normal Values

Adults:	4–9.5 µg/dL	SI = 51–122 nmol/L
Females taking estrogen:	6.5–12.5 µg/dL	SI = 84–161 nmol/L

Description

The T₄-RIA test measures the level of total circulating thyroxine using a radioimmunoassay procedure. It provides an accurate result even if organic iodine in a contrast dye has been used in a recent radiograph.

Clinical Implications

➤ **More** than 95% of total thyroxine (T₄) is bound to thyroxine-binding globulin (TBG) and to prealbumin and albumin. The remaining T₄ is in the free or unbound (biologically active) form. Thus, it is necessary to have an assessment of free thyroxine (along with TSH) in a thyroid disease workup.
➤ **Increased** values are associated with hyperthyroidism, acute thyroiditis, pregnancy, early hepatitis, idiopathic TBG elevation, and estrogen use.
➤ **Decreased** values are associated with hypothyroidism, thyroiditis, nephrosis, cirrhosis, hypoproteinemia, malnutrition, and idiopathic TBG decrease. Values will be decreased with use of anabolic steroids, salicylates, phenytoin, or propranolol.
➤ **Administration** of traces of radioactive iodine within 48 hours before testing will interfere with the results.

FREE THYROXINE (FREE T₄)

Free thyroxine can be assessed in one of two ways. First, equilibrium dialysis to assess T₄ not bound to proteins can be used. Second, a measure called the free thyroxine index can be obtained indirectly by measuring total T₄ and also assessing the binding capacity of thyroid-binding globulin as described below under T₃UR.

Normal Values
Normal values for free T_4 by equilibrium dialysis:

> 0.8–2.7 ng/dL   SI = 0.010–0.035 nmol/L

TRIIODOTHYRONINE UPTAKE RATIO (T_3UR)

Normal Values
> T_3U = 25–35%   SI = 0.25–0.35

Description
The measurement of T_3UR is an indirect measurement of unsaturated thyroxin-binding globulin (TBG) in the blood. Low T_3UR levels are indicative of situations that result in elevated levels of TBG. Despite the name, the main use of T_3UR is to help provide an indirect measure of free T_4, as described above.

Clinical Implications
➤ **Measurement** of T_3UR with total T_4 provides a measure of free T_4, which is necessary to diagnose hypothyroidism along with measurement of TSH.
➤ **Increased** levels are associated with hyperthyroidism, nephrosis, severe liver disease, metastatic malignancy, pulmonary insufficiency, thyroxine and desiccated thyroid therapy, heparin, androgens, anabolic steroids, phenytoin, and large doses of salicylates.
➤ **Decreased** levels are associated with hypothyroidism, pregnancy, hyperestrogenic status, and T_3 treatment for hypothyroidism.

TRIIODOTHYRONINE (T_3)

Normal Values
> 45–137 ng/dL   SI = 0.69–2.10 nmol/L

Description
T_3 is more metabolically active than T_4 but has a shorter half-life. In the serum, there exists less T_3 than T_4, which is bound less firmly to thyroid-binding globulin. T_3 testing is of little value in diagnosing hypothyroidism. The T_3 test is a diagnostic test for hyperthyroidism and T_3 thyrotoxicosis

(i.e., elevated T_3 levels will be seen with normal T_4 levels in T_3 thyrotoxicosis).

Clinical Implications

➤ **Increased** values are associated with hyperthyroidism, T_3 thyrotoxicosis, daily dosage of >25 μg T_3 (liothyronine), acute thyroiditis, idiopathic TBG elevation, daily dosage of 300 μg of levothyroxine (T_4), pregnancy, estrogen use, and oral contraceptives.

➤ **Decreased** values are associated with hypothyroidism (although some clinically hypothyroid patients will have normal levels), starvation, idiopathic TBG depression, acute illness, anabolic steroids, androgens, large doses of salicylates, and phenytoin.

Adrenal Gland

PLASMA CORTISOL

Normal Values

Morning:	6–24 μg/dL	SI = 165–662 nmol/L
Evening:	3–12 μg/dL	SI = 83–331 nmol/L

Description

Cortisol affects the metabolism of proteins, carbohydrates, and lipids and inhibits the effect of insulin. It stimulates gluconeogenesis by the liver and decreases the rate of glucose use by the cells.

In the healthy person with normal diurnal rhythms, the secretion rate of cortisol is higher in the early morning (6–8 A.M.) and lower in the evening (4–6 P.M.).

Clinical Implications

➤ **Extreme** increases in the morning and no variation later in the day suggest carcinoma.

➤ **Decreased** levels are expected in liver disease, Addison's disease, anterior pituitary hyposecretion, and hypothyroidism.

➤ **Increased** levels are found in hyperthyroidism, stress (circadian variation less apparent in this setting), obesity, Cushing's syndrome, pregnancy, and the use of spironolactone and/or oral contraceptives.

HEMOGLOBIN AIC (HGB A₁C)

Normal Values

4.3–6% of total hemoglobin   SI = 0.043–0.06 fraction
of total Hgb

Description

Glycosylated hemoglobin measures the blood glucose bound to hemoglobin. The more glucose the RBC is exposed to, the higher the percentage of glycosylated hemoglobin.

Hemoglobin A_1 undergoes glycosylation by a slow nonenzymatic process within the RBC, has a life span of 120 days, and is dependent on available glucose. The measure of hemoglobin A_1C reflects the average blood sugar level in the 2–3 months preceding the test and allows for assessment of blood glucose control during that time. An elevated hemoglobin A_1C indicates that glucose was not under good control over the 2–3 months before the level was obtained.

Clinical Implications

➤ **A** diabetic patient whose disease has only recently come under good control may still have a high Hbg A_1C.
➤ **Values** vary among laboratories; therefore, assessments should be based on a single laboratory consistently performing the test.

> ### HEMATOLOGIC DIAGNOSTIC TESTS

Anemias

IRON (FE)

Normal Values

Newborn:	100–250 µg/dL	SI = 18–45 µmol/L
Infant:	40–100 µg/dL	SI = 7–18 µmol/L
Child:	50–120 µg/dL	SI = 9–21 µmol/L
Adult male:	50–160 µg/dL	SI = 9–29 µmol/L
Adult female:	40–150 µg/dL	SI = 7–27 µmol/L

Description

Serum iron measures the amount of iron bound to transferrin.

Clinical Implications

➤ **Serum** iron is increased in hemolytic anemia, pernicious anemia, thalassemia, acute hepatitis, acute porphyria, hemochromatosis, pyridoxine deficiency, excessive iron therapy, repeated transfusions, and nephritis.

➤ **Serum** iron is decreased in iron-deficiency anemia, remission of pernicious anemia, kwashiorkor, some systemic infections, idiopathic pulmonary hemosiderosis, hypothyroidism, paroxysmal nocturnal hemoglobinuria, pregnancy (third trimester), and rheumatoid arthritis.

➤ **Iron** is a frequent cause of accidental poisonings, especially in children.

➤ **Iron** levels in many patients with iron-deficiency anemia may remain in the low normal range (false-negative results). Diurnal and day-to-day variations of as much as 30% may occur; therefore, the serum iron value alone is not useful. Better diagnostic information is obtained when serum iron is elevated along with the total iron binding capacity (TIBC).

FERRITIN

Normal Values

Newborn:	25–200 ng/mL	SI = 25–200 µg/L
1 month:	200–600 ng/mL	SI = 200–600 µg/L
2–5 months:	50–200 ng/mL	SI = 50–200 µg/L
6 months– 15 years:	7–140 ng/mL	SI = 7–140 µg/L
Adult male:	15–200 ng/mL	SI = 15–200 µg/L
Adult female:	12–150 ng/mL	SI = 12–150 µg/L

Description

Ferritin is a measure of the body's iron stores and reflects storage of iron in the reticuloendothelial system.

Clinical Implications

➤ **Increased** levels are seen in hemochromatosis, hemosiderosis, liver diseases, certain malignancies, hyperthyroidism, non–iron-deficiency anemias, and chronic inflammation.

➤ **Decreased** levels are found in iron-deficiency anemia.
➤ **Levels** return to normal within a few days of the start of iron therapy unless the patient is noncompliant or continuing to lose iron.

TRANSFERRIN

Normal Values
212–360 mg/dL   SI = 2.12–3.6 g/L

Description
Transferrin is a serum protein (β-globulin) synthesized in the liver and reticuloendothelial system. It binds and transports ferric iron between tissues (primarily liver) and bone marrow, where the iron is incorporated into the RBCs' hemoglobin.

Clinical Implications
➤ **Transferrin** is increased in iron-deficiency anemia, estrogen therapy, pregnancy, and hypoxia as well as with the use of oral contraceptives.
➤ **Transferrin** is decreased in nephrotic syndrome, chronic renal failure, GI losses, severe burns, chronic infections, malnutrition, genetic deficiency (atransferrinemia), kwashiorkor, severe liver diseases, certain inflammatory conditions, and iron overdose.
➤ **Transferrin** is usually approximately 30% saturated with iron. The remaining 70%, which is unsaturated, reflects the body's TIBC.
➤ **Transferrin** is one of several proteins that may reflect nutritional status.

TOTAL IRON BINDING CAPACITY (TIBC)

Normal Values
Children 3+   250–400 μg/dL   SI = 44.8–71.6 μmol/L
  years and
  adults:

Description
TIBC is an indirect measure of serum transferrin. It is determined by adding an excess of iron to plasma to saturate all transferrin with iron. After removing excess iron, the iron bound to transferrin is determined.

Clinical Implications

➤ TIBC is increased in iron-deficiency anemia, acute and chronic blood loss, acute liver damage, and pregnancy as well as with the use of oral contraceptives.

➤ TIBC is decreased in hemochromatosis, anemias (of chronic diseases and infections), nephrosis, thalassemia, and other non–iron-deficiency anemias.

➤ TIBC is less sensitive to changes in iron stores than serum ferritin.

GLUCOSE-6-PHOSPHATE DEHYDROGENASE (G6PD) IN ERYTHROCYTES

Normal Value

4.6–13.5 IU/g hemoglobin

Description

G6PD in RBCs maintains reduced glutathione to prevent oxidation of hemoglobin to methemoglobin. Reduced levels of G6PD may cause hemolytic anemia.

Clinical Implications

➤ G6PD is decreased in 13% of U.S. black males and in 3% of U.S. black females, with about 20% carriers. G6PD is decreased in about 50% of Sardinians, Greeks, and Kurdish Jews. Decreased enzyme levels are also seen in Chinese persons.

➤ **Increased** G6PD may be seen in pernicious and other megaloblastic anemias, thrombocytopenia purpura, chronic blood loss, hyperthyroidism, and MI.

➤ **Class I** deficiency is the most severe and presents as chronic hemolysis in the absence of oxidative stress.

➤ **Class II** deficiency has levels of G6PD <10% of normal; however, it is associated with severe episodic hemolysis rather than chronic hemolysis.

➤ **Class III** deficiency is associated with occasional hemolytic episodes with identifiable precipitating factors.

➤ **Class IV** is normal.

➤ **Precipitating** factors include 4- and 8-aminoquinoline antimalarials, para-amino salicylates, methylene blue, aspirin, quinine, quinidine, large doses of ascorbic acid,

nitrofurantoin, some sulfonamides and sulfones, fava beans, infections, and diabetic ketoacidosis.
➤ **The** degree of hemolysis is dependent on the extent of deficiency and the dose of the precipitating agent. Hemolysis generally occurs by the third day of drug exposure.

Coagulation Tests

ACTIVATED PARTIAL THROMBOPLASTIN TIME (aPTT) AND PROTHROMBIN TIME (PT)

Normal Values
aPTT: 25–35 sec
PT: 11–13 sec

Description
The aPTT is used to detect deficiencies of the components of the intrinsic thromboplastin system. It is used for monitoring heparin therapy.

The PT is used to directly measure a defect in Stage II of the clotting cascade and the ability of prothrombin, fibrinogen, Factor V, Factor VII, and Factor X. It has been used for monitoring warfarin therapy. However, patients taking warfarin are now being monitored by the INR, and some laboratories do not report PT but only INR (see below).

Clinical Implications
➤ **The** aPTT is prolonged in coagulation defects of Stage I von Willebrand's disease, hemophilia, liver disease, or disseminated intravascular coagulopathy (DIC).
➤ **The** aPTT is the preferred test to monitor heparin therapy.
➤ **PT** is prolonged in prothrombin deficiency, vitamin K^+ deficiency, hemorrhagic disease of the newborn, liver disease, or salicylate intoxication.
➤ **aPTT** can also be used to determine the presence of circulating anticoagulants (antibodies induced in hemophiliacs by plasma transfusions).
➤ **Heparin** is used for the treatment of deep vein thrombosis (DVT) as a primary agent because it works rapidly and prevents fibrin clot formation, inhibits thrombosis

formation, and may inhibit extension of existing thrombi.
➤ **Warfarin** may prolong the aPTT because of its effects on Factors II, IX, and X.
➤ **Warfarin** acts in the liver to delay coagulation by interfering with the gamma-carboxylation of vitamin K^+-dependent Factors (II, VII, IX, X).
➤ If the PT is significantly prolonged, it is necessary to evaluate the patient for bleeding.
➤ **Green** leafy vegetables contain vitamin K^+ and can antagonize the effect of warfarin.
➤ **Variations** exist in reporting methods. The clinician should check with the laboratory.

International Normalized Ratio (INR). The INR is the result of efforts made to standardize the PT. To convert a PT ratio to an INR, the sensitivity of the thromboplastin reagent used in the laboratory must be known. The sensitivity should be expressed as an international sensitivity index (ISI). The ISI often falls in the 1.1–2.6 range, depending on the source of thromboplastin. The patient's PT is measured, and at the same time, PT is also measured on control or normal serum from other individuals not taking warfarin. The INR is calculated as follows:

$$INR = \frac{PT \; patient^{ISI}}{PT \; control}$$

The goal of warfarin therapy is to have a therapeutic INR of 2–3 except for those patients with mechanical prosthetic valves, for which the INR should be maintained in the 2.5–3.5 range.

FIBRIN DEGRADATION PRODUCTS (FIBRIN SPLIT PRODUCTS, FDP, FSP, D DIMER)

Normal Values

Negative: <0.25 μg/mL

Description

Formed by the fibrinolytic action of plasmin on abnormal fibrin deposition within the vasculature.

Clinical Implications

➤ **Serum** levels are elevated in (1) venous thrombosis and pulmonary embolus, which indicate the clot has begun to dissolve; and (2) disseminated intravascular coagulation (DIC).

➤ **Elevated** urine levels suggest renal disease or rejection crisis following renal transplant.

➤ **False** elevations are caused by exercise, stress, and traumatic venipuncture.

➤ **FDP** is one of the most sensitive and specific tests for DIC.

➤ In DIC, FDPs usually begin to fall within 1 day. If levels are very high, it may take a week or longer to return to normal.

THROMBIN TIME (TT)

Normal Values

Within 3 seconds of control value is considered normal (usual control range is 17.5–23.5 sec)

Description

TT tests the fibrinogen to fibrin conversion, a late phase of coagulation. TT is affected by the concentration of fibrinogen and plasmin, and the presence of fibrin degradation products (FDP) and antithrombotic agents.

Clinical Implications

➤ **TT** is elevated in DIC in approximately 60% of cases. It is a less sensitive and specific test for DIC than other tests. TT is also elevated in deficiencies of fibrinogen and in the presence of inhibitors of thrombin or fibrinogen. Unfortunately, it will not differentiate DIC from primary fibrinolysis. It is also elevated with heparin (most methods), urokinase, streptokinase, and asparaginase therapy.

➤ **TT** is not elevated in the presence of heparin when assayed by the reptilase method.

FACTOR V

Normal Values

65–100% of the normal pooled plasma (NPP)

Description

Factor V is one of the cofactors in the transformation of prothrombin to thrombin.

Clinical Implications

➤ **Defects** in Factor V result in increased PT and PTT values, but not bleeding time.

➤ **Factor** V is usually decreased in DIC, along with Factors VIII and XIII, but is not usually used for primary diagnosis of DIC due to time and technical difficulties.

➤ **Circulating** anticoagulants interfering with Factor V are associated with SLE and streptokinase or urokinase administration.

FACTOR VIII

Normal Values

60–180% of normal pooled plasma (NPP)

Description

Factor VIII is one of the cofactors in the activation of Factor X by the intrinsic pathway. Hemophilia A (classic hemophilia) is the hereditary deficiency of Factor VIII. The gene for Factor VIII is located on the X chromosome. Factor VIII has a serum half-life of 8–12 hours.

Clinical Implications

➤ **Factor** VIII levels may be decreased in DIC, along with Factors V and XIII. The consumption of these factors is due to the abnormal clot formation in the microvasculature. Factor VIII assays are not usually used for the primary diagnosis of DIC.

➤ **Defects** in factor VIII activity will result in increased PTT and coagulation time but a normal PT and bleeding time.

➤ **Circulating** anticoagulants interfering with Factor VIII activity are associated with the following conditions: SLE, rheumatoid arthritis, drug reaction, postpartum period, advanced age, and following replacement therapy for hereditary deficiency.

ANTITHROMBIN III (ATIII)

Normal Values

Age 6+ months: >75% normal pooled plasma (NPP)
   Reference ranges differ for the many methods available. The clinician should check with the laboratory.

Description

ATIII is a naturally occurring thrombin inhibitor, which also inactivates the activated forms of factors XII, XI, IX, X, and probably VII.

Clinical Implications

➤ **Heparin's** anticoagulant activity results from accelerating the inhibitory activity of ATIII. A decrease in AIII may predispose patients to thrombus formation and failure of heparin anticoagulation.

➤ **Increased** ATIII may be seen in acute hepatitis, in vitamin K^+ deficiency, following renal transplant, with inflammation, and during menstruation.

➤ **Decreased** ATIII may be seen in DIC; in congenital deficiency; following liver transplant and partial hepatectomy; in cirrhosis, chronic liver failure, and other liver diseases; with nephrotic syndrome; in carcinoma; during the last trimester of pregnancy and in the early postpartum period; and during the midperiod of the menstrual cycle.

➤ **Test** interferences include anabolic steroids, warfarin, heparin, asparaginase, estrogens, and oral contraceptives.

> INFECTIOUS DISEASE/
> IMMUNOLOGIC/
> RHEUMATOLOGIC DIAGNOSTIC
> TESTS

Human Immunodeficiency (HIV) Tests

Description

HIV is a retrovirus (RNA-containing virus) that invades cells of the immune system, specifically CD4+ T lymphocytes, weakens host defenses, and leads to opportunistic infections and full-blown acquired immune deficiency syndrome (AIDS) in almost all cases.

Some of the tests described below are used for a patient possibly infected with the HIV virus. Most patients with AIDS are anergic, with moderate anemia (Hgb, 7–12 g/dL), moderate thrombocytopenia, moderate leukopenia ($1000–3000/mm^3$), and lymphocytes $<1200/mm^3$.

ENZYME-LINKED IMMUNOSORBENT ASSAY (ELISA) OR ENZYME IMMUNOASSAY (EIA)

Description

Screening test for the antibody to the virus causing AIDS, HIV-1 (formerly HTLV-III). Most screening tests also pick up HIV-2. It takes 4–8 weeks after infection for antibody to appear. If a person has the antibody in their blood, it will react and bind to the HIV antigen that is bound to a surface. The antigen-antibody binding triggers a color reaction that is then evaluated as negative, positive, or in some cases indeterminate. Positive test results and indeterminate results must be repeated and then confirmed with a Western blot test.

Clinical Implications

A confirmed positive test (see below) indicates that the person is infected or potentially infectious and has a high risk of developing symptomatic illness within several years. The sensitivity of ELISA for HIV is approximately 99.5%, so there are few false-negative results. However, if a person is tested soon after being infected, before antibodies are made, a false-negative result can occur. If such an individual is truly infected, retesting at a later date will provide a positive result. ELISA also produces some false-positive results, so that noninfected individuals appear to be infected. For this reason, all positive test results using ELISA or EIA should be confirmed with another test (Western blotting).

WESTERN BLOT

A series of proteins unique to the HIV virus is separated by molecular weight using electrophoresis and bound to test strips. Strips are incubated with patient serum. If the patient serum contains antibody to the HIV antigens on the strip, it will bind and trigger a reaction that is read as positive.

Clinical Implication

A positive Western blot confirms the fact that the person is infected with HIV.

HIV ANTIGEN TEST

An infected person may not have antibody in the bloodstream (e.g., early in infection) but he or she will have HIV antigens (proteins) in the circulation. This test is not ordinarily used to screen individual patients for HIV, but instead is used to screen blood donations.

HIV RNA BY POLYMERASE CHAIN REACTION (PCR)

Description

This test measures viral load (number of virus particles) in the bloodstream. First, the viral RNA is converted into DNA. The PCR step then uses small primer segments of DNA that match parts of the viral sequence, plus DNA polymerase, an enzyme that can replicate DNA. In this assay, called polymerase chain reaction (PCR), one can detect very small quantities of nucleic acid in a test specimen. This is because the test will only create multiple copies of the particular test sequence if the sample contains a match to that sequence (in other words, contains virus).

Clinical Implications

When a patient sample is tested with PCR and there is no virus within the sample, then no copies will be made and the test is negative. If the person is infected, however, copies will be made and can then be detected. The presence of HIV viral DNA means the person is infected, and the viral load provides an indication of the progress of disease.

The main use of PCR in HIV is for monitoring the course of therapy.

CD4+ T-CELL COUNTS

Normal Values

Age 18+:

	%	Absolute number/mm^3
CD3:	58–82	690–1900
CD3+CD4+:	38–64	500–1300
CD3+CD8+:	15–33	210–690
CD3−CD19+:	4–16	65–300

| CD3−CD16 +CD56+: | 2–23 | 35–420 |

Description

The CD4+ cell count is the product of the total lymphocyte count and the percentage of CD4+ cells.

Before the development of viral load assays, CD4+ cell count was used to monitor disease course and treatment. CD4+ T lymphocytes are essential to combat infection, as they are necessary for responding to foreign antigens and encouraging formation of antibodies against antigens by B lymphocytes.

Clinical Implications

CD4+ lymphocytes are decreased in AIDS, and the CD4+ cell count provides an indicator of the immunologic competence of the patient. As CD4+ T lymphocytes decline, the risk of opportunistic infections increases.

Patients with CD4+ cell counts below 200 are at high risk for infection with *Pneumocystis carinii*. Those with CD4+ T cell counts <100 are at high risk from cytomegalovirus and the Mycobacterium avium-intracellular complex.

OTHER DIAGNOSTIC TESTS RELATED TO IMMUNOLOGIC/ RHEUMATOLOGIC DISEASE AND INFECTIOUS DISEASE

Erythrocyte Sedimentation Rate (ESR, Sed Rate)

Normal Values (Westergren Method)

Men:
 18–50 years 0–15 mm/hr
 50+ years 0–20 mm/hr
Women:
 18–50 years 0–20 mm/hr
 50+ years 0–30 mm/hr

Description

A nonspecific test that may be useful for monitoring infections and inflammatory diseases.

Clinical Implications

➤ **Increased** ESR is seen in conditions that have increased plasma fibrinogen, globulin or cholesterol, infections (e.g., tuberculosis), inflammatory diseases (e.g., rheumatoid arthritis), and tissue destruction (e.g., acute MI, neoplasms).

➤ **Decreased** ESR may be seen in polycythemia vera, sickle cell anemia, and congestive heart failure.

➤ **ESR** is useful for following certain diseases (e.g., MI, rheumatic fever, rheumatoid arthritis, tuberculosis).

Beta$_2$-Microglobulin (B$_2$M)

Normal Values

Urine: <120 µg/24 hr
Serum: 1.2–2.5 mg/L

Description

B$_2$M is a cell-membrane–associated, 100 amino acid protein that is increased during inflammatory reactions and in active chronic lymphocytic leukemia. This protein is readily filtered by the glomerular basement membrane and almost completely reabsorbed by the proximal renal tubular. Serum B$_2$M values depend on glomerular filtration rate (GFR), whereas urinary B$_2$M values vary with the functional activity of proximal renal tubular cells. Therefore, in glomerular disease, B$_2$M is increased in the serum and decreased in the urine. In tubular dysfunction, the opposite is true. It is useful for evaluating kidney allograft rejection in transplant patients and will often change in advance of serum creatinine values.

Clinical Implications

➤ **Serum** B$_2$M monitoring may allow diagnosis of renal graft rejection before changes in serum creatinine are seen, allowing for earlier treatment.

➤ **During** the treatment of acute rejection, serum B$_2$M often drops faster than serum creatinine.

➤ **In** aminoglycoside toxicity, B_2M levels become abnormal before the serum creatinine does so.

Hepatitis Panel

Normal Values

Negative

Description

There are at least four different types of viral hepatitis. These forms are clinically similar but differ with respect to immunology, epidemiology, prognosis, and prophylaxis. The specific types of viral hepatitis are as follows: (1) hepatitis A: infectious hepatitis; (2) hepatitis B: serum or transfusion hepatitis; (3) hepatitis D: always associated with hepatitis B; and (4) hepatitis C (formerly nonA/nonB): viral hepatitis caused by hepatitis C virus.

Persons at risk for hepatitis infection include renal dialysis patients, hematology/oncology patients, hemophiliacs, IV drug abusers, and homosexuals.

Serologic Markers

➤ Hepatitis A

- **The** HAV-Ab/IgM is detected 4–6 weeks after the infection. It indicates acute stage hepatitis A.
- **The** HAV-Ab/IgG is detected 8–12 weeks after infection. The presence indicates previous exposure/immunity to hepatitis A.

➤ Hepatitis B

- **HBs-Ag** hepatitis B surface antigen occurs 4–12 weeks after infection. A positive result indicates acute stage hepatitis B (acute and chronic infection).
- **Hbe-Ag** is present 4–12 weeks after infection. The presence indicates acute active stage (highly infectious).
- **HBc-Ab** hepatitis B core antibody occurs 6–14 weeks after infection. Its presence indicates past infection. It is a life-long marker.
- **Hbe-Ab** antibody is present 8–16 weeks after infection. Its presence indicates resolution of acute infection.
- **A** positive result of the HBs-Ab antibody to hepatitis

B surface antigen occurs 2–10 months after infection. It indicates previous exposure/immunity to hepatitis B but not necessarily to other types of viral hepatitis. It is also an indicator of clinical recovery. It will also be seen in individuals who have been successfully immunized with hepatitis B vaccine.

- **Measurement** of viral DNA by PCR can be used to monitor the course of HBV therapy with antiviral agents.

Infectious Mononucleosis (IM) Monospot

Normal Values
Negative

Description
The IM Monospot is a serologic test used for the diagnosis of infectious mononucleosis.

Clinical Implications
➤ **A** negative test result indicates the absence of significant IM-specific heterophile antibodies. False-negative results occur a very small percentage of the time.
➤ **False-positive** results can occur.
➤ **Acute** and convalescent (2–3 weeks after onset) titers should be obtained. A four-fold increase in titers from acute to convalescent titers is considered diagnostic.
➤ **The** highest incidence of IM occurs in whites aged 15–24 years. Clinical IM is associated with exposure to Epstein–Barr Virus (EBV) in the teenage years.

Venereal Disease Research Laboratory (VDRL)

Normal Values
Negative

Description
VDRL is a slide flocculation test used in diagnosing and staging syphilis.

Clinical Implications

➤ **The** test result does not become positive until 4–6 weeks after infection (1–3 weeks after the development of chancres). Positive tests should be confirmed with fluorescent treponemal antibody absorbed (FTA-ABS) testing.

➤ **False-positive** results may occur in pregnancy, drug addiction, infectious mononucleosis, leprosy, malaria, and collagen diseases such as rheumatoid arthritis and SLE.

➤ **Up** to 25% of patients may be nonreactive in early primary, late latent, and late syphilis. It is negative in more than 25% of patients with syphilitic aortitis.

➤ **Titers** may be helpful in following the disease. A decrease in titer may indicate response to treatment.

➤ **Titers** fall over 6–12 months with treatment of primary syphilis. Titers fall over 12–18 months with treatment of secondary syphilis. Some may remain positive for several years. Those with late latent or tertiary syphilis have titers that may gradually decrease over years. Increased titers indicate relapse or reinfection.

➤ **Titers** >1:16 are high and usually indicate active disease. Titers of less than 1:8 may be false-positive results or occasionally active disease.

➤ **Some** patients with primary or secondary syphilis may have high titers but the undiluted serum is nonreactive. Diluted serum will be positive in these patients.

➤ **Serial,** quantitative VDRLs are helpful in the diagnosis and assessment of response of congenital syphilis.

➤ **Cerebrospinal** fluid samples tested for VDRL are used to determine the presence of neurosyphilis. These should always be quantified.

NUTRITIONAL DIAGNOSTIC TESTS

Albumin

Normal Values

0–1 year of age:	3.4–5.0 g/dL	SI = 34–50 g/L
1+ year of age:	3.9–5.0 g/dL	SI = 39–50 g/L

Description

Albumin is formed in the liver and helps maintain normal water distribution (colloidal osmotic pressure). It aids in the transport of blood constituents (e.g., ions, bilirubin, hormones, enzymes, and drugs).

Clinical Implications

➤ **Increased** albumin levels are generally not observed. However, albumin may increase with IV infusions and dehydration.

➤ **Decreased** albumin levels are associated with inadequate iron intake, severe liver disease, malabsorption, severe burns, starvation states, nephrotic syndrome, diabetes, and SLE.

➤ **Decreased** serum albumin may result in an increase in free drug (and increased effect) for those agents that are highly protein bound (i.e., phenytoin, aspirin, valproate).

Zinc, Serum

Normal Values

Men:	75–291 μg/dL	SI = 11.5–44.5 μmol/L
Women:	65–256 μg/dL	SI = 9.95–39.2 μmol/L

Description

Approximately 80% of the total zinc in whole blood is in the erythrocytes. Zinc is a cofactor of many enzymes (e.g., alkaline phosphatase, lactic dehydrogenase).

Clinical Implications

➤ **Decreased** levels of zinc usually occur because of abnormal losses such as in Crohn's disease, pregnancy, fistulas, and malabsorption. Primary losses are in pancreatic and intestinal secretions. Decreased levels may be seen in patients who are alcoholics; obese patients who are fasting; patients with renal disease, diabetes, liver disease, porphyria, proteinuria, trauma, sickle cell disease, infection, hypoalbuminemia, and stress; and patients undergoing prolonged parenteral nutrition.

➤ **Increased** levels of zinc are rare but may be seen with tissue injury, hemolysis, and contaminated collection tubes.

➤ **Signs** of deficiency include dermatitis, hair loss, diarrhea, depression, and hypogeusia.

➤ **Serum** concentrations undergo circadian variations, with peaks around 9 A.M. and again around 6 P.M..

BODY FLUID ANALYSIS

Cerebrospinal Fluid (CSF) Examination

Normal Values

Glucose:	40–80% of serum glucose	
Appearance:	Clear, colorless, no clot	
Opening pressure:	70–180 mm water	
Protein		
Ventricular:	5–15 mg/dL	SI = 0.05–0.15 g/L
Cisternal:	10–25 mg/dL	SI = 0.1–0.25 g/L
Lumbar:	15–45 mg/dL	SI = 0.15–0.45 g/L
WBC:	0–10 cells/mm^3	

Description

Collection of CSF may be obtained via lumbar, cisternal, or ventricular puncture. The gross appearance and laboratory analysis of the fluid are important for differential diagnosis.

Clinical Implications

➤ **The** appearance may be purulent, opalescent, or turbid in cases of meningitis. Bloody CSF may be seen in cases of subarachnoid hemorrhage, traumatic tap, head trauma, and subdural hematoma.

➤ **Opening** pressure may be increased in cases of meningitis, encephalitis, brain tumor, head trauma, subarachnoid hemorrhage, and uremia.

➤ **Protein** may be increased in meningitis, encephalitis, tumor (brain and spinal cord), or a traumatic tap.

➤ **Fasting** glucose is usually normal in CSF. It may be increased in diabetic coma and sometimes in uremia.

➤ **WBC** may be increased in meningitis, encephalitis, and tumor (brain and spinal cord). WBC will be the same as that in the blood of patients with bloody CSF taps.

Glucose (in CSF)

Normal Values

Adult: 40–80% of serum glucose

Description

The measurement of CSF glucose is helpful in determining impaired transport of glucose from plasma to CSF and increased use of CNS, leukocytes, and microorganisms. The CSF glucose value varies with blood glucose levels and is usually 40–80% of the blood glucose value.

Clinical Implications

➤ **Decreased** glucose levels are associated with infection, tuberculosis, and the spread of lymphomas or leukemias into the meninges. All types of organisms consume glucose, and decreased glucose reflects bacterial activity.
➤ **Increased** glucose levels are associated with diabetes.

Acknowledgments

The previous authors Richard C. Christopherson and Karen E. Vick Smith are acknowledged for their primary work on this chapter.

Suggested Readings

Anonymous. Laboratory Handbook, Standard Edition. Madison, WI: University of Wisconsin Hospitals & Clinics; 2000.

Beers MH, Berkow R, eds. The Merck Manual of Diagnosis and Therapy. 17th ed. Whitehouse Station, NJ: Merck & Co., Inc.; 2000.

Braunwald E et al. Harrison's Principles of Internal Medicine. 14th ed. New York, NY: McGraw-Hill; 1999.

Condon RE. Manual of Surgical Therapeutics. 8th ed. Boston, MA: Little Brown & Co.; 1993.

DiPiro JT et al., eds. Pharmacotherapy: A Pathophysiologic Approach. 4th ed. Stamford, CT: Appleton & Lange; 1999.

Fischbach F. A Manual of Laboratory Diagnostic Tests. 6th ed. Philadelphia, PA: JB Lippincott; 2000.

Henry JB. Clinical Diagnosis and Management by Laboratory Methods. 19th ed. Philadelphia, PA: WB Saunders; 1996.

Kratz A, Lewandrowski KB. Case records of the Massachusetts General Hospital. Weekly clinicopathological exercises. Normal reference laboratory values. N Engl J Med. 1998;339:1063–72.

Macklis RM. Introduction to Clinical Medicine. 3rd ed. Boston, MA: Little Brown & Co.; 1994.

Malarkey LM, McMorrow ME. Nurse's Manual of Laboratory Tests and Diagnostic Procedures. 2nd ed. Philadelphia, PA: WB Saunders; 2000.

Ravel R. Clinical Laboratory Medicine—Clinical Application of Laboratory Data. 6th ed. St. Louis, MO: Mosby; 1995.

Sacher RH, McPherson RA. Widmann's Clinical Interpretation of Laboratory Tests. 11th ed. Philadelphia, PA: FA Davis; 2000.

Systeme International (SI) Units Conversion Table for Common Laboratory Tests. Ann Pharmacother. 1995;29:818–25.

Tierney LM, McPhee SJ, Papadakis MA, eds. Current Medical Diagnosis and Treatment. 39th ed. Stamford, CT: Appleton & Lange; 2000.

Tietz NW. Clinical Guide to Laboratory Tests. 3rd ed. Philadelphia, PA: WB Saunders; 1995.

Tietz NW (ed), Fundamentals of Clinical Chemistry. 4th ed. Philadelphia, PA: WB Saunders; 1996.

Tilkian SM. Clinical and Nursing Implications of Laboratory Tests. 5th ed. St. Louis, MO: CV Mosby; 1995.

Traub SL, ed. Basic Skills in Interpreting Laboratory Data. 2nd ed. Bethesda, MD: ASHP, 1996:245–80.

Wallach J. Interpretation of Diagnostic Tests. 6th ed. Boston, MA: Little Brown & Co.; 1996.

Young DS, Huth, EJ, eds. SI Units for Clinical Measurement. Philadelphia, PA: American College of Physicians; 1998.

Younossi ZM. Evaluating asymptomatic patients with mildly elevated liver enzymes. Cleveland Clin J Med. 1998;65:150–8.

Chapter 7

Diagnostic Procedures

Robert M. Breslow

Chapter Roadmap

GENERAL PROCEDURES
  Biopsy
  Computed Tomography (CT)
  Gallium Scan
  Magnetic Resonance Imaging (MRI)
  Ultrasonography

ALLERGY/IMMUNOLOGY
  Candida, Histoplasmin, and Mumps Skin Test
  Tuberculin Skin Test (PPD)

CARDIOLOGY
  Cardiac Catheterization
  Echocardiography
  Electrocardiography (ECG)
  Electrophysiology Study (EPS)
  Exercise Electrocardiography (Stress Test)
  Holter Monitoring
  MRI of the Heart
  Multiple Gated Acquisition Scan (MUGA)
  Myocardial Biopsy
  Swan-Ganz Catheterization
  Thallium Stress Test/Scan

ENDOCRINOLOGY
  Adrenocorticotropic Hormone Stimulation Test
    (Cosyntropin)
  Dexamethasone Suppression Test (DST)
  Oral Glucose Tolerance Test (OGTT)
  Thyroid Uptake/Scan
  Thyrotropin Releasing Hormone Test (Protirelin)

GASTROENTEROLOGY
  Abdominal Radiograph (KUB)
  Barium Enema
  Barium Enema with Air Contrast
  Enteroclysis

Barium Swallow (Upper GI with Small Bowel Follow
   Through [UGI/SBFT])
Cholangiography (Percutaneous Transhepatic)
Cholangiography (T-Tube)
CT of the Abdomen
Endoscopy
   Colonoscopy
   Endoscopic Retrograde Cholangiopancreatography
      (ERCP)
   Esophagogastroduodenoscopy (Upper Endoscopy)
   Proctoscopy
   Sigmoidoscopy (Flexible)
Hepatobiliary Scintigraphy (Hida, Papida, or Disida Scan)
Laparoscopy
Liver Biopsy
MRI of the Abdomen
Paracentesis
Small Bowel Series
Small Bowel Biopsy
Ultrasonography of the Abdomen
Urea Breath Test

GYNECOLOGY
   Breast Biopsy (Needle and Open)
   Colposcopy
   Hysterosalpingography
   Laparoscopy
   Mammography
   Ultrasonography of Pelvis, Uterus, and Ovaries

HEMATOLOGY
   Bone Marrow Aspiration and Biopsy

INFECTIOUS DISEASE
   Gram's Stain
   Indium-Labeled WBC Scan (Indium-111 Leukocyte Total
      Body Scan)

NEPHROLOGY
   Renal Biopsy
   Renal Scan

NEUROLOGY
   Brainstem Auditory Evoked Response (BAER)

CT of the Head
Electroencephalography (EEG)
Electromyography (EMG)
Lumbar Puncture (LP)
MRI of the Head
Muscle Biopsy
Myelography
Nerve Biopsy
Nerve Conduction Study
Visual Evoked Response (VER)

OPHTHALMOLOGY
Ophthalmoscopy
Slit Lamp Examination
Tonometry

ORTHOPEDICS
Arthroscopy
Arthrography
Bone Densitometry
Bone Scan

OTOLARYNGOLOGY
Laryngoscopy

PULMONOLOGY
Bronchial Alveolar Lavage (BAL)
Bronchoscopy
Chest Radiograph
CT of the Chest
Pulmonary Function Tests (PFTS)
Pulse Oximetry
Sweat Test
Thoracentesis
Ventilation-Perfusion Scintigraphy (V-Q Scan)

UROLOGY
Cystometrography (CMG)
Cystoscopy
Intravenous Pyelography (IVP)
Kidneys, Ureters, Bladder (KUB)
Retrograde Pyelography
Voiding Cystourethrography

VASCULAR
  Arteriography/Venography
  Doppler Studies
  Impedance Plethysmography (Occlusive Cuff)
  Lymphangiography (Lymphography)
  Magnetic Resonance Angiography (MRA)

Diagnostic procedures are an integral part of the clinical approach to patient care. The physical examination and patient history, clinical laboratory test results, and diagnostic procedures are key elements in making or confirming a diagnosis. All these diagnostic building blocks can influence a patient's pharmaceutical care. For example, if a patient is admitted to the hospital after experiencing abdominal pain with "coffee ground" emesis and the clinical laboratory test results demonstrate decreased hematocrit and hemoglobin levels and guaiac-positive stools, there is a high suspicion of upper gastrointestinal (GI) bleeding. As confirmation, an endoscopic procedure would assist in determining this diagnosis and could ultimately influence the choice and duration of drug therapy. Further or repeat diagnostic procedures can be useful for follow-up assessment to evaluate the success or failure of an intervention intended for a specific therapeutic outcome.

This chapter provides a general overview of diagnostic procedures and the role of these diagnostic procedures in patient care, the pharmacotherapy treatment plan, and patient outcome. It is organized by organ systems rather than diagnostic procedure classes. This format allows the reader to identify quickly the pertinent diagnostic procedures that apply to specific experiential settings. each diagnostic procedure section consists of a description of the procedure, the procedure's intended purpose, the normal and abnormal findings, and the procedure's pharmacy practice implications. These implications may be drug related or may prompt the monitoring of specific laboratory tests that may affect, or be affected by, the performance or outcome of a particular diagnostic procedure.

GENERAL PROCEDURES

Biopsy[1,2]

Description

A biopsy is performed by means of an aspiration or cutting needle, fine needle, scalpel, or punch. Biopsies may be closed (i.e., not requiring a surgical incision) or open (i.e., requiring a surgical incision). The technique and equipment used are dependent on the location and type of tissue to be sampled. Common biopsy sites include the bone marrow, breast, bone, cervix, liver, lung, lymph node, muscle, myocardium, nerve, pleura, prostate, kidney, skin, small bowel, and thyroid. A local or general anesthetic may be administered before the procedure. Diagnostic modalities such as radiographs, computed tomography (CT), and ultrasound (US) are used to guide the needle to the appropriate site.

Purpose

The purpose of a biopsy is to gather a small piece of tissue for microscopic analysis (either histologic or cytologic) to determine if the tissue is cancerous or noncancerous, to determine if infection is present, or to determine if other diagnostic findings are due to inflammation, scarring, or organ rejection. Biopsy usually follows other diagnostic procedures, such as CT or magnetic resonance imaging (MRI), that can identify changes but cannot diagnose the cause of those changes.

Findings

Normal and abnormal findings are dependent on the histology or cytology of the specific tissue undergoing biopsy.

Pharmacy Implications

➤ Patients may require sedation with a parenteral benzodiazepine such as midazolam or diazepam. Patients should be monitored for oversedation and respiratory depression.
➤ If a local anesthetic such as lidocaine or bupivacaine is to be used, the patient should be asked about a history of allergic reactions.

➤ In those patients requiring general anesthesia, an anticholinergic such as parenteral atropine or glycopyrrolate, a sedative such as diazepam or midazolam, or an analgesic such as morphine or meperidine may be required 15–30 minutes before anesthesia.

➤ It is recommended that antiplatelet agents should be discontinued before open and needle biopsies. Aspirin should be discontinued 7–10 days before the procedure. Nonsteroidal antiinflammatory drugs (NSAIDs) (e.g., ibuprofen, naproxen) that reversibly inhibit the enzyme cyclooxygenase should be discontinued 2–4 days before the procedure. Based on early evidence, it appears that COX-2 inhibitors may not require discontinuation before biopsy.

Computed Tomography (CT)[3–7]

Description

Computed tomography (CT or CAT), is a painless, noninvasive method for obtaining a three-dimensional picture of body structures using cross-sectional (transverse) slice x-rays. A complete scan consists of many pictures.

When performing a CT scan, an x-ray source or beam, together with a gamma ray detector, rotates around the patient in a 360° arc. The x-ray beam is very narrow, allowing little internal scatter of radiation. The detector simultaneously measures the intensity of radiation. A computer calculates the amount of radiation absorbed by each volume of tissue and assigns a Gray scale number to it. The computer analyzes the numbers and reconstructs a cross-sectional picture that can be displayed on a screen or produced as a hard copy for a permanent record and later interpretation.

Contrast media such as diatrizoate, iohexol, iopamidol, iothalamate, metrizoate, or metrizamide may be injected intravenously to enhance the images of brain, abdominal structures, and vasculature. Several doses of oral contrast media (diatrizoate) as a 2% solution (4 mL/200 mL H_2O) is administered before abdominal CT scans to provide contrast enhancement of certain abdominal structures.

Purpose

CT scans can confirm the diagnosis of suspected malignancies, assist in determining the staging and extent of neoplastic disease, and determine the effectiveness of therapy. CT scans of the brain and skull (cranial CT) may be performed to define the nature of head trauma, hydrocephalus, increased intracranial pressure, cerebrovascular lesions, degenerative brain diseases, and infections. CT scans of the body (body CT) which examine the neck, thorax, abdomen, and extremities may provide information on the cause of jaundice, inflammatory processes, pleural or chest wall abnormalities, and suspected abnormal collections of blood or fluid. A spinal CT is performed to evaluate disorders of the spine and spinal cord.

Findings

Normal and abnormal findings are dependent on the organs being evaluated.

Pharmacy Implications

➤ Because patients must lie completely still for an extended period, uncooperative patients are sedated with benzodiazepines (e.g., midazolam, diazepam, or lorazepam) or a sedative such as chloral hydrate. The typical sedative doses for these agents are as follows:

- *Midazolam.* Children: 0.05–0.1 mg/kg via an intravenous (IV) route or 0.1 mg/kg via an intramuscular (IM) route. Adults: 0.05–0.1 mg/kg IV or 0.07–0.08 mg/kg IM.
- *Diazepam.* Adults: 0.1–0.3 mg/kg IV.
- *Lorazepam.* Adults: 0.04 mg/kg IV or 0.5 mg/kg IM up to 4 mg.
- *Chloral Hydrate.* Children: 50–70 mg/kg up to 2.5 g.

➤ IV iodine contrast media should be used cautiously in patients with known or suspected hypersensitivity to iodine. Ionized contrast media are more likely to produce hypersensitivity reactions. Non-ionized products rarely produce reactions and are used in patients with previously documented histories of iodine hypersensitivity.

Gallium Scan[4,6–8]

Description

Radioactive gallium citrate (Ga^{67}) is administered intravenously 24–48 hours before the scan. The gallium scan is performed over the entire body by the use of a gamma scintillation camera or a rectilinear scanner. The scanning device measures the radiation emissions of Ga^{67} and shows the distribution or uptake patterns of Ga^{67} throughout the body. These emissions are converted into images that can be displayed in a video format or can be photographed for later use and interpretation. The degree of radioactivity Ga^{67} possesses is minimal and not harmful. A complete scan takes approximately 30–60 minutes.

Purpose

Gallium scans are used to detect or evaluate primary or metastatic neoplasms; inflammatory lesions of bacterial, autoimmune, or other origin; malignant lymphoma or recurrent tumors after chemotherapy or radiation therapy; and lung cancer. In addition, these scans aid in the diagnosis of focal defects in the liver.

Findings

NORMAL

Ga^{67} uptake is seen in the liver, spleen, bones, and large bowel.

ABNORMAL

Ga^{67} uptake is seen in abscesses, inflamed tissues, and some tumors.

Pharmacy Implications

Ga^{67} is excreted into the feces. This could interfere with the detection of inflammatory or neoplastic diseases of the colon. Therefore, a cleansing enema should be administered before the scan. Patients do not need to restrict food or fluid intake before the scan.

Magnetic Resonance Imaging (MRI)[4,9–14]

Description

With conventional MRI, the patient is placed inside a large circular magnet. The magnetic field causes the protons inside the body's atoms to spin in the same direction. A radio frequency signal is then beamed into the magnetic field which causes the protons to move out of alignment. When the radio signal is terminated, the protons move back into the position produced by the magnetic field, releasing energy as this occurs. A receiver coil measures the energy released and the time it takes for the protons to return to the aligned position. This provides information about the type and condition of the tissue from which the energy emanates. A computer then processes all the information and constructs a two- or three-dimensional picture of the tissues examined which appears on a television screen. A permanent copy of this image is produced on film or magnetic tape.

Open MRI uses the same technology as conventional MRI but does not have a closed tube into which the patient is placed to perform the imaging. This open technology is advantageous for the patient who experiences claustrophobia in narrow closed spaces.

MRI combines the advantage of anatomic imaging with excellent soft tissue characterization. Although MRI does not use ionizing radiation and does not require a contrast agent to identify vascular structures, a specialized contrast material such as gadolinium is now being used in certain circumstances to enhance MRI images.

Purpose

MRI is especially useful for diagnosis of brain and nervous system disorders, cardiovascular disease, and cancer. MRI provides very precise and detailed images of internal organs.

Findings

Normal and abnormal findings are dependent on the anatomy being evaluated.

Pharmacy Implications

➤ Successful imaging requires patients to lie very still. Uncooperative patients, patients who are claustrophobic, and children should be sedated (see CT scan recommendations). No contrast media are required.

➤ MRI is contraindicated in patients with cardiac pacemakers, surgically inserted metal hardware such as aneurysm clips, intrauterine devices, and recently inserted metal prostheses.

Ultrasonography [4,15]

Description

Ultrasound (US) is a noninvasive, nontoxic (without dyes) diagnostic procedure that examines internal structures by using high-frequency sound waves. As sound travels through the body tissues, it is modified (weakened as it goes through tissues) and travels at different speeds depending on the density and elasticity of the tissues. This is referred to as the acoustic impedance of the tissue.

In ultrasonography, a transducer produces short pulses of sound. When the sound wave produced by the transducer encounters an interface (the border between two adjacent structures), some of the waves are reflected (echoed) back to the transducer and an electric current is produced. The current is amplified, and the resultant image is displayed on a cathode ray tube (CRT).

US produces a good image when there are small differences in tissue density of the adjacent structures. However, when there are large differences, as between bone and soft tissue or air-filled spaces and soft tissue, the image is unintelligible because most of the sound waves are reflected back.

Traditionally, US could not be used to evaluate bone or air-filled spaces. A new generation of equipment used to screen for osteoporosis uses US principles to assess bone density. Because US can measure sound frequency shifts due to motion, US can be used to evaluate blood flow, free fluid, and amniotic fluid.

Purpose

➤ Examine internal soft tissue organs and structures including the eye, thyroid, breast, heart, liver, spleen, gallbladder, bile ducts, pancreas, uterus, ovary, bladder, and kidneys.
➤ Detect and evaluate masses, abscesses, stones, motion, fluid, and other reasons for obstruction.
➤ Determine size, shape, and position of the organ under study.
➤ Differentiate solid, cystic, and complex masses.

Several enhancement techniques are now used to provide better contrast and visualization of various body structures and to provide more recognizable images with greater detail.

Findings

NORMAL

Absence of masses, obstructions, and abscesses. Normal shape, size, and position of organs.

ABNORMAL

Presence of masses, obstructions, or abscesses. Abnormal size, shape, or location of organs.

Pharmacy Implications

None.

ALLERGY/IMMUNOLOGY

Candida, Histoplasmin, and Mumps Skin Test[4,16,17]

Description

Skin testing is a method of detecting an individual's sensitivity to certain allergens (antigens) or microorganisms responsible for disease. Skin testing may also be used to assess the integrity of a person's cell-mediated immune system. Three types of skin tests are generally used: scratch, patch, and intradermal tests. Reaction to a skin test demonstrates a hypersensitivity to the tested antigen. This indicates immunity to a disease or product or can indicate the presence of the active or inactive disease being studied.

An antigen is made from serum in which the organism responsible for the respective infection is present. The antigen is injected (0.1 mL) intradermally as a bleb on the volar (flexor) surface of the forearm by use of a tuberculin syringe and a small (25- to 27-gauge) needle. Tests are usually evaluated at 48–72 hours.

Purpose

Although each test can be used by itself to determine whether a patient has had the respective infection, the primary purpose of these recall antigens (those to which a patient has had, or may have had, previous exposure or sensitization) is to evaluate the competence of the cell-mediated immune system by attempting to provoke an immune response These skin tests are referred to as "controls" because they are used to determine whether a negative response to a skin test (e.g., tuberculin) is the result of negative exposure to the antigen or to incompetent cell-mediated immunity.

Findings

NORMAL

A positive reaction indicates previous exposure and resistance to the antigen. A positive test is observed when an induration greater than or equal to 10 mm in diameter appears after injection of the antigen.

ABNORMAL

A negative reaction indicates that the patient has not been exposed to the antigen or is suggestive (more likely) of a compromised immune system (anergy). No erythema and a lesion less than 10 mm in diameter indicates a negative test.

Pharmacy Implications

Skin tests are refrigerated before use. Concurrent or recent use of corticosteroids can produce a false-negative result due to suppression of the cell-mediated (delayed hypersensitivity) immune response. Antihistamines and H_2-blockers interfere with the cutaneous histamine response of the immunoglobulin E (IgE)-mediated immediate hypersensitivity reaction and can produce false-negative results.

Tuberculin Skin Test (PPD)[4,7,16]

Description

Tuberculin is a protein fraction (purified protein derivative) of the soluble growth product of *Mycobacterium tuberculosis* or *Mycobacterium bovis*. The antigen is administered intradermally (0.1 mL), creating a bleb at the intradermal injection site (usually the volar or dorsal aspect of the forearm). The antigen is available in three concentrations described as tuberculin units (TU): 1 TU, 5 TU, and 250 TU. The test is evaluated within 48–72 hours.

Purpose

The tuberculin antigen is administered to determine if the patient has active or dormant tuberculosis. However, the test cannot differentiate active from dormant infections.

Findings

NORMAL

Absence of redness or induration. This is referred to as a negative skin test.

ABNORMAL

Induration of the skin, erythema, edema, and central necrosis. The larger the wheal diameter in millimeters around the injection site, the more positive is the result (negative, <5 mm; doubtful or probable, 5–9 mm; positive, ≥10 mm). A positive skin test indicates prior exposure to the tubercle bacilli (TB) or previous bacille Calmette-Guérin (BCG) vaccination.

Pharmacy Implications

PPD is refrigerated and must be drawn up just before use. The 5-TU concentration is used most frequently; however, the 1-TU concentration is sometimes used as initial screening in patients with suspected tuberculosis to lessen the severity of the reaction. The 250-TU concentration, although rarely used, can be utilized when tuberculosis is suspected and a state of anergy may be present.

Concurrent or recent use of corticosteroids and other immunosuppressive agents can produce false-negative results due to suppression of the cell-mediated (delayed hypersensitivity) immune system. Antihistamines and H_2-blockers interfere with the cutaneous histamine response of the IgE-mediated immediate hypersensitivity reaction and can produce false-negative results. Lymphoid disease can produce a false-positive result. Viral and certain bacterial infections can cause false-negative results due to suppression of the delayed hypersensitivity reaction. Prior administration of BCG vaccine and recent vaccination with attenuated live virus vaccines can result in a false-positive reaction.

CARDIOLOGY

Cardiac Catheterization[11,12]

Description

Cardiac catheterization is performed by inserting a catheter (a thin, flexible tube) through a small incision made in an artery or vein in the neck, arm, or groin after administration of a local anesthetic at the intended insertion site to minimize patient discomfort. The catheter is then threaded into the right or left side of the heart with the assistance of fluoroscopy to help guide the placement of the catheter. Patients are mildly sedated before the test but remain awake throughout the procedure. Cardiac catheterization is usually performed in conjunction with coronary angiography, which uses an IV contrast material to visualize the coronary arteries. Fluoroscopy provides immediate visualization of the coronary circulation.

Purpose

Cardiac catheterization is performed to evaluate cardiac valvular disease, heart function, and congenital heart anomalies as well as to determine the need for cardiac surgery. When combined with angiography, the coronary arteries can be evaluated for obstruction (occlusion) to assess patient risk for myocardial infarction (MI). Catheterization can also be used to perform angioplasty and place stents to open up and prevent reocclusion of coronary arteries.

Findings

NORMAL

Heart size, motion, thickness, blood supply, and blood pressure within normal limits.

ABNORMAL

Presence of coronary artery disease, valvular heart disease, ventricular aneurysms, or enlargement of the heart.

Pharmacy Implications

➤ Patients receiving daily digoxin should receive their dose on the day of the procedure.

➤ It is likely that patients will receive diazepam or lorazepam 30 minutes before the procedure.
➤ Patients should be evaluated for a history of sensitivity to local anesthetics or IV contrast material.

Echocardiography[4,7,11,12,15,18,19]

Description

This is a specialized two-dimensional ultrasonographic technique by which a transducer is placed on the chest where there is no bone or lung tissue. High-frequency sound waves are directed at the heart. The heart reflects these waves (echoes) back to the transducer. These sound waves are then converted to electrical impulses and relayed to an echocardiography machine, which creates a diagram on an oscilloscope.

Conventional (transthoracic echocardiography) is performed by placing the transducer on the exterior chest wall. The problem encountered with this technique is a degraded heart image due to bony structures (sternum and ribs) and an extensive lung interface. Transesophageal echocardiography was developed to overcome these barriers to image quality. This technique involves the placement of an echo transducer on the tip of a gastroscope. Following administration of a local anesthetic spray to the back of the throat, a gastroscope is advanced orally into the esophagus, permitting placement of the transducer in closer proximity to the heart. This approach serves to eliminate chest cage and lung interference seen with the conventional technique. Because the transducer can be placed closer to the heart, transesophageal echocardiography can use higher-frequency transducers that significantly improve the resolution of the images. Two-dimensional conventional or transesophageal echo can be complemented with the addition of three-dimensional Doppler echocardiography, which is used to gather hemodynamic information because of its ability to measure the velocity of the red blood cells.

Purpose

➤ Diagnose or rule out valvular abnormalities or pericardial effusion.
➤ Measure the size of heart chambers.

➤ Evaluate chambers and valves of the heart.
➤ Detect atrial tumors and cardiac thrombi.
➤ Evaluate cardiac function or wall motion after MI.
➤ Evaluate blood flow through the heart chambers and valves.

Findings

NORMAL

No mechanical or gross anatomic abnormalities. Normal cardiac function. Normal blood flow patterns and blood velocity through the heart chambers and valves.

ABNORMAL

Abnormal motion, pattern, and structure of the four cardiac valves, left ventricular dysfunction, valve abnormalities, wall thickening, tumors or thrombi in the heart, abnormal size of the heart or chamber, or pericardial effusion. Abnormal blood flow.

Pharmacy Implications

CONVENTIONAL ECHOCARDIOGRAPHY

None.

TRANSESOPHAGEAL ECHOCARDIOGRAPHY

➤ Patients should be questioned about allergies to topical anesthetic spray.
➤ Patient will require parenteral sedation (e.g., midazolam) and analgesia (e.g., morphine).
➤ Patients at risk for bacterial endocarditis should receive appropriate antibiotic prophylaxis according to the newest American Heart Association bacterial endocarditis guidelines.

Electrocardiography (ECG)[4,7,11,12,16,20]

Description

ECG is a graphic recording of the electrical impulses of the heart that tracks the cardiac cycle from depolarization through repolarization. The electrical current generated by myocardial depolarization is naturally conducted to the surface of the body, where it is detected by electrodes placed on the patient's limbs and chest. The waves produced by this electrical activity are amplified for greater visibility before being printed on a moving graph paper strip. To capture the multidirectional electrical activity, 12 ECG leads are used simultaneously to achieve a comprehensive view of the electrical activity of the heart. Leads I, II, III, AVF, AVL, and AVR are attached to the limbs and provide an electrical view of the frontal plane of the heart; leads V1, V2, V3, V4, V5, and V6 are attached to the chest and produce a horizontal view of the heart's electrical activity. The tracing produced by the ECG shows the voltage of the waves, the time duration of waves, and the interval between them.

Purpose

ECG is used in the diagnosis of coronary artery disease, MI, pericardial effusion, pericarditis, rhythm disturbances as a result of ischemia or electrolyte abnormalities, and disorders of impulse formation and conduction. It is also helpful for evaluation of the effect of drugs on the heart.

Findings

NORMAL
See Table 7-1.

Table 7-1. Description of ECG Wave and Normal Findings

Wave/Interval	Explanation	Normal Finding
P wave	Impulse from SA node to atria (atrial depolarization)	Normal size, shape, and deflection
PR interval	P wave to QRS complex	0.1–0.2 sec
QRS complex	Depolarization of the ventricle	<0.12 sec
ST segment	Interval between depolarization and repolarization	No elevation or depression
T wave	Recovery phase after contraction (ventricular polarization)	No inversion

ABNORMAL

Abnormal heart rate, rhythm, axis, or position of the heart; myocardial hypertrophy; or MI. Conclusions can be reached about heart function after comparing the waves and intervals of the particular tracing against a normal tracing. However, this information cannot be used to depict the actual mechanical state of the heart or the integrity of the heart valves.

Pharmacy Implications

Cardioactive drugs (e.g., digoxin, quinidine, beta blockers) have various specific effects on the ECG tracing.

Electrophysiology Study (EPS)[16,18,21]

Description

Solid electrode catheters are most commonly inserted into the venous system and advanced into the right atrium, across the septal leaflet of the tricuspid valve and into the right ventricle in a fashion similar to cardiac catheterization. Discrete conduction intervals are measured by recording electrical conduction during the slow withdrawal of a bipolar or tripolar electrode catheter from the right ventricle through the HIS bundle to the sinoatrial (SA) node. As part of the study, ECG leads are attached to the patient's chest. After baseline values have been determined, pacing (electrical stimulation of the heart) is used to induce arrhythmias. When an ectopic site takes over as pacemaker, EPS can help pinpoint its origin. If a sustained arrhythmia is induced, an attempt will usually be made to capture the heart by pacing to terminate the arrhythmia. If the patient's cardiovascular system cannot compensate for the arrhythmia, the patient may require cardioversion to convert the dysrhythmia into a normal sinus rhythm (NSR).

Purpose

➤ To aid in the diagnosis of disorders of the heart's conduction system. EPS can also provide insight into the etiology and mechanism of ventricular arrhythmias and other disturbances within the atrioventricular (AV) conduction system.
➤ To aid in the selection of an antiarrhythmic drug and/or evaluation of the effectiveness of antiarrhythmic drug therapy.

➤ To assess the need for an implanted pacemaker in some patients.
➤ To perform a work-up for patients with syncope and sick sinus syndrome.

Findings

NORMAL

Normal conduction intervals, refractory periods, recovery times, and absence of arrhythmias. Normal conduction intervals in adults are: H-V interval 35–55 msec; A-H interval 45–150 msec; P-A interval 20–to 40 msec.

ABNORMAL

Prolonged conduction intervals (Table 7-2), abnormal refractory periods, abnormal recovery times, and induced arrhythmias.

Pharmacy Implications

➤ Patients are not permitted to have food or fluids for at least 6 hours before the study.
➤ EPS is contraindicated in patients with severe coagulopathy, recent thrombophlebitis, and acute pulmonary embolism.

Table 7-2. Conduction Intervals and Potential Causes

Interval Prolonged[a]	Possible Cause
H-V	Acute or chronic disease
A-H	Atrial pacing, chronic conduction system disease, carotid sinus pressure, recent MI, and drugs
P-A	Acquired, surgically induced, congenital atrial disease, and atrial pacing

[a] H-V, time from the onset of Bundle of His deflection to ventricular activation; A-H, time from atrial activation to onset of His deflection; P-A, time from onset of the p wave on the ECG to atrial deflection.

Exercise Electrocardiography (Stress Test)[4,7,11,12,18]

Description

Electrical cardiac principles are the same as for the ECG; however, the exercise stress test requires more preparation and patient participation. The electrode sites are shaved if necessary, and the skin is cleansed to remove the superficial epidermal skin layer and excess skin oil. The chest electrodes are placed according to the lead system selected to provide the desired tracing. Electrodes are held in place by adhesive or a rubber belt. The lead wire cable is draped over the patient's shoulder, with the lead wires connected to the previously placed electrodes. A baseline rhythm strip is run and checked for dysrhythmias. Blood pressure is checked, and a stethoscope is used to listen for the presence of S_3 and S_4 gallops or chest rales. The patient then steps onto a treadmill moving at a slow speed. A monitor is continuously observed for any changes in cardiac electrical activity, and a rhythm strip is checked at preset intervals for any abnormalities as the treadmill speed is increased. Blood pressure is monitored at predetermined intervals, and changes in systolic blood pressure are recorded. The speed and incline of the treadmill are increased every 2–3 minutes. The test is terminated when the maximum (target) heart rate is reached or if unstable changes occur pertaining to the ECG, blood pressure, heart rate, or patient status (i.e., exhaustion or angina). Once the exercise stops, the patient lies down and an ECG tracing is recorded every minute for 5 minutes or until ischemic changes have returned to normal or until the heart rate has returned to normal.

Purpose

➤ Test cardiac reaction to increased demands for oxygen.
➤ Help diagnose the source of chest pain or other cardiac pain.
➤ Help determine the functional capacity of the heart after cardiac surgery or MI.
➤ Screen for coronary artery disease.
➤ Establish the limits of an exercise program.
➤ Identify dysrhythmias.
➤ Evaluate the effectiveness of antiarrhythmic or antianginal drug therapy.

Findings

NORMAL
A normal ECG tracing with expected wave forms and intervals (see ECG).

ABNORMAL
The most prominent abnormal findings are a flat or downsloping ST segment depression and an up-sloping but depressed ST segment.

Pharmacy Implications

➤ Use of beta-adrenergic blockers may make the stress test difficult to interpret because the heart will be prevented from reaching the maximal target rate.
➤ If possible, digoxin should be discontinued for 3 days before stress testing due to the negative chronotropic effect of the drug.

Holter Monitoring[3, 7]

Description
Holter monitoring, also known as ambulatory electrocardiography, continuously records heart rate and rhythm for a period of time (24–72 hours). Although a Holter monitor is primarily used by ambulatory patients, it also can be used by patients restricted to bed. Three to five electrodes are placed on the chest, and heart rate and rhythm are recorded on magnetic tape. The tape is then analyzed for evidence of cardiac arrhythmias that would normally not have been present during a routine ECG test.

Purpose
➤ Diagnosis supraventricular and ventricular cardiac arrhythmias.
➤ Evaluate therapy (drugs and pacemakers) for cardiac arrhythmias.
➤ Identify asymptomatic patients at high risk for sudden cardiac death.
➤ Evaluate syncopal episodes in which arrhythmias are not evident.
➤ Detect myocardial ischemia.

Findings

Holter monitoring can demonstrate the relationship between symptoms such as syncope, palpitations, or shortness of breath and a cardiac arrhythmia. Unfortunately, symptom(s) and the Holter monitor abnormality must occur during the same testing period.

Pharmacy Implications

Patients keep a diary of all activities and symptoms during the period tested. All medications are recorded at the exact time taken.

MRI of the Heart

See General Procedures, Magnetic Resonance Imaging (MRI).

Multiple Gated Acquisition Scan (MUGA)[4,21–23]

Description

Most commonly, erythrocytes labeled with a radioactive isotope (technetium 99-m pertechnetate) are injected into the patient's venous circulation. As the isotope-labeled erythrocytes pass through the ventricle of the heart, a scintillation camera, triggered by and synchronized with the patient's ECG signals, records 14–64 points of a single cardiac cycle. This produces sequential images that can be viewed like a motion picture film. A MUGA scan allows evaluation of ventricular performance including wall motion, ejection fraction (EF), and other indices of cardiac function. The MUGA scan can also be performed after exercise. When compared to the results at rest, changes in ejection fraction and cardiac output (CO) can be assessed. The test is also known as cardiac blood pool scanning, because the blood, not the heart itself, is imaged.

Purpose

➤ Evaluate left ventricular function to assess prognosis in patients after acute MI.
➤ Evaluate the efficacy of coronary artery disease therapies.
➤ Differentiate ventricular hypokinesis from left ventricular aneurysms.

➤ Detect intracardiac shunting in patients with congenital heart disease or septal rupture after MI.
➤ Detect right ventricular failure.
➤ Provide useful information in patients with aortic regurgitation.

Findings

NORMAL

The left ventricle contracts symmetrically and the isotope appears evenly distributed in the scans. EF (amount of blood in the left ventricle propelled forward with each contraction) is 50–65%.

ABNORMAL

Asymmetric blood distribution in the myocardium, the presence of coronary artery disease as seen by segmental abnormalities of ventricular motion, the presence of cardiomyopathies as seen by globally reduced EFs, right to left shunting as seen by early arrival of activity in the left ventricle or aorta, and the presence of aneurysms in the left ventricle.

Pharmacy Implications

None.

Myocardial Biopsy[7,11,12,24]

Description

Myocardial biopsy is performed similarly to or as part of cardiac catheterization (see cardiac catheterization). When myocardial biopsy is performed alone, the jugular vein in the neck is the most common point of insertion for the IV catheter. The catheter is carefully threaded into the right side of the heart through the superior vena cava by using fluoroscopy. A local anesthetic may be used to minimize patient discomfort. Once in the right ventricle of the heart, a cutting instrument is used to remove heart muscle for analysis.

Purpose

Diagnose cardiac disease (e.g., cardiomyopathy, myocarditis, cardiac amyloid) and assess suspected rejection of a transplanted heart.

Findings

NORMAL

Normal pathology and histology.

ABNORMAL

➤ Signs of rejection in a transplanted heart. These are graded 0 through 4 based on the degree of interstitial lymphocytic infiltration.
➤ Presence of amyloid protein.
➤ Bacterial, viral, or parasitic causes of myocarditis.

Pharmacy Implications

➤ Antiplatelet agents are discontinued before the procedure. Aspirin should be stopped 7–10 days before, and other NSAIDs should be stopped 2–4 days before the procedure.
➤ As with cardiac catheterization, patients are assessed for sensitivity to local anesthetics.

Swan-Ganz Catheterization[7]

Description

Swan-Ganz catheterization can be performed by using the internal jugular vein, subclavian vein, femoral vein, or brachial vein as the point of insertion. The procedure should be performed in a setting in which vital signs and heart rhythm can be monitored closely. The procedure may be performed with or without the use of fluoroscopy. The skin at the insertion site is prepared with an antiseptic such as Betadine. If the internal jugular or subclavian veins are used, the patient is often placed in a Trendelenburg position to increase central venous distension. Sedation may be necessary if the patient is unable to cooperate. A local anesthetic, such as lidocaine, is injected into the subcutaneous layer and deeper tissues to provide patient comfort. A thin gauged needle (21-gauge, 1.5") is usually attached to a 5-mL syringe and used to locate the vessel of interest. Once the vessel has been located, a large-gauge needle (16- or 18-gauge) is attached to a syringe and placed into the vessel, following the course of the "finder needle." When blood is aspirated easily into the syringe, the syringe is disconnected from the needle and a flexible guidewire is threaded through the needle into the vein. The guidewire must be controlled carefully to prevent serious complications and death if lost in the patient. Once the needle is removed, a dilator is advanced over the guidewire and through the skin, to facilitate passage of a venous introducer. The introducer should be flushed with heparinized saline before insertion to avoid air emboli. Once the tract along the guidewire is dilated, the dilator should be slipped off the guidewire (maintaining guidewire position in the vein). The introducer and dilator can then be put together as a unit (dilator within introducer) and slid over the guidewire into the vein, again taking care to control the tip of the guidewire outside the patient's body. After the placement of the introducer and guidewire assembly, the guidewire and dilator should be removed from the patient. This leaves only the venous introducer sheath within the patient. At this point, if the introducer has a side-port lumen, venous blood should be aspirated and the introducer then flushed. If blood cannot be aspirated via a side-port lumen, the introducer is incorrectly placed and must be reinserted. No blood should come from the center of the introducer since this piece is usually accompanied by a one-way ball valve that does not allow blood leakage. The introducer is secured to the patient's skin with sutures. When the venous introducer has been placed, the Swan-Ganz catheter can then be inserted. The catheter can then be guided via the introducer, through the central venous system, through the right atrium, right ventricle, pulmonary artery, and into the wedge position. The catheter usually passes smoothly through the circulation, with the aid of the inflated balloon at its tip. The catheter should never be withdrawn with the balloon inflated. Catheter position can be ascertained by pressure wave forms, although fluoroscopy can be quite helpful in guiding the catheter into the wedge position. A chest radiograph is usually obtained after catheter insertion to verify position and to rule out the possibility of pneumothorax if the subclavian or internal jugular approach was used.

Purpose

➤ Monitor acute MI with hemodynamic instability.
➤ Evaluate severe hypotension of unknown etiology.
➤ Monitor selected cases of septic shock.

➤ Confirm the diagnosis of noncardiogenic pulmonary edema (normal "wedge" pressure).
➤ Aid in fluid and ventilator management of patients with adult respiratory distress syndrome.
➤ Confirm the diagnosis of cardiac tamponade, monitor hemodynamics during pericardiocentesis, and follow response to therapy.
➤ Evaluate suspected papillary muscle rupture.
➤ Diagnose possible ventricular septal defect or atrial septal defect following MI.
➤ Monitor congestive heart failure responding poorly to diuretics, especially when intravascular volume status is uncertain.
➤ Provide intraoperative monitoring of patients undergoing open heart surgery, particularly coronary artery bypass procedures involving multiple vessels; patients undergoing abdominal aortic aneurysm repair may also benefit from pulmonary artery (PA) catheterization perioperatively.
➤ Monitor drug overdose, especially when the risk of acute lung damage is high (e.g., heroin, aspirin).
➤ Monitor exacerbations of chronic obstructive lung disease requiring intubation; hemodynamic monitoring may detect occult or superimposed causes of respiratory failure not suspected clinically (e.g., left ventricular dysfunction).
➤ Evaluate and monitor end-stage liver failure with deteriorating renal function.
➤ Diagnose pulmonary hypertension.

Findings
See Table 7-3.

Pharmacy Implications
➤ Patients should be evaluated for hypersensitivity to local anesthetics.
➤ Sedation may be induced by a benzodiazepine such as midazolam or a parenteral analgesic such as morphine or meperidine.
➤ Aspirin and NSAIDs should be discontinued in advance of the procedure. However, use of these agents is not an absolute contraindication to performing the procedure.
➤ The effects of heparin or warfarin should be reversed before catheterization.

Table 7-3. Normal Findings for Swan-Ganz Catheterization

Parameter of Interest	Normal Resting Hemodynamic Value
Right atrium	Mean: 0–8 mm Hg; A wave: 2–10 mm Hg; V wave: 2–10 mm Hg
Right ventricle	Systolic: 15–30 mm Hg; End diastolic: 0–8 mm Hg
Pulmonary artery	Systolic: 15–30 mm Hg; end diastolic: 3–12 mm Hg
Wedge	A wave: 3–15 mm Hg; V wave: 3–12 mm Hg; mean: 5–12 mm Hg
AVO$_2$ difference (mL/L)	30–50
Cardiac output (L/min)	4.0–6.5 (varies with patient size)
Cardiac index (L/min/m^2)	2.6–4.6
Pulmonary vascular resistance (dynes/sec/cm^2)	20–130
Systemic vascular resistance (dynes −sec/cm^2)	700–1600

Thallium Stress Test/Scan[7,25,26]

Description

This nuclear medicine study can be performed while the patient is at rest or while exercising on a tread mill. The procedure incorporates the radionuclide thallium[201], which has biologic properties similar to potassium. These similarities account for its intracellular uptake when administered intravenously. Blood flow then distributes the radionuclide to the myocardium and other organs. A gamma camera is used to measure the radioactivity throughout the myocardium. Healthy myocardium rapidly takes up the thallium, whereas areas of infarcted myocardium show little or no radioactivity.

The stress test is performed using a multi-stage treadmill test and ECG monitoring with thallium[201] being administered at the time of peak exercise. The patient exercises for an additional 30–60 minutes with imaging performed immediately after. Three hours later, the myocardium is reimaged, and myocardial perfusion is further assessed following redistribution of the thallium. For those patients unable to exercise, adenosine, dipyridamole, or dobutamine is administered intravenously along with the thallium to simulate the change in cardiac blood flow that would normally occur with exercise.

Purpose

➤ Evaluate regional myocardial perfusion.
➤ Detect evidence of recent or remote MI.
➤ Identify viable myocardium in a previously infarcted portion of the myocardium.

Findings

NORMAL
Homogeneous distribution of thallium throughout the myocardium.

ABNORMAL
A thallium defect demonstrates a region of decreased myocardial blood flow. Infarcted areas can be demonstrated on the images immediately after injection and at the time of delayed imaging. Ischemic areas are detected on the early images as defects but disappear with delayed imaging due to thallium redistribution.

Pharmacy Implications

➤ Patients should not eat for several hours before the test to prevent increased distribution of the thallium to the gut. Caffeine and theophylline products should be withheld for 36–48 hours before dipyridamole and for 12 hours before adenosine.
➤ Beta-adrenergic blockers should be withheld for 24–48 hours before the test if exercise is to be performed to prevent a blunted response to exercise. Calcium channel blockers (diltiazem and verapamil) can also blunt maximal heart rate and should be withheld for 24–48 hours before the examination.
➤ Angiotensin-converting enzyme inhibitors should be withheld for 24–48 hours and nitrates for 6 hours before dobutamine.

➤ Chest pain, headache, nausea, and dizziness occur frequently with dipyridamole. Chest pain, headache, and flushing are common with adenosine. Chest pain, palpitations, arrhythmia, and flushing are common with dobutamine.

➤ IV aminophylline can be administered (75–250 mg) to counteract the systemic adverse effects of IV dipyridamole.

➤ The dobutamine dose is 10 μg/kg/min titrated up to 40 μg/kg/min.

➤ The adenosine dose is 50–140 μg/kg/min given over 6 minutes (21–60 mg).

➤ A typical dipyridamole dose for a 70-kg adult is 40 mg given over 4 minutes.

ENDOCRINOLOGY

Adrenocorticotropic Hormone Stimulation Test (Cosyntropin)[4,27–29]

Description

Cosyntropin (a synthetic derivative of adrenocorticotropic hormone [ACTH]) 250 μg IM or IV (preferred route) is administered following baseline blood sampling to measure the patient's cortisol level. Additional blood samples are drawn at 30 and 60 minutes after the cosyntropin has been administered, and serum cortisol concentrations are determined from these samples by radioimmunoassay.

Purpose

The ACTH stimulation test is a useful screening test to aid in the differentiation of primary and secondary adrenal failure and is used to diagnose adrenal insufficiency.

Findings

NORMAL

Serum cortisol will rise at least 10 μg/dL above the baseline determination. Generally, a doubling of the baseline level is a normal response. Baseline determinations are affected by the time of day due to diurnal variation.

ABNORMAL

Baseline cortisol level will be low and will display an in-adequate response by rising <10 µg/dL over the baseline. This does not fully differentiate primary (adrenal) failure from secondary (pituitary) failure. Further testing is necessary.

Pharmacy Implications

➤ The patient may fast overnight, but this is not always done.
➤ If cosyntropin is to be given intravenously, the injection time should not exceed 2 minutes.
➤ Estrogens, spironolactone, cortisone and its analogues, lithium, amphetamines, vasopressin, insulin, and metyrapone can interfere with the test.
➤ Dexamethasone does not affect the test due to its nonin-terference with the assay technique.
➤ Smoking, obesity, and alcohol can produce increased cortisol levels.

Dexamethasone Suppression Test (DST)[4, 11,12,27–31]

Description

The low-dose dexamethasone suppression test involves the administration of 1 mg of dexamethasone at midnight. At 8:00 AM the following morning, a blood sample is drawn to measure the plasma cortisol level. Variants of this low-dose study include dexamethasone 500 µg every 6 hours for 2 days or 2 mg every 6 hours for 2 days. In both cases, the plasma cortisol level is measured on the second day. The RIA method of measuring the plasma cortisol concentra-tion is generally preferred. For use in evaluating depression, 1 mg of dexamethasone is administered at 11:00 PM and cortisol levels are measured at 4:00 PM and 11:00 PM the following day.

Purpose

➤ The DST is a screening test for the presence of Cushing's syndrome. It is most useful for ruling out Cushing's syn-drome as the diagnosis. The overnight test does not eas-ily differentiate among pituitary, adrenal, or ectopic etiologies. The 2-day test provides more information and may be more diagnostic with respect to etiology. Nevertheless, it is performed less frequently due to the time required.

➤ The DST also aids in the diagnosis of major endogenous depression.

Findings

NORMAL
Plasma cortisol <5 μg/dL.

ABNORMAL

➤ Failure to suppress (cortisol >5 μg/dL) suggests that the pituitary-adrenal axis is not suppressible and Cushing's disease may be present.
➤ Failure to suppress appears in only approximately 50% of patients with major depression. Consequently, the usefulness of the DST as a screening test for depression is limited.
➤ Patients with significant psychiatric disorders, thyrotoxicosis, obesity, or acromegaly; pregnant patients; and alcoholic patients often have elevated plasma cortisol levels. This may confound the screening test. Diurnal rhythm (time of day) can also influence the result.

Pharmacy Implications

➤ The patient must fast overnight.
➤ ACTH, cortisone, estrogens, hydrocortisone, oral contraceptives, ethanol, lithium, or methadone taken 2 weeks before testing increases plasma test results. Phenytoin and androgenic steroids may decrease plasma cortisol levels.

Oral Glucose Tolerance Test (OGTT)[4,11,12,32–34]

Description

A blood sample to determine the fasting (baseline) blood glucose for the patient is drawn first. Then, the patient drinks a highly concentrated glucose solution (75 g/300 mL for nonpregnant adults and 100 g/400 mL for pregnant women). Subsequently, a timed series of blood glucose tests is performed at 30, 60, 90, and 120 minutes for nonpregnant adults and 1, 2, and 3 hours for pregnant women to determine the rate of removal of glucose from the bloodstream. This test is not performed if the fasting blood sugar is >126 mg/dL in nonpregnant adults, because virtually all such patients will have blood glucose determinations that meet or exceed the diagnostic criteria for diabetes mellitus.

Purpose

Diagnose or rule out overt diabetes, glucose intolerance, Cushing's syndrome, and acromegaly.

Findings

NORMAL—ADULT (NONPREGNANT)

Fasting blood glucose: 70–110 mg/dL

After 75 g of oral glucose:

30 minutes	<200 mg/dL
60 minutes	<200 mg/dL
90 minutes	<200 mg/dL
120 minutes	<140 mg/dL)
180 minutes	70–110 mg/dL

ABNORMAL—ADULT

➤ *Diabetes Mellitus.*

  • Sustained elevated blood glucose levels during at least two OGTTs.
  • Two-hour sample, ≥200 mg/dL.

➤ *Impaired Glucose Tolerance.* Two-hour OGTT blood glucose level ≥140 and <200 mg/dL.

➤ *Impaired Fasting Glucose.* Fasting plasma glucose of ≥110 mg/dL and <126 mg/dL.

➤ *Gestational Diabetes* (following administration of 100 g of anhydrous glucose). This diagnosis may be made if two blood glucose values equal or exceed the following values:

Fasting	105 mg/dL
1 hour	190 mg/dL
2 hours	165 mg/dL
3 hours	145 mg/dL

Pharmacy Implications

➤ The patient should be instructed to fast overnight (12 hours).

➤ Seventy-five grams of glucose (Glucola) are given to nonpregnant adults and 100 g are given to pregnant women on the morning of the test.

➤ Insulin or oral hypoglycemic agents should not be taken until the test is completed.

➤ The following drugs should be discontinued at least 3 days before the test: hormones (including oral contraceptives), alcohol, salicylates, indomethacin, diuretics (especially higher dose thiazides), guanethidine, hypoglycemic agents, beta-adrenergic blockers, corticosteroids, monoamine oxidase inhibitors (MAOIs), lithium, nicotinic acid, phenothiazines, ascorbic acid, amphetamines, benzodiazepines, diazoxide, epinephrine, and phenytoin.

Thyroid Uptake/Scan[7]

Description

UPTAKE

Radioactive iodine (I^{131} or I^{123}) is ingested by the patient in either solid oral dosage form or as an oral liquid. Six hours and 24 hours after ingestion, a gamma probe placed over the thyroid measures the amount of radioactivity in the thyroid gland. This result is compared against the dose of radioactive iodine administered to the patient, and a percent uptake is calculated.

SCAN

Technetium-99m pertechnetate is administered intravenously and is concentrated in the thyroid gland like iodine. A gamma camera is used to scan the thyroid gland approximately 30 minutes after injection. The information gathered by the scanner is sent to a computer, which creates a two-dimensional image of the thyroid gland and thyroid nodules on x-ray film or as a computer printout. Alternatively, the patient can ingest I^{131} or I^{123} as in the thyroid uptake test. Six and 24 hours later, the thyroid gland is scanned and two-dimensional images produced.

Purpose

UPTAKE

To evaluate thyroid function when blood tests of thyroid function are abnormal. The test is able to detect and quantify the extent of thyroid disease and can be useful in distinguishing between primary and secondary thyroid disease.

SCAN

To evaluate the location, size, anatomy, and function of the thyroid gland.

Findings

NORMAL

Percent uptake of radioactive iodine is in the normal range at 6 and 24 hours. The thyroid gland is of normal size, shape, location, and color. There is a homogeneous and symmetrical distribution of radioactive material throughout the thyroid gland.

ABNORMAL

The percent of radioactive iodine uptake is less than or greater than the range for normal. This will indicate either hypothyroid or hyperthyroid disease. Scanning can reveal a thyroid tumor, goiter, thyroid nodules, thyroiditis, or ectopic thyroid tissue. The color of the thyroid gland will appear lighter or darker than the normally expected color.

Pharmacy Implications

➤ Barbiturates, estrogen, lithium, and phenothiazines can increase iodine uptake.

➤ ACTH, antihistamines, corticosteroids, Lugol's solution, nitrates, potassium iodide solution, thyroid drugs, antithyroid drugs, tolbutamide, iodinated contrast agents, and cough syrups containing iodine compounds suppress radioactive iodine uptake.

➤ Patients should discontinue thyroid and antithyroid drugs 1–2 weeks before uptake or scanning studies.

Thyrotropin Releasing Hormone Test (Protirelin)[35,36]

Description

The test is performed by administering IV protirelin (TRH) 500 μg over 15–30 seconds following pretest blood sampling to determine the patient's baseline thyroid stimulating hormone (TSH). Plasma TSH levels are drawn 30 and 60 minutes after TRH is administered.

Purpose

➤ Diagnose suspected hyperthyroidism in individuals whose routine thyroid function tests are not fully diagnostic.
➤ Assess the integrity of the pituitary thyrotropes to aid in differentiating hypothyroidism due to intrinsic pituitary disease from hypothalamic dysfunction.
➤ Aid in the diagnosis of mild hypothyroidism.

Findings

NORMAL

TSH rise >5 µU above the baseline TSH excludes the diagnosis of hyperthyroidism.

ABNORMAL

➤ *Hyperthyroidism.* No TSH rise or <5 µU rise.
➤ *Primary Hypothyroidism.* Initially high baseline levels of TSH (exaggerated response).
➤ *Secondary Hypothyroidism.* Little or no response when pituitary failure is present.
➤ *Hypothalamic Hypothyroidism.* TSH will rise at 45 or 60 minutes after TSH.

Pharmacy Implications

➤ Results can be affected by patients receiving thyroid supplementation.
➤ A 14-hour overnight fast is recommended.

GASTROENTEROLOGY

Abdominal Radiograph (KUB)[4,7,37,38]

Description

The patient lies on his or her back, and a radiograph is taken of the kidneys, ureters, and bladder (KUB). A KUB radiograph is also called a "scout film." No contrast media are used for this study. When performed in the erect position, gas fluid levels within the small and large intestine and free air in the peritoneum can be better visualized. Patients who cannot stand can be placed on their side (lateral decubitus position). A posterior-anterior (PA) view of the chest is sometimes done along with the KUB to evaluate pulmonary pathology as a possible cause of abdominal pain.

Purpose

➤ Diagnose intraabdominal abnormalities such as nephrolithiasis, intestinal obstruction, tissue masses, abnormal accumulation of gas, free air in the abdomen, or enlargement or perforation of the tissues.
➤ Evaluate size, shape, and position of the liver, spleen, and kidneys.

Findings

NORMAL

No masses, smooth peritoneal space, and normal size and position of organs. Right kidney is slightly lower than the left.

ABNORMAL

Foreign bodies, abnormal fluid, ascites, abnormal kidney location or shape, urinary calculi, calcification of blood vessels, cysts, or tumors.

Pharmacy Implications

➤ Normally, there is no patient preparation.
➤ The presence of feces or gas can obscure the film, which may necessitate the administration of a laxative (milk of magnesia) at bedtime the night before the examination or 75 mL of senna fruit concentrate at 4:00 PM on the day before the film. However, this is not frequently done.
➤ The presence of barium obscures the clarity of the film. The KUB should be scheduled before examinations requiring the administration of oral contrast media.

Barium Enema[11,12,39,40]

Description

Barium contrast is instilled through the rectum by inserting a rectal tube up to the ileocecal valve. The rectal tube remains in place while the films are taken. The rectal tube may be equipped with a small balloon at the tip, which can be inflated to prevent leakage of the barium. Examination of the large intestine is performed using x-ray and fluoroscopy. These show position, filling, and movement of the colon. The barium contrast opacifies the bowel mucosa and outlines folds of the large intestine.

Abdominal CT scan or US are now considered first-line procedures for the initial evaluation of suspected abdominal masses.

Purpose

➤ Diagnose colorectal masses and inflammatory bowel diseases such as ulcerative colitis.
➤ Detect the presence of polyps or diverticula.
➤ Evaluate the structure of the large intestine.
➤ Diagnose intestinal stricture or obstruction.

Findings

NORMAL
Normal position, contour, filling, rate of passage of barium, movement, and patency of colon.

ABNORMAL
Presence of tumors, diverticula, obstructions, inflammation, or other abnormal findings.

Pharmacy Implications

A typical procedure protocol includes the following:

TYPICAL PROCEDURE VARIANT 1
➤ Ingesting a liquid diet 2 days before procedure.
➤ Drinking 32 oz of water the day before the examination (from noon to 11:00 PM).
➤ Drinking 300 mL magnesium citrate at 5:00 PM the day before the procedure. If severe renal disease is present, the patient should drink 1 bottle (75 mL) senna fruit concentrate.

TYPICAL PROCEDURE VARIANT 2
➤ Taking 4 5-mg bisacodyl tablets at 7:00 PM the day before the procedure. Tablets should be swallowed whole and should not be taken within 1 hour of antacids or milk.

TYPICAL PROCEDURE VARIANT 3
➤ Taking metoclopramide 10 mg by mouth or intravenously IV at 3–4 PM the day before the procedure.

➤ Ingesting GI lavage solution 240 mL orally every 10 minutes up to 4 L or until the evacuated fluid is clear. When using GI lavage solution, the patient should be evaluated for preexisting fluid overload conditions or fluid restrictions.

➤ Ingesting no food or drink after midnight the night before the procedure.

➤ Performing a 2000-mL cleansing enema before the procedure.

➤ Taking 30 mL milk of magnesia orally as a cathartic after the procedure. In a patient with compromised renal status, 30 mL sorbitol 70% should be given orally after the procedure.

Use of magnesium citrate or magnesium hydroxide cathartics should be avoided in patients with renal failure.

Barium Enema with Air Contrast [4,39,40]

Description

This test is often referred to as double contrast barium enema or pneumocolon. It involves the same principles as a standard barium enema but includes the instillation of air into the bowel in addition to the contrast medium. This method improves detection of subtle changes in the colon but is not as thorough an examination as a colonoscopy.

Purpose

See Gastroenterology, Barium Enema.

Findings

See Gastroenterology, Barium Enema.

Pharmacy Implications

See Gastroenterology, Barium Enema.

Enteroclysis [11,12,41–43]

Description

Enteroclysis is a radiographic examination of the small bowel performed by delivering barium directly into the jejunum by way of an orogastric or nasogastric tube (12- or 14-gauge French catheter), followed by a radiolucent methylcellulose solution. Enterolysis provides an improved and more detailed view of the entire small bowel compared with the standard small bowel series. It is the procedure of choice in evaluating suspected small bowel malabsorption.

Purpose

Evaluate malabsorption, inflammatory bowel disease, and the presence of a small bowel obstruction. It should be performed only after other diagnostic procedures have been attempted or performed.

Findings

NORMAL

The presence of normal-appearing bowel mucosa, small bowel wall thickness, and normal fluid transit time. The absence of lesions, obstructions, or fistulas.

ABNORMAL

Inflamed mucosa, motility disorder, presence of masses, obstruction, narrowed lumen, fistulas, and small bowel bleeding.

Pharmacy Implications

➤ See Gastroenterology, Barium Enema.
➤ Metoclopramide 10 mg IV may be administered 20–30 minutes before the procedure to aid in intubation of the small bowel.
➤ Apprehensive patients may benefit from administration of a low-dose anxiolytic such as diazepam or lorazepam to aid in intubation.

Barium Swallow (Upper GI with Small Bowel Follow Through [UGI/SBFT])[4,41,42]

Description

A fluoroscopic radiographic examination of the pharynx, esophagus, stomach, duodenum, and upper jejunum comprises the upper GI portion of the examination. An oral contrast medium (barium) is swallowed, permitting visualization of the lumen in these areas. To evaluate the remainder of the jejunum and the ileum (small bowel follow through), a series of hourly films may be required to track the contrast medium through the small bowel. This portion of the examination is complete when the ileocecal valve has filled with the contrast material.

Purpose

Detect or diagnose congenital abnormalities of the bowel, esophageal stricture, esophageal cancer, tumors, pyloric stenosis, varices, diverticula, ulcers, polyps, hiatal hernia, gastritis, regional enteritis, malabsorption, gastroesophageal reflux, obstruction, and motility disorders.

Findings

NORMAL
Normal size, contour, motility, and peristalsis.

ABNORMAL
Deformed contour from intrinsic tumor, filling defects, or stenosis with dilation. Ulcers and other irregularities also may be seen.

Pharmacy Implications

➤ Barium sulfate or diatrizoate meglumine (Gastrografin) must be given during procedure.
➤ No oral ingestion (including medications, antacids) after 10:00 PM the day before the examination.
➤ Administration of 30 mL of milk of magnesia after the procedure as a cathartic. In a patient with compromised renal status, 30 mL sorbitol 70% should be given after the procedure.

Cholangiography (Percutaneous Transhepatic)[7,11,12,44–46]

Description

With the patient lying supine, a local anesthetic is administered in the right upper quadrant of the abdomen. A 20- to 22-gauge, 6-inch long flexible needle is used to puncture the skin and is passed into the intrahepatic biliary tree with the help of fluoroscopy. Contrast material is then administered via this needle into the biliary tree. A fluoroscopic examination is performed, and individual radiographs are taken.

Purpose

➤ Aid in the diagnosis of obstructive jaundice (differentiate intrahepatic and extrahepatic causes of cholestasis).
➤ Outline the detail of the intrahepatic and extrahepatic ducts and the biliary tree.
➤ Identify the presence of stones, tumors, lesions, strictures, and biliary duct fistula.

Findings

NORMAL

Normal sized ducts and duct anatomy (duct is smooth). Absence of stones or lesions.

ABNORMAL

Extrahepatic obstructive jaundice is associated with dilated ducts with an accompanying biliary system obstruction caused by stones, biliary carcinoma, sclerosing cholangitis, stricture, cholangiocarcinoma, gallbladder carcinoma, or pancreatic carcinoma impinging on the common bile duct.

Intrahepatic cholestasis is associated with normal sized ducts and no obstruction.

Pharmacy Implications

➤ The patient should take nothing by mouth (NPO) 4 hours before the procedure.
➤ Contrast dye may produce a hypersensitivity reaction.
➤ The patient may receive a parenteral benzodiazepine anxiolytic before the procedure.
➤ Prophylactic antibiotics may be administered (e.g., ampicillin, an aminoglycoside, cefoxitin or cefotetan, cefoperazone or ceftriaxone) before and after the procedure to prevent infection from Enterobacteriaceae, enterococci, and bacteroides.
➤ Aspirin should be discontinued 7–10 days before the procedure and NSAIDs 2–4 days before the procedure.
➤ Patients should be evaluated for non–drug-related impaired coagulopathy.
➤ If the international normalized ratio (INR) is abnormal, oral or parenteral (preferably subcutaneous [SC] or IM) vitamin K may be given daily before the procedure. Alternatively or in addition, fresh frozen plasma (FFP) as a source of vitamin K and clotting factors can be administered to correct coagulopathy.

Cholangiography (T-Tube) [4,7]

Description

An iodine contrast dye is injected into a T-tube (a self-retaining drainage tube attached to the common bile duct during gallbladder surgery), and a fluoroscopic examination is made. The T-tube is then unclamped and the contrast material drains out. This test is often referred to as postoperative cholangiography.

Purpose

Evaluate the patency of the common bile duct following gallbladder surgery and evaluate the presence of an extrahepatic obstruction.

Findings

NORMAL
Patent common bile duct with no obstructions.

ABNORMAL
Extrahepatic obstruction noted.

Pharmacy Implications

Contrast dye may produce a hypersensitivity reaction.

CT of the Abdomen

See General Procedures, Computed Tomography (CT).

Endoscopy[4,11,12,47]

Endoscopy is the visual examination of various internal body structures using a fiber-optic instrument. The fiber-optic instrument is composed of a flexible tube and a lighted mirror lens system. The diameter of the endoscope will vary depending on the orifice into which the endoscope is inserted. Endoscopy can be used for diagnostic purposes, because the device allows direct visualization. Endoscopy can be used to perform therapeutic procedures and tissue biopsies.

COLONOSCOPY[7,11,12]

Description

Colonoscopy is examination of the colon and terminal ileum by use of a flexible fiber-optic endoscope. Following cleansing of the bowel the evening before or morning of the procedure, the patient is placed on his or her left side with knees drawn up toward the abdomen. The colonoscope is inserted through the anus and advanced to the terminal small bowel. To aid in direct observation of the bowel, air is inserted through the scope. Suction is used to keep the bowel clear of secretions. Better views of the bowel occur during withdrawal of the scope, permitting a more careful examination of the bowel during this phase of the procedure. Colonoscopy is considered more sensitive for early detection of select abnormalities than colon x-ray procedures.

Purpose

➤ Further evaluate an abnormal barium enema result.
➤ Help determine the cause of lower GI bleeding.
➤ Screen (serve as surveillance) for the presence of cancer.
➤ Evaluate patients with colonic cancer or inflammatory bowel disease.
➤ Determine the cause of unexplained diarrhea.
➤ Perform polypectomy.
➤ Arrest the bleeding from lesions.
➤ Decompress a dilated colon, reduce an intestinal volvulus, or dilate strictures.
➤ Remove foreign objects from the large bowel.
➤ Perform tissue biopsies to aid in the diagnosis of suspected disease.

Findings

NORMAL
Absence of inflammation, normal mucosa, and normal anatomy.

ABNORMAL
Presence of polyps or tumors, areas of inflammation, signs of bleeding, presence of foreign objects, and abnormal anatomy.

Pharmacy Implications

➤ Preparation for colonoscopy with lavage is thought to be more effective than standard cathartics (either evening before or morning of colonoscopy) and includes:

- Metoclopramide 10 mg (IM, IV, or by mouth [PO]) 30 minutes before GI lavage solution.
- GI lavage solution (polyethylene glycol-electrolyte solution) 1.2–1.8 L/hr until bowel evacuations are clear (usually 4 L). Lavage is stopped if the patient develops vomiting or severe abdominal pain. If the patient is unable to tolerate the solution by mouth, a nasogastric tube may need to be placed.

➤ Alternate preparation for a typical procedure protocol includes:

- A clear liquid diet 2 days before the procedure.
- On the evening before the procedure: administration of magnesium citrate 300 mL PO at 5:00 PM (senna concentrate 75 mL is used instead of magnesium citrate in patients with renal disease); administration of a bisacodyl tablet 10 mg PO at 7:00 PM; encouragement of clear fluids; and NPO after midnight.
- On the morning of procedure: administration of a 1500 mL saline enema. Repeat the enema one time. Administration of meperidine IM on call or 30 minutes before the procedure.

If a biopsy or other surgical procedure is to be performed, antibiotic prophylaxis of bacterial endocarditis for susceptible individuals (e.g., patients with prosthetic heart valves, congenital cardiac malformations, valvular disease, and history of endocarditis) should be administered before the procedure. Ampicillin 2 g plus gentamicin 1.5 mg/kg IV (maximum: 80 mg per AHA guidelines) is the recommended regimen. Vancomycin can be substituted for ampicillin if the patient is allergic to penicillin. Either regimen may be repeated 8 hours after the initial dose.

ENDOSCOPIC RETROGRADE CHOLANGIOPANCREATOGRAPHY (ERCP)[4,7,11,12,48,49]

Description

Following administration of a local anesthetic spray to the pharynx with the patient lying in the left lateral decubitus position, a special side-viewing flexible duodenoscope is passed orally into the duodenum and advanced to the Papilla of Vater (the point of junction where the pancreatic duct and the common bile duct enter into the duodenum). A catheter (cannula) is then placed into the papilla, and a radiographic contrast medium is injected. Radiographs are taken of the ducts. Areas visualized include the common bile duct, intrahepatic ducts, gallbladder, and pancreatic ducts. This direct diagnostic method is thought to be the most reliable approach to evaluating pancreatic and biliary tract disease. Other techniques such as ultrasonography and CT do not provide as detailed a view of the ductal anatomy and specific pathology.

Purpose

➤ Aid in the diagnosis and treatment of certain biliary tree and pancreatic diseases by helping to differentiate surgical from nonsurgical disease.
➤ Evaluate the anatomy of the pancreas and ductal system prior to possible therapeutic intervention in patients with suspected obstructive jaundice, disease of the biliary system, pancreatic cancer, and recurrent pancreatitis.
➤ Place biliary stents (devices used to keep the biliary or pancreatic duct open).
➤ Perform sphincterotomy, remove common duct gallstones, and perform other minor surgical procedures related to the pancreatic and common bile duct.

Findings

NORMAL

Normal ductal anatomy (pancreatic duct and common bile duct) and the absence of lesions, stones, and other causes of obstruction.

ABNORMAL

Ductal dilation and/or strictures as well as presence of stones or tumors.

Pharmacy Implications

➤ IM atropine is administered 30 minutes before the procedure to decrease secretions and to prevent a vagal response due to stimulation from the endoscope.
➤ IM meperidine is administered 30 minutes before the procedure to reduce pain perception. Meperidine is thought to have less of an effect on the Sphincter of Oddi compared with other narcotic analgesics. The clinical significance of this finding is unclear. Morphine or hydromorphone can be administered as alternatives.

➤ IV benzodiazepines (diazepam, midazolam, or lorazepam) are sometimes used to alleviate anxiety and provide an amnesic effect.

➤ If minor surgery is anticipated, ampicillin 2 g (vancomycin 1 g if the patient is allergic to penicillin) and gentamicin 1.5 mg/kg IV (maximum: 120 mg per AHA guidelines) are administered just before the procedure as a prophylactic measure to prevent infection from enterococci and gram-negative rods. These agents may be continued after the procedure if necessary. This regimen is also used as prophylaxis of bacterial endocarditis in susceptible individuals. If used, it is followed by ampicillin 1 g IM/IV or amoxicillin 1 g orally 6 hours after the initial dose.

➤ Aspirin should be discontinued 5 days before the procedure and NSAIDs 2 days before, especially if biopsy or sphincterotomy are planned.

➤ Glucagon in 0.2-ml doses may be given to decrease motility and improve visualization.

➤ Contrast dye may produce a hypersensitivity reaction.

ESOPHAGOGASTRODUODENOSCOPY (UPPER ENDOSCOPY) [4,11,12,50]

Description

Esophagogastroduodenoscopy is direct visual examination of the esophagus (esophagoscopy), stomach (gastroscopy), and duodenum (duodenoscopy) using an endoscope. Following the application of a local anesthetic spray to the throat to prevent gagging, the endoscope is placed through the mouth and throat and passed along the esophagus into the stomach and duodenum. Air is placed into the esophagus and stomach for better visualization.

Purpose

➤ Determine the cause of upper GI bleeding.
➤ Determine the presence of inflammation, ulcerations, tumors, and esophageal strictures.
➤ Visualize directly abnormalities seen on an upper GI series.
➤ Evaluate ulcer healing following pharmacotherapy.
➤ Investigate gastric emptying and swallowing abnormalities.

➤ Perform polypectomy, sclerotherapy of esophageal varices, esophageal and gastric dilation, and tissue biopsies.
➤ Remove foreign objects.
➤ Coagulate bleeding sites.
➤ Place feeding tubes and percutaneous gastrostomy tubes.

Findings

NORMAL
Absence of inflammation, lesions, and bleeding. Mucosa and anatomy appear normal.

ABNORMAL
Inflammation (reddened mucosa) of the examined structures, identified area of bleeding (hemorrhage), hiatal hernia, lesions (benign or malignant), visible ulcers, and esophageal narrowing.

Pharmacy Implications

➤ NPO for at least 6 hours before the examination.
➤ No antacids after 10:00 PM on the day before the examination, or before the examination if being performed on an emergency basis.
➤ IM atropine is administered 30 minutes before the procedure to decrease secretions and prevent reflex bradycardia secondary to vagal stimulation from insertion of the scope. Caution is required when giving IM injections to a patient who has a low platelet count, has a bleeding disorder, or is receiving anticoagulant therapy.
➤ Parenteral narcotics and benzodiazepines (e.g., midazolam) may be administered just before the examination to produce sedation, reduce anxiety, and decrease the perception of discomfort. The patient must be alert enough to assist in swallowing.
➤ Local anesthetics may be used to anesthetize the throat. If used, the patient should not eat or drink for 1–2 hours after the procedure to reduce the risk of aspiration when swallowing. Initially, clear liquids are administered and the patient is closely observed for swallowing difficulties.
➤ If a biopsy is to be performed, parenteral antibiotic prophylaxis for bacterial endocarditis, in susceptible individuals, should be administered 30 minutes before the

procedure: ampicillin 2 g IV (vancomycin 1 g IV if the patient is allergic to penicillin) plus gentamicin 1.5 mg/kg IV (maximum: 120 mg per AHA guidelines). Ampicillin 1 g IM/IV or amoxicillin 1 g orally may be repeated 6 hours after the initial dose.

PROCTOSCOPY[4,51]

Description

Proctoscopy, also known as anoscopy, is direct instrumental examination of a 12-inch area of the rectum and anal canal using a proctoscope. A proctoscope is a rigid metal or plastic tube with a lighted mirror and lens at the end.

Purpose

➤ Confirm or rule out ulcerative, pseudomembranous, or granulomatous colitis.
➤ Examine the rectosigmoid area for the presence of tumors, polyps, hemorrhoids, foreign bodies, suspected anal or rectal fissures, perianal abscesses, and fistulae.
➤ Aid in the diagnosis of irritable bowel syndrome and Crohn's disease.
➤ Evaluate rectal bleeding.
➤ Perform a biopsy.

Findings

NORMAL
No tumors or inflammation. Rectal mucosa is smooth and pink. The rectum has normal anatomy.

ABNORMAL
Edematous, red, or denuded mucosa. Presence of grainy-like minute masses. The tissue is easily broken or pulverized. Visible ulcers or pseudomembranes. Spontaneous bleeding on examination.

Pharmacy Implications

➤ Laxatives and an enema (tap water or phosphate) are given the evening before the procedure.
➤ One or two phosphate enemas or a suppository (bisacodyl) may be given 1 hour before the procedure.
➤ Barium administered within the previous week could interfere with the examination.

➤ The patient should take nothing by mouth 2 hours before the examination.

➤ If a biopsy is planned, parenteral antibiotic prophylaxis for bacterial endocarditis, in susceptible individuals, should be administered 30 minutes before the procedure: ampicillin 2 g IV (vancomycin 1 g IV if the patient is allergic to penicillin) plus gentamicin 1.5 mg/kg IV (maximum: 120 mg per AHA guidelines). Ampicillin 1 g IM/IV or amoxicillan 1 g orally may be repeated 6 hours after the initial dose.

SIGMOIDOSCOPY (FLEXIBLE)[4,7,11,12,52]

Description

Sigmoidoscopy is direct visual examination of the distal 60 cm (24 inches) of the rectum and sigmoid colon using a flexible fiber-optic scope. The patient is placed in the left lateral decubitus position. After lubricating the sigmoidoscope, it is inserted into the rectum and advanced to the sigmoid colon. Air is introduced into the bowel to aid in visualization. This diagnostic procedure may be preferable to rigid proctoscopic examination. However, anoscopy is thought to be superior to sigmoidoscopy for visualization of the rectum and anal canal.

Purpose

➤ Visualize and biopsy abnormalities in the rectosigmoid area.

➤ Evaluate lesions seen on radiographs.

➤ Evaluate patients who have undergone bowel resection and the cause of bloody diarrhea or rectal bleeding.

➤ Diagnose and monitor inflammatory bowel disease and the effectiveness of therapy.

➤ Reduce a sigmoid volvulus.

➤ Screen for colon cancers and monitor patients with a history of colon cancer.

Findings

NORMAL

Absence of inflammation, bleeding, and lesions. Normal anatomy.

ABNORMAL

Reddened or bleeding mucosa, presence of neoplastic disease.

Pharmacy Implications

➤ No preparation for patients who present with a primary complaint of diarrhea, who are suspected of having inflammatory bowel disease, or have a history of acute bright red rectal bleeding.

➤ Usual preparation includes withholding breakfast on the morning of the procedure and the rectal administration of two phosphate enemas (130 mL each) given 30 minutes before the procedure.

➤ If a biopsy is planned, antibiotic prophylaxis of bacterial endocarditis, in susceptible individuals, is recommended: ampicillin 2 g IV/IM (vancomycin 1 g IV if the patient is allergic to penicillin) plus gentamicin 1.5 mg/kg IV (maximum: 120 mg per AHA guidelines) 30 minutes before the procedure. Ampicillin 1 g IM/IV or amoxicillin 1 g orally may be repeated 6 hours after the initial dose.

Hepatobiliary Scintigraphy (HIDA, PAPIDA, or DISIDA SCAN)[4,53]

Description

A radionuclide tracer, (^{99m}Tc) IDA (technetium labeled iminodiacetic acid derivatives), is injected intravenously, undergoes uptake by the liver, and is excreted into the biliary tree. Using a scintillation camera, serial images are taken (an image every 5 minutes for 1 hour) that show the radioactivity in the liver, bile ducts, gallbladder, and duodenum.

Purpose

➤ Diagnose cholecystitis, biliary tract stones, tumors, cancer, obstruction, leaks, and anatomic anomalies of the biliary tree.

➤ Evaluate the biliary ducts for patency after surgical intervention.

➤ Evaluate liver function and determine liver rejection after transplantation.

Findings

NORMAL

The gallbladder, bile ducts, liver, and portion of the small bowel are visualized within 1 hour of radionuclide administration showing normal size, shape, and function of the biliary system.

ABNORMAL

Radioactivity in the liver, but little or none in the gallbladder and duodenum, indicates biliary obstruction. Decreased or absent radioactivity in the gallbladder, bile ducts, and duodenum or delayed uptake by the liver indicates hepatocellular disease.

Pharmacy Implications

Administration of cholecystokinin or sincalide intravenously may be used to improve the procedure by stimulating contraction of the gallbladder to hasten movement of the tracer into the bile ducts. The dose of sincalide is 0.02 μg/kg administered over a 30- to 60-second interval. A second dose of 0.04 μg/kg may be administered if the first dose does not produce satisfactory results.

Laparoscopy

See Gynecology, Laparoscopy.

Liver Biopsy[4,7,47,54]

Description

This procedure is performed at bedside and uses a percutaneous needle aspiration of a core of tissue from the liver via a Menghini needle (a long, large-bore needle), the Jamshidi, or the Tru-Cut needle. The needle is inserted through an intercostal space anterior to the midaxillary line just below the point of maximal dullness on expiration. The biopsy may be guided by using US or CT. The biopsied tissue is then sent for histologic analysis.

Purpose

➤ Diagnose the cause of hepatocellular disease such as cirrhosis or hepatitis.
➤ Confirm alcoholic liver disease.
➤ Assess the cause of persistently elevated liver function tests such as AST, ALT, bilirubin, and alkaline phosphatase.
➤ Assess the cause of cholestasis of unknown origin after other testing has been inconclusive.
➤ Assess the course of and response to therapy of various hepatic cellular diseases.
➤ Assist in diagnosing and staging lymphomas and other malignancies.

➤ Assist in the diagnosis of metabolic disease, multisystem disease, and granulomatous infections.
➤ Assess the effect of hepatotoxic drugs (e.g., methotrexate).
➤ Evaluate suspected rejection of a transplanted liver.

Findings

NORMAL

Presence of normal pathology and histology.

ABNORMAL

Presence of tumors or cysts, hepatic cellular changes consistent with cirrhosis or hepatitis, signs of organ rejection, and signs of drug toxicity.

Pharmacy Implications

➤ It is recommended that antiplatelet agents be stopped before open and needle biopsies. Aspirin should be discontinued 7–10 days before the procedure. NSAIDs (e.g., ibuprofen, naproxen) that reversibly inhibit the enzyme cyclooxygenase should be discontinued 2–4 days before the procedure.
➤ Preprocedure medications such as parenteral analgesics (e.g., meperidine, morphine) and parenteral sedatives/anxiolytics (e.g., lorazepam, diazepam, midazolam) may be administered.
➤ A local anesthetic (e.g., lidocaine) may be necessary. The patient's history should be checked for allergic reactions.

MRI of the Abdomen

See General Procedures, Magnetic Resonance Imaging (MRI).

Paracentesis[4,7,55]

Description

Paracentesis is the puncture of any cavity for the aspiration of fluid; however, the withdrawal of fluid from the abdomen (abdominal paracentesis) is the most commonly encountered. First, the patient is asked to empty his or her bladder. Second, the area between the umbilicus and the pubis is prepared with iodine and anesthetized with a local anesthetic such as lidocaine. Third, a long 22-gauge needle is inserted through the abdominal wall into the peritoneum 1–2 inches below the umbilicus. For diagnostic purposes, 50–100 mL of fluid are aspirated and sent to the laboratory for analysis. When performed for therapeutic purposes, fluid volumes of 1.5–5 L may be removed.

Purpose

➤ Aid in the diagnosis of a suspected infection (peritonitis) or malignancy.
➤ Assess the electrolyte and protein make-up of the fluid.
➤ Remove ascitic fluid therapeutically from the abdomen of patients with cirrhosis or abdominal malignancy.
➤ Determine if abdominal bleeding is present.

Findings

NORMAL
Peritoneal fluid: see Table 7-4.

ABNORMAL
Cloudy or turbid appearance, elevated protein content, elevated glucose, presence of RBCs or bloody fluid, WBCs >300/mL, and cytology positive for malignant cells.

Pharmacy Implications

The patient should be assessed for allergies to local anesthetics and iodine.

Small Bowel Series[11,12]

See Gastroenterology, Barium Swallow (Upper GI With Small Bowel Follow Through [UGI/SBFT]).

Table 7-4. Normal Paracentesis Findings	
Appearance	Clear and yellowish
Volume	<50 mL
Protein content	0.3–4.1 g/dL
Glucose	70–100 mg/dL
RBCs	None
WBCs	<300/mL
Bacteria and fungi	None
Cytology	No malignant cells

Small Bowel Biopsy[4,7,47,56]

Description

Small bowel biopsy is usually performed using a suction apparatus called the Rubin tube. It is passed orally into the small bowel, and a piece of jejunal tissue is harvested or duodenal fluid is aspirated. Alternatively, a Carey capsule directed by gravity may be used to perform the biopsy. The specimen obtained with this device is more broad and less deep than the samples obtained with the Rubin tube. Fluoroscopy is used to check the position of the tube. However, biopsy samples are obtained in a blind fashion. Histologic, microbiologic, and fluid analysis are performed on the samples. A similar procedure can be undertaken with upper endoscopy permitting direct visualization of the small bowel. However, the endoscope can only reach the duodenum, thus limiting its usefulness when sampling of the ileum or jejunum must be performed.

Purpose

➤ Determine the cause of malabsorption or diarrhea.
➤ Assess response to drug or non–drug-therapies.
➤ Verify a suspected malignancy.
➤ Diagnose and assess inflammatory bowel disease
➤ Collect pancreatic fluid and bile fluid for analysis to assess gallbladder disease.
➤ Diagnose bacterial overgrowth or giardiasis.

Findings

NORMAL

Presence of normal pathology, histology, and fluid composition.

ABNORMAL

Presence of histologic changes characteristic of inflammatory bowel disease or malignancy, the presence of Giardia or bacterial overgrowth, or the presence of cholesterol crystals and WBCs in bile fluid.

Pharmacy Implications

➤ The patient should take nothing by mouth for at least 6–8 hours before the procedure.

➤ The patient's throat is sprayed with a local anesthetic (e.g., benzocaine, Cetacaine, or lidocaine) to reduce the likelihood of gagging when the tube is passed.

➤ Preprocedure medications such as parenteral analgesics (e.g., meperidine) and parenteral sedatives/anxiolytics (e.g., lorazepam, diazepam, or midazolam) may be administered. However, the patient needs to be cooperative and somewhat alert to be able to swallow the tube.

➤ Metoclopramide 10 mg PO or IV may be used to help advance the tube or capsule into the small bowel.

➤ Antiplatelet agents such as aspirin and other NSAIDs should be discontinued at least 5 days in advance of the biopsy. Anticoagulants such as warfarin may be a contraindication to this test.

➤ An elevated PT or aPTT for a non–drug-related reason is a contraindication to performance of this procedure unless coagulopathy can be corrected in advance of the procedure.

Ultrasonography of the Abdomen

See General Procedures, Ultrasonography.

Urea Breath Test[57–59]

Description

The breath test is used to detect urease, which is an enzyme produced by *Helicobacter pylori*, the bacteria thought to be responsible for peptic ulcer disease. The breath test is a reliable alternative to serologic testing or biopsy (histologic examination or a rapid urease test such as the CLOtest). Two versions of the breath test are in commercial use.

The carbon-14 test requires the patient to swallow a capsule containing 1 mCi of carbon-14 labeled urea. After 10 minutes, the patient breathes into a bag. A scintillation counter is used to measure the amount of carbon-14 radioactively labeled carbon dioxide.

In the carbon-13 method, the patient eats a small container of pudding and then breathes into a bag. This breath sample serves as a baseline for test comparison because carbon-13 may be present in low concentrations in food. Next, the patient drinks a container of fluid containing carbon-13–enriched urea and water. If *H. pylori* is present, urease hydrolyzes the labeled urea releasing carbon-13 labeled carbon dioxide. Thirty minutes after drinking the labeled urea, the patient breathes into a bag. The baseline and post-urea breath samples are transferred to test kit breath tubes. The samples are sent to a test center for analysis using gas isotope ratio mass spectometry, which measures the ratio of carbon-13 labeled carbon dioxide to carbon-12 labeled carbon dioxide. The carbon-13 method does not expose the patient to radioactive material.

Purpose

➤ Diagnose *H. pylori* infection as the cause of peptic ulcer disease symptoms.
➤ Monitor response to anti-*H. pylori* treatment.

Findings

NORMAL

Absence of carbon-13 or carbon-14 labeled carbon dioxide denotes absence of *H. pylori*.

ABNORMAL

Sufficient amounts of carbon-13 or carbon-14 labeled carbon dioxide positively diagnose *H. pylori* infection.

Pharmacy Implications

➤ Antibiotics, proton pump inhibitors, bismuth subsalicylate, and sucralfate should be withheld for 2 weeks before the test to prevent false-negative results.
➤ A positive breath test will generally lead to antimicrobial therapy against *H. pylori*.
➤ The patient should be evaluated for allergies to antimicrobial agents used to treat *H. pylori*.

GYNECOLOGY

Breast Biopsy (Needle and Open)[4,11,12,60]

Description

NEEDLE

A needle is introduced into the breast mass where fluid (if present) is aspirated. Tissue obtained from the biopsy is sent for cytologic study. Diagnostically, this procedure is limited by the small tissue sample obtained from a needle biopsy; it may not be representative of the entire breast mass. There is also an increased risk of "seeding" the needle tract with potentially malignant cells, thus causing further spread of the disease. Therefore, a needle biopsy is generally reserved for a fluid-filled cyst or an advanced malignant lesion.

OPEN

In an open biopsy of the breast, an incision is made to expose the breast mass. If the mass is small enough (<2 cm) and looks benign, the mass is excised. If the mass is larger or looks malignant, a representative amount of tissue is incised from the mass. This complete or partial excision of the mass is called lumpectomy. The tissue is sent for receptor assay analysis and frozen section. Frozen section involves quick freezing of the tissue sample so it can be cut into microscopic sections and examined by the pathologist to determine if the tissue is malignant and if the tissue margins indicate adequate excision. This entire process takes 10–15 minutes and provides valuable information on whether more malignant tissue needs to be excised or if the wound can be closed.

Purpose

Needle and open breast biopsies are performed to determine if breast tumors are benign or malignant. Receptor assays are done on malignant tissues to determine if the tumor is estrogen-receptor (ER) and/or progesterone-receptor (PR) positive or negative. ER(+) and PR(+) tumors will respond best to hormonal chemotherapy such as tamoxifen or anastrazole.

Findings

NORMAL

Results from a breast biopsy will reveal adequate amounts of cellular and noncellular connective tissue with proper development of tissue.

ABNORMAL

Presence of a benign tumor (such as adenofibroma) or presence of a malignant tumor (such as adenocarcinoma, inflammatory carcinoma, or sarcoma). Plasma cell mastitis or the presence of intraductal papilloma.

Pharmacy Implications

➤ Local anesthetics are administered before needle and some open breast biopsies. Some open biopsies require the use of a general anesthetic, in which case the patient is not to eat or drink after midnight the night before the procedure.

➤ A penicillinase-resistant antibiotic (e.g., dicloxacillin, cephradine, cefazolin, ampicillin/sulbactam) is sometimes used after an open breast biopsy as prophylaxis against penicillinase-producing staphylococcal infections.

Colposcopy[4,11,12]

Description

Colposcopy is a visual examination of the cervix and vagina by using a colposcope, an instrument containing a magnifying lens and a light. A speculum is used to open the birth canal. The cervix is swabbed with acetic acid to remove the surface layer of mucus and to highlight abnormal tissue if present. The colposcope is placed at the opening of the vagina, and the entire area is examined. Biopsies of abnormal tissue may be performed.

Purpose

➤ Observe the cervix and vagina directly.
➤ Perform a tissue biopsy of the cervix and vagina.
➤ Confirm intraepithelial neoplasia or invasive carcinoma.
➤ Evaluate other vaginal or cervical lesions.
➤ Monitor antineoplastic therapy.

Findings

NORMAL
Vaginal and cervical mucosa and epithelium of normal color and appearance.

ABNORMAL
Presence of color tissue changes or lesions.

Pharmacy Implications

The patient may be instructed to take an over-the-counter NSAID (such as ibuprofen 400–600 mg or naproxen

125–250 mg) the night before the procedure to minimize the cramping that can occur with the colposcopy and biopsy.

Hysterosalpingography[4,7]

Description

Hysterosalpingography, also known as a uterogram, is a radiographic examination performed to visualize the outline of the uterine cavity and the fallopian tubes by means of a contrast medium injected through a cannula inserted into the cervix. The uterus and fallopian tubes are viewed under fluoroscopy, and radiographs are taken.

Purpose

Evaluate tubal patency as part of an infertility work-up or to evaluate the fallopian tubes following tubal ligation or reconstruction.

Findings

NORMAL

Normal anatomy with no tubal or uterine abnormalities.

ABNORMAL

Tubal adhesions or occlusions. Uterine abnormalities including foreign bodies, fibroid tumors, congenital malformations, or fistulas.

Pharmacy Implications

A sedative may be administered before the procedure.

Laparoscopy[4,8]

Description

A laparoscopy is the direct visual examination of the peritoneal cavity (omentum, liver peritoneum, gallbladder, portions of the spleen, diaphragm, and serosal surfaces of the small bowel and colon) with an endoscope (laparoscope) through the anterior abdominal wall. In women, the ovaries, uterus, and fallopian tubes can be evaluated. A small incision is made at the level of the umbilicus with the patient under local or general anesthesia. A special needle is inserted, and approximately 2 L of carbon dioxide or nitrous oxide is instilled into the abdominal cavity to distend the abdominal wall and provide organ-free space to aid in visualization. The laparoscope is then advanced into the peritoneal cavity. The gas is removed after the examination is completed. If fallopian tube patency is being evaluated, a dye is injected through the cervix and observed before gas removal.

Purpose

➤ Perform procedures such as lysis of adhesions, ovarian biopsy, tubal ligation, removal of foreign bodies, or cholecystectomy.
➤ Detect ectopic pregnancy, endometriosis, pelvic inflammatory disease, or appendicitis.
➤ Evaluate pelvic masses.
➤ Examine the fallopian tubes of infertile women.
➤ Harvest eggs (ovum) for in vitro fertilization.
➤ Evaluate ascites of unknown origin.
➤ Evaluate liver disease of unknown etiology. This can add diagnostic accuracy to a blind liver biopsy.
➤ Evaluate abdominal trauma.

Findings

NORMAL

Uterus, ovaries, and fallopian tubes are of normal size and shape without adhesions, cysts, or presence of endometriosis. Normally appearing liver, spleen, and peritoneum.

ABNORMAL

Presence of cysts, adhesions, fibroids, endometriosis, ectopic pregnancy, infection, abscess, or trauma.

Pharmacy Implications

➤ The patient should not eat or drink after midnight the night before the procedure.
➤ The patient should avoid aspirin for 7–10 days before the procedure and should avoid NSAIDs 2–4 days before the procedure.
➤ Pelvic or abdominal postoperative discomfort may require analgesics.

Mammography[4,7]

Description

A mammogram is a radiograph of the breast. A low-energy x-ray beam (0.1–0.8 rads) delineates the breast on mammograms. A frontal view and a lateral view are taken.

Purpose

➤ Screen for breast cancer and investigate or detect masses missed during physical examination of the breast.
➤ Help differentiate benign from malignant masses identified by other means.

Findings

NORMAL

No calcification, no abnormal mass, and normal duct contrast with narrowing of ductal branches.

ABNORMAL

A poorly outlined, irregularly shaped, and opaque lesion suggests malignancy. Malignant cysts are usually solitary and unilateral and contain an increased number of blood vessels. Benign cysts are usually round and smooth with definable edges.

Pharmacy Implications

➤ No medications/preparations are needed.
➤ The American Cancer Society recommends a baseline mammogram for all women between 35 and 40 years of age, an annual or biannual mammogram for ages 40–49, and a yearly mammogram after age 50. Routine breast self-examination is recommended.

Ultrasonography of Pelvis, Uterus, and Ovaries

See General Procedures, Ultrasound.

HEMATOLOGY

Bone Marrow Aspiration and Biopsy[4,7,8]

Description

ASPIRATION

The preferred site is the posterior superior iliac spine (PSIS), but this may also be performed at the sternum. The skin is prepared with povidone-iodine, and the area is anesthetized with lidocaine including deeper structures down to the periosteum. A small incision is made over the PSIS extending down to the periosteum. A special aspiration needle (Illinois) is directed into the cortex of the PSIS. Once in the marrow, a sample of 4–5 mL is aspirated for microscopic examination.

BIOPSY

A biopsy of the bone marrow is most commonly obtained from the posterior superior iliac spine (preferred site), the spinous process, or the tibia. Preparation of the site follows the same procedure as aspiration biopsy. A large-bore hollow needle (Jamshidi) is then inserted through the skin, through the subcutaneous fatty tissues, and into the cortex of the bone being sampled. With this large-bore needle, a back and forth rotary motion is used to harvest a bone marrow core from the cortex of the bone. Unlike aspiration, biopsy preserves the marrow architecture for histologic evaluation.

Purpose

➤ Diagnose disorders such as anemias, thrombocytopenia, leukemias, and granulomas.
➤ Distinguish between primary and metastatic tumors.
➤ Determine the cause of bone infection.
➤ Aid in the staging of neoplastic disease.
➤ Evaluate the effectiveness of chemotherapy and monitor myelosuppression.

Findings

NORMAL

Normal hematologic analysis with differential count. Normal relative amounts of fat and hemopoietic cells and normal number of megakaryocytes, immature platelets, plasma, and mast cells.

ABNORMAL

Detection of osteoclasts or osteoblasts, groups of malignant cells in the marrow, granulomas, and cells with indistinct margins indicating marrow necrosis.

Pharmacy Implications

Patients may require sedation before bone marrow aspiration or biopsy with an IM or IV narcotic analgesic and/or an IM or IV benzodiazepine.

INFECTIOUS DISEASE

Gram's Stain[11,12,61]

Description

Gram's stain is a procedure whereby a specimen or sample of a body fluid (e.g., blood, sputum, urine, or wound aspirate) is fixed to a slide stained with a crystal violet solution; rinsed, then flooded with Gram's Iodine Solution; rinsed, decolorized with a mixture of ethanol and/or acetone; rinsed, then counterstained with safranin; rinsed, and then allowed to dry. This is a relatively quick screening method for identifying infecting bacteria. The composition of the cell wall appears to be the key element in the staining and differentiation of organisms.

Purpose

Classify bacterial organisms into gram-positive or gram-negative cocci or rods.

Findings

➤ Gram-positive organisms retain the primary dye and appear dark purple.
➤ Gram-negative organisms will appear pinkish-red following decolorization and counterstaining.

Pharmacy Implications

The ability to differentiate gram-positive and gram-negative organisms and the knowledge of their antibiotic sensitivity patterns aids in the selection of appropriate empiric antibiotic therapy until the final identification of the organism occurs.

Indium-Labeled WBC Scan (Indium-111 Leukocyte Total Body Scan)[4,7,11,12,16]

Description

Approximately 40 mL of blood is taken from the patient for labeling of the WBCs with radioactive Indium-111. The labeled WBCs are intravenously reinjected into the patient.

The radioisotope-labeled WBCs concentrate in areas of inflammation or infection. At 6 and 24 hours after reinjection, imaging studies are performed on the patient. The scanner detects radiation that is emitted from the radioisotope-tagged WBCs. It takes approximately 1 hour for each imaging study. The radiation from this test is equivalent to one abdominal radiograph.

Purpose

Diagnose infectious and inflammatory processes.

Findings

NORMAL

Results will show high concentrations of the labeled WBCs in the liver, spleen, and bone marrow.

ABNORMAL

Results will show high concentrations of the labeled WBCs outside the liver, spleen, and bone marrow, such as in an abscess formation, acute and chronic osteomyelitis, orthopedic prosthesis, infection, and active inflammatory bowel disease.

Pharmacy Implications

Hyperalimentation, steroid therapy, and long-term antibiotic therapy can produce false-negative results because of their ability to change the chemotactic response of WBCs.

NEPHROLOGY

Renal Biopsy[3,4]

Description

The safest method is percutaneous needle biopsy using a 6-inch, 20-gauge needle. After placing the patient in the prone position, US or anatomic landmark identification is used to locate the ideal site for biopsy. The skin is prepared with povidone iodine and a local anesthetic is used to anesthetize the skin. A small incision is made, and the deeper tissues are also anesthetized with a local anesthetic. The biopsy needle is then advanced toward the kidney, where a biopsy core is extracted and the needle is withdrawn. If a tissue sample from a solid lesion is necessary, an open biopsy may need to be performed.

Purpose

➤ Diagnose diseases that alter the structure of the glomerulus.
➤ Evaluate proteinuria of unknown origin.
➤ Determine the nature of a renal mass identified by other diagnostic techniques.
➤ Determine the cause of acute renal failure when other etiologies have been ruled out.
➤ Monitor the course of chronic renal disease.
➤ Evaluate suspected cases of renal dysfunction secondary to inflammatory vasculitides.
➤ Evaluate suspected rejection of a transplanted kidney.

Findings

NORMAL
Normal pathology and histology.

ABNORMAL
Presence of a tumor, clot, or renal stone. Presence of histologic changes characteristic of lupus erythematosus, amyloid infiltration, glomerulonephritis, renal vein thrombosis, pyelonephritis, and renal transplant rejection.

Pharmacy Implications

It is recommended that antiplatelet agents be stopped before open and needle biopsies. Aspirin should be discontinued 7–10 days before the procedure. NSAIDs (e.g., ibuprofen, naproxen) that inhibit the enzyme cyclooxygenase should be stopped 2–4 days before the procedure.

Renal Scan[4,7]

Description

A radioactive tracer, technetium-99m, is injected intravenously. A scanning camera then takes images of the blood flow to and through the kidneys. During the first stage of scanning, images are taken in rapid succession to evaluate renal perfusion. During the second stage, several still images are taken over a 30- to 45-minute period to evaluate renal function.

Purpose
➤ Detect or rule out masses.
➤ Investigate kidney function.
➤ Evaluate kidney transplant viability and renal blood flow.

Findings

NORMAL
Normal size, shape, position, and function of the kidneys.

ABNORMAL
Tumors (irregular masses) within the kidney, obstructions, decreased renal perfusion, abnormal kidneys (shape or size), and presence of rejection.

Pharmacy Implications
None.

NEUROLOGY

Brainstem Auditory Evoked Response (BAER)[7,62,63]

Description
Electrodes are placed on the scalp to obtain baseline electrical activity. An electrode is also placed on the earlobe of the ear to be tested. Then a large number of click stimuli (10 clicks/sec for about 1000 clicks) are delivered to one ear and then the other by using earphones and a tone stimulator. White noise is presented to the ear that is not being tested to isolate the ear that is being tested. The clicks induce electrical activity (evoked response) in the auditory pathways which is then detected by the electrodes. A computer enhances the electrical activity and records it as wave activity. This activity is translated into seven discrete waves (I-VII) that correspond to specific anatomic structures.

Purpose
➤ Diagnose cerebral deficiencies of the eighth cranial nerve.
➤ Diagnose brainstem lesions such as multiple sclerosis, brainstem infarction, brainstem gliomas, and disorders of the central nervous system (CNS).

➤ Diagnose posterior fossa tumors and acoustic neuromas.
➤ Assess coma and cerebral death when EEG findings are inconclusive.
➤ Assess a factitious hearing loss.
➤ Evaluate hearing loss in a child or newborn.

Findings

It takes about 10 msec for a sound stimulus to reach the cerebral cortex. Lesions at different sites in a tract along the eighth cranial nerve through the brainstem and into the cerebral cortex will alter these waves in different ways, providing a method of locating a suspected brainstem lesion.

Pharmacy Implications

None.

CT of the Head

See General Procedures, Computed Tomography (CT).

Electroencephalography (EEG)[4,7,16,64,65]

Description

Electrodes are placed on the scalp in the form of small discs. They are fastened to the scalp after an electrical conduction paste has been applied to the scalp/electrodes. The electrodes are connected by wires to an amplifier and are arranged in one of several patterns on the scalp. Electrical impulses from the brain (alpha, beta, and delta waves) are recorded on a moving paper tape. This tape is then compared against a standardized normal tape and against tapes showing patterns for specific pathologies. A period of hyperventilation and light stimulation at different frequencies is used to stimulate the brain. The EEG may be done under normal conditions in a sleep-induced state or in a sleep-deprived state. Both of these states have characteristic electrical patterns.

Purpose

➤ Measure and record electrical impulses in the brain to diagnose seizure disorders. An EEG should be performed while the patient is having a seizure or as soon after the seizure as possible. Simultaneous video monitoring and EEG monitoring may be necessary to classify the seizure.
➤ Evaluate suspected pseudoseizures.

➤ Aid in identifying brain tumors, abscesses, and subdural hematomas.
➤ Ascertain information about the possibility of other cerebrovascular diseases, such as cerebral infarcts and intracranial hemorrhage, and cerebral diseases, such as advanced cases of multiple sclerosis, narcolepsy, and acute delirium.
➤ Diagnose infections of the CNS such as herpes simplex encephalitis and Creutzfeldt-Jakob disease.
➤ Determine brain death.
➤ Aid in the diagnosis and characterization of sleep apnea or other sleep disorders.

Findings

NORMAL

The EEG tracing produces a tape that is consistent with normal electrical brain activity in the awake and sleep state.

ABNORMAL

Brain wave activity consistent with a seizure disorder or other cerebral disease or lesion. A flat EEG results from cerebral hypoxia or ischemia from which there is no neurologic recovery.

Pharmacy Implications

➤ A sleep EEG patient receives chloral hydrate 1–2 g PO before the test to promote rest and sleep.
➤ Caffeine-containing drinks should be withheld for 8 hours before the test.
➤ Drugs altering brain wave activity (e.g., anticonvulsants, sedatives, tranquilizers) will interfere with an accurate tracing. A physician may choose to stop anticonvulsant therapy before the EEG.

Electromyography (EMG)[4,7,16,64,66]

Description

A needle electrode is inserted through the skin and into the muscle to measure the electrical activity of skeletal muscle. This electrical activity (muscle action potential) is amplified and displayed on a cathode-ray oscillograph, and a permanent record is obtained by recording on magnetic tape. To evaluate physiologic function fully, the electrical activity of the muscle is measured at three activity levels: rest, mild contraction, and maximal contraction. The muscle is not electrically stimulated during this test.

Purpose

The amplitude, duration, number, and configuration of the muscle action potentials aid in differentiating neurogenic pathology from myogenic involvement. The procedure is used to evaluate the integrity of the nervous system, the neuromuscular junction, and the muscle itself. EMG by itself is not considered diagnostic for any specific disease.

Findings

NORMAL

A normally relaxed muscle is electrically silent at rest. During voluntary contraction, electrical activity increases significantly.

ABNORMAL

Waveforms that are different from normal muscle are evaluated to differentiate a muscle disorder from a denervation disorder. These results can aid in the diagnosis of muscular dystrophies, myopathies from a variety of causes, amyotrophic lateral sclerosis, peripheral nerve disorders, myasthenia gravis, and certain corticospinal tract tumors.

Pharmacy Implications

Drugs that affect the nerve-muscle junction such as cholinergics, anticholinergics, and skeletal muscle relaxants can interfere with test results.

Lumbar Puncture (LP)[16,67]

Description

The patient lies on either side at the edge of a firm surface with knees drawn up and head bent forward to put the spine in hyperflexion. The usual site of puncture is between the 3rd and 4th (or 4th and 5th) lumbar vertebrae. The area is cleaned with an antiseptic and locally anesthetized. The lumbar puncture needle (3 to 4 inches in length) is inserted through the skin in the midline between the vertebra, perpendicular to the surface of the back and diverted slightly upward toward the patient's head. When the needle penetrates the dura and enters the spinal canal, a slight decrease in resistance can be felt. Once the spinal canal has been penetrated, cerebrospinal fluid (CSF) is removed.

Purpose

➤ Obtain a CSF specimen for diagnostic study.
➤ Aid in the diagnosis of suspected meningitis, intracranial hemorrhage, and CNS involvement from malignant disease (e.g., leukemia, lymphoma).
➤ Determine the CSF pressure to document impairment of flow or to lessen pressure by removing a volume of fluid.
➤ Diagnose organic CNS disease (e.g., multiple sclerosis and Guillain-Barré syndrome).
➤ Evaluate certain electrolyte disturbances.
➤ Remove blood or exudate from the subarachnoid space.
➤ Administer x-ray contrast media (e.g., myelogram) or to give drugs intrathecally (e.g., antibiotics and antineoplastic agents).

Findings

NORMAL

Normal appearance, consistency, expected cell composition, absence of bacteria, normal chemistry of the fluid, and normal pressure (see the section on cerebrospinal fluid examination in Chapter 6, "Interpretation of Clinical Laboratory Results").

ABNORMAL

See Table 7-5.

Table 7-5. Abnormal CSF Fluid

Apperance	Cloudy fluid
Protein content	>50 mg/dL
Glucose concentration	<30 mg/dL or >70 mg/dL
WBCs	>10/mm^3
pH of fluid	< or >7.3
Bacteria or virus	Present
RBCs	Present

Pharmacy Implications

➤ Patients may experience a headache after removal of CSF and require treatment with an analgesic.
➤ Patients should lie flat for up to 8 hours after the procedure.

MRI of the Head

See General Procedures, Magnetic Resonance Imaging (MRI).

Muscle Biopsy[11,12,69,70]

Description

A muscle biopsy can be performed by making a small incision through the skin and into the muscle. A sample of the desired muscle segment is excised (open biopsy). An alternate method is percutaneous by means of a biopsy needle. The needle is inserted into the muscle, and a small plug of muscle tissue is removed when the needle is withdrawn. In most cases the biopsy can be performed using a local anesthetic.

Purpose

➤ Investigate the origin of muscle weakness (neurogenic or myogenic).
➤ Diagnose localized or diffuse inflammatory disease of the muscle and suspected genetic diseases of the muscle.
➤ Assist in the diagnosis of diffuse vascular, connective tissue, and metabolic diseases.
➤ Evaluate suspected myopathy.

Findings

NORMAL
Presence of normal pathology and histology.

ABNORMAL
Presence of myogenic or myopathic changes.

Pharmacy Implications

➤ Antiplatelet agents should be discontinued before open and needle biopsies. Aspirin should be discontinued 7–10 days before the procedure. NSAIDs (e.g., ibuprofen, naproxen) that reversibly inhibit the enzyme cyclooxygenase should be stopped 2–4 days before the procedure.

➤ Preprocedure medications such as parenteral analgesics (e.g., meperidine, morphine) and parenteral sedatives/anxiolytics (e.g., lorazepam, diazepam, midazolam) may be administered.

➤ A local anesthetic such as lidocaine may be necessary.

Myelography[4,7,68]

Description

Myelography is a radiographic examination of the cervical, thoracic, and/or lumbar spinal cord and the space around the spinal cord. A local anesthetic is administered at the needle insertion site. Using fluoroscopy, a spinal needle is guided into the subarachnoid space. A nonionic water-soluble contrast dye is then injected. With the patient tilted upward, x-ray films of the lumbar spine are taken. The patient is tilted downward to take x-ray films of the thoracic and cervical spine. Generally, a sample of spinal fluid is collected before administration of the contrast media and is sent for laboratory analysis.

This test is sometimes followed or replaced by CT scanning, which can improve visualization.

Purpose

Visualize spinal cord abnormalities.

Findings

NORMAL

Normal outline of spinal cord and normal nerve structures. Contrast medium flows freely through the subarachnoid space. No evidence of spinal cord abnormalities

ABNORMAL

Presence of a herniated disc, spinal cord compression, nerve root injury, degenerative spur, vascular abnormalities, CSF leakage, dural tear, traumatic injury, neoplasm, or mass.

Pharmacy Implications

➤ No food or fluids 4 hours before the examination.

➤ A local anesthetic, such as lidocaine, is used to anesthetize the area at the site of spinal needle insertion.

➤ The procedure should not be performed if the patient is receiving anticoagulants.

➤ Medications that can lower the seizure threshold, such as phenothiazines, MAOIs, tricyclic antidepressants, and CNS stimulants, should be discontinued at least 48 hours before and at least 24 hours after myelography.

➤ The use of phenothiazine antiemetics should be avoided.

Nerve Biopsy[11,12,71]

Description

The sural nerve (situated in the lower leg near the Achilles tendon), the deep peroneal nerve (located in the area of the calf below the knee), or the superficial radial nerve are the sites most commonly used for nerve biopsy. An incision is made, the nerve is exposed, and by sharp dissection a 3- to 4-cm length of nerve or nerve tissue is removed for evaluation. A nerve deficit may be a complication resulting from the biopsy.

Purpose

Diagnose neuropathic disorders and distinguish between demyelinating disease versus axon degeneration disease.

Findings

NORMAL
Presence of normal pathology and histology.

ABNORMAL
Presence of polyarteritis nodosa, amyloidosis, sarcoidosis, vasculitis, various neuropathies, mononeuritis multiplex, specific nerve (radial, distal median, tibial) dysfunction, leprosy, metachromatic leukodystrophy, Krabbe's disease, ataxia telangiectasia, giant axonal neuropathy, and genetically determined pediatric neurologic disorders.

Pharmacy Implications

It is recommended that antiplatelet agents be stopped before open and needle biopsies. Aspirin should be stopped 7–10 days before the procedure. NSAIDs (e.g., ibuprofen, naproxen) that reversibly inhibit the enzyme cyclooxygenase should be discontinued 2–4 days before the procedure.

Nerve Conduction Study[7]

Description

Peripheral nerves are electrically stimulated using EMG equipment in combination with a nerve stimulator. This produces action potentials that travel through the nerve to distant sites and are detected by surface electrodes. These evoked action potentials are displayed on an oscilloscope screen, which enables the investigator to see the amplitude and duration of the action potential. By knowing the time interval between applying the electrical stimulus and the initiation of the action potential along with the maximum nerve conduction velocity, objective information about nerve conduction can be obtained. Nerve conduction testing is the preferred test for evaluating patients with peripheral nerve dysfunction. This testing may be done at the same time as EMG to differentiate peripheral nerve disease from myogenic disease. Nerves commonly tested include the median, ulnar, radial, peroneal, tibial, superficial peroneal, and sural.

Purpose

➤ Confirm a sensory deficit and distinguish from a motor deficit.
➤ Evaluate the extent and severity of polyneuropathy.
➤ Differentiate muscle disease from neuropathic disease, and demyelinating disease from axonal disease.
➤ Confirm the diagnosis of Guillain-Barré syndrome, mononeuritis multiplex, and other demyelinating diseases.
➤ Assess nerve entrapment, such as carpal tunnel syndrome, and differentiate from diffuse neuropathy.

Findings

NORMAL

Action potential amplitude, conduction velocity, and latency (nerve conduction time plus the time to muscle action potential after the distal electrode senses the electrical stimulus) are all within normal ranges.

ABNORMAL

Slowing of conduction velocity, delayed distal latency, and decreased amplitude of the action potential compared with normal are signs of nerve dysfunction.

Pharmacy Implications

Cisplatin, carboplatin, vincristine, paclitaxel, docetaxel, metronidazole, foscarnet, ganciclovir, lamivudine, didanosine, ritonavir, and stavudine are known causes of neuropathy.

Visual Evoked Response (VER)[7,62,63]

Description

EEG electrodes are placed on the scalp over the occipital or visual cortex area. Baseline electrical activity is recorded. The patient is instructed to fix on a point. A visual stimulus such as flashes of light or a sudden change of a checkerboard pattern is administered. First one eye is stimulated, then the other. The time interval between the stimulus and the response is recorded and displayed.

Purpose

VER aids in diagnosing lesions of the optic nerve or confirming the diagnosis of multiple sclerosis. It may also be used to rule out hysterical blindness, to monitor surgery of the optic nerve, and to assess visual acuity in special circumstances.

Findings

NORMAL

No evidence of optic nerve damage.

ABNORMAL

A difference in the responses between the left and right eye, with an increased latency and duration in one eye, indicates a lesion in that optic nerve. Both optic nerves can be involved. VER is abnormal with optic neuritis, pseudotumor cerebri, toxic amblyopias, nutritional amblyopias, neoplasms interfering with the optic pathway, sarcoidosis, pernicious anemia, and Friedreich's ataxia.

Pharmacy Implications

None.

OPHTHALMOLOGY

Ophthalmoscopy[11,12,72,73]

Description

The inner eye is viewed using an ophthalmoscope, an instrument with a special illumination system. A strong light is directed into the patient's eye by reflection from a small mirror. The light is reflected from the fundus of the eye back through the ophthalmoscope to the examiner. The opening of the instrument is held as close as possible to the patient's and the examiner's eyes.

Purpose

Examine the fundus of the eye including the optic disk, macula, retina, retinal vessels, choroid, and sclera. Baseline and follow-up ophthalmoscopy is recommended when hypertension or diabetes is present or when certain drugs are being taken.

Findings

NORMAL

Optic disk is normal size, color, and vascularity. Macula is devoid of blood vessels and darker than surrounding retina. Retina is attached and has normal vascularity and color. Choroid and sclera should not be visualized.

ABNORMAL

➤ Two descriptive approaches for staging or grading of retinopathy are used. The choice of grading methods for retinal vascular changes is influenced by the underlying disease (Table 7-6).

➤ Optic disk has abnormal vascularity, elevation (bulging), small hemorrhages, and abnormal color. The macula is edematous and ischemic with degeneration appearing as a round white mass. Blood vessels of the choroid and sclera can be visualized. Malignant melanoma appears as a pigmented elevated mass.

Pharmacy Implications

➤ Drugs affecting the retina include chloroquine, hydroxychloroquine, phenothiazines, penicillamine, isoniazid, ethambutol, and indomethacin.

Table 7-6.	Retinal Vascular Grading Systems

Hypertensive Retinopathy (Keith-Wagner Method)

Grade I	Constriction of retinal arterioles only
Grade II	Constriction and sclerosis of retinal arterioles
Grade III	Hemorrhages and exudates in addition to vascular changes
Grade IV	Papilledema (edema of the optic disk)

Diabetic Retinopathy (Retinal Changes Fall Into Two Categories)

Background retinopathy

➤ Multiple microaneurysms appear
➤ Veins dilate, multiple dot and blot hemorrhages occur, and hard waxy white and yellow exudates may leak from the retinal vasculature in the area of the macula
➤ Cotton-wool patches (microinfarcts of the retinal nerve fiber layer) appear in the superficial retina; hard exudates may form what is described as the macular star

Proliferative retinopathy

➤ Neovascularization occurs
➤ Neovascularization of the optic disk occurs
➤ End-stage of retinopathy with organized vitreous hemorrhage, fibrosis, and retinitis proliferans (detached retina) leading to blindness.

➤ Dilating eye drops may be used to improve visualization of eye structures.

Slit Lamp Examination[72,74]

Description

Slit lamp examination involves the combination of a light and microscopic examination of the eye. Dilation of the pupil using a mydriatic and cycloplegic agent facilitates viewing.

Purpose

The slit lamp allows for examination of the lids, cornea, anterior chamber of the eye, and transparent and nearly transparent ocular fluids and tissues.

Findings

NORMAL

Clear, avascular vitreous fluid.

ABNORMAL

Vitreous disease including retraction, condensation, and shrinkage. Presence of blood and floaters. Presence of cataracts or corneal deposits.

Pharmacy Implications

Slit lamp examination may be needed to evaluate drug-induced ocular toxicity associated with indomethacin, clofazimine, allopurinol, corticosteroids, gold salts, chloroquine, hydroxychloroquine, griseofulvin, chlorambucil, cytosine arabinoside, mitotane, tamoxifen, amiodarone, quinidine, phenothiazines, phenytoin, and isotretinoin.

Tonometry[7,72,73,75]

Description

There are three types of tonometers: indentation, applanation and noncontact. In the case of indentation and applanation, these tonometers make contact with the eye. The most commonly used contact tonometer is the applanation (Goldman) tonometer. After first anesthetizing the eye with a topical anesthetic, fluorescein is dripped in the eye to outline the corneal rings (standard area of the cornea). The applanating prism mounted at the end of an arm projecting vertically from a black box is placed in contact with the patient's cornea. A knob on the black box actuates a spring-loaded device that allows the examiner to increase or decrease the pressure necessary to flatten a standard area of cornea. The pressure needed for flattening to occur is read off a scale on the knob.

Noncontact tonometry is performed by directing a puff of air at the cornea to determine eye pressure. This method is less reliable when the pressure in the eye is at a higher pressure range, when the cornea is abnormal, or when the patient is unable to establish visual fixation.

Purpose

Measure the eye's intraocular pressure.

Findings

NORMAL

Ten to 20 mm Hg (16 mm average).

ABNORMAL

Greater than 24 mm Hg is diagnostic for glaucoma.

Pharmacy Implications

Drugs that may increase intraocular pressure include anticholinergics, corticosteroids, and sympathomimetics.

ORTHOPEDICS

Arthroscopy[4,8,11,12,16]

Description

Arthroscopy is visual examination of a joint (most commonly the knee and less commonly the shoulder) using a special fiber-optic endoscope called an arthroscope. Arthroscopy is performed using a local anesthetic. However, general or spinal anesthesia may be used if surgery is anticipated. For knee arthroscopy, approximately 75–100 mL of normal saline solution is injected into the joint to distend it. The arthroscope is then inserted close to the knee tendon and upper tibia. All parts of the knee are examined at various degrees of flexion and extension, and joint washings are examined. Arthroscopy usually follows arthrography, because arthroscopy is an invasive procedure.

Purpose

➤ Diagnose athletic injuries.
➤ Differentiate and diagnose acute and chronic disorders of the knee and other large joints.
➤ Perform joint surgery.
➤ Monitor progression of disease and effectiveness of therapy.

Findings

NORMAL

Normal joint vasculature, normal color of synovium, normal ligaments, normal cartilage, and undamaged suprapatellar pouch.

ABNORMAL

Torn and displaced cartilage and meniscus, trapped synovium, loose fragments of bone or cartilage, torn ligaments, chronic inflammatory arthritis, chondromalacia of bone, secondary osteoarthritis, presence of cysts or foreign bodies, torn rotator cuff, or rotator cuff tendonitis.

Pharmacy Implications

➤ Patient should take nothing by mouth from midnight the night before the procedure.

➤ A sedative is usually given before the examination.

➤ Analgesics may be given after the procedure as needed for pain. NSAIDs are commonly used along with narcotic analgesics.

Arthrography[4,7,76]

Description

An arthrogram is a radiograph of a joint following injection of contrast media into the synovium. If fluid is present in the joint space, a sample is aspirated and sent to the laboratory to detect the presence of bacteria and/or chemicals. The aspiration is performed before injecting the contrast medium into the joint. Using a fluoroscope, contrast material and air are injected into the joint space. The joints most often examined in this manner are the knee, hip, and shoulders.

Purpose

Elucidate soft tissue injury in cartilage and ligaments surrounding the joint that cannot be seen with conventional x-ray techniques.

Findings

NORMAL

Normal anatomy and condition of the joint supportive tissues.

ABNORMAL

Ligamentous and cartilaginous tears or injuries.

Pharmacy Implications

Hypersensitivity reactions to the iodine dye are less likely to occur due to the small amount of iodine present in the synovial space.

Bone Densitometry[7,77]

Description

A number of noninvasive techniques are used to measure bone density. They include single photon absorptiometry (SPA), dual photon absorptiometry (DPA), dual energy x-ray absorptiometry (DXA), and quantitative computed tomography (QCT). DPA, DXA, and QCT can be used to measure the bone density of the femoral neck and the lumbar spine. However, SPA can only measure bone mineral density of the radius. Unlike SPA, DPA, and DXA, QCT can be used to measure bone density in other peripheral bones. All the techniques measure cortical and trabecular bone. Because the bone density of the radius may not accurately reflect the density of the femur or spine, SPA has limited usefulness. DXA is considered the gold standard for bone mineral density measurement.

SPA, DPA, and DEXA use much less radiation than QCT and can be performed in a shorter period. Furthermore, the non-QCT techniques use a narrow beam of radiation.

Method	Radiation Source
SPA	I-125
DPA	Gd153
DXA	X-ray
QCT	X-ray

With recent advances in bone mineral density equipment, two types of portable equipment are now available that measure the bone mineral density of the heel. One of these technologies uses radiation, whereas the other uses ultrasound.

The T-score (number of standard deviations the bone density is above or below the mean for young, normal subjects) is used to determine fracture risk and the need for treatment. There is approximately a 10% reduction or increase in bone mineral density for each standard deviation below or above zero.

Purpose

Bone mineral density is the major determinant of fracture risk. Bone density studies are used to identify patients who are at risk for developing osteoporosis, to evaluate fracture risk, and to evaluate the patient's response to osteoporosis therapy.

Findings

NORMAL

A T-score greater than −1.

ABNORMAL

A T-score of −1 to −2.5 indicates osteopenia. A T-score less than −2.5 indicates osteoporosis.

Pharmacy Implications

➤ If a patient's T-score is less than −2, recommendations should be made about treatment.
➤ If a patient's T-score is less than −1.5 and the patient smokes tobacco, has had a fracture, has a first-degree relative with a fracture history, or is of low body weight (<57.7 kg), treatment should be initiated.
➤ For those patients undergoing treatment, follow-up bone scans should be performed on an annual or biannual basis.

Bone Scan[7]

Description

A bone scan is a radiograph of the whole body after IV injection of Tc-99m methylene diphosphate. The radionuclide has particular affinity for bone and collects in areas of abnormal metabolism. There is a 2- to 3-hour waiting period after injection of the tracer to allow for full concentration in the bone.

Purpose

➤ Determine the site of bone and bone marrow biopsy.
➤ Diagnose myeloproliferative disorders.
➤ Identify focal defects in bone and bone marrow.
➤ Stage lymphoma or Hodgkin's disease or find cancer metastases.
➤ Aid in the diagnosis of bone pain and inflammatory processes (e.g., infection or osteomyelitis).

Findings

NORMAL

The radioisotope is distributed evenly throughout the bone. No "hot spots" (concentrated areas of uptake) are noted.

ABNORMAL

Presence of "hot spots" indicating increased concentration of the radioactive compound at sites of abnormal metabolism (e.g., infection, fracture, degenerative bone disease, failing bone grafts). Bone marrow depression following radiation or chemotherapy. Nonvisualization in myelofibrosis. Sites of primary bone tumors and bone metastases from other malignancies.

Pharmacy Implications

None.

OTOLARYNGOLOGY

Laryngoscopy[78,79]

Description

Three types of examination can be performed:

➤ *Indirect.* This involves the placement of a laryngeal mirror in the mouth and a light source to visualize the back of the tongue, the epiglottis, valleculae, the pyriform fossae, and the structures of the larynx.

➤ *Direct, Involving the Use of a Flexible Fiber-Optic Nasolaryngoscope.* The scope is passed through the locally anesthetized nasal cavity and then suspended above the larynx to provide a direct view of the nose, nasopharynx, larynx, and adjacent structures.

➤ *Direct, Involving the Use of a Rigid, Lighted Laryngoscope.* This technique requires the patient to undergo general anesthesia. The scope is inserted through the mouth and passed through the throat to expose the larynx and its structures.

Purpose

➤ Examine the visible structures for disease, trauma, and strictures.

➤ Detect and remove foreign bodies.

➤ Perform tissue biopsies of suspicious lesions to aid in the diagnosis of cancer.

Findings

NORMAL

Normal position, color, and anatomy of the examined area. Absence of lesions, strictures, inflammation, and foreign bodies.

ABNORMAL

Color changes of laryngeal and adjacent structures. Position changes, presence of lesions, strictures, or foreign bodies.

Pharmacy Implications

INDIRECT LARYNGOSCOPY

None.

DIRECT FIBER-OPTIC LARYNGOSCOPY

A sedative/anxiolytic (e.g., midazolam, diazepam) may be administered before the procedure.

DIRECT RIGID LARYNGOSCOPY

An IM anticholinergic (e.g., atropine or glycopyrrolate) and an IM sedative/anxiolytic (e.g., midazolam) may be administered 30 minutes before the procedure.

PULMONOLOGY

Bronchial Alveolar Lavage (BAL)

See Pulmonology, Bronchoscopy.

Bronchoscopy[7,80]

Description

Bronchoscopy is the examination of the inside of the tracheobronchial tree by direct visualization. After first anesthetizing the throat with a local anesthetic, a flexible fiber-optic bronchoscope is inserted through an oral endotracheal tube and advanced into the tracheobronchial tree. An eyepiece at the proximal end of the bronchoscope allows viewing of fourth to sixth division of the bronchi, the upper airway, and the vocal cords. A camera can also be attached to the eye piece.

If bronchial alveolar lavage is to be performed, 100 mL of normal saline is instilled into the lung through the bronchoscope. Approximately 30–60 mL of fluid is aspirated for cytologic, microbiologic, and cell count analysis.

If brush biopsy is to be performed, the brush is passed through the bronchoscope to the lesion to be biopsied. The lesion is brushed, and the brush is withdrawn. An optional technique is to leave the brush in place at the tip of the bronchoscope and withdraw the bronchoscope slowly. With either technique, the material collected on the brush is transferred to glass slides where is prepared for viewing under the microscope.

Purpose

➤ View nasopharyngeal and laryngeal lesions and visualize the source of hemoptysis.

➤ Further evaluate a patient with positive sputum cytology and suspected interstitial lung disease.

➤ Perform transbronchial biopsy of the lung and bronchial alveolar lavage (BAL).

➤ Assess recurrent nerve paralysis.

Findings

NORMAL
No malignancies, lesions, source of bleeding, or infection.

ABNORMAL
Presence of malignancies, infections, or other abnormal findings as stated above.

Pharmacy Implications

➤ Patient should not eat or drink after midnight the evening before the procedure.

➤ A parenteral skeletal muscle relaxant (e.g., a benzodiazepine) and an anticholinergic (e.g., atropine) should be administered to dry up secretions 30–60 minutes before the procedure. A narcotic analgesic may also be administered IM or IV before the procedure.

➤ The patient should not eat or drink for 1–2 hours after the procedure to reduce the risk of aspiration. Clear liquids should be administered initially, and the patient should be observed for swallowing difficulties.

Chest Radiograph[4,7,16]

Description
A radiograph of the chest from the front, side, and some-times back. It is best performed with the patient in the standing position.

Purpose
Chest radiographs are useful in the diagnosis of pul-monary, mediastinal, and bony thorax disease. The stand-ing position demonstrates the presence of fluid levels.

Findings

NORMAL
Absence of fluids, masses, and infection. Air-filled spaces appear black.

ABNORMAL
The film will have opacities (shadowy or white areas) sug-gestive of the presence of fluid, tumors and other lesions, in-fectious processes, unusual air in the lungs, or a collapsed lung. Spinal deformities, bone destruction, and trauma can be observed.

Pharmacy Implications
None.

CT of the Chest
See General Procedures, Computed Tomography (CT).

Pulmonary Function Tests (PFTs)[81,82]

Description
Using spirometry, a patient is instructed to inhale and then exhale as rapidly as possible. As the patient exhales into the spirometer, he or she displaces a bell and the pen deflection records the volume of air entering or exiting the lung (Fig. 7-1).

The tidal volume or the volume of air being inhaled and exhaled during normal breathing can be recorded. The vital capacity (VC) is the amount of air being moved during maximal inhalation and exhalation. Residual volume (RV) reflects the volume of air left in the lung after maximal expiration. Total lung capacity (TLC) is the sum of the vital capacity and the residual volume. Patients with restrictive lung disease often display a decrease in all lung volumes, whereas those individuals with obstructive disease often have normal TLC but decreased VC and increased RV.

In evaluating the performance of the lung, forced expiration techniques together with a spirometer can measure lung volumes and air flow, providing useful information in graphic form (Figs. 7-2 and 7-3). The forced expiratory volume (FEV) measures the amount of air the patient can exhale after a maximal inhalation, often over a set period such as 1 second (FEV_1). Together with the forced vital capacity (FVC), which measures the maximum volume of air exhaled with maximally forced effort after a maximal inhalation effort, these values can provide important performance measures of the lung. The peak expiratory flow rate (PEFR) measures the maximal flow that can be produced during the forced expiration. Generally, this measurement provides similar information as the FEV_1 but is less reproducible. Portable peak flow meters are in common use by patients

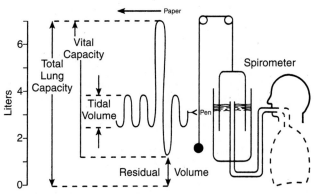

Figure 7-1.   Spirometric graphics during quiet breathing and maximal breathing. Reprinted with permission from Young LY, Koda-Kimble MA. Applied Therapeutics: The Clinical Use of Drugs. 6th ed. Vancouver, WA: Applied Therapeutics, Inc.; 1995.

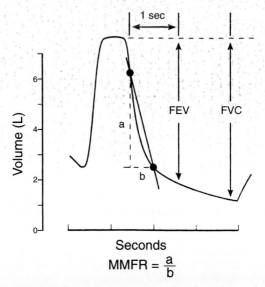

Figure 7-2. Volume versus time curve resulting from a forced expiratory volume (FEV) maneuver. Reprinted with permission from Young LY, Koda-Kimble MA. Applied Therapeutics: The Clinical Use of Drugs. 6th ed. Vancouver, WA: Applied Therapeutics, Inc.; 1995.

with reactive airway disease to assist patients and medical providers in following variations in airway tone throughout the day. Another measurement is the forced expiratory flow, which occurs during the middle 50% of the expiratory curve ($FEF_{25\%-75\%}$, $FEF_{50\%}$ or maximal midexpiratory flow rate [MEFR]). This measure is helpful for patients with emphysema, because it represents the elastic recoil force of the lung and is less dependent on the patient's expiratory effort.

Spirometry can also be used to establish the reversibility of airway disease. The use of bronchodilators can be administered after baseline pulmonary function tests to determine the degree of reversibility. Generally, a significant clinical reversibility is defined as a 15–20% improvement in the FEV_1 after administration of the bronchodilator.

Arterial blood gases ($PaCO_2$, pH, PaO_2) are often measured at the same time as spirometry to assess the degree of blood oxygenation. The use of the carbon monoxide diffusing capacity (D_{co}) can help determine whether the ventilatory change is due to poor diffusion or ventilation. This test involves the inspiration of a small amount of carbon monoxide (CO) that is then held for 10 seconds while the blood CO test is measured. A reduction is seen in emphysema, pulmonary edema, and pulmonary fibrosis and is normal in asthma and pneumonia. For a more complete discussion, see Chapter 6, "Interpretation of Clinical Laboratory Results."

Purpose

The respiratory system is responsible for the exchange of carbon dioxide (CO_2) and oxygen (O_2). Together with the

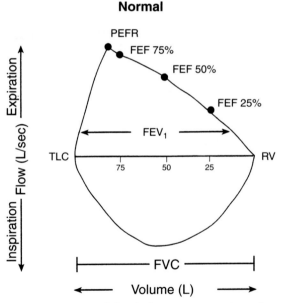

Figure 7-3. A normal flow/volume curve resulting from a forced expiratory maneuver. Adapted with permission from Young LY, Koda-Kimble MA. Applied Therapeutics: The Clinical Use of Drugs. 6th ed. Vancouver, WA: Applied Therapeutics, Inc.; 1995.

circulatory system, body tissues can exchange CO_2 and receive adequate O_2. A variety of disease processes alter the exchanges of these gases between the alveoli and the bloodstream. Pulmonary function tests are performed to provide an objective measurement of the respiratory system.

Pulmonary disorders are often classified as restrictive or obstructive. Typical air flow and volume curves can assist in classifying a disorder, as shown in Figure 7-4.

Findings

NORMAL
FEV_1/FVC, 75–80%.

ABNORMAL

➤ In the obstructive pattern that reflects limitations to airflow during expiration, the expiratory flow rate is de-

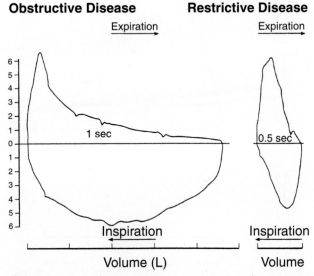

Figure 7-4. Flow/volume curve showing a typical pattern for obstructive and restrictive diseases. Adapted with permission from Young LY, Koda-Kimble MA. Applied Therapeutics: The Clinical Use of Drugs. 6th ed. Vancouver, WA: Applied Therapeutics, Inc.; 1995.

creased. In later stages of the disease, the FEV_1/ FVC and $FEF_{25\%-75\%}$, are also reduced. The TLC may be normal or increased and the RV is elevated due to trapping of air during expiration. The ratio of RV/TLC is often increased.

➤ A restrictive pattern of lung disease that closely corresponds to impairment in inhalation (e.g., bronchitis, asthma) will present as a decrease in lung volumes, primarily TLC and VC.

Pharmacy Implications

➤ Bronchodilators should be administered before the procedure to evaluate the degree of reversibility.
➤ No preparation is needed before or after the procedure, unless bronchodilators are used.

Pulse Oximetry[7]

Description

A spectrophotometric sensor is placed (clipped) on the finger, toe, ear, or bridge of the nose. Light at two different wavelengths are passed through the pulsing capillary bed. The light sensed on the other side of the site is proportional to the amount of oxyhemoglobin present in the arterial capillary bed relative to the amount of hemoglobin available for binding with oxygen. The test may not be as sensitive as arterial blood gas because it does not take into consideration total hemoglobin, carboxyhemoglobin, or methemoglobin. Consequently, pulse oximetry may overestimate the oxygen content of the blood. Poor circulation to the tested area will produce an inaccurate result. Skin pigmentation can also affect the measurement. Advantages of the test include noninvasiveness, portability, and an immediate result.

Purpose

Measure the level of arterial oxygenation at rest, during exercise, when undergoing a surgical procedure, during bronchoscopy, when providing ventilator support, and when evaluating the need for and flow rate of supplemental oxygen therapy.

Findings

NORMAL
Oxyhemoglobin saturation ≥95%.

ABNORMAL
Oxyhemoglobin saturation <93%.

Pharmacy Implications
None.

Sweat Test[4,11,12,83]

Description
Pilocarpine solution is applied topically to the forearm. Three mA of current applied for 5–12 minutes cause the pilocarpine to penetrate into the skin, thus stimulating the sweat glands. The area is then washed with distilled water. Preweighted filter paper is placed over the area, covered with paraffin to prevent evaporation, and left in place for 30–60 minutes. The filter paper is removed, weighed, and diluted in distilled water. A chloridometer is used to determine the concentration of chloride. A minimum of 50–100 mg of sweat must be collected for an accurate result.

Purpose
Diagnose cystic fibrosis (CF) in conjunction with one or more other symptoms (i.e., documented exocrine pancreatic insufficiency, chronic obstructive airways disease, or a positive family history).

Findings

NORMAL
Chloride value in children is <40 mEq/L and in healthy adults may be up to 80 mEq/L.

ABNORMAL

➤ Chloride >60 mEq/L is diagnostic for CF if one or more of the above symptoms are present up to age of 20 years. Chloride levels of 40–60 mEq/L may be suggestive of CF in those patients who tend to have relatively normal pancreatic function.
➤ Other conditions that may cause elevations of sweat chloride include untreated adrenal insufficiency, ectodermal dysplasia, glucose-6-phosphatase deficiency, hy-

pothyroidism, hypoparathyroidism, familial cholestasis, pancreatic insufficiency, mucopolysaccharidosis, fucosidosis, and malnutrition.

Pharmacy Implications

None.

Thoracentesis[4,7,55,84]

Description

Thoracentesis can be performed for diagnostic purposes (50- to 100-mL sample) or for therapeutic purposes (1000- to 1500-mL sample). It involves the insertion of a needle into the pleural space. The patient should be seated and leaning forward, with arms crossed in front and resting on an object such as a bedside table or back of a chair. If unable to sit and lean, the patient may lay supine in bed with the affected side elevated. A site at the fourth or fifth intercostal space along the posterior axillary line is generally selected. The intercostal space that is finally chosen should be one space below the highest level of pleural effusion. The skin is prepared with an antiseptic, and then the skin, subcutaneous tissues, and intercostal space are anesthetized with a local anesthetic. Type of equipment will dictate how a pleural fluid sample is collected. One option is to advance a large-gauge aspiration needle that has a catheter inside of it. Once the pleura is penetrated and fluid can be aspirated, the inner catheter is advanced into the pleural space and the outer needle is withdrawn. The catheter is attached to a 50-mL syringe and one or more 50-mL samples of fluid are collected. An alternate technique involves attaching the catheter to connecting tubing, which is in turn connected to glass vacuum bottles that can hold up to 1 L of fluid. As much as 1 L or more of fluid can be collected using this technique. Heparin must be added to glass tubes or bottles used for cytology samples.

Purpose

➤ Remove pleural fluid for culture, cell count, specific gravity, chemical analysis, and cytology for characterization as either a transudate (due to abnormalities of hydrostatic or osmotic pressure) or an exudate (due to increased vascular permeability or trauma). Transudate fluid can be differentiated from exudate fluid by protein content, the ratio of pleural to serum protein, the LDH content, and the ratio of pleural LDH to serum content.

➤ Tap pleural effusions to make the patient more comfortable.

➤ Inject sclerosing agents such as antibiotics or cytotoxic agents into the pleural space to prevent further effusions.

Findings

NORMAL

No pleural fluid.

ABNORMAL

Blood in the pleural space (hemothorax) is generally a sign of a traumatic injury. Large volumes of pleural fluid due to inflammatory lung disease or neoplasms may be encountered. Cells may be found that will confirm the cell type of a malignancy. Infectious organisms may be found in the pleural fluid.

Pharmacy Implications

➤ Drugs such as bleomycin (60 U in 50 mL normal saline solution) or doxycycline (500 mg in 30 mL normal saline solution) may be instilled into the pleural space as sclerosing agents.

➤ Patients may require a sedative such as a benzodiazepine and/or an opiate analgesic 30–45 minutes before the procedure.

➤ A local anesthetic such as lidocaine should be available to anesthetize the skin and deeper tissues.

➤ Heparin 5000–10,000 units must be added to containers used for cytology specimens.

Ventilation-Perfusion Scintigraphy (V-Q Scan)[4,85–87]

Description

The perfusion portion of the study requires aggregates of albumin labeled with technetium (Tc-99m) to be injected intravenously. These particles lodge in capillaries and precapillaries of the lung. The lungs are viewed with a gamma camera immediately after injection for perfusion. The ventilation portion of the study involves the breathing of air mixed with radioactive (Xenon) gas. A nuclear scanner monitors the distribution of the gas in the lungs.

Purpose

Diagnose and monitor pulmonary embolism and to a lesser extent bronchiectasis, bronchial obstruction, and bronchopleural fistula. Ventilation by itself can be useful in quantifying ventilation status in patients with obstructive pulmonary disease. Ventilation-perfusion scans can also be used to assess pulmonary function in patients undergoing lung resection.

Findings

NORMAL

Normal perfusion and normal ventilation.

ABNORMAL

Normal areas of regional ventilation combined with segmental perfusion defects indicating pulmonary embolus.

Pharmacy Implications

Findings consistent with a diagnosis of pulmonary embolism will generally necessitate initiation of anticoagulants or fibrinolytic agents if no contraindications are present.

UROLOGY

Cystometrography (CMG)[4,7,11,12,88]

Description

A cystometrogram can be either simple or complex.

SIMPLE

This version of the procedure can be completed at bedside. The patient is asked to empty his or her bladder. With a special device, the amount of urine, rate of flow of the urine, and time needed to void are all measured. Additional information gathered includes the time required to initiate voiding, the size of the urine stream, the continuity (single continuous stream versus interrupted stream), and the presence of urinary hesitancy, straining, or dribbling. A Foley or 14-

French straight catheter is placed through the urethra into the bladder. Any remaining urine is measured. Thermal sensations are then measured by first instilling room temperature sterile water or sterile saline solution into the bladder followed by warm sterile water or saline. The patient is asked to report sensations such as discomfort, the need to void, flushing, sweating, or nausea. The fluid is then drained from the bladder and the catheter is connected to a cystometer used to measure pressure in the bladder. In small increments (approximately 50 mL) the bladder is filled with sterile water or normal saline. Alternatively, carbon dioxide gas can be used. The patient is instructed to report when the need to void is felt. Pressures and volumes are automatically recorded and plotted on a graph. When the patient's bladder becomes full, the patient must void and the pressures are recorded.

COMPLEX

This procedure is usually performed in urodynamics laboratory. A triple or double lumen Foley catheter is inserted into the bladder. Residual urine volume is measured in the same fashion as in simple cystometry. The patient is instructed to relax the bladder and avoid abdominal contractions. One lumen of the catheter is connected to an infusion pump and another lumen is connected to a microtip transducer or fluid-filled catheter/transducer set-up. An anal probe is inserted, and intraabdominal pressures are continuously recorded. The infusion pump instills room temperature sterile water into the bladder at a constant rate (slow, medium, or rapid). Simultaneously, bladder and anorectal pressures are recorded. The patient is instructed to report the first sensation of bladder fullness and the first strong urge to void. Filling of the bladder continues until the patient reports discomfort or an involuntary contraction is recorded. Alternatively, carbon dioxide gas can be substituted for fluid, but volume measurements may not be as accurate as fluid nor can gas be used for voiding cystometry. On some occasions the procedure continues by having the patient void as vigorously and as completely as possible. The catheter with the transducer measures bladder pressure during emptying. A variety of provocative tests can be performed to add to the diagnostic utility of the test. For example, cholinergic and anticholinergic drugs may be instilled into the bladder to assess its function by altering neurostimulation to the bladder.

Purpose

➤ Assess the integrity of neuroanatomic connections between the spinal cord and the bladder.
➤ Differentiate a flaccid bladder from an obstructed bladder.
➤ Document bladder muscle (detrusor) instability.
➤ Assess suspected bladder sensory or motor dysfunction.
➤ Evaluate postprostatectomy incontinence and possibly stress urinary incontinence.

Findings

NORMAL

Bladder wall activity demonstrates appropriate motor and sensory function with a normal bladder filling pattern.

ABNORMAL

Findings reveal either an uninhibited, reflex, or autonomous neurogenic bladder or a sensory or motor paralytic bladder. Each dysfunction is associated with specific neurons from the spinal cord.

Pharmacy Implications

All drugs that can affect bladder function or patient reporting (sedatives, cholinergic, anticholinergic, anxiolytics, or pain medications) should be withheld before the procedure.

Cystoscopy[4,11,12,78]

Description

Direct visual examination of the entire surface of the urethra, prostate (in men), and bladder by use of a rigid or flexible fiber-optic scope. This examination is also known as cystourethroscopy.

Purpose

➤ Evaluate patients with hematuria, voiding problems, history of bladder tumors, chronic urinary tract infections, or abnormalities revealed by other studies.
➤ Perform biopsies and extract stones from the lower ureters and from the bladder.
➤ Perform bladder irrigation and instill drugs.
➤ Perform resection and fulguration of bladder tumors and transurethral resection of the prostate.

Findings

NORMAL

Normal anatomy; absence of strictures, stones, and tumors.

ABNORMAL

Presence of stones, obstruction, stricture, tumors, signs of inflammation and infection, and sites of bleeding.

Pharmacy Implications

➤ Cystoscopy can be performed with a local anesthetic (e.g., lidocaine gel instilled into the urethra).
➤ A benzodiazepine such as diazepam, lorazepam, or midazolam may be administered before the procedure.
➤ Cystoscopy may be performed under general anesthesia, in which case an analgesic such as morphine and an anticholinergic such as atropine may be administered preoperatively.

Intravenous Pyelography (IVP)[4,7,89]

Description

IVP is visualization of the kidneys and collecting system both intrarenal (renal calices) and extrarenal (ureter and bladder) by administration of an iodine contrast dye through a vein, followed by radiographs taken at 5, 10, 15, and 20 minutes after the injection of dye. The term intravenous pyelography inaccurately describes the extent of this procedure because it limits the anatomy studied to the renal pelvis and calyceal system. The study examines anatomy beyond the scope of this term and should more appropriately be referred to as urography.

Purpose

➤ Detect congenital abnormalities, kidney obstruction, and changes in renal size.
➤ Determine the presence of renal masses (tumors, cysts, abscesses, or stones).
➤ Assess the extent of renal damage after traumatic injury.
➤ Evaluate a unilateral nonfunctioning kidney.

Findings

NORMAL

No anatomic defects, no obstructions, no masses, and a functional collecting system.

ABNORMAL

Presence of obstruction, masses, stones, signs of trauma to the kidney, or compromised function of the collecting system.

Pharmacy Implications

➤ Senna fruit concentrate (75 mL) should be administered at 4:00 PM the day before the procedure.
➤ The patient should only have clear liquids after the senna.
➤ The patient should not eat or drink on the morning of the examination.
➤ Patient allergies should be assessed due to the potential for hypersensitivity reactions to the contrast dye.
➤ IVPs should not be performed in patients whose creatinine clearance is <25 mL/min.
➤ Adequate hydration (IV or PO) should be maintained after the procedure to prevent renal injury from the dye.

Kidneys, Ureters, Bladder (KUB)

See Gastroenterology, Abdominal Radiograph (KUB).

Retrograde Pyelography[4,7,16,90]

Description

A ureter is catheterized by means of a cystoscope, and dye is injected in a retrograde direction (opposite the normal flow of urine). A radiograph is taken to visualize the ureters.

Purpose

Retrograde pyelography allows visualization of the collecting structures of the kidney (renal pelvis) and ureters, which together comprise the upper urinary tract. It is also used to confirm IVP findings.

Findings

NORMAL

Normal anatomy of the ureters and kidney pelvis.

ABNORMAL

Intrinsic disease of ureters and pelvis of the kidneys. Diseases of the ureters including obstructive tumors or stones.

Pharmacy Implications
See Urology, Cystoscopy.

Voiding Cystourethrography[4,7,91]

Description
Contrast medium is instilled into the bladder via a Foley catheter. Radiographs are taken as the bladder fills and when the patient voids.

Purpose
➤ Determine potential causes of chronic urinary tract infections (UTIs), bladder emptying dysfunction, and incontinence.
➤ Evaluate congenital abnormalities of the lower urinary tract.
➤ Evaluate and perform follow-up for patients with spinal cord injuries who have voiding difficulties.
➤ Evaluate prostatic hypertrophy in males and suspected strictures of the urethra.
➤ Evaluate a patient before renal transplantation.

Findings
NORMAL
Appropriate bladder and urethra structure and function.

ABNORMAL
Urethral strictures and diverticula, ureteroceles, prostatic enlargement, vesicoureteral reflux, or neurogenic bladder.

Pharmacy Implications
Iodine contrast medium may produce a hypersensitivity reaction. Special precautions should be taken in patients with known hypersensitivities to iodine compounds.

VASCULAR

Arteriography/Venography[7,55]

Description
An iodine contrast dye is injected into an artery (arteriogram) or a vein (venogram) by means of a needle or

catheter to outline and view a portion of the arterial or venous system. The arteries or veins are then observed using fluoroscopy and x-rays.

Purpose

Examine and evaluate the arterial or venous system of a particular organ or area of the body and evaluate the flow into or out of that area. This allows for the detection of lesions and abnormalities of flow. It can also allow for surgical correction if possible. Fluoroscopy is used to guide the catheter to the desired location for dye administration.

Findings

NORMAL

No flow abnormalities.

ABNORMAL

Presence of clots, strictures, obstructions, lesions, incompetent valves, aneurysms, embolism, thrombosis, fistulas, atherosclerosis, trauma, vasculitis, or congenital abnormalities.

Pharmacy Implications

➤ Iodine contrast dye may produce hypersensitivity reactions or anaphylaxis. Special precautions should be taken in patients with known hypersensitivities to iodine compounds.
➤ When necessary, diphenhydramine, ranitidine, and prednisone may be started at least 12 hours before the procedure to prevent or reduce the severity of the hypersensitivity reaction.
➤ A local anesthetic is used to anesthetize the area of the puncture site.
➤ Adequate IV hydration should be provided to reduce the risk of renal injury from the contrast media.

Doppler Studies[4,7,11,12,64,92]

Description

DOPPLER ULTRASOUND[11,12]

Doppler ultrasound is employed as a blood flow detector that is sensitive to frequency shifts reflected from moving blood cells. The Doppler transducer is placed over the area to be evaluated (e.g., peripheral artery, peripheral vein, or the common carotid, internal carotid, and external carotid). The probe (transducer) directs high-frequency sound waves through tissue and hits RBCs in the blood-stream. The frequency of sound waves changes in proportion to the flow velocity of RBCs. The transducer then amplifies the sound waves which permits direct listening. A graphic recording of the blood flow can be made from the sound waves.

Systolic pressures using compression maneuvers are also measured. To evaluate arterial disease in the lower extremities, a pressure cuff is placed around the calf and inflated. A systolic pressure over the dorsalis pedis and posterior tibial arteries is obtained and waveforms are recorded. The cuff is then wrapped around the thigh, and the procedure is repeated over the popliteal artery. The entire process allows segmental evaluation of the arterial tree in the lower extremities to aid in localizing the area of disease. An evaluation of the upper extremities can be performed in a similar fashion using forearm and upper arm compression taking ulnar, radial, and brachial artery readings. The transducer is placed near the cuff. The pressure in the cuff is slowly released. When a "swishing" noise is heard, the pressure is recorded as the systolic blood pressure.

The pressures and waveforms from the ankle and brachial arteries can be compared in the tested individual, and an ankle-arm pressure index is calculated. Pulse volume recording (PVRs) can be done concurrently to quantitate blood volume or flow in an extremity.

DUPLEX DOPPLER ULTRASOUND[7,11,12]

The Technique is the same as standard Doppler ultrasound. However, with the duplex method, the sound waves can be used to create an image that is recorded on x-ray film.

COLORFLOW DOPPLER ULTRASOUND[7,11,12]

Colorflow Doppler enhances standard Doppler ultrasound by providing flow data from the studied vessel. A variety of colors displayed on a screen represent different velocities and direction of blood flow.

Purpose

Doppler studies allow the detection of arterial or venous obstruction or thrombi. They are also used to monitor patients who have had reconstructive or peripheral artery by-pass surgery.

Findings

NORMAL

Veins will make a "swishing" sound and there is no evidence of narrowing. Flow should be spontaneous and phasic with respiration (venous). For arteries, blood pressure is normal and has a multiphasic signal with prominent systolic sound and one or more diastolic sounds. Signals should fluctuate with respiration, not heart beat. The ankle-arm pressure index (API), the ratio between ankle systolic pressure and brachial systolic pressure, is >1. Proximal thigh pressure is greater than arm pressure by 20–30 mm Hg. There is increased flow velocity with compression of vessels.

ABNORMAL

➤ Evidence of arterial or venous occlusion or blood clots.
➤ API is <1 (see Table 7-7 for severity ranking). Arm pressure is changed. Diminished or absent blood flow velocity signal. Calcified and noncompressible vessels produce unreliable measurements.

Pharmacy Implications

None.

Impedance Plethysmography (Occlusive Cuff)[4,93]

Description

Plethysmography is a noninvasive test that detects blood volume changes in the leg. A pneumatic cuff is placed around the mid thigh and inflated to occlude venous return.

Table 7-7.	Relationship of Ankle-Arm Pressure Index (API) and Disease Severity
API	**Severity of Disease**
1–0.7	Mild ischemia
0.75–0.5	Claudication
0.5–0.25	Pain at rest
0.25–0	Pregangrene

Occlusion is maintained for a minimum of 45 seconds and the cuff is then rapidly deflated. Electrodes placed around the calf detect changes in electrical resistance (impedance) due to alteration in blood volume distal to the cuff. The impedance changes occurring during inflation and deflation of the cuff are recorded on an ECG paper strip. The changes in impedance during cuff inflation and deflation are compared against a discriminant line that separates the normal from the abnormal graph.

Purpose

Detect thrombi that produce obstruction to venous outflow. The test is sensitive and specific for occlusive thrombosis of the popliteal, femoral, or iliac veins. The test is relatively insensitive to calf vein thrombosis. Diagnostic accuracy nears 90%. The test is unable to distinguish between thrombosis and nonthrombotic obstruction.

Findings

NORMAL

The graph for the patient will fall above the discriminant line (i.e., the test will be negative for proximal vein thrombi). However, false-negative results can occur in patients with extensive collateral circulation, which allows for adequate venous outflow, and in patients in whom proximal vein thrombosis is not occlusive.

ABNORMAL

The graph will fall below the discriminant line (i.e., positive for proximal vein thrombosis). False-positive results can occur when nonthrombotic occlusion (mechanical) is present and when arterial inflow disease limits the amount of venous filling, decreasing venous return.

Pharmacy Implications

None.

Lymphangiography (Lymphography)[8,11,12,94]

Description

Lymphography is the radiographic examination of the lymphatic system after radioactive material is injected into a lymphatic vessel in each foot (alternately, the hand, mastoid area, or spermatic cord can be used). Fluoroscopy is used to monitor the spread of the contrast media through the lymphatic system of the legs, groin, and the back of the abdominal cavity. Radiographs are taken of the legs, pelvis, abdomen, and chest. Twenty-four hours later, additional radiographs are taken to compare and evaluate contrast distribution.

Purpose

➤ Detect obstruction, disease, or neoplasm in the lymphatic system.
➤ Stage lymphoma.
➤ Distinguish between primary and secondary lymph edema.
➤ Evaluate the need for surgical treatment.
➤ Assess the results of previous chemotherapy or radiation therapy.

Findings

NORMAL
Homogeneous and complete filling of the lymphatic system with the radioactive contrast material on the initial films.

ABNORMAL
Presence of enlarged, foamy-looking nodes indicate lymphoma. Filling defects or lack of opacification of vessels indicate metastatic involvement of nodes by neoplasm. The number of nodes, the unilateral versus bilateral location of the nodes, and the extent of extranodal involvement determine staging of neoplastic disease.

Pharmacy Implications
The patient should be evaluated for hypersensitivity to iodine or other contrast media.

Magnetic Resonance Angiography (MRA)[7,95]

Description
MRA uses the same hardware technology as standard MRI [see Magnetic Resonance Imaging (MRI)]. Large magnets and radio waves are used to create an image of the vascular anatomy being investigated. This noninvasive test can

produce information about the vascular system (head and neck, abdomen, chest, and peripheral) comparable to the information provided by standard angiography. Although MRA can generally be performed without the use of contrast agent, gadolinium may need to be administered to increase the accuracy of the test. The patient must remain very still during MRA and is placed in a narrow tube to perform the test. Patients who are unable to lie still or who are claustrophobic may require sedation. Certain implanted metallic objects are absolute or relative contraindications for performing MRA.

Purpose

Diagnose vascular abnormalities such as vascular malformations, aneurysms, vertebrovascular and carotid atherosclerosis, thrombosis, and evidence of peripheral vascular disease.

Findings

NORMAL
Absence of atherosclerosis, aneurysm, AV malformation, or occlusive disease.

ABNORMAL
Presence of vascular malformation, occlusive vascular disease, aneurysm, and atherosclerosis.

Pharmacy Implications

➤ Use of a sedating benzodiazepine such as midazolam, lorazepam, or diazepam may be required to keep the patient still and to manage claustrophobia.
➤ Patients receiving gadolinium should be monitored for hypersensitivity reactions.

References

1. Kline TS, ed. Handbook of Fine Needle Aspiration Biopsy Cytology. 2nd ed. New York, NY: Churchill Livingstone;1988:9–16.
2. Teplick SK, Haskin PK. Imaging modalities. In: Kline TS, ed. Handbook of Fine Needle Aspiration Biopsy Cytology. 2nd ed. New York, NY: Churchill Livingstone; 1988:17–48.

3. Michaels D, ed. Procedures requiring the use of contrast media. In: Diagnostic Procedures: The Patient and the Health Care Team. New York, NY: John Wiley and Sons; 1983:274–9.

4. Ford RD, ed. Diagnostic Tests Handbook. Springhouse, PA: Springhouse Corporation; 1987.

5. Taub WH. Relative strengths and limitations of diagnostic imaging studies. In: Straub WH, ed. Manual of Diagnostic Imaging. Boston, MA: Little, Brown and Company; 1989:13–5.

6. Grossman ZD et al., eds. The Clinicians Guide to Diagnostic Imaging Cost Effective Pathways. 2nd ed. New York, NY: Raven Press; 1987.

7. Golish JA, ed. Diagnostic Procedures Handbook. Hudson (Cleveland), OH: Lexi-Comp, Inc.;1994. Available at: http://www.healthgate.com/dph/html. Accessed February 27, 2000.

8. Hamilton HK, Cahill M, eds. Diagnostics. Springhouse, PA: Springhouse Corporation; 1986.

9. Edelman RR et al. Basic principles of magnetic resonance imaging. In: Edelman RR, Hesselink JR, eds. Clinical Magnetic Resonance Imaging. Philadelphia, PA: WB Saunders; 1990:3–38.

10. Lufkin RB. The MRI Manual. Chicago, IL: Yearbook Medical Publishers;1990:21–41.

11. Adam.com Encyclopedia. Available at: http://www.adam.com/dir/Tests/Tests.htm. Accessed March 6, 2000.

12. Zaret BL, ed. The Yale University School of Medicine Patient's Guide to Medical Tests. Boston, MA: Houghton Mifflin; 1997. Available at: http://health.excite.com/yale_books_a_to_z/asset/yale_books_a_to_z/a_to_z/A. Accessed March 6, 2000.

13. Wellness Web. Magnetic Resonance Imaging. Available at: http://www.wellweb.com/diagnost/arnief/mri.htm. Accessed March 6, 2000.

14. Rodriguez P. MRI Indications for the Referring Physician. Garden City, KS: Aurora Publishing Company; 1995. Available at: http://www.gcnet.com/maven/aurora/mri/mra.html. Accessed March 6, 2000.

15. Hagen–Ansert SL. Textbook of Diagnostic Ultrasonography. 3rd ed. St. Louis, MO: CV Mosby; 1989:594–624.

16. Fischbach FT. A Manual of Laboratory Diagnostic Tests. 4th ed. Philadelphia, PA: JB Lippincott; 1992.

17. Webb DR. Diagnostic methods in allergy. In: Altman LC, ed. Clinical Allergy and Immunology. Boston: GK Hall Medical Publishers; 1984:149–68.

18. Timmis A. Essentials of Cardiology. Oxford: Blackwell Scientific Publications; 1988:40–5.

19. Gazes PC. Clinical Cardiology. 3rd ed. Philadelphia, PA: Lea & Febiger; 1990.

20. Conover MB. Understanding Electrocardiography. 3rd ed. St. Louis, MO: CV Mosby; 1980.

21. DaCunha JP, ed. Diagnostics: Patient Preparation Interpretation Sources of Error, Post Test Care. 2nd ed. Springhouse, PA: Springhouse; 1986:947–8.

22. Michaels D, Willis K. Noninvasive cardiovascular procedures. In: Michaels D, ed. Diagnostic Procedures: The Patient and The Health Care Team. New York, NY: John Wiley & Sons; 1983:441–2.

23. Alpert JS, Rippe JM, eds. Manual of Cardiovascular Diagnosis and Therapy. 2nd ed. Boston, MA: Little, Brown and Co.; 1985:21.

24. Tilkian AG, Daily EK. Endomyocardial biopsy. In: Cardiovascular Procedures: Diagnostic Techniques and Therapeutic Procedures. St. Louis, MO: CV Mosby; 1986:180–203.

25. Howard PA. Intravenous Dipyridamole: Use in Thallous Chloride TL 201 Stress Imaging. Ann Pharmacother. 1991;25:1085–91.

26. Anonymous. Persantine IV. Hosp Pharm. 1991;26:356, 361–366.

27. Carpenter PC. Diagnosis of adrenocortical disease. In: Mendelsohn G, ed. Diagnosis and Pathology of Endocrine Diseases. Philadelphia, PA: JB Lippincott; 1988:179–97.

28. Stern N, Griffon D. Protocols for stimulation and suppression tests commonly used in clinical endocrinology. In: Lavin N, ed. Manual of Endocrinology and Metabolism. 1st ed. Boston, MA: Little, Brown and Company; 1986:703–20.

29. Merkle WA. Secretion and metabolism of the corticosteroids and adrenal function and testing. In: Degroot LJ, ed. Endocrinology. Philadelphia, PA: WB Saunders; 1989:2;1610–32.

30. Fitzgerald PA. Pituitary disorders. In: Fitzgerald PA, ed. Handbook of Clinical Endocrinology. Greenbrae, CA: Jones Medical Publications; 1986:1–63, 450.

31. Carpenter PC. Cushing's syndrome: update of diagnosis and management. Mayo Clin Proc. 1986;61:49–58.

32. Larenzi M. Diabetes mellitus. In: Fitzgerald PA, ed. Handbook of Clinical Endocrinology. Greenbrae, CA: Jones Medical Publications; 1986:337–406.

33. Stern N, Griffin D. Protocols for stimulation and suppression tests commonly used in clinical endocrinology. In: Lavin N, ed. Manual of Endocrinology and Metabolism. Boston: Little, Brown and Co.; 1986:703–19.

34. American Diabetes Association. Clinical Practice Recommendations 1999. Screening for Type 2 Diabetes. Diabetes Care. 1999;22(suppl 1S):205–35.

35. Singer PA. Thyroid function tests and effects of drugs on thyroid function. In: Manual of Endocrinology and Metabolism. 1st ed. Boston: Little, Brown, and Company; 1986:341–54.

36. Safrit HF. Thyroid disorders. In: Fitzgerald PA, ed. Handbook of Clinical Endocrinology. Greenbrae, CA: Jones Medical Publications; 1986:122–69.

37. Field S. The acute abdomen—the plain radiograph. In: Grainger RG, Allison DJ, eds. Diagnostic Radiology: An Anglo-American Textbook of Imaging. Edinburgh: Churchill Livingstone; 1986;2:719–42.

38. Rice RP. The plain film of the abdomen. In: Taveras JM, Ferrucci JT, eds. Radiology: Diagnosis-Imaging-Intervention. Philadelphia, PA: JB Lippincott; 1990:4;1–21.

39. Bartram CI. The large bowel. In: Grainger RG, Allison DJ, eds. Diagnostic Radiology: An Anglo-American Textbook of Imaging. Edinburgh: Churchill Livingstone; 1986:2;859–95.

40. Kressel HY, Laufer I. Double contrast examination of the gastrointestinal tract. In: Taveras JM, Ferrucci JT, eds. Radiology: Diagnosis-Imaging-Intervention. Philadelphia, PA: JB Lippincott; 1990:4;1–21.

41. Nolan DJ. The small intestine. In: Grainger RG, Allison DJ, eds. Diagnostic Radiology: An Anglo-American Textbook of Imaging. Edinburgh: Churchill Livingstone; 1986:2;833–58.

42. Maglinte DDT. The small bowel: anatomy and examination techniques. In: Taveras JM, Ferrucci JT, eds. Radiology: Diagnosis-Imaging-Intervention. Philadelphia, PA: JB Lippincott; 1990:4;1–7.

43. Virtual Hospital: Iowa Health Book: Diagnostic Radiology: Enteroclysis. University of Iowa Health Care. Available at: http://www.vh.org/Patients/IHB/Rad/DRad/Enteroclysis.html. Accessed March 6, 2000.

44. Levinson SC. Percutaneous transhepatic cholangiography. In: Drossman DA, ed. Manual of Gastroenterologic Procedures. 2nd ed. New York, NY: Raven Press; 1987:162–8.

45. Bowley NB. The biliary tract. In: Grainger RG, Allison DJ, eds. Diagnostic Radiology: An Anglo-American Textbook of Imaging. Edinburgh: Churchill Livingstone; 1986:2;955–87.

46. Simeone JF. The biliary ducts: anatomy and examination technique. In: Taveras JM, Ferrucci JT, eds. Radiology: Diagnosis-Imaging-Intervention. Philadelphia, PA: JB Lippincott; 1990:4;1–11.

47. Drossman DA. Colonoscopy. In: Drossman, DA, ed. Manual of Gastroenterologic Procedures. 2nd ed. New York, NY: Raven Press; 1987:110–8.

48. Bozynski EM. Endoscopic retrograde cholangiopancreatography. In: Drossman DA, ed. Manual of Gastroenterologic Procedures. 2nd ed. New York: Raven Press; 1987:103–9.

49. Shapiro HA. Diagnostic and Therapeutic Procedures II. Endoscopic Retrograde Cholangiopancreatography (ERCP). Manchester, MA: American Society for Gastrointestinal Endoscopy. Available at: http://www.asge.org/resources/manual/185.html. Accessed March 6, 2000.

50. Sartar RB. Upper gastrointestinal endoscopy. In: Drossman DA, ed. Manual of Gastroenterologic Procedures. 2nd ed. New York, NY: Raven Press; 1987:90–7.

51. Powell DW. Anoscopy and rigid sigmoidoscopy. In: Drossman DA, ed. Manual of Gastroenterologic Procedures. 2nd ed. New York, NY: Raven Press; 1987:125–32.

52. Sandler RS. Flexible sigmoidoscopy. In: Drossman DA, ed. Manual of Gastroenterologic Procedures. 2nd ed. New York, NY: Raven Press; 1987:119–24.

53. Drane WE. Radionuclide imaging of the liver, biliary system, and gastrointestinal tract. In: Chobanian SJ, Van Ness MM, eds. Manual of Clinical Problems in Gastroenterology. Boston, MA: Little, Brown, and Company; 1988:290–6.

54. Tao LC, Kline TS. Liver. In: Kline TS, ed. Handbook of Fine Needle Aspiration Biopsy Cytology. 2nd. ed. New York, NY: Churchill Livingstone; 1988:343–63.

55. Corbett JV. Diagnostic Procedures in Nursing Practice. Norwalk, CT: Appleton and Lange; 1987.

56. Weinstein WM, Hill TA. Gastrointestinal mucosal biopsy. In: Berk JE, ed. Gastroenterology. 4th ed. Philadelphia, PA: WB Saunders; 1985:1;626–44.

57. On Health Gastrointestinal Center. Urea Breath Test. Available at: http://onhealth.com/ch1/condctr/gastro/item. 38639.asp. Accessed March 6, 2000.

58. Sutton FM. Diagnosis of *H. pylori* infection. Infect Med [serial on line]. 1998;15:331–6. Available at: http://www.medscape.com/SCP/IIM/1998/v15.n05/m3285. sutt/m3285.sutt-01.html Accessed March 6, 2000.

59. MERETEK Physician Information. The MERETEK UBT® Breath Test for *H. pylori* with Pranactin®. Available at http://www.meretek.com/phyin.htm. Accessed March 6, 2000.

60. Paulfrey ME. Histology: breast biopsy. In: Hamilton HK, Cahill M, eds. Diagnostics. Springhouse, PA: Springhouse Corporation; 1986:467–73.

61. Larson E. Clinical Microbiology and Infection Control. Boston, MA: Blackwell Scientific Publications; 1984: 527–77.

62. Adams RD, Victor M. Principles of Neurology. 3rd ed. New York, NY: McGraw-Hill; 1985:27–8.

63. Pryse-Phillips W, Murray TJ. Essential Neurology. 3rd ed. New York, NY: Medical Examination Publishing Co.; 1986:103–4.

64. Berkow R, ed. The Merck Manual of Diagnosis and Therapy. 14th ed. Rahway, NJ: Merck Sharp & Dohme Research Laboratories; 1982.

65. Coniglio AA, Garnett WR. Status epilepticus. In: Dipiro JT et al, eds. Pharmacotherapy: A Pathophysiologic Approach. New York, NY: Elsevier Science Publishing Company; 1989:599–610.

66. Vander AJ et al., eds. Human Physiology: The Mechanisms of Body Function. 4th ed. New York, NY: McGraw-Hill; 1985:690–1.

67. Rotschafer JC, Humphrey ZZ, Steinberg I. Central nervous system infection. In: Dipiro JT et al., eds. Pharmacotherapy: A Pathophysiologic Approach. New York, NY: Elsevier Science Publishing Co; 1989:1074–88.

68. Virtual Hospital: Iowa Health Book: Diagnostic Radiology: Myelogram. University of Iowa Health Care. Available at: http://www.vh.org/Patients/IHB/Rad/Drad/Myelogram.html. Accessed March 6, 2000.

69. Kakulas BA, Adams RD, eds. Diseases of Muscle. Philadelphia, PA: Harper and Row; 1985:771–86.

70. Anderson JR. Atlas of Skeletal Muscle Pathology. Lancaster: MTP Press Limited; 1985:11–17.

71. Connolly ES. Techniques of diagnostic nerve and muscle biopsies. In: Wilkins RA, ed. Neurosurgery. New York: McGraw-Hill; 1985:2;1907–8.

72. Vaughn D, Asbury T. General Ophthalmology. 10th ed. Los Altos, CA: Lange Medical Publications; 1983.

73. Peters HB, Bartlett JD. Optical fundus in diagnosis. In: Physifax: Physicians Pocket Compendium of Normal Values, Tests, Diagnostic Criteria, Drug Therapy, and Other Useful Data. Montclair: Medication International, Ltd; 1984:97–120.

74. Lesar TS. Drug-induced ear and eye toxicity. In: DiPiro JT et al., eds. Pharmacotherapy: A Pathophysiologic Approach. New York, NY: Elsevier; 1989:919–31.

75. Phillips CI. Basic Clinical Ophthalmology. London: Pitman Publishing; 1984:55–86.

76. Stoker DJ. Arthrography. In: Harris NH, ed. Postgraduate Textbook of Clinical Orthopaedics. Bristol: Wright-PSG; 1983:882–90.

77. Osteoporosis Education System. Bone mass measurement techniques (module 5). Whitehouse Station, NJ: Merck & Co., Inc. Available at: http://www.merck.com/pro/osteoporosis/inde113.htm. Accessed March 6, 2000.

78. Karmody CS. Textbook of Otolaryngology. Philadelphia, PA: Lea & Febiger; 1983.

79. Barton RP. Endoscopy. In: Keer Ag, Stell PM, eds. Scott-Brown's Otolaryngology: Laryngology. 5th ed. London: Butterworth's; 1987:31–41.

80. Ebadort AM. Bronchoscopy. In: Michaels D, ed. Diagnostic Procedures: The Patient and the Health Care Team. New York, NY: John Wiley and Sons; 1983:493–506.

81. Menendez R, Kelly HW. Pulmonary-function testing in the evaluation of bronchodilator agents. Clin Pharm. 1983;2:120–8.

82. Kelly HW. Asthma. In: Koda-Kimble MA, Young LY eds. Applied Therapeutics: The Clinical Use of Drugs. 5th Ed. Vancouver: Applied Therapeutics; 1992:15-1–4.

83. Behrman RE, Vaughn VC. Nelson Textbook of Pediatrics. 13th ed. Philadelphia, PA: WB Saunders; 1987:928–9.

84. Lim RC. Surgical diagnosis and therapeutic procedures. In: Dunphy JE, Way LW, eds. Current Surgical Diagnosis and Treatment. Los Altos, CA: Lange Medical Publications; 1981:1085–97.

85. Sullivan D. Radionuclide imaging in lung disease. In: Putman C ed. Pulmonary Diagnosis: Imaging and Other Techniques. New York, NY: Prentice-Hall; 1981:67–78.

86. Bell WR, Simon TL. Current status of pulmonary thromboembolic disease: pathophysiology, diagnosis, prevention, and treatment. Am Heart J. 1982;103:239–62.

87. Hull DR et al. Pulmonary angiography, ventilation lung scanning, and venography for clinically suspected pulmonary embolism with abnormal perfusion lung scan. Ann Intern Med. 1983;98:891–9.

88. Blavis JG. Cystometry. In: deVere RW, Palmer JM, eds. New Techniques in Urology. New York, NY: Futura Publishing Corporation; 1987:193–219.

89. Friedenberg RM. Excretory urography in the adult. In: Pollack HM, ed. Clinical Urography. Philadelphia, PA: WB Saunders; 1990:101–243.

90. Imray TJ, Lieberman RP. Retrograde pyelography. In: Pollack HM, ed. Clinical Urography. Philadelphia, PA: WB Saunders; 1990:244–55.

91. Hertz M. Cystourethrography. In: Pollack HM, ed. Clinical Urography. Philadelphia, PA: WB Saunders; 1990:256–95.

92. Bastarche MM et al. Assessing peripheral vascular disease: noninvasive testing. AJN. 1983;85:1552–6.

93. Hirsch J. Natural history and diagnosis of venous thrombosis. Paper presented at a symposium sponsored by the Page and William Black Post-Graduate School of Medicine of the Mount Sinai School of Medicine, New York, New York, October 30, 1981.

94. Bryan GT. Diagnostic Radiography: A Concise Practical Manual. 4th ed. Edinburgh: Churchill Livingstone; 1987:289–96.

95. Smith PL. Magnetic Resonance Angiography (MRA). Midsouth Imaging and Therapeutic, P.A. Memphis, TN. Available at: http://www.msit.com/ra-mra.htm. Accessed October 30, 2000.

Chapter 8

Home Test Kits and Monitoring Devices

Beth A. Martin and Denise L. Walbrandt Pigarelli

Chapter Roadmap

Home self-test kits and monitoring devices are valuable aides that can reduce health care costs and have become increasingly easier to use. The kits and devices provide patients with an opportunity to participate actively in early disease detection and monitoring. Pharmacists play an essential role in helping patients select self-test kits and monitoring devices, counseling them on appropriate use, interpreting results, and identifying limitations. Pharmacists should help consumers make educated choices regarding product selection for home testing and monitoring. Accuracy, reliability, and product utility must be considered.

To achieve an appropriate rate of accuracy and to ensure safety and efficacy, the pharmacist should assess and counsel the patient on the following points:

➤ These products are for self-*testing*, not self-*diagnosing*. In general, positive results should be reported to a health care practitioner immediately, and negative results should be questioned if the patient is experiencing symptoms of a suspected condition. Some test results need to be reported whether they are positive or negative because they convey useful information.

➤ It should be determined whether the patient is capable of performing and interpreting test results. A family member, friend, or caregiver may need to assist.

➤ General questions[1] to consider in patient assessment include the following:

- What is the purpose of using this product?
- What chronic medical conditions does the patient have?
- What prescription or nonprescription medications or herbal products is the patient taking?
- Does the patient have any visual (i.e., difficulty reading, difficulty with color vision) or physical (i.e., arthritis, peripheral neuropathies) limitations? If so, please describe.
- Has the patient ever used a product like this? If so, which one?
- What other health care practitioners have been consulted?

➤ The patient should be instructed to consider the following factors when selecting a product: complexity of the test procedure, ease of reading the results, presence of a control to determine if the test is functioning appropriately, and price.

The patient should be instructed on the following guidelines[2]:

➤ Check the test kit expiration date and follow the manufacturer's instructions for storage.

➤ Read the instructions entirely before attempting to perform a test. Note the time of day the test is to be

conducted, necessary equipment, and length of time required.
➤ Use an accurate timing device that measures seconds if needed.
➤ Follow directions exactly and in sequence. A toll-free number is often available for assistance.

This chapter focuses on those products most commonly available: pregnancy tests, ovulation tests, urinary tract infection tests, thermometers, fecal occult blood tests, illicit drug tests, HIV tests, blood glucose monitors, urine ketone tests, cholesterol tests, blood pressure monitors, and peak flow meters. Each section begins with an overview that describes the intent of the test and important background information. Tables of representative products provide a comparison of specific parameters. Patient counseling tips highlight important steps for appropriate use. Considerations include points to aid in product selection (because availability varies) and how to interpret results.

The products listed in this chapter are representative but not exhaustive of those currently available. The selection of medical devices should be guided by product reliability, specificity, and sensitivity as well as professional judgment.

PREGNANCY TESTS

Additional Questions to Ask in Patient Assessment

1. How late is your period?
2. Have you ever used a pregnancy test? If so, which one?

Overview

At-home tests for detection of pregnancy are indicated for use as early as the first day of a missed period, ideally using first morning urine. The most current products available (Table 8-1) use monoclonal antibodies specific for detecting the hormone human chorionic gonadotropin (hCG), which the body produces during pregnancy. When hCG is detected, a color change or symbol is elicited on the indicator

Table 8-1. Selected Pregnancy Tests

Product/Tests per Kit	Number of Steps	Reaction Time	Positive Indicator
Answer/1	2	3 min	Two pink lines
Answer Quick & Simple/2	1	2 min	Two pink lines
Clearblue Easy/2	1	1–3 min	Blue line
Confirm/2	1	5 min	Blue line
e.p.t. Quick Stick/1–2	1	3 min	Pink/purple line
Early Pregnancy Test/1–2	1	3 min	Two purple-pink lines
Fact Plus/1	2	5 min	Pink-red + sign
First Response/2	1	1–3 min	Two pink lines
Precise/1	2	1 min	Blue check mark

strip. Newer technology offers several advantages, including improved sensitivity, up to 99% accuracy, rapidity in obtaining results, and ease of use. Urine tests are the most common pregnancy test used in health care settings. However, blood tests are also available and have two advantages. They can detect a pregnancy earlier than a urine test (usually 6–8 days after ovulation) and can measure the concentration of hCG hormone in the blood. Blood tests are useful for the health care provider in tracking certain problems of early pregnancy. A pregnancy blood test is needed if a urine test result is negative but a woman has signs of pregnancy (a missed period, breast tenderness, morning sickness, or fatigue).

Considerations

➤ Kits with fewer steps and a control window reduce the chance of false results.
➤ Patients with a color vision defect may have difficulty interpreting the results.
➤ False-positive results can occur if:

  • The patient has had a recent birth or miscarriage. This is due to residual levels of hCG.

- There are elevated luteinizing hormone (LH) levels, notably in postmenopausal women.
- There is ectopic production of hCG, such as that seen with small cell carcinoma of the lung, hydatiform mole, and choriocarcinoma.
- The patient is receiving hCG injections, usually for induction of ovulation.

➤ False-negative results are a concern because of delays in obtaining prenatal care and appropriate behavior modification. In addition, the safety and feasibility of pregnancy termination is also affected. Although the potential for a false-negative result is virtually zero, it can result if the test was used too soon after conception and if the patient performed the test incorrectly.

➤ Price range: $8–30 (higher price reflects kits with two tests).

Patient Counseling

➤ Most tests can be done on the first day of a missed period, ideally using first morning urine. The patient should avoid drinking large amounts of fluids before testing, because the concentration of hormone in the urine can become diluted and more difficult to detect.

➤ Some tests require urine collection in a cup and then either dipping the test stick into the cup or adding urine to a well on the end of the stick with a dropper. One-step tests require holding the test stick under the stream of urine.

➤ If the collected urine cannot be tested within 1 hour, it should be stored in the refrigerator and allowed to come to room temperature (approximately 30 minutes) before testing.

➤ A positive result indicates conception, and a health care practitioner should be contacted to confirm pregnancy and begin prenatal care. Prenatal care may include a prenatal vitamin with adequate amounts of folic acid and any appropriate lifestyle modifications.

➤ If there is a negative result, it should be verified that the test was performed correctly. If symptoms that mimic pregnancy persist despite a negative result, a health care practitioner should be contacted.

OVULATION PREDICTION TESTS

Additional Questions to Ask in Patient Assessment

1. Have you consulted a physician who specializes in fertility problems?
2. Are your periods regular?
3. Have you ever used an ovulation prediction test? If so, which one?

Overview

Ovulation prediction tests aid in the prediction of ovulation for persons trying to conceive. Ovulation prediction products (Table 8-2) measure levels of LH in the urine. LH levels peak approximately 24–36 hours before ovulation and usually around day 15 of the menstrual cycle. Most tests rely on an indicator color change to document increased LH concentrations in the urine. The newest product, ClearPlan Easy Fertility Monitor, uses monoclonal technology to detect LH and estrone 3-glucuronide (E3G), a metabolite of estradiol, in the urine. E3G reflects changes of estradiol in the plasma, thus enabling earlier detection of the fertile period, because serum estradiol levels peak approximately 3 days before serum LH concentrations.[3]

Considerations

➤ Reported 96–99% accuracy.
➤ Kits include a chart to determine on which day of the cycle to begin testing.
➤ It is recommended that basal body temperature be monitored for 2 months before beginning the test to determine when ovulation occurs.
➤ Patients with a color vision defect may have difficulty interpreting the results.
➤ Once LH surge is detected (i.e., a change in color intensity), ovulation will occur in 24–48 hours. Patients should have intercourse during this time to maximize their chance of becoming pregnant.
➤ Results may not be accurate if the patient is using infertility medications, experiencing menopause, has ovarian cysts, or has had an abortion in the past month.
➤ Price range: $15–40; $190 (fertility monitor).

Table 8-2. Selected Ovulation Prediction Kits

Product	Test Days per Kit	Time for Procedure	Indicator (First Significant Increase in Color Intensity)
Answer Ovulation Test Kit	5	5 min	Presence of two similar lines in result window (have *not* reached LH surge if presence of one or two lines, with the test line lighter than the reference line)
ClearPlan Easy Ovulation Test	5	5 min	Color line in a window
ClearPlan Easy Fertility Monitor Kit	Monitor can store 6 months of cycle data	5 min	Monitor displays fertility status as low, high, or peak (uses urine test sticks)
OvuQuick One-Step	6	3 min	Color line in a window
First Response 1-Step Ovulation Predictor Test	5 (3/refill)	5 min	Two similar purple lines in result window (LH surge *not* reached if only one line present or test line is lighter than the reference line)

Patient Counseling

➤ Patients should be advised that the tests are an aid for conception and not intended as contraceptive devices.

➤ Consistent collection time and early morning urine recommended. Urine should be tested immediately after collection. If unable to perform the test within 1 hour, the sample should be refrigerated and allowed to reach room temperature (approximately 30 minutes) before testing.

➤ For the ClearPlan Easy Monitor, the patient should switch the monitor to the on position and hold the urine test stick in the stream of urine for 3 seconds when indicated. A cap is then placed over the wet end of the test stick and inserted into the machine when a red light on the unit flashes.

THERMOMETERS: ORAL, RECTAL, EAR, AND BASAL BODY

Additional Questions to Ask in Patient Assessment

1. Have you ever used a product like this? If so, which one?
2. What is the purpose of this product's use?
3. What is the age of the patient for whom this product is intended?

Overview: Oral, Rectal, and Ear Thermometers

Measuring body temperature is useful in detecting a fever and in determining when a woman is ovulating (see "Basal Body Temperature" for more information on determining ovulation).

Fever is the body's normal response to infection. A "normal" oral temperature is 98.6° F or 37° C (see Box 8.1 for temperature conversions). Although "normal" means "average," each person has their own normal temperature, which may be slightly higher or lower than the average. Temperature also varies throughout the day and is usually lower on awakening, with a diurnal variation of approximately 1° C (1.8° F). Normal temperature variations occur with physical activity, stress, environmental conditions, and ovulation.

Box 8.1   Conversion of Temperatures
98.6°F = 37°C
100.4°F = 38°C
102.2°F = 39°C
104°F = 40°C

Temperatures can be measured in different ways and with different types of thermometers. Factors to consider when choosing a route are ease of use, comfort, safety, accuracy, reliability, and cost. Skin thermometers/temperature strips are less accurate and reliable than other available devices and will not be discussed in this chapter. The rectal route is considered the gold standard because it is not affected by environmental factors, is accurate, and is reproducible.

Rectal temperatures are approximately 1° higher than oral temperatures and 2° higher than axillary temperatures (Box 8.2). Axillary temperatures are about 1° lower than oral temperatures. The newer ear thermometers are calibrated to provide an equivalent oral or rectal temperature.

GLASS THERMOMETERS

➤ Rectal thermometers: shorter tip (security bulb) than oral thermometers. Can be used to measure temperature by the rectal, oral, and axillary (under the arm) routes.
➤ Oral thermometers: only used with the oral and axillary routes.
➤ Mercury thermometers: may pose a risk if broken and the spill is improperly contained. If this occurs, the local poison control center should be contacted immediately for appropriate guidance.
➤ Cleaning: cool soapy water or alcohol wipes should be used preferably before and after each use. To avoid contamination, wipe away from the end of the thermometer being held and down to the bulb in one motion.

ELECTRONIC (DIGITAL) THERMOMETERS

These are easier and quicker to use than glass thermometers, and there is less chance for breakage. Infrared tym-

Box 8.2	Normal Body Temperature Based on Route	
Route	"Normal" Temperature	Fever
Oral	98.6°F (37°C)	≥100°F (37.8°C) or ≥99°F (37.2°C) in early morning
Rectal	99.5°F (37.5°C)	≥100.4°F (38°C)
Axillary	97.5°F (36.4°C)	≥99°F (37.2°C)

panic membrane thermometers measure the naturally emitted infrared energy from the surface of the tympanic membrane and surrounding tissue. Although tympanic membrane thermometers offer greater convenience, the devices are more expensive. Studies have documented significant temperature differences between glass and electronic thermometers. Ease of use should be weighed against the need for reliable and accurate data.[4]

Probe covers should be changed with each use. A damp towel or alcohol wipe can be used to clean the device itself.

Considerations

➤ Digital and tympanic thermometers require batteries.
➤ Mercury-in-glass thermometers have the risk of breakage and present a potential hazard. Newer models contain no absorbable mercury and are nontoxic.
➤ Glass thermometers require more time to obtain an accurate reading, can be difficult to read, and must be cleaned with each use.
➤ Price range: $3–80.

Patient Counseling: Glass Thermometers

RECTAL

➤ The thermometer is shaken down to 96° or lower, and the tip is lubricated with petroleum jelly.
➤ The buttocks are separated with the thumb and first finger of one hand, and the thermometer is gently inserted to depth of about 1 inch with the other (if being used in an infant, the thermometer should be inserted only the length of the security bulb).
➤ The buttocks are pinched closed, and the thermometer is held in place for 3–5 minutes.
➤ The thermometer is removed, and the temperature is recorded (subtract 1° to compare with an oral temperature).

ORAL

➤ Smoking or drinking liquids (hot or cold) should be avoided at least 15 minutes before measuring a temperature orally.
➤ The thermometer is shaken down to 96° or lower. The bulb end is placed under the tongue and slightly to one side of the mouth.

➤ The mouth and lips are gently closed around the thermometer without biting down.
➤ The patient should keep the mouth shut for 3–5 minutes before reading the temperature.
➤ The thermometer is removed, and the temperature is recorded.
➤ This route is not recommended if the patient is uncooperative, asleep, or lethargic. Mercury-in-glass thermometers are not recommended for oral use in children younger than 3 years of age, and a child should never be left unattended with a thermometer in his or her mouth.

AXILLARY

➤ Although this route may not be as accurate or reliable, it may be more tolerable for some children.
➤ The thermometer is shaken down to 96° or lower.
➤ The bulb of the thermometer is placed at the midpoint in the axilla (armpit), and the child's arm is held firmly against the side of the body for at least 5 minutes.
➤ The thermometer is removed, and the temperature is recorded (adding 1° to compare with an oral temperature).

Patient Counseling: Digital Thermometers

RECTAL, ORAL, AND AXILLARY

➤ Probe covers should be applied when applicable.
➤ The "On" button should be pushed, and the instrument placed appropriately at the site of the measurement.
➤ Most digital displays will flash and/or beep when the peak temperature has been reached (approximately 30 seconds).
➤ Temperature should be recorded after the thermometer is removed.

EAR

➤ The probe cover is applied, and the probe is placed into the ear canal. The probe tip is aligned toward the patient's opposite eye.
➤ Firm pressure is applied gently (with a slight twist) to seal the ear canal from ambient air.
➤ The temperature button is pressed and released, and the probe is held in place until the temperature reading is displayed (approximately 3 seconds).

➤ The thermometer is removed, and the temperature is recorded.
➤ An additional reading on the opposite ear may be useful, because measurement can vary by 1° with repeated tympanic readings.

BASAL BODY TEMPERATURE

Overview

Basal body temperature (BBT) is the temperature of the body at rest. BBT can be measured using either a glass or digital basal thermometer. The basal thermometer has an expanded scale measuring to one-tenth of a degree, ranging from 95–100°. Charting BBT helps identify when a woman is ovulating or possibly pregnant. It also helps to identify conditions such as anovulation, low progesterone, or thyroid dysfunction. Fertility specialists require a woman to chart her BBT for at least 3 consecutive months or menstrual cycles to aid in identifying cyclic patterns.

Considerations

➤ By the time the rise in basal temperature is detected, the opportunity to become pregnant has probably passed. BBT can assist in determining a biphasic temperature pattern that can indicate "normal" ovulation. By assessing the length of the phases, a hormonal imbalance may be suspected.
➤ Price range: $5–12.

Patient Counseling

MEASUREMENT

➤ Before using the basal thermometer to predict ovulation, the package insert should be read thoroughly.
➤ The thermometer should be cleaned with rubbing alcohol or cool, soapy water.
➤ The thermometer should be shaken down to 96° or below and placed on the night stand (or within easy reach of the patient while still in bed) before the patient goes to bed.

➤ At the same waking time each morning, after at least 3 consecutive hours of sleep, the BBT is taken orally, vaginally, or rectally for 5 minutes. The same route of measurement should be used for the entire cycle.

➤ Any activity (including sexual activity, eating, drinking, or smoking) may raise the BBT, so it should be taken before getting out of bed. BBT should be taken every morning, even during menstruation.

➤ It is estimated that the normal variation in BBT is 0.2° per hour (lower by 0.2 if time of measurement is earlier, and higher if measurement is later than the usual wake time).

CHARTING

➤ The BBT reading is recorded on a chart, with notations regarding the day of the cycle (day 1 is the first day of menses) and the time of the measurement. Days when the woman has sexual intercourse, any illnesses, any medications, and menses are also noted, as are any obvious reasons for temperature variations (travel, stress, interrupted sleep) and changes in cervical mucus.

➤ In addition to BBT, cervical mucus observations can be helpful in determining when ovulation has occurred. During ovulation, increases in estrogen levels prepare the uterus for pregnancy by causing the inner lining of the uterus to build up. During the fertile period, the discharge changes from a sticky substance to a more fluid and copious substance, similar to raw egg whites.

➤ The charted dots for each consecutive day are connected (day 1 to day 2, day 2 to day 3, etc.).

INTERPRETING RESULTS

➤ The BBT before ovulation (follicular phase) is slightly lower than the basal temperature after ovulation (luteal phase). After ovulation, the BBT will rise approximately 0.4° and remain in that temperature range until the next menstrual cycle begins. The amount of rise over the baseline (preovulatory) temperatures should be noted. The actual temperature at ovulation and maximum temperature are not important.

➤ The most probable time that conception will occur is during the 2–3 days before the rise in basal temperature and the day of ovulation itself.

➤ A postovulatory rise in BBT sustained for 18 or more days is a good indicator of pregnancy.[5]

FECAL OCCULT BLOOD TESTS

Additional Questions to Ask in Patient Assessment

1. Have you ever used a product like this? If so, which one?
2. What is the purpose of this product's use?
3. What type of diet do you follow?

Overview

The fecal occult blood test (FOBT) (Table 8-3) is used to find occult (hidden or not detectable on visual inspection) blood in feces. Blood vessels at the surface of colorectal adenomas or cancers, if damaged by the passage of stool, release a small amount of blood into the feces. If the FOBT is positive, additional testing is needed because colorectal cancer is not the only condition that can cause blood in the stool. Other sources of bleeding, such as hemorrhoids, diverticulitis, or peptic ulcers, may be present. The FOBT can also produce false-negative results and miss some adenomas and cancers. Therefore, the American Cancer Society (ACS) recommends using the FOBT in conjunction with invasive tests (such as a flexible sigmoidoscopy, digital rectal examination, and/or contrast barium enema) to screen for colorectal cancer. Two studies recently concluded that colonoscopic screenings were able to detect many advanced colonic neoplasms that were undetected with sigmoidoscopy in asymptomatic adults,[6,7] thus pointing toward potential benefits of colonoscopy versus sigmoidoscopy for colorectal cancer screening.

The American Cancer Society guidelines recommend annual fecal occult blood tests for men and women 50 years of age and older. Earlier and/or more frequent screening is recommended for those who have any of the following:

➤ A strong family history of colorectal cancer or polyps (cancer or polyps in a first-degree relative younger than 60 years or in two first-degree relatives of any age).

Table 8-3. Selected Fecal Occult Blood Test Kits

Product	Reaction Time	Number of Tests	Special Considerations
ColoCARE (OTC product)	30 sec	• 3 test pads • Each test pad has three reaction sites: 1 large square for test area and 2 smaller squares as control pads	Contains a test result card to be mailed to the clinician's office Blue/green color change All three stool tests should be completed even if first two produce negative results
EZ Detect (OTC product)	2 min	5 test pads and control package to test water quality	Results not affected by red meat or vitamin C Contains a test result card to be mailed to a clinician's office Blue/green color change Three stool tests should be completed even if first two produce negative results
Hemoccult II and Hemoccult II Sensa	Developer solution: up to 30 sec	3 test windows, control strip on back of card	Must be returned to clinician's office to be processed Blue color change

➤ Families with hereditary colorectal cancer syndromes (familial adenomatous polyposis and hereditary non-polyposis colon cancer).

➤ A personal history of colorectal cancer or adenomatous polyps, or a personal history of chronic inflammatory bowel disease (ulcerative colitis or Crohn's disease).

Stool guaiac tests are colorimetric assays for hemoglobin. The guaiac-based slide tests detect the presence of blood by the oxidation of colorless phenolic compounds present in guaiac. The hematin portion of the hemoglobin in the occult blood catalyzes the release of oxygen from the hydrogen peroxide, which in turn causes the oxidation of guaiac and results in the production of a blue color. Quality control strips/boxes on the guaiac slide indicate if the test is functioning correctly. The two nonprescription products available contain a reagent layer chemically treated with a chromogenic dye (tetramethylbenzidine) and peroxide sandwiched between two layers of biodegradable paper. Sensitivity for the products listed in Table 8-3 is 2 mg hemoglobin per 100 mL water.

Considerations

➤ Patients with a color vision defect may have difficulty interpreting the results.

➤ The nonprescription test kits are not intended to be diagnostic, and patients should be encouraged to send results to their clinician and consult them for a thorough work-up when needed.

➤ Other resources: http://www.cancer.org.

Patient Counseling

➤ Instructions should be read and followed carefully and completely.

➤ Tests should not be performed during, or until 4 days after, known bleeding such as hemorrhoidal or menstrual bleeding.

➤ A well-balanced diet with the following modifications should be followed 3 days before and during the test period:

• Vitamin C in excess of 250 mg/day (from all sources) should be omitted because it can produce a false-negative test result.

• Red meat (rare, cooked, and processed beef, lamb, and liver) and broccoli, cauliflower, horseradish, parsnips, radishes, turnips, and melons should be omitted because they can produce false-positive test results.

• Dietary fiber intake should be increased for several day before testing to stimulate bleeding from lesions and to increase frequency of bowel movements. Suggested foods in moderation are as follows: vegetables (raw and cooked), fruits (especially apples, grapes, plums, and prunes), peanuts, popcorn, and a serving of bran cereal per day.

➤ Medications that can cause gastritis (aspirin, nonsteroidal anti-inflammatory drugs, other antiplatelet drugs, sulfinpyrazone, rectal products) should be avoided for 7 days before testing. The patient's health care provider should be consulted before discontinuing any prescribed medication. A positive test result while taking medications should not be attributed solely to the medications and warrants repeating the test after the medicines have been stopped.

➤ Toilet bowl cleaners may affect the results, so they should be removed from the toilet tank. The toilet should be flushed at least two times before conducting an FOBT. The over-the-counter test pads may be flushed with the bowel movement after observing the test results.

➤ Tests should be repeated for three consecutive bowel movements because lower intestinal bleeds may not occur all the time. Diarrhea will not affect the accuracy of the test.

➤ The stool specimen may be collected from the toilet bowl, toilet paper, or a clean cup.

➤ For Hemoccult products, the test kit is distributed by health care providers with instructions that explain how to take a stool sample at home. The kit is then returned to the clinic or a medical laboratory for testing. The cover flap of slides should be kept closed when not in use. The applicator stick is used to obtain stool samples from two different areas of the stool specimen, and the sample should be applied as a thin smear to each of the slide windows.

➤ Positive results indicate the presence of occult blood in the stool, not necessarily the presence of cancer. A single positive result is enough to warrant further investigation.

➤ Negative results indicate there was no evidence of occult blood in the stool specimen. This does not absolutely confirm the absence of colorectal disease or other gastrointestinal disorders. Any new signs or symptoms, including changes in bowel habits, should be reported to the patient's health care provider.

PEAK FLOW METERS

Additional Questions to Ask in Patient Assessment

1. Have you ever used a product like this? If so, which one?

2. What is the purpose of its use?
3. What is your current asthma management plan?

Overview

For additional information, see Chapter 7, "Diagnostic Procedures."

DEFINITIONS

➤ Peak expiratory flow rate (PEFR): a measure of the force with which a breath is expelled from the lungs.
➤ Forced vital capacity (FVC): a measure of the maximal volume of air forcibly exhaled from the point of maximal inhalation.[8]
➤ Forced expiratory volume in 1 second (FEV_1): volume of air exhaled during the first second of the FVC which, when reduced, indicates an airflow obstruction.

INDICATION

Used to measure lung function for patients with moderate to severe persistent asthma. Ambulatory peak expiratory flow (PEF) monitoring is recommended in national guidelines as a useful self–management activity for patients with asthma. Emphasis is placed on using the peak flow meter (Table 8-4) as a monitoring tool and not as a diagnostic device. Spirometry (a precise pulmonary function test) measures FVC, FEV_1, and FEV_1/FVC. Although PEF and FEV_1 are closely correlated ($r = 0.85$), this correlation is not sufficient to allow PEF to substitute for spirometry.[9]

PEF monitoring can be used as a tool to:

➤ Determine the severity of asthma.
➤ Check response to treatment during an acute asthma episode.
➤ Monitor progress in treatment of chronic asthma and provide objective information for any possible adjustments in therapy.
➤ Detect worsening lung function and thereby avoid a possible serious incident with early intervention.
➤ Identify the relationship between changes in PEF and exposure to allergens, irritants, and other triggers.
➤ Establish the patient's personal best PEF.

A patient's personal best value is the highest reading achieved over a 2- to 3-week period when their asthma is considered well controlled. An unusually high PEF value can be obtained if the patient "spits" or coughs into the peak flow meter, so judgment must be used in determining

Table 8-4. Selected Peak Flow Meters[a]

Product & PEF Range	Comments
AirWatch Airway Monitoring System 50–875 L/min	Measures both PEF and FEV_1 Records/stores up to 500 measurement pairs (PEF and FEV_1) Batteries required; requires some set-up Able to enroll in reporting system program Tracks green-yellow-red zones
Assess-Low Range 0–390 L/min Assess-Full Range 60–880 L/min	Includes two mouthpieces and daily chart
Astech 60–800 L/min	Red, yellow, and green indicators and daily record book
Mini Wright-Standard Range 60–800 L/min Mini Wright-Low Range 30–370 L/min	Includes mouthpieces
Personal Best-Low Range 50–390 L/min Personal Best-Full Range 60–810 L/min	Red, yellow, and green indicators
Truzone 60–800 L/min	Unique shape is easy for children to hold

[a] Currently, all peak flow meters include the prescription legend and therefore require an authorized prescription to be dispensed. The FDA Panel has OTC labeling guidelines that allow manufacturers who meet the criteria to relabel the products for nonprescription sale. Those guidelines specify that the device only measure peak flow, is not programmable, does not require health care provider adjustment, and does not alert the patient to take medication. (http://www.fda.gov)

if the outlying value should be used to establish a personal best.

The personal best value is used to calculate three zones adapted to a traditional traffic light system: red, yellow, green (described below). Each patient should have a written, individualized action plan similar to the example in Box 8.3.

The measurement of PEF is dependent on effort and technique. Training patients on proper technique and frequent review of technique are extremely important. Patient education should include basic facts about asthma, goals of

---

Box 8.3   Sample Individualized Action Plan

Green zone—Peak expiratory flow rate (PEFR) 80–100% of personal best
All systems "go." Patient is relatively symptom-free and can maintain current asthma management program. If patient is taking continuous medication and the peak flow is constantly in the green zone with minimal variation, the health care provider may consider gradually decreasing daily medication.

Yellow zone—PEFR 50–80% of personal best
"Caution," as asthma is worsening. Health care provider should be contacted to fine-tune therapy. A temporary increase in asthma medication is indicated. If patient is on chronic medications, maintenance therapy will probably need to be increased.

Red zone—PEFR below 50% of personal best
"Danger," asthma management and treatment program are failing to control symptoms. Patient should use inhaled bronchodilator. If peak flow readings do not return to at least the yellow zone, the health care provider should be contacted. Aggressive therapy needs to be started. Maintenance therapy will have to be increased.

Adapted from the Expert Panel Report 2: Guidelines for the Diagnosis and Management of Asthma. Bethesda, MD: National Asthma Education and Prevention from Program, National Heart, Lung, and Blood Institute; 1997.

therapy, role of peak flow monitoring, assessment of skill for meter use, how to keep a daily asthma diary (include symptoms, peak flow, medication use, and restricted activity), and a written asthma care plan.

Patient Counseling

MEASUREMENT

➤ Step 1: Before each use, the marker or arrow should be at the zero or bottom position of the numbered scale (for the AirWatch, manufacturer instructions should be followed). Gum or food should be removed from the mouth.

➤ Step 2: The patient must stand up straight (if unable to stand, he or she should sit with good posture).

➤ Step 3: The patient should take a deep breath, filling the lungs completely.

➤ Step 4: The patient should put the mouthpiece in his or her mouth and close the lips tightly around it, making sure to keep the tongue away from the mouthpiece (this will generate unusually high readings).

➤ Step 5: The patient should blow out as fast and hard as possible. He or she should be instructed to "blow a fast, hard blast" rather than "slowly blowing." The force of the breath will move the marker.

➤ Step 6: The number is noted.

➤ If the patient coughed or made a mistake, the number is not recorded. The test is repeated.

➤ Steps 1–6 are repeated two more times (the closer the readings, the more accurate), and the highest of the three ratings is recorded. An average should not be calculated.

➤ Patients should use the meter when they sense that their asthma is getting worse and to determine if the treatment plan is working.

CLEANING

Peak flow meters should be cleaned weekly with hot, soapy water. Some meters can be put in the dishwasher. If the patient has a cold or other respiratory infection, the peak flow meter should be cleaned more frequently. For AirWatch, the mouth pieces should be cleaned as instructed.

ROUTINE

➤ The patient should measure the PEF close to the same time each day. One suggestion is to measure peak flow twice daily: on rising (7–9 AM) and in the evening (6–8 PM), preferably before using asthma medications. If once-a-day monitoring is required, the peak flow meter is used when the patient wakes up, before taking medicine.

➤ The patient should maintain an asthma diary. He or she should chart the highest of the three readings and include symptoms, medication use, and any restricted activity.

PERSONAL BEST

➤ Patients should take peak flow readings when their asthma is under good control. Measurements should be taken at least twice a day for 2–3 weeks, either on waking and between noon and 2 PM or before and after taking short-acting inhaled beta$_2$-agonist for relief, as instructed by the clinician.

➤ The personal best is used to calculate three zones of measurement for the asthma action plan.

Considerations

➤ Children younger than 4 years of age and as old as 7 may have difficulty using a peak flow meter.

➤ Validity and reliability of the PEF measurements depend on correct technique and maximal effort.

➤ It is recommended that patients use the same brand of peak flow meter because individual PEF measurements may vary between different brands.

➤ Some insurance plans cover all or part of the cost of peak flow meters under prescription or durable medical supply deductibles.

➤ Monitoring devices may fail or wear out over time. Periodic comparisons should be made with the PEF measured by spirometry. The values may not be the same but should be consistent.

➤ Patients may not record values correctly. The electronic peak flow meter is capable of data storage and eliminates the need for keeping a manual record.

➤ As with other devices, some patients have difficulty adhering to regular self-monitoring. Motivation and a specific treatment plan may help maintain adherence.

➤ National guidelines for the diagnosis and management of asthma are available at: http://www.nhlbi.nih.gov /guidelines/asthma/asthgdln.htm.

➤ An example of a peak flow chart is available at http://www.lungusa.org/asthma/astpeakchrt.html.

BLOOD PRESSURE MONITORS

Additional Questions to Ask in Patient Assessment

1. Have you ever used a product like this? If so, which one?
2. What is the purpose of its use?
3. What is your current blood pressure and goal blood pressure?

Overview

Monitoring blood pressure is indicated for patients who have high blood pressure or at risk for high blood pressure. Blood pressure monitoring can help identify whether drug treatment and lifestyle changes are effective in achieving desired outcomes. For monitoring purposes, patients should know their treatment goals for hypertension[10]:

Uncomplicated hypertension:	<140/90 mm Hg
Diabetes or renal disease:	<130/85 mm Hg
Renal disease with >1 g/24 hr proteinuria:	<125/75 mm Hg

High blood pressure is a risk factor for many serious conditions including coronary heart disease, congestive heart failure, stroke, kidney disease, and eye problems. Monitoring blood pressure at home may be beneficial for patients who experience "white coat hypertension," a phenomenon in which a patient's blood pressure increases when in a clinician's office. Blood pressure generally increases with age and is associated with diurnal variation—it tends to be higher during the day and normalizes during sleep.

Blood pressure is typically measured when seated, although standing and supine positions are useful in monitoring orthostatic hypotension. Heart rate (pulse) should be measured each time a blood pressure reading is obtained. An average resting heart rate is 60–80 beats/min.

To measure blood pressure at home, a sphygmomanometer (blood pressure device) is used. Three types of blood pressure devices are available: mercury, aneroid, and automatic.

Overview: Mercury Sphygmomanometer

➤ Works by gravity and is typically wall-mounted. It looks like an oversized thermometer.
➤ Used in clinics and hospitals and provides the most accurate and consistent readings.
➤ Requires good hand strength, hearing, and vision.
➤ Does not require calibration.
➤ Not recommended for home use because of expense and the risk of a mercury hazard.

Overview: Aneroid Sphygmomanometer

➤ Requires manual inflation and has a dial gauge attached to the cuff or a digital display. In some cases, the stethoscope is attached to the cuff. This makes it easier for patients to measure their own pressure, because they do not need to hold the stethoscope in place.
➤ Requires good hand strength, hearing, and vision.
➤ Over time the aneroid monitor can lose accuracy, although the gauge can be recalibrated with a mercury gauge.
➤ Least expensive type of device.

Overview: Automatic Monitor

DIGITAL

➤ Most popular because it is the easiest to use.
➤ Requires less manual dexterity and is a good choice for hearing impaired.
➤ Digital displays are easy to read for those with visual problems.
➤ The error indicator will register an irregular heart rate or arm movement during measurement.
➤ Some models have a memory function for logging recent blood pressures.
➤ Monitors are two to three times more expensive than aneroid monitors.

FINGER AND WRIST

➤ Finger monitors are considered inaccurate and should be avoided.

➤ Wrist monitors are accurate as long as the cuff size is appropriate and the wrist is at heart-level during measurement. This is a good choice for those with large upper arms.

COMPUTER SOFTWARE

➤ Requires more hardware and is the most expensive blood pressure monitor.
➤ Useful for pharmacy monitoring services with multiple user profiles and trend analysis.

Considerations

➤ All devices (Table 8-5) come with a manufacturer's warranty and may require maintenance.

Table 8-5. Selected Blood Pressure Monitors

Product	Comments
Manual Inflation with Standard Cuff Lumiscope Standard Cuff Lumiscope Self-taking Kit	Includes standard cuff, aneroid gauge, bulb, stethoscope, and recording chart Cuff sizes: large D-ring mikeless cuff, child/small adult cuffs, and thigh cuffs available for obese arms Not recommended for patients with visual, hearing, or physical limitations
Manual Inflation with Digital Display BD Assure Manual Inflate Omron Manual Inflation	Includes stethoscope attached to cuff, bulb, easy-to-read display, chart, and case
Automatic Inflation BD Automatic and Automatic Deluxe Lumiscope Digital Omron Automatic	BD: Automatic—require batteries, 7 reading memory plus average; Deluxe—includes AC adaptor

Table 8-5. *Continued*

Product	Comments
Automatic **Inflation** (cont'd) Inflation Samsung Automatic with Heart Sense Samsung with Adjustable Inflation	Lumiscope require: one 9V battery; displays error codes and BP measurement Omron requires 4 AA batteries, memory button recalls the previous reading (BP and pulse), adjustable inflation control Samsung "senses" how high to inflate arm cuff, displays BP and pulse, requires 4 AA batteries
Automatic Inflation **with Printer** Omron BP Monitor Printer	Prints blood pressure and pulse measurements, requires 4 AA batteries
Digital Wrist BD Assure Automatic Wrist Cuff BD Assure Portable Wristwatch Omron Automatic Digital Wrist Samsung Wrist with Heart Sense	All display BP and pulse measurements, lightweight BD: Automatic—7 reading memory plus average; Portable—last reading Omron requires 4 AA batteries Samsung requires 2 AAA batteries, 8 reading memory
Computer Software DynaPulse Software	System includes user's guide, DynaPulse unit, standard adult cuff, air hose with pressure bulb and connector, communication cable, and DynaPulse software (diskettes)

➤ Some insurance plans cover all or part of the cost of monitors under prescription or durable medical supply deductibles.

➤ It is important to choose an appropriate cuff size. Choosing too small of a cuff may result in a falsely higher blood pressure reading. The circumference of the arm or wrist is measured to determine proper cuff size. Cuff sizes available (arm circumference) are as follows: child/small adult (7–10.25″), standard (9–13″), large (13–17″), and thigh (15–20″). Wrist cuff fits wrist 5.25–7.75″ in circumference.

➤ A systolic pressure can be palpated in patients with an unknown blood pressure or used in patients with poorly audible heart sounds (caused by vascular disease, poor peripheral blood flow, or extremely low blood pressures). See proper procedure below.

➤ Periodically check equipment and tubing for cracks or leaks. The results of aneroid or automatic monitors should be compared with a mercury gauge at least once a year.

➤ Further information on blood pressure can be found at the American Heart Association web site: http://www.americanheart.org/hbp/.

➤ JNC-VI guidelines (Table 8-6) are available at http://www.nhlbi.nih.gov/guidelines/hypertension/jncintro.htm.

➤ Blood pressure tracker is available at: http://www.mayohealth.org/mayo/0001/htm/bloodpressureread.htm.

➤ Price range: $20–500.

Patient Counseling

GENERAL ISSUES IN BLOOD PRESSURE MEASUREMENT

➤ The patient should rest for 5–10 minutes and use the restroom if needed. Caffeine, nicotine, and vigorous exercise are avoided for 30 minutes before the blood pressure measurement.

➤ The patient should be seated and rest his or her arm on a table or pillow so that it is level with heart.

➤ The cuff is positioned on the bare upper arm approximately 1–2 inches above the bend of the elbow. Blood flow may be restricted by a rolled-up sleeve; therefore, the patient may have to remove the article of clothing. The cuff can be applied over a thin shirt. The cuff should be snug but not too tight. The tubing from the cuff

Table 8-6.   JNC-VI[a] Criteria for Classifying Adult Hypertension

Category	Systolic (mm Hg)	Diastolic (mm Hg)
Optimal	<120	<80
Normal	<130	<85
High normal	130–39	85–89
Hypertension		
Stage 1 (mild)	140–159	90–99
Stage 2 (moderate)	160–179	100–109
Stage 3 (severe)	180–209	110–119
Stage 4 (very severe)	>209	>119

[a] The Sixth Report of the Joint National Committee on Prevention, Detection, Evaluation and Treatment of High Blood Pressure (JNC-VI). Arch Intern Med 1997;157:2413–46.

should be pointing downward toward the hand and aligned with the inside of the elbow. If the cuff has an arrow on it, it is aligned over the brachial artery (felt over medial side of biceps tendon).

MANUAL MEASUREMENT TECHNIQUES

➤ The stethoscope ear pieces are placed in the ears (tips facing forward) and the bell or diaphragm is placed over the brachial pulse, avoiding interference with the tubing or cuff. The dial gauge is marked off in increments of 2 mm Hg and should be in a location for easy view (many can clip to the cuff). The inflation valve should be turned clockwise just enough to close the valve, but easy to open with a single finger movement.

➤ The cuff is inflated 20–30 mm Hg above the last systolic reading. Inflating the cuff too slowly will cause a false reading.

➤ The valve is opened slightly to release air at a rate of 2–3 mm Hg per second.

➤ The systolic pressure is noted when the first thumping sounds or continuous heart beats are heard.

➤ As the cuff continues to deflate, the thumping will increase and then muffle just before the diastolic pressure is reached.

➤ Blood pressure is recorded as follows: systolic/diastolic (e.g., 118/72 mm Hg).
➤ The radial pulse is palpated (located with second and third fingers on the inner wrist at the base of the thumb) and the heart rate is calculated. This is recorded with the blood pressure.

AUTOMATIC

➤ The power is turned on and, if applicable, inflation setting is chosen 20–30mm Hg above the last systolic pressure measured.
➤ The button to initiate inflation is pushed. On the semi-automatic models, the cuff is inflated by squeezing the rubber bulb. After the cuff is inflated, the automatic mechanism will slowly reduce the cuff pressure.
➤ The display window will show systolic and diastolic pressures. Some models will show pulse. All measurements should be recorded.
➤ The exhaust button is pressed to release the air from the cuff. The cuff is removed, and the machine is turned off.

DYNAPULSE SOFTWARE

The following steps should be followed.

Step 1: Add a New User

➤ Select *Add* from the *Patient* menu.
➤ Enter an appropriate identification number, patient name, and data pathway.

OR
Step 1: Select User

➤ Select *Find* or *Select* from the *Patient* menu.

Step 2: Take a Test Measurement

➤ Select *Start* from the *Measure* menu.
➤ Place the cuff on the arm when prompted. Slide the cuff over the arm with the tube pointing toward the hand and aligned with the inside of the elbow (over the brachial artery). Tighten the cuff so it is snug but does not cut off circulation.
➤ Adjust the Air Release knob on the unit to the Air Release Index provided. Click *OK*.
➤ Close the release valve when prompted by turning clockwise until it stops and select *OK*.
➤ A mercury column appears with instructions to *Pump* up the cuff. Pump cuff until instructed to *Stop Pumping*.

➤ *Measuring* message will appear while measurement is taken. Instruct patient not to talk or move while the Measuring message is displayed. Air release is done automatically.
➤ After the diastolic pressure is measured, a *Release Air* message is displayed. Turn the air release valve on the inflation bulb counterclockwise.
➤ Measurement result will appear on the screen.

Step 3: Take and Save Several Measurements

➤ Additional measurements can be taken at this point. Save measurements by selecting *Save* from the *File* menu. Comments can be added at this time (i.e., arm used, patient position, medications/changes). Comments will appear on the Trend Display when the measurement is highlighted and on the Tabular Report.

ADDITIONAL READINGS

➤ Repeated deep breaths, coughing, sneezing, talking, or arm movement may affect a blood pressure reading.
➤ For greater accuracy, two or three consecutive measurements should be averaged (waiting 3–5 minutes between each) and compared with personal blood pressure goals.
➤ Blood pressure should be checked and results should be logged once or twice a day.
➤ Blood pressure medicines should not be self-adjusted based on home measurements unless instructed to do so by a health care provider.
➤ Dangerously high blood pressure requires immediate medical attention.

SYSTOLIC PRESSURE BY PALPATION

➤ The cuff is applied and then inflated until a radial pulse is no longer felt.
➤ The pressure in the cuff is slowly released, and the point at which a pulse is first felt is noted. This is the systolic pressure and is recorded as, "Systolic blood pressure 126 mm Hg by palpation."

DIABETES MONITORING

Additional Questions to Ask in Patient Assessment

1. Do you have diabetes? Type 1 or Type 2?
2. What diabetes home monitoring systems/tests have you used?

3. How frequently will you monitor your diabetes?
4. Do you have any manual dexterity difficulties?

Overview

Home monitoring of diabetes has evolved from urine glucose testing to sophisticated blood glucose meters (Table 8-7), urine ketone testing, and home test kits for glycosylated hemoglobin. Tailoring a home monitoring system is essential to assist the patient in achieving optimal outcomes. Patients with diabetes should be encouraged to keep daily records of all monitoring results to facilitate routine reflection of disease control.

The blood glucose goals for home monitoring are 80–120 mg/dL preprandially and 100–140mg/dL at bedtime.[11] Certain factors such as severe cardiovascular disease, advanced age, severe renal disease, and others may require alteration of these goals for specific patients.

Blood Glucose Testing

Two methods are available to monitor blood glucose: visual glucose strips and glucose meters.

The most commonly used visual glucose strips are the Chemstrip bG strips, which are available in quantities of 50 and 100 per vial. To use visual strips, a drop of blood is placed on a reagent pad on the strip and then wiped off after a specified amount of time. The color change of the reagent pad is then compared with the color chart on the vial label to determine the glucose range.

Considerations

➤ Requires a single fingerstick to obtain a blood sample.
➤ Anemia can cause false-positive results. Polycythemia can cause false-negative results.
➤ Visually read strips only provide information about a broad range of glucose values rather than a specific number. Visually read strips require good color vision.
➤ Glucose meters provide actual blood glucose values and may have features such as audio readout, digital readout, memory, and printout capability.
➤ Whole blood glucose determinations are approximately 12% lower than those obtained using serum or plasma in a commercial laboratory.

Table 8-7. Selected Home Blood Glucose Meters

Meter	Time to Result (sec)	Whole Blood/Plasma	No. of Readings in Memory	Comments
Simplest to use/basic models				
One Touch Basic	45	Whole blood	See comments	Large display; English/Spanish can download; last result retrievable manually; last 75 results retrievable via download
ExacTech RSG	30	Whole blood	Not available	No calibration
Glucometer Elite Basic	30	Plasma	20	No buttons; no cleaning required
Accu-Chek Simplicity	25	Whole blood	30	Very similar to Accu-Chek Instant
One Touch FastTake	15	Plasma	150	Large display; no cleaning; can download

continued

Table 8-7. *Continued*

Meter	Time to Result (sec)	Whole Blood/Plasma	No. of Readings in Memory	Comments
More sophisticated models				
Accu-Chek Advantage	40	Whole blood	100	No cleaning; can download; Voicemate available
Glucometer Elite XL	30	Plastma	120	Large display; can download
Precision QID	20	Either	10/125	Large display; strips available for either whole blood or plasma; no cleaning required. 10 readings retrievable by the patient; 125 readings downloadable
Most sophisticated models				
Accu-Chek Complete	40	Whole blood	1000	Graphic and other reports displayed on meter screen; no cleaning; can download
Glucometer DEX	30	Plasma	100	Uses cartridge with built-in-strips; can download
One Touch Profile	45	Whole blood	250	User can record events such as meals, insulin dosing/timing, and others; multilingual; can download

➤ Blood drop sample size varies with each meter.
➤ Range of glucose detection varies with each meter. In general, the range is 10 or 20 mg/dL to 500 or 600 mg/dL.
➤ This is more expensive than urine glucose testing. Visual strip prices: $35–40 per 50 strips. Meter prices: $37–150. Meter strip prices: $25–35 per 50 strips.
➤ Some insurance plans cover all or part of the cost of monitors and/or strips under prescription or durable medical supply deductibles.

Patient Counseling

➤ Supplies needed: strips, lancet and lancing device as well as glucose meter (if used).
➤ The patient must understand the technique for using visually read strips or glucose meters before obtaining the blood sample.
➤ The blood glucose meter must be calibrated if required.
➤ Quality control must be performed as recommended by the meter manufacturer.
➤ Hands must be properly washed and thoroughly dried before obtaining a blood sample.
➤ A finger is lanced to obtain the blood sample.
➤ Drop size and sample placement must be in accordance with manufacturer's specifications.
➤ The patient must understand how to dispose of lancets and strips properly.
➤ The test kit/system must be stored at room temperature; it cannot be frozen.
➤ Medications for diabetes should not be self-adjusted based on home glucose measurements unless instructed to do so by a health care provider.
➤ Dangerously high or low glucose levels require immediate medical attention.

Urine Glucose Testing

Urine glucose testing was the only method available to monitor diabetes control until approximately 15 years ago. Surprisingly, only urine glucose testing has been shown in clinical trials to affect disease state outcomes favorably; there is no such data for blood glucose testing. However, urine glucose testing has several drawbacks. First, urine glucose measurements correspond to blood glucose concentrations from several hours before the measurement is taken. Second, great variability exists from patient to patient for the renal threshold of spilling glucose into the urine. Many texts state that patients will spill glucose into the urine when the serum glucose is approximately 180 mg/dL or greater, but this threshold varies significantly from person to person and changes with age and renal function. Third, urine glucose testing is of no value to monitor diabetes control for individuals who desire routine blood glucose values of 80–120mg/dL; therefore, this would eliminate urine glucose monitoring as an option for most patients with diabetes.

Urine glucose testing may have a niche for patients unable to afford the supplies/meters for home glucose testing (Table 8-8) or for patients for whom less than optimal blood glucose control is acceptable (e.g., an elderly patient with multiple diseases who either is not capable of monitoring blood glucose or has a limited longevity and the goal is to allow some hyperglycemia and to eliminate episodes of hypoglycemia).

Considerations

➤ Urine glucose test strips use either a copper reduction or a glucose oxidase test for urine glucose detection.

➤ Fluid intake affects results.

➤ Some common medications that cause false-positive results with the copper reduction test include the following: ascorbic acid, cephalosporins, chloral hydrate, isoniazid, levodopa, methyldopa, high dose penicillins, probenecid, and salicylates.

➤ Some common medications that cause false-negative results with the glucose oxidase test are as follows: ascorbic acid, aspirin, iron, levodopa, and methyldopa.

➤ Advantages of urine glucose testing include lower expense than blood glucose testing with a meter, no pain inflicted by testing process, and the noninvasive nature of the test.

➤ Disadvantages of urine glucose testing include time lag behind blood glucose, inability to detect hypoglycemia, medication interferences with urine tests, the need for intact color vision, and results reported as ranges rather than specific values.

➤ Price range: approximately $6–8 per 50 strips.

Table 8-8. Selected Urine Glucose Tests

Product	Detection Method	No. of Color Blocks Used to Interpret Results	Comments
Clinistix	Glucose oxidase	3	Reagent strips; must wet test strip pad with urine, time carefully and observe color change; qualitative result
Clinitest	Copper sulfate	4	Reagent tablets; must drop specified number of urine drops on tablet, time carefully and wait for color change; semiquantitative result
Diastix	Glucose oxidase	5	Reagent strips; must wet test strip pad with urine, time carefully and observe color change; semiquantitative result
Multistix	See Table 8-9		

Patient Counseling

➤ The expiration date on test strip vial should be checked.
➤ The patient must understand the technique for using urine glucose strips before performing the urine glucose test.
➤ If using a strip, it should be held in the urine for the amount of time specified by the manufacturer.

➤ Good color vision is essential for proper urine glucose result interpretation.
➤ The test should be timed carefully and the result read at the appropriate time. Continuing color changes may occur within seconds of one another.
➤ Strips should be stored as recommended by the manufacturer. A desiccant packet should never be removed from a strip vial.

Urine Ketone Testing

In the absence of insulin, the body begins to oxidize fat; ketones are by-products of this process. Ketones (acetoacetic acid, acetone, and beta-hydroxybutyric acid) accumulate in the blood and spill into the urine, where their presence can signal the onset of ketoacidosis.

Considerations

➤ The urine ketone testing product (Table 8-9) should be tailored to each patient's needs.
➤ Price range: approximately $8–30 per 50 strips.

Patient Counseling

➤ Urine ketone testing should be performed whenever patients who use insulin measure a blood glucose concentration of >240 mg/dL and/or are experiencing any of the following: extreme stress, pregnancy, and symptoms such as diarrhea, vomiting, loss of appetite, increased urine production, fruity-smelling breath, or high fever. If moderate or large amounts of ketones are present, the patient should seek medical attention immediately.

Table 8-9.   Urine Ketone Testing Products

Product	Substances Detected
Ketostix	Ketones
Keto-Diastix	Glucose, ketones
Multistix	Bilirubin, glucose, ketones, occult blood, pH, protein, and urobilinogen

➤ Test strips are visually read with color comparison blocks/result ranges or plus signs, as listed on the product packaging.
➤ Excessive water intake decreases urine concentration, potentially resulting in a false-negative result.
➤ The wait time for results ranges from 15 seconds to 2 minutes.
➤ The product must be stored according to the manufacturer's instructions.
➤ The product expiration date should be checked before each use.

Hemoglobin A1c Testing

Hemoglobin A1c testing provides information about blood glucose control over the past 3 months, which makes it a useful tool in addition to home blood glucose monitoring. Glucose binds to hemoglobin on red blood cells, and the lifespan of a red blood cell is approximately 3 months. Approximate normal values for hemoglobin A1c are 4–6%. The goal for patients with Type 1 or Type 2 diabetes (as established by the Diabetes Control and Complications Trial[12] and the United Kingdom Prospective Diabetes Study)[13] is 7%, although this may need to be altered for certain patients.

Considerations

➤ Hemoglobin A1c testing may have been conducted at a provider's request at a laboratory; patients should inquire about laboratory results before purchasing a home A1c test kit (Box 8.4).
➤ Price range: approximately $37–40 per kit.

Patient Counseling

➤ Hemoglobin A1c testing should be conducted in addition to (not instead of) home blood glucose monitoring.

Box 8.4	Selected Home Hemoglobin A1c Tests
Accu-Chek Hemoglobin A1c Test	
Biosafe Hemoglobin A1c Test Kit	

➤ It requires a fingerstick.
➤ Samples must be mailed to a laboratory for processing.
➤ According to the American Diabetes Association, the recommended frequency of A1c testing is as follows:

- Glycemic control at goal and stable medication doses: once every 6 months.
- Glycemic control not at goal or recent medication dose adjustment: once every 3 months.[14]

HIV TESTING

Additional Questions to Ask in Patient Assessment

1. Have you been previously tested for HIV?
2. Have you been in contact with blood or other body secretions from another person you suspect might be infected with HIV?

Overview

Detection of human immunodeficiency virus (HIV) type-1 in those individuals carrying or at risk for the infection may help to slow the spread of acquired immunodeficiency syndrome (AIDS). Any interaction with a patient desiring information about or wanting to purchase a home HIV test kit (Table 8-10) should be tactful and sensitive to the patient's concerns and needs.

Considerations

➤ Products are approved by the FDA for use by individuals older than 18 years of age.
➤ The specimen is screened using an enzyme-linked immunoabsorbent assay (ELISA) test. If the screen is positive, an immunofluorescence assay (IFA) is used to confirm the result.
➤ The accuracy of the home test kits equals that of a laboratory test conducted using a venipuncture blood sample.
➤ Price range: approximately $40 for the 1-week-to-results kit; approximately $50 for the 3-days-to-results kit.

Table 8-10. Currently Available Home HIV Test Kits

Product	Number of Tests in Kit	Sample Mailed to Company for Processing	Time to Result Availability
Home Access HIV-1 Test System	1	Yes	One week
Home Access HIV-1 Express Test System	1	Yes	Three days (except Sunday or holidays

Patient Counseling

➤ Test kit lancets should be used only by the person using the HIV test kit, and they should be disposed in the container provided with the kit.
➤ A complete sample should be provided on the specimen collection card.
➤ Testing is anonymous and confidential; the test result is identified only by a test kit code number.
➤ Test results, counseling, and referrals are available via telephone 24 hours a day.
➤ Patients with hemophilia or receiving anticoagulation therapy should not use this kit.
➤ Kit contents must be kept dry before and after use.

ILLICIT DRUGS

Additional Questions to Ask in Patient Assessment

1. What is the age of the individual(s) to be tested?
2. During what time period do you suspect the drug use occurred?

Overview

Testing for illicit drugs may be accomplished using urine, hair, or saliva samples. The standard for this drug testing is urine sample testing, but hair and saliva tests are now available as well (Table 8-11). In addition to home use, it is becoming acceptable to use such kits in the workplace and in schools.

Considerations

➤ Urine testing does not indicate duration of drug use. Samples may be tampered with by sample collector and are often viewed as offensive to collect.
➤ Drug residues in the hair cannot be removed by washing, coloring, or other processing. Hair grows approximately 0.5 inches per month; a 1-inch sample provides information about drug use over the past 2 months.
➤ Saliva testing offers a less offensive method for sample collection.
➤ Possible interferences with illicit drug testing (Table 8-12).
➤ Price range: $40–60.

Patient Counseling

➤ Only a parent or legal guardian may obtain a sample for illicit drug testing from a child.
➤ Urine sample collection should be directly observed if feasible to minimize the possibility of sample tampering.
➤ Test kit directions should be read carefully before sample collection and should be followed exactly. Toll-free telephone numbers are provided with the kits if questions exist concerning sample collection, processing, or results notification.
➤ Hair samples should not be collected from a hairbrush. Hair from multiple individuals may be entwined in the brush bristles. Also, hairs may be present on the brush which do not contain "recent" drug residues.

Table 8-11. Drugs of Abuse Testing

	Drugs Detected (Examples)	Drug Use Detection Window	Selected Drugs of Abuse Detection Kits	Time to Available Test Results	Home/Send-Out
Hair	Amphetamine, barbiturates, benzodiazepines, cocaine, marijuana, methamphetamine, opiates, PCP	7–90 days	PDT-90 Personal Drug Testing Service	3–7 days	Send-out
Saliva	Amphetamine, cocaine, marijuana, methamphetamine, opiates	0–36 hr	The Oral Screen	10 min	Home
Urine	Amphetamine, barbiturates, benzodiazepines, cocaine, marijuana, methamphetamine, methadone, opiates, PCP	4 hr to 3 days	Rapid Drug Screen	3 min	Home
			Parent's Alert	3–5 days	Home

Table 8-12. Possible Factors That Contribute False-
Positive or False-Negative Results

	False-Positive Results	False-Negative Results
Hair	None known	Automobile exhaust exposure
Saliva	A very heavily poppy-seeded bagel immediately before sample collection—rare chance	None known
Urine	Amphetamines: diphenoxylate, ephedrine, phenylpropanolamine, pseudoephedrine (within 24–48 hr of ingestion)	Fentanyl
	Methadone: high doses of chlorpromazine dextromethorphan, promethazine	Use of someone else's urine
	PCP: procainamide	Diuretics/excessive fluid intake
	Narcotics in general: poppy seeds (2–3 dinner rolls covered with 2 g of poppy seeds each[11]), diphenhydramine, doxylamine, thioridazine	Additives to the sample: bleach, lemon juice, salt, soap, or vinegar

➤ If a positive or "nonnegative" test result is obtained (Table 8-12), the result should be confirmed with a second test (preferably a urine test in a laboratory).
➤ Open communication and discussion regarding test results are best conducted in a nonthreatening manner.

URINARY TRACT INFECTION TESTS

Additional Questions to Ask in Patient Assessment

1. Have you experienced a urinary tract infection? How recently?
2. What symptoms are you having?
3. Do you currently have any hemorrhoidal or menstrual bleeding?

Overview: Utility

At-home test for detection of urinary tract infection (Table 8-13). May also be used to confirm resolution of a urinary tract infection after treatment. Symptoms that may suggest the presence of a urinary tract infection include frequency,

Table 8-13. Selected Available Urinary Tract Infection Tests

Product	No. of Tests in Package	Reaction Time	Positive Indicator
AZO	3	2 min	Test dipstick color change
First Response Uriscreen	2	2 min	Presence of foam in sample tube
HealthCheck Uri-Test Urinary Tract Infection Screening Test	3	1 min	Test dipstick color change
UTI Home Screening	6	<1 min	Test dipstick color change

urgency, and burning with urination. Current products rely on a test dipstick color change or the presence of foam in a sample tube to indicate a positive result.

Considerations

➤ False-negative results can occur if:

- The urine is alkaline.
- The organisms present do not convert nitrate to nitrite.
- There are inadequate nitrates in food consumption (vegetarian meal plans).
- There is inadequate bladder dwell time.

➤ False-positive results can occur if:

- The urine is discolored from medications or foods (such as phenazopyridine or beets).
- There is gross hematuria present.

➤ Price range: $9–12.

Patient Counseling

➤ A patient without a history of urinary tract infection should always be referred to a health care practitioner for evaluation of symptoms.

➤ The urinary tract screening test is for use in adults only.

➤ Urine must dwell in the bladder from 4 hours to overnight (preferred) for proper testing.

➤ The expiration date on the test kit box should be checked before use.

➤ If a patient presents with symptoms of a urinary tract infection as noted above but also has fever, chills, or gross hematuria, he or she should be referred immediately to a health care practitioner for assessment.

➤ If urinary tract infection symptoms are present, the patient should be advised to contact his or her health care practitioner to report either negative or positive test kit results.

➤ The use of nonprescription phenazopyridine by consumers should be discouraged unless a health care practitioner has recommended use of this drug.

➤ Consumption of cranberry juice has been shown to be beneficial in postmenopausal women with asymptomatic bacteriuria. No study has shown efficacy for use in men or younger women.[12]

➤ To aid in prevention of future urinary tract infections, the patient should be instructed to:

- Assure adequate daily water intake (8 glasses).
- Empty the bladder at regular intervals throughout the day; urine should not be retained in the bladder for extended periods.
- (for women) (1) void after intercourse, (2) consider birth control options other than a diaphragm or spermicide, and (3) wipe from front to back to keep genital areas clean

FUTURE INNOVATIONS

A multitude of products and home test kits are in development or will soon be brought to the U.S. marketplace. Many of these products and kits were previously available via commercial laboratories and are now being developed for home use. These new technologies have been created in response to increased patient demand for self-management tools. Products are currently in development for the following:

➤ Cancer of the colon, lung, breast, cervix, and prostate.
➤ Infectious diseases such as hepatitis C, *Helicobacter pylori*, *Streptococcus group A*, herpes simplex virus, *Chlamydia trachomatis*, and yeast infections.
➤ Allergies.
➤ Glaucoma.
➤ Kidney and liver disease.

New hand-held monitors, with a simple change of an encoded computer chip, may test various blood chemistries, such as international normalized ratio (INR), lipids, glucose, hemoglobin A1c, fructosamine, ketones, liver enzymes, and proteins. Other analyzers for home use may allow for therapeutic drug monitoring by patients.

References

1. Limon L, Cimmino A, Lakamp J, eds. APhA Nonprescription Products: Patient Assessment Handbook. Washington, DC: American Pharmaceutical Association; 1997:25, 201.

2. Munroe WP. Home diagnostic kits. Am Pharm. 1994;34 (2):50–9.

3. Newton GD et al. New OTC drugs and devices 1999: a selective review. J Am Pharm Assoc. 2000;40(2):222–33.

4. Smith J. Are electronic thermometry techniques suitable alternatives to traditional mercury in glass thermometry techniques in the paediatric setting? J Adv Nurs. 1998;28(5):1030–9.

5. Hatcher et al. Contraceptive Technology. 17th ed. New York, NY: Ardent Media, Inc; 1998:319.

6. Imperiale TF et al. Risk of advanced proximal neoplasms in asymptomatic adults according to the distal colorectal findings. N Engl J Med. 2000;343:169–74.

7. Lieberman DA et al. Use of colonoscopy to screen asymptomatic adults for colorectal cancer. N Engl J Med. 2000;343:162–8.

8. Expert Panel Report 2: Guidelines for the Diagnosis and Management of Asthma. Bethesda, MD: National Asthma Education and Prevention Program, National Heart, Lung, and Blood Institute; 1997.

9. Connelly CK, Chan NS. Relationship between different measurements of respiratory function in asthma. Respiration. 1987;52:22–33.

10. The Sixth Report of the Joint National Committee on Prevention, Detection, Evaluation and Treatment of High Blood Pressure (JNC-VI). Arch Intern Med. 1997;157:2413–46.

11. American Diabetes Association. Standards of medical care for patients with diabetes mellitus. Diabetes Care. 2000;23(1 suppl):S32–S42.

12. The Diabetes Control and Complications Trial Research Group. The effect of intensive treatment of diabetes on the development and progression of long-term complications in insulin-dependent diabetes mellitus. N Engl J Med. 1993;329:977–986.

13. UK Prospective Diabetes Study Group. Intensive blood-glucose control with sulphonylureas or insulin compared with conventional treatment and risk of complications in patient with type 2 diabetes (UKPDS 33). Lancet. 1998;352:837–853.

14. American Diabetes Association. Tests of glycemia in diabetes. Diabetes Care. 2000;23(1 suppl):S80–S82.

15. ElSohly HN, ElSohly MA, Stanford DF. Poppy seed ingestion and opiates urinalysis: a closer look. J Anal Toxicol. 1990;14:308–310.

16. Stapleton A. Prevention of urinary tract infection. Infect Dis Clin North Am. 1997;11(3):719–33.

Chapter 9

Drug Administration

Susan M. Stein

A question often asked of practitioners and students in pharmacy is, "How does one determine the most appropriate route of administration for a specific patient and/or medication?" Many factors are involved in this decision-making process. This chapter presents various routes of administration and provides a selection process to determine the most appropriate drug/dosage formulation and route.

Technological advances continually provide greater variety for administration of medications. New delivery systems can often expand the therapeutic indication or decrease the adverse effects of an older drug. For example, Amphotericin B recently became available as a parenteral lipid emulsion. This form decreased the incidence of nephrotoxicity, thereby increasing usage and patient tolerability.

Common routes of drug administration are oral and parenteral. Topical and rectal administration are less common routes. Site-specific routes also exist, such as ophthalmic and otic administration. The nature of the drug may dictate the dosage form and route available. Often, a drug will initially be available parenterally to avoid complications involving metabolism. A drug with solubility concerns may only be available orally as a tablet. In this case, the route of administration is not an issue, as the available formulation is limited.

PATIENT ASSESSMENT

When determining an appropriate route of administration, assessing the patient's clinical health status provides valuable information. In addition, the seriousness of the condition being treated can assist in selection of the route of administration. Examples of various patient conditions and resulting administration routes are described in Table 9-1.

Table 9-1. Examples of Recommended Routes of Administration for Various Patient Conditions

Patient Status	Recommended Route
Oral intake	Oral, topical
Nothing by mouth (NPO)	Parenteral, rectal, topical
Critical condition	Parenteral
Chronic condition	Oral, rectal, topical
Severe hypokalemia (potassium level <3 mEq/L)	Parenteral
Nausea, vomiting	Parenteral, rectal

ROUTES OF ADMINISTRATION

When selecting an appropriate route of administration, available forms of the desired drug should be reviewed. Various references may be used, including *Drug Facts and Comparisons, USPDI,* and *AHFS.* It is important to investigate the availability of new dosage forms. Micromedex, an on-line resource updated frequently, is valuable for locating up-to-date drug formulations. In addition, it may be feasible to compound a commercially unavailable product. A literature review is useful to locate compounded drug formulations. Maintaining this information for future reference is advised. Issues relating to various dosage formulations are described in Table 9-2.

There are other limitations to consider when determining the most appropriate dosage form. The administration route available will often change as the patient's condition changes. Factors involving these choices are shown in Table 9-3. Each highlights some of the major routes of administration available.

ORAL MEDICATIONS

In general, oral administration is often the most desired route of administration despite limitations. Additional considerations involving oral medications pertain to the ability

Table 9-2. Issues Relating to Various Dosage Formulations

Route	Dosage Form	Comments
Oral	Solid—capsule, tablet, powder packet, lozenge, pastille	Limited strengths available
	Solution	May titrate dose
	Suspension	"Shake well" to resuspend
	Emulsion	Oil-in-water more palatable
Parenteral (drug only)	Solution	Evaluated ease of preparation
		Sterility issues
	Reconstitutable	Diluent/stability issues
		Sterility issues
	Dispersion (liposomal)	Restricted availability
		Sterility issues
Topical	Bulk—cream, lotion ointment, emulsion powder	Flexibility in compounding formulations
	Transdermal—patch	Controlled release
Rectal/ vaginal	Suppositories	Good absorption
		Compounding flexibility
		Temperature dependant
	Cream	Applicator for administration
Ophthalmic	Solution	Soluble product
		Sterility issues
	Suspension	"Shake well" to resuspend
		Sterility issues
	Ointment	Difficult to apply
Otic	Solution	Soluble product
	Suspension	"Shake well" to resuspend

Table 9-3. Comparison of Advantages and Disadvantages of Various Dosage Formulations

Route	Advantage	Disadvantage
Oral	Functional gastrointestinal maintained Ease of administration Less expensive	Slower time to effect First-pass metabolism Bioavailability issues
Parenteral	Rapid time to effect No bioavailability issues Ability to titrate dose	Costly preparation issues Costly administration issues Sterility and stability issues Compatibility issues Safety issues (related to route of administration) Painful administration
Topical	Localized effect Little systemic absorption Few adverse reactions Controlled absorption (transdermal) No first-pass metabolism	Difficult to measure dose Irritation at site of application Response altered with various physiologic changes (blood pressure, temperature) Increased absorption in elderly patients or exposed skin May stain clothing
Rectal/vaginal	Well-absorbed No first-pass metabolism Generally inexpensive form	Socially unacceptable Few drugs available rectally May stain clothing Indication/route potentially unrelated
Ophthalmic	Localized effect Little systemic absorption	Difficult self-administration Contamination possible
Otic	Localized effect Little systemic absorption	Difficult self-administration

---

Box 9.1   Types of Medications That Should Not Be Divided or Crushed

---

Extended Release tablets: exceptions include Calan SR, Isoptin SR, Imdur, Sinemet CR, and MS Contin

Enteric-coated tablets

Sublingual tablets[a]

Buccal tablets[a]

[a] Source: McPherson ML. Don't crush that tablet! Am Pharm. 1994;NS34:57–8.

---

to crush or divide a tablet to increase dosing flexibility. Due to continually changing formulations, it is vital to clarify this information for each specific manufacturer for a particular formulation. Box 9.1 and Table 9-4 provide information regarding these issues.

MONITORING PARAMETERS

It is vital to monitor the patient's condition to evaluate the effectiveness of drug therapy (see Chapter 15, "Clinical Drug Monitoring," for a more detailed discussion). Parameters range from the signs of an infection (redness, warmth, fever) to the appearance of an allergy to the medication (rash). Table 9-5 contains a sample of monitoring parameters that pertain to major routes of administration.

PARENTERAL ADMINISTRATION

Parenteral delivery of medications is a common form of drug administration in hospitals, long-term care facilities, and more recently the patient's home. Solutions delivered vascularly replenish fluid requirements, deliver medications, and even supplement nutritional needs. Direct access, whether by bloodstream, spinal fluid, or peritoneal fluid, eliminates one of the human body's primary defense

(text continues on page 399)

Table 9-4. Oral Dosage Forms That Should not Be Crushed

Drug Product	Manufacturer	Dosage Forms	Reasons/Comments
Accutane	Roche	Capsule	Mucous membrane irritant
Actified 12 Hour	Glaxo Wellcome	Capsule	Slow release[b]
Acutrim (various)	Novartis Customer Health		Slow release
Adalat CC	Bayer Corp	Tablet	Slow release
Aerolate SR, JR, III	Fleming & Co.	Capsule	Slow release[a, b]
Afrinol Repetabs	Schering Plough	Tablet	Slow release
Allegra-D	Hoechst Marion Roussel	Tablet	Slow release
Allerest 12 Hour	Novartis	Capsule	Slow release
Ammonium Chloride Extended Release	Various	Tablet	Enteric-coated
Artane Sequels	ESI-Lederle	Capsule	Slow release[a, b]
Arthritis Bayer Time Release	Bayer Corp	Capsule	Slow release
Arthrotec	Searle	Tablet	Enteric-coated
ASA Enseals	Lilly	Tablet	Enteric-coated
Asacol	Proctor & Gamble	Tablet	Slow release
Ascriptin A/D	Rhone Ponlenc Rorer	Tablet	Enteric-coated

Ascriptin Extra Strength	Rhone Ponlenc Rorer	Tablet	Enteric-coated
Atrohist LA	Adams	Tablet	Slow release[b]
Atrohist Plus	Adams	Tablet	Slow release[b]
Atrohist Sprinkle	Adams	Capsule	Slow release[a, b]
Azulfidine Entabs	Pharmacia and Upjohn	Tablet	Enteric-coated
Baros	Lafayette	Tablet	Effervescent tablet[f]
Bayer Low Adult 81-mg Strength	Bayer Corp	Tablet	Enteric-coated
Bayer Regular Strength (325-mg Caplets)	Bayer Corp	Tablet	Enteric-coated
Bayer Enteric-coated Caplets	Bayer Corp	Caplet	Enteric-coated
Betachron E-R	Inwood	Capsule	Slow release
Betapen-VK	Bristol-Myers Squibb	Tablet	Taste[e]
Biohist-LA	Wakefield	Tablet	Slow release[b]
Bisacodyl	Various	Tablet	Enteric-coated[c]
Bontril SR	Carnrick	Capsule	Slow release
Breonesin	Sanofi Winthrop	Capsule	Liquid-filled[d]
Brexin LA	Savage	Capsule	Slow release[b]
Bromfed	Muro	Capsule	Slow release[b]
Bromfed-PD	Muro	Capsule	Slow release[b]

continued

Table 9-4. *Continued*

Drug Product	Manufacturer	Dosage Forms	Reasons/Comments
Calan SR	Searle	Tablet	Slow release[b]
Cama Arthritis Pain Reliever	Novartis	Tablet	Multiple compressed
Carbatrol	Athena Neurosciences	Capsule	Slow release[a]
Carbiset-TR	Nutripharm	Tablet	Slow release
Cardizem	Marion-Merrell	Tablet	Slow release
Cardizem CD	Marion-Merrell Dow	Capsule	Slow release[a]
Cardizem SR	Marion-Merrell Dow	Capsule	Slow release[a]
Carter's Little Pills	Carter	Tablets	Enteric-coated
Ceclor CD	Lilly	Tablet	Slow release
Celtin	Glaxo Wellcome	Tablet	Taste[b] Note: use suspension for children
CellCept	Roche	Capsule	Teratogenic potential[i]
Charcoal Plus	Kramer	Tablet	Enteric-coated
Chloral Hydrate	Various	Capsule	Note: product is in liquid form within a special capsule[b]
Chlorpheniramine Maleate Time Release	Various	Capsule	Slow release

Chlor-Trimeton 8-Hour, 12-Hour	Schering Plough	Tablet	Slow release[b]
Choledyl SA	Parke-Davis	Tablet	Slow release[b]
Cipro	Bayer Corp	Tablet	Taste[e]
Claritin-D	Schering Plough	Tablet	Slow release
Claritin-D 24 Hour	Schering Plough	Tablet	Slow release
Codimal-LA	Schwarz Pharma	Capsule	Slow release
Codimal-LA Hall	Schwarz Pharma	Capsule	Slow release
Colace	Bristol-Myers	Capsule	Taste[e]
Comhist LA	Roberts	Capsule	Slow release[a]
Compazine Spansule	SmithKline Beecham	Capsule	Slow release[b]
Congress SR, JR	Fleming & Co.	Capsule	Slow release
Contac 12-Hour	SmithKline Beecham	Capsule	Slow release[a, b]
Contac Maximum Strength	SmithKline Beecham	Capsule	Slow release[a, b]
Cotazym S	Organon Teknita	Capsule	Enteric-coated[a]
Covera-HS	Searle	Tablet	Slow release
Creon 10, 20, 25	Solvay	Capsule	Enteric-coated[a]
Cystospaz-M	PolyMedica	Capsule	Slow release
Cytoxan	Mead Johnson Oncology	Tablet	Note: drug may be crushed but maker recommends using injection

continued

Table 9-4. Continued

Drug Product	Manufacturer	Dosage Forms	Reasons/Comments
Cytovene	Roche	Capsule	Skin irritant
D.A. II	Dura Pharm	Tablet	Slow release[b]
Dallergy	Laser	Capsule	Slow release
Dallergy-D	Laser	Capsule	Slow release
Dallergy-JR	Laser	Capsule	Slow release
Deconamine SR	Bradley	Capsule	Slow release[b]
Deconstal II	Adams	Tablet	Slow release
Deconhist-LA	Zenith Goldline	Tablet	Slow release
Defen-LA	Horizon	Tablet	Slow release[b]
Depakene	Abbott	Capsule	Slow release mucous membrane irritant
Depakote	Abbott	Capsule	Enteric-coated
Desoxyn Gradumets	Abbott	Tablet	Slow release
Desyrel	Bristol Myers	Tablet	Taste[e]
Dexatrim, Max. Strength	Thompson Medical	Tablet	Slow release
Dexedrine Spansule	SmithKline Beecham	Capsule	Slow release
Diamox Sequels	ESI Lederle	Capsule	Slow release

Dilacor XR	Rhone-Poulenc Rorer	Capsule	Slow release
Dilatrate-SR	Schwarz Pharma	Capsule	Slow release
Dimetane Extentab	Robins	Tablet	Slow release[b]
Dimetapp Extentabs	Robins	Tablet	Slow release
Disobrom	Geneva	Tablet	Slow release
Disophrol Chronotab	Schering Plough	Tablet	Slow release
Dital	UAD	Capsule	Slow release
Ditropan XL	Alza	Tablet	Slow release
Dolobid	Merck	Tablet	Slow release
Donnatal Extentab	Robins	Tablet	Irritant
Donnazyme	Robins	Tablet	Slow release[b]
Drisdol	Sanofi Winthrop	Capsule	Enteric-coated
Drixoral	Schering Plough	Tablet	Liquid-filled[d]
Drixoral Plus	Schering Plough	Tablet	Slow release[b]
Drixoral Sustained Action	Schring Plough	Tablet	Slow release
Dulcolax	Novartis Consumer	Tablet	Slow release
Duratuss	Whitby	Tablet	Enteric-coated[c]
Dura-Vent/A	Dura	Tablet	Slow release[b]
Dura-Vent/DA	Dura	Tablet	Slow release[b]
Dynabac	Sanofi Winthrop	Tablet	Slow release[b]
DynaCirc CR	Novartis	Tablet	Enteric-coated
			Slow release

continued

Table 9-4. Continued

Drug Product	Manufacturer	Dosage Forms	Reasons/Comments
Easprin	Parke-Davis	Tablet	Enteric-coated
EC-Naprosyn	Syntex	Tablet	Enteric-coated
Ecotrin Adult Low Strength	SmithKline Beecham	Tablet	Enteric-coated
Ecotrin Maximum Strength	SmithKline Beecham	Tablet	Enteric-coated
Ecotrin Regular Strength	SmithKline Beecham	Tablet	Enteric-coated
E.E.S. 400	Abbott	Tablet	Enteric-coated[b]
Efidac/24	Novartis	Tablet	Slow release
Efidac/24 chlorpheniramine	Novartis	Tablet	Slow release
Effexor XR	Wyeth Ayerst	Capsule	Slow release
E-Mycin	Pharmacia & Upjohn	Tablet	Enteric-coated
Endafed	Forest	Capsule	Slow release
Entex LA	Procter & Gamble	Tablet	Slow release[b]
Entex PSE	Procter & Gamble	Tablet	Slow release
Equanil	Wyeth-Ayerst	Tablet	Taste[e]
Egomar	Lotus	Tablet	Sublingual form[g]
Eryc	Warner-Chilcott	Capsule	Enteric-coated[a]
Ery-Tab	Abbott	Tablet	Enteric-coated

Erythrocin Stearate	Abbott	Tablet	Enteric-coated
Erythromycin Base	Various	Tablet	Enteric-coated
Eskalith CR	SmithKline Beecham	Tablet	Slow release
Exgest LA	Schwarz Pharma	Tablet	Slow release
Extendryl JR	Fleming	Capsule	Slow release[b]
Extendryl S-R	Fleming	Capsule	Slow release[b]
Fedahist Gyrocaps	Schwarz Pharma	Capsule	Slow release[b]
Fedahist Timecaps	Schwarz Pharma	Capsule	Slow release[b]
Feldene	Pfizer	Capsule	Mucous membrane irritant
Feocyte	Dunhall	Tablet	Slow release
Feosol	SmithKline Beecham	Tablet	Enteric-coated[b]
Feosol Spansule	SmithKline Beecham	Capsule	Slow release[a, b]
Feretab	Upsher-Smith	Tablet	Enteric-coated[b]
Fergon	Bayer	Capsule	Slow release[a]
Fero-Grad 500 mg	Abbott	Tablet	Slow release
Feverall Sprinkle	Upsher-Smith	Capsule	Taste[a] Note: capsule contents intended to be placed in a teaspoonful of water or soft food
Flomax	Boehringer Ingelheim	Capsule	Slow release

continued

Table 9-4. *Continued*

Drug Product	Manufacturer	Dosage Forms	Reasons/Comments
Fumatinic	Laser	Capsule	Slow release
Gastrocrom	Meveda	Capsule	Note: contents may be dissolved in water for administration
Geocillin	Roerig	Tablet	Taste
Glucotrol XL	Pfizer	Tablet	Slow release
Gris-Peg	Allergan	Tablet	Note: crushing may result in precipitation as larger particles
Guaifed	Muro	Capsule	Slow release
Guaifed-PD	Muro	Capsule	Slow release
Guaifenex LA	Ethex	Tablet	Slow release[b]
Guaifenex PPA	Ethex	Tablet	Slow release
Guaifenex PSE	Ethex	Tablet	Slow release[b]
Guiamax-D	Schwarz Pharma	Tablet	Slow release
Humabid	Adams	Tablet	Slow release
Humabid DM Sprinkle	Adams	Capsule	Slow release[a]

Humabid LA	Adams	Tablet	Slow release
Humabid Sprinkle	Adams	Capsule	Slow release[a]
Hydergine L-C	Sandoz	Capsule	Note: product is in liquid form within a special capsule[b]
Hydergine Sublingual	Sandoz	Tablet	Sublingual route[b]
Hytakerol	Sanofi Winthrop	Capsule	Liquid-filled[b, d]
Iberet	Abbott	Tablet	Slow release[b, d]
Iberet 500	Abbott	Tablet	Slow release[b]
ICaps Plus	Ciba Vision	Tablet	Slow release
ICaps Time Release	Ciba Vision	Tablet	Slow release
Ilotycin	Dista	Tablet	Enteric-coated
Imdur	Key	Tablet	Slow release[b]
Inderal LA	Wyeth Ayerst	Capsule	Slow release
Inderide LA	Wyeth Ayerst	Capsule	Slow release
Indocin SR	MSD	Capsule	Slow release[a,b]
Ionamin	Medeva	Capsule	Slow release
Isoptin SR	Knoll	Tablet	Slow release
Isordil Sublingual	Wyeth Ayerst	Tablet	Sublingual form[g]
Isordil Tembid	Wyeth Ayerst	Tablet	Slow release
Isosorbide Dinitrate Sublingual	Various	Tablet	Sublingual form[g]

continued

Table 9-4. Continued

Drug Product	Manufacturer	Dosage Forms	Reasons/Comments
Isosorbide Dinitrate SR	Various	Tablet	Slow release
K + 8	Alra	Tablet	Slow release[b]
K + 10	Alra	Tablet	Slow release[b]
Kadian	Zeneca	Capsule	Slow release[a]
K + Care	Alra	Tablet	Effervescent tablet[b, f]
Kaon CL	Pharmacia & Upjohn	Tablet	Slow release[b]
K-Dur	Key	Tablet	Slow release
K-Lease	Pharmacia & Upjohn	Capsule	Slow release[a, b]
Klor-Con	Upsher-Smith	Tablet	Slow release[b]
Klor-Con/EF	Upsher-Smith	Tablet	Effervescent tablet[b, f]
Klorvess	Novartis	Tablet	Effervescent tablet[b, f]
Klotrix	Bristol-Myers Squibb	Tablet	Slow release[b]
K-Lyte	Bristol-Myers Squibb	Tablet	Effervescent tablet[f]
K-Lyte CL	Bristol-Myers Squibb	Tablet	Effervescent tablet[f]
K-Lyte DS	Bristol-Myers Squibb	Tablet	Effervescent tablet[f]
K-Tab	Abbott	Tablet	Slow release[b]
Levbid	Schwarz Pharma	Tablet	Slow release[b]

Levsinex Timecaps	Schwarz Pharma	Capsule	Slow release
Lexxel	Merck	Tablet	Slow release
Lithobid	Solvay	Tablet	Slow release
Lodrane LD	ECR Pharmaceuticals	Capsule	Slow release[a]
Mag-Tab SR	Niche	Tablet	Slow release
Mestinon Timespan	Zeneca	Tablet	Slow release[b]
Mt-Cebrin	Lilly	Tablet	Enteric-coated
MI-Cebrin T	Lilly	Tablet	Enteric-coated
Micro K	Robins	Capsule	Slow release[a, b]
Monafed	Monarch	Tablet	Slow release
Monafed DM	Monarch	Tablet	Slow release
Motrin	Ortho-McNeil	Tablet	Taste[e]
MS Contin	Purdue Frederick	Tablet	Slow release[b]
Muco-Fen-LA	Wakefield	Tablet	Slow release[b]
Naldecon	Apothecon	Tablet	Slow release[b]
Naprefan	Wyeth Ayerst	Tablet	Slow release
Nasatab LA	ECR Pharmaceutical	Tablet	Slow release[b]
Niaspan	KOS	Tablet	Slow release[i]
Nico 400	Jones Medical	Capsule	Slow release[i]
Nicotinic Acid	Various	Capsule	Slow release
Nitro Bid Plateau	Hoechst-Marion Roussel	Capsule	Slow release[a]

continued

Table 9-4. Continued

Drug Product	Manufacturer	Dosage Forms	Reasons/Comments
Nitroglyn	Key	Capsule	Slow release[a]
Nitrong	Wharton	Tablet	Sublingual route[g]
Nitrostat	Parke-Davis	Tablet	Sublingual route[g]
Nitro-Time	Time-Cap Labs	Capsule	Slow release
Nolamine	Carnrick	Tablet	Slow release
Nolex LA	Carnrick	Tablet	Slow release
Norflex	3M	Tablet	Slow release
Norpace CR	Searle	Capsule	Slow release form within a special capsule
Novafed A	Hoechst Marion Roussel	Capsule	Slow release
Ondrox	Unimed	Tablet	Slow release
Optilets 500 filmtab	Abbott	Tablet	Enteric-coated
Optilets-M 500 filmtab	Abbott	Tablet	Enteric-coated
Oragrafin	Bristol-Myers Squibb	Capsule	Note: product is in liquid form within a special capsule
Oramorph SR	Roxane	Tablet	Slow release[b]
Ornade Spansule	SmithKline Beecham	Capsule	Slow release

OxyContin	Purdue Frederick	Tablet	Slow release
Pabalate	Robins	Tablet	Enteric-coated
Pabalate SF	Robins	Tablet	Enteric-coated
Pancrease	Ortho McNeil	Capsule	Enteric-coated[a]
Pancrease MT	Ortho McNeil	Capsule	Enteric-coated[a]
Panmist Jr, LA	Pan American Lab	Tablet	Slow release[b]
Panmycin	Pharmacia & Upjohn	Capsule	Taste
Pannaz	Pan American Lab	Tablet	Slow release[b]
Papaverine Sustained Action	Various	Capsule	Slow release
Pathilon Sequels	ESI Lederle	Capsule	Slow release[a]
Pavabid Plateau	Hoescht Marion Roussel	Capsule	Slow release[b]
PBZ-SR	Novartis	Tablet	Slow release
Pentasa	Hoescht Marion Roussel	Tablet	Slow release
Perdiem	Novartis	Granules	Wax-coated
Penitrate SA	Parke-Davis	Tablet	Slow release[b]
Permitl Chronotab	Schering Plough	Tablet	Slow release[b]
Phazyme	Schwarz Pharma	Tablet	Slow release
Phazyme 95	Schwarz Pharma	Tablet	Slow release
Phenergan	Wyeth Ayerst	Tablet	Taste[b, c, e]
Phyllocontin	Purdue Frederick	Tablet	Slow release
Plendil	Astra Merck	Tablet	Slow release

continued

Table 9-4. *Continued*

Drug Product	Manufacturer	Dosage Forms	Reasons/Comments
Pneumomist	ECR Pharmaceutical	Tablet	Slow release[b]
Polaramine Repetabs	Schering Plough	Tablet	Slow release[b]
Posicor	Roche	Tablet	Mucous membrane irritant
Prelu-2	Boehringer Ingelheim	Capsule	Slow release
Prevacid	TAP Pharmaceutical	Capsule	Slow release
Prilosec	Astra Merck	Capsule	Slow release
Pro-Banthine	Schiapparelli Searle	Tablet	Taste
Procanbid	Parke-Davis	Tablet	Slow release
Procainamide HCL SR	Various	Tablet	Slow release
Procardia	Pfizer	Capsule	Delays absorption[b, e]
Procardia XL	Pfizer	Tablet	Slow release Note: AUC is unaffected
Profen II	Wakefield	Tablet	Slow release[b]
Profen-LA	Wakefield	Tablet	Slow release[b]
Pronestyl SR	Bristol-Myers Squibb	Tablet	Slow release

Propecia	Merck	Tablet	Note: crushed or broken tablets should not be handled by women who are or may become pregnant
Proscar	Merck	Tablet	Note: crushed or broken tablets should not be handled by women who are or may become pregnant
Proventil Repetabs	Schering Plough	Tablet	Slow release[b]
Prozac	Lilly	Capsule	Slow release[a]
Quibron-T SR	Roberts	Tablet	Slow release[b]
Quinaglute Dura-Tabs	Berlex	Tablet	Slow release
Quinidex Extentabs	Robins	Tablet	Slow release
Quin-Release	Major	Tablet	Slow release
Respa-1st	Respa	Tablet	Slow release[b]
Respa-DM	Respa	Tablet	Slow release[b]
Respa-GF	Respa	Tablet	Slow release[b]
Respahist	Respa	Capsule	Slow release[a]
Respaire SR	Laser	Capsule	Slow release
Respbid	Boehringer Ingelheim	Tablet	Slow release
Ritalin SR	Novartis	Tablet	Slow release

continued

Table 9-4. *Continued*

Drug Product	Manufacturer	Dosage Forms	Reasons/Comments
Robimycin	Robins	Tablet	Enteric-coated
Rondec TR	Dura Pharma	Tablet	Slow release[b]
Ru-Tuss DE	Knoll	Tablet	Slow release
Sinemet CR	DuPont Pharm	Tablet	Slow release
Singlet for Adults	SmithKline Beecham	Tablet	Slow release
Slo-bid Gyrocaps	Rhone-Poulenc Rorer	Capsule	Slow release[a]
Slo-Niacin	Upsher Smith	Tablet	Slow release[b]
Slo-Phyllin GG	Rhone-Poulenc Rorer	Capsule	Slow release[b]
Slo-Phyllin Gryocaps	Rhone-Poulenc Rorer	Capsule	Slow release[a, b]
Slow-FE	Novartis	Tablet	Slow release[b]
Slow-FE with Folic Acid	Novartis	Tablet	Slow release
Slow-K	Novartis	Tablet	Slow release[b]
Slow-Mag	Searle	Tablet	Slow release
Sorbitrate SA	Zeneca	Tablet	Slow release
Sorbitrate Sublingual	Zeneca	Tablet	Sublingual route
Sparine	Wyeth-Ayerst	Tablet	Taste[e]

S-P-T	Fleming	Capsule	Note: liquid gelatin thyroid suspension
Sudafed 12 hour	Warner Lambert	Capsule	Slow release[b]
Sudal 60/500	Atley	Tablet	Slow release
Sudal 120/600	Atley	Tablet	Slow release
Sudex	Roberts	Tablet	Slow release[b]
Sular	Zeneca	Tablet	Slow release
Sustaire	Pfizer	Tablet	Slow release[b]
Syn-RX	Adams Lab	Tablet	Slow release
Syn-RX DM	Adams Lab	Tablet	Slow release
Tavist-D	Novartis	Tablet	Multiple compressed tablet
Teczam	Hoechst Marion Roussel	Tablet	Slow release
Tedral SA	Parke-Davis	Tablet	Slow release[b]
Tegretol-XR	Novartis	Tablet	Slow release
Teldrin Maximum Strength	SmithKline Beecham	Capsule	Slow release[a]
Tepanil Ten-Tab	3M Pharmaceutical	Tablet	Slow release
Tessalon Perles	Forest	Capsule	Slow release
Theo-24	UCB	Tablet	Slow release[b]
Theobid Duracaps	Ross	Capsule	Slow release[a, b]
Theoclear LA	Schwarz Pharma	Capsule	Slow release[b]
Theochron	Inwood	Tablet	Slow release

continued

Table 9-4. *Continued*

Drug Product	Manufacturer	Dosage Forms	Reasons/Comments
Theo-Dur	Key	Tablet	Slow release[b]
Theo-Dur Sprinkle	Key	Capsule	Slow release[a, b]
Theolair SR	3M Pharmaceuticals	Tablet	Slow release[b]
Theo-Sav	Savage	Tablet	Slow release[b]
Theo-Span-SR	Laser	Capsule	Slow release
Theo-Time SR	Major	Tablet	Slow release
Theo-X	Schwarz Pharma	Tablet	Slow release
Theovent	Schering Plough	Capsule	Slow release[b]
Thorazine Spansule	SmithKline Beecham	Capsule	Slow release
Toprol XL	Astra	Tablet	Slow release[b]
Touro A&D	Dartmouth	Capsule	Slow release
Touro EX	Dartmouth	Tablet	Slow release
Touro LA	Dartmouth	Tablet	Slow release
T-Phyl	Purdue Frederick	Tablet	Slow release
Trental	Hoechst Marion Roussel	Tablet	Slow release
Triaminic	Novartis	Tablet	Enteric-coated[b]

Triaminic 12	Novartis	Tablet	Slow release[b]
Triaminic TR	Novartis	Tablet	Multiple compressed tablet[b]
Tri-Phen-Chlor Time Released	Rugby	Tablet	Slow release
Tri-Phen-Mine SR	Zenith Goldline	Tablet	Slow release
Triptone Caplets	Del	Tablet	Slow release
Tuss LA	Hyrex	Tablet	Slow release
Tuss Ornade Spansule	SmithKline Beecham	Capsule	Slow release
Tylenol Extended Relief	McNeil Consumers	Capsule	Slow release
ULR-LA	Geneva	Tablet	Slow release
Ultrase	Scandipharm	Capsule	Enteric-coated[a]
Ultrase MT	Scandipharm	Capsule	Enteric-coated[a]
Uni-Dur	Key	Tablet	Slow release
Uniphyl	Purdue Frederick	Tablet	Slow release
Urocit-K	Mission	Tablet	Wax-coated
Verelan	ESI Lederle	Capsule	Slow release[a]
Volmax	Muro	Tablet	Slow Release
Wellbutrin SR	GlaxoWellcome	Tablet	Anesthetize mucous membrane
Wygesic	Wyeth Ayerst	Tablet	Taste
ZORprin	Knoll	Tablet	Slow release

continued

Table 9-4. *Continued*

Drug Product	Manufacturer	Dosage Forms	Reasons/Comments
Zyban	GlaxoWellcome	Tablet	Slow release
Zymase	Organon Teknika	Capsule	Enteric-coated[a]

Reprinted with permission from Mitchell JF. Oral dosage forms that should not be crushed: 2000 update. Hospital Pharm. 2000;35:553–67.

[a] Capsule may be opened and the contents taken without crushing or chewing; soft food such as applesauce or pudding may facilitate administration; contents may generally be administered via nasogastric tube using an appropriate fluid provided entire contents are washed down the tube.

[b] Liquid dosage forms of the product are available; however, dose, frequency of administration, and manufacturers may differ from that of the solid dosage form.

[c] Antacids and/or milk may prematurely dissolve the coating of the tablet.

[d] Capsule may be opened and the liquid contents removed for administration.

[e] The taste of this product in a liquid form would likely be unacceptable to the patient; administration via nasogastric tube should be acceptable.

[f] Effervescent tablets must be dissolved in the amount of diluent recommended by the manufacturer.

[g] Tablets are made to disintegrate under the tongue.

[h] Tablet is scored and may be broken in half without affecting release characteristics.

[i] Skin contact may enhance tumor production; avoid direct contact.

[j] Discontinued by the manufacturer but supplies may still be available.

Table 9-5. Examples of Monitoring Parameters Pertaining to Major Routes of Administration

Route	Monitoring Parameters	Examples
Oral	Nausea, pain relief, respiratory status	Acetaminophen with codeine
Parenteral	Redness at site, line infiltration	Erythromycin infusion
Topical	Skin irritation, blood pressure	Clonidine transdermal patch

mechanisms. Therefore, sterility is of utmost importance when dealing with parenteral administration.

Medications intended for parenteral administration are most often delivered subcutaneously, intramuscularly, or intravenously. Other, less common methods of administration are also available. The following discussion describes these routes in more detail. Figure 9-1 provides a visual display of these routes.

Subcutaneous and Intramuscular Routes

Subcutaneous and intramuscular routes of parenteral administration are used more often. A subcutaneous (SQ or SC) injection is delivered directly under the skin, between the dermal layer and the muscle. This route results in slow, steady drug absorption. Conversely, an intramuscular (IM) injection delivered directly into the muscle produces more rapid drug absorption.[2] Because both methods involve absorption before systemic circulation of the drug, drug effect is delayed.[3] Not all parenteral drugs may be given by SQ, IM, and intravenous (IV) routes. Table 9-6 lists a few examples.

When using the SQ route of administration, it is important to alleviate patient discomfort whenever possible. A small needle is generally used. Needle sizes are characterized by bore size or gauge (abbreviated as "G") as well as

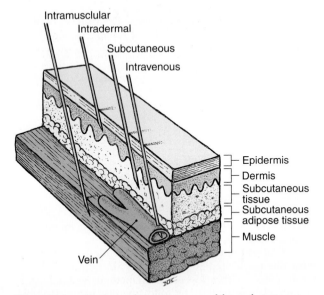

Figure 9-1. Diagram of various routes of drug administration.

length in inches. A smaller-gauge needle is reflected by a larger number size, with gauges ranging from 14–32. The length of the needle reflects the depth of the target tissue, with lengths ranging from 0.5–1.5 inches. A longer needle

Table 9-6. Examples of Drugs Restricted to Specific Routes of Administration

Drug	SQ	IM	IV	Comments
Insulin	Yes	Yes	Yes	Better absorption via SQ
Filgrastim	Yes	No	No	Not given IV
Erythropoetin	Yes	No	Yes	IV also available
Heparin	Yes	No	Yes	Hematomas and pain result from IM
Calcitriol	Yes	No	Yes	IV also available

is used for a deeper injection. For SQ administration, a 24-
to 27-G, 5/8-inch needle is often used. The volume administered should be less than or equal to 1 mL.

IM injections, conversely, require a much longer needle
to access the muscle tissue. Again, patient comfort is of utmost importance. A typical needle used is 21- to 23-G, 1.5
inch.[4] The volume of medication is determined by the age
of the patient and the muscle selected. Table 9-7 specifies
these limitations.

When administering an IM injection, the needle should
enter the muscle at a 90° angle.[5] If the bone is contacted, the
needle should be withdrawn a small distance. Another concern regarding IM administration involves the possibility of
aspiration. This can be avoided by pulling the plunger of
the syringe back slightly, piercing the tissue. If no blood is
present, the needle is not in a vein and the medication may
be administered. Typical rate of IM administration is approximately 1 mL every 10 seconds.[2]

A highly recommended method of IM administration is
the Z track method. Before injection, the skin is displaced
downward approximately 1–2 cm. The injection is then

Table 9-7. **Volume Limitations of Intramuscular Administration**

Muscle Group	Birth–1.5 yr (mL)	1.5–3 yr (mL)	3–6 yr (mL)	6–15 yr (mL)	15 yr to Adult (mL)
Deltoid	Not recommended	Not recommended; if no other sites, 0.5	0.5	0.5	1
Gluteus maximus	Not recommended	Not recommended; if no other sites, 1	1.5	1.5–2	2–2.5
Ventrogluteal	Not recommended	Not recommended; if no other sites, 1	1.5	1.5–2	2–2.5
Vastus lateralis	0.5 to 1	1	1.5	1.5–2	2–2.5

Source: Howry LV, Bindler RM, Tso Y. Pediatric Medications.
Philadelphia, PA: JB Lippincott; 1981:62.

given. After 10 seconds, the needle is removed and the skin is released. The skin movement allows the tissue to close over the site of entry after administration to decrease drug loss. This method decreases pain for the patient as well.[2]

Intradermal Route

Intradermal (ID) injection is a less common method of drug administration. An ID injection is delivered directly under the dermis layer of the skin. ID administration is generally restricted to diagnostic skin testing. A few vaccines may be administered ID as well. To administer an ID injection, a 25-G needle is inserted at a 10–15° angle into the dermis, the layer immediately below the epidermis. The volume administered is restricted to less than 0.5 mL for patient comfort.[2]

IV Administration

Administration of a medication directly into a vein is an intravenous (IV) infusion. Drug administered by rapid infusion will mix with the blood and reach maximum concentration in 4 minutes.[3]

IV administration delivers the medication into the bloodstream through direct push, intermittent, or continuous infusion methods. Direct push administration is a very short infusion, usually lasting a few minutes, with the intent of producing a high drug concentration swiftly. The drug is concentrated, often removed from the vial immediately before administration. Intermittent infusions involve dilute drug solutions, which are given periodically throughout the day. These solutions may be infused over 30 minutes to a few hours. Continuous infusion generally refers to large volume (250–1000 mL) solutions, with or without drug, running IV uninterrupted.[6] Figure 9-2 shows examples of various IV delivery systems available.

Multiple factors influence the most suitable method of infusion for a particular medication. Table 9-8 presents some examples of each method of IV infusion.

Vascular Access

Vascular access for IV infusion is accomplished by using vascular access devices (VADs). Generally, either needles or catheters are used. Needles are placed peripherally and used

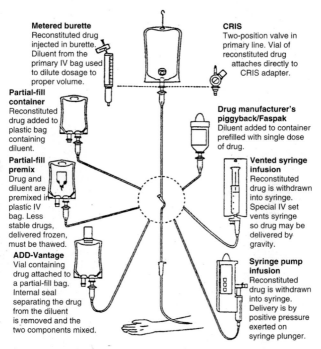

Metered burette
Reconstituted drug injected in burette. Diluent from the primary IV bag used to dilute dosage to proper volume.

Partial-fill container
Reconstituted drug added to plastic bag containing diluent.

Partial-fill premix
Drug and diluent are premixed in plastic IV bag. Less stable drugs, delivered frozen, must be thawed.

ADD-Vantage
Vial containing drug attached to a partial-fill bag. Internal seal separating the drug from the diluent is removed and the two components mixed.

CRIS
Two-position valve in primary line. Vial of reconstituted drug attaches directly to CRIS adapter.

Drug manufacturer's piggyback/Faspak
Diluent added to container prefilled with single dose of drug.

Vented syringe infusion
Reconstituted drug is withdrawn into syringe. Special IV set vents syringe so drug may be delivered by gravity.

Syringe pump infusion
Reconstituted drug is withdrawn into syringe. Delivery is by positive pressure exerted on syringe plunger.

Figure 9-2. Intravenous delivery systems. Reprinted with permission from Pleasants RA. Intravenous Delivery Systems: Overview of Systems and Patient Care Implications. Research Triangle Park, NC: Glaxo, Inc.; 1989.

short term. Catheters provide peripheral or central access and may be used short or long term. Peripheral catheters are placed in the dorsal metacarpal or cephalic vein in the arm, whereas central catheters span a small distance from the skin to the intravascular space. Entrance points for central catheters are usually the subclavian or external jugular vein. This additional distance from the point of entry to placement results in lower infections and longer patency. Figure 9-3 is a diagram depicting catheter locations. Various types of catheters are available, each able to deliver medications and fluids to specific targets. These lines must

Table 9-8. Examples of Various Methods of IV Infusion

Drug	IV Infusion	Concentration	Indication
Epinephrine	Push (1–2 min)	1 mg/mL	Cardiac emergency
Total parenteral nutrition	Continuous	Varies	Nutrition
Sodium chloride	Continuous	0.9%	Hydration
Vancomycin	Intermittent (over 1 hr)	1 g/100 mL	Antibiotic
Fluoruracil	Intermittent (over 15–30 min)	30 mg/mL	Chemotherapy

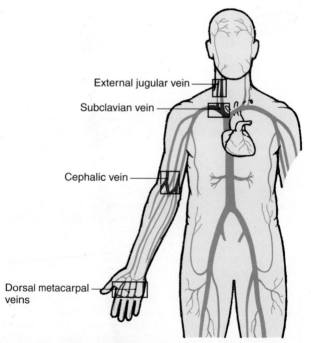

Figure 9-3. Possible catheter access and location.

be flushed with dilute heparin or saline to maintain patency. Frequency of flushing catheters ranges from twice daily to once weekly, and volumes administered range from 5–20 mL. Supplementary information regarding catheters is provided in Table 9-9, and various placements are shown in Figure 9-4.

Extravasation, which is unintentional leakage of IV fluid into interstitial tissue, is a major concern when dealing with

Table 9-9. Issues Relating to Various Types of Catheters

Access	Types	Comments	Use
Peripheral	Needle, butterfly needle, short plastic catheters	Catheters more comfortable than needles; flush every 6–8 hr	Short-term IVs (<60 days)
Central—Nontunneled	Subclavian	Short distance to exit site results in higher risk of infections; flush heparin every 12 hr; single or double lumen	Short-term IVs (<60 days)
Central—tunneled (in-dwelling)	Hickman, Broviac, Corcath, Raaf, Hemed	Inserted centrally (surgically); long distance to exit site, lower infection; flush bi-weekly with heparin when not using daily; single, double, or triple lumen	Long-term IVs (1–2 yr), total parenteral nutrition, Chemotherapy
	Groshong	See above; also contains a three-position valve and closed tip; flush well with saline	Infusions and blood draws

continued

Table 9-9. *Continued*

Access	Types	Comments	Use
Central—PICC	Intrasil, C-PICs, Per-Q-Cath	Inserted peripherally (no surgery); increased phlebitis risk; flush every 12 hr; single or double lumen	Long-term IVs (weeks to months)
Implantable	Port-A-Cath, Infus-A-Port, Medtronic, Cath Link	Implanted SC (surgically— usually chest wall); very low risk of infection; flush monthly	Long-term IVs

Sources: Lindley CM, Deloatch KH. Infusion Technology Manual: A Self-Instructional Approach. Bethesda, MD: ASHP Special Project's Division; 1993: 37–50. LaRocca JC, Otto SF. Mosby's Pocket Guide to Intravenous Therapy. 3rd ed. St. Louis, MO: Mosby; 1997:42–60.

IV administration of particular drugs. Box 9.2 lists drugs considered vesicants by many institutions. Vesicants require close monitoring due to their tendency to produce serious consequences such as necrosis and severe irritation on extravasation.

Unconventional Routes

Available routes for parenteral administration of medications have evolved in recent years. In many cases, the drug can be delivered directly to the target tissue or organ. Table 9-10 describes some of these alternative routes of administration.

Flow Rate

When medications are given by intermittent or continuous infusion, the flow of the solution is regulated. The rate at which the solution is administered to the patient is considered the flow rate. Flow rates vary depending

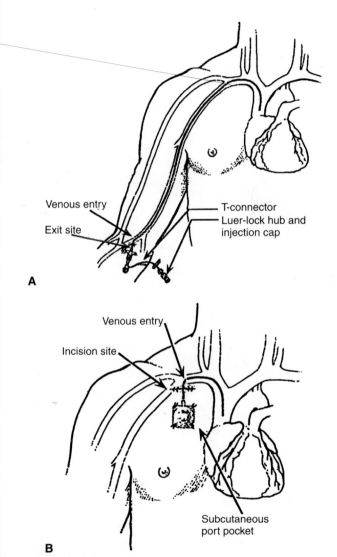

Venous entry

Exit site

T-connector

Luer-lock hub and
injection cap

A

Venous entry

Incision site

Subcutaneous
port pocket

B

Figure 9-4.   Catheter placements. **A**. PICC placement. **B**. SC port implanted in chest wall.

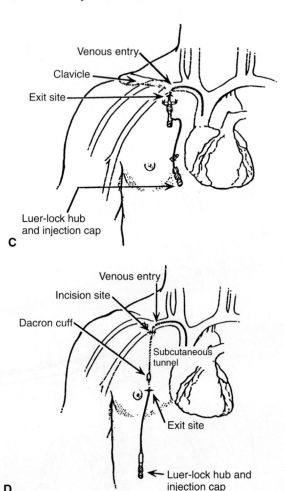

Figure 9-4. *(Continued)* **C.** Nontunneled central venous catheter placement. **D.** Tunneled central venous catheter placement. Adapted with permission from Wickham R. Techniques for long-term venous access. Presented at the Fifth National Conference on Cancer Nursing, ACS, with Association of Pediatric Oncology Nurses and Oncology Nursing Society, September 1987; 1988.

Dactinomycin
  (Actinomycin D)
Daunorubicin
  (Daunomycin)
Doxorubicin
  (Adriamycin)
Epirubicin (Pharmorubin)
Esorubicin
  (4-Deoxyrubicin)
Idarubicin (Idamycin)
Mechlorethamine
(Nitrogen Mustard)

Menogaril (Tomasar)
Mitomycin (Mutamycin)
Piroxantrone (Oxantrazole)
Plicamycin (Mithramycin,
  Mithracin)
Vinblastin (Velban)
Vincristine (Oncovin)
Vindestine (Eldisine)
Vinorelbine (Navelbine)

Sources: Phillips LD. Manual of I.V. Therapeutic. 2nd ed. Philadelphia, PH: FA Davis Company; 1997: 513. LaRocca JC, Otto SF. Mosby's Pocket Guide to Intravenous Therapy. 3rd ed. St. Louis, MO: Mosby; 1997: 252.

Table 9-10.   Examples of Unconventional Routes of Administration

Route	Location	Drug Treatment
Intradermal	Superficial skin layer	Diagnostic test, vaccines
Intraarterial catheter	Hepatic, celiac, or carotid artery	Chemotherapy
Intraosseous needle	Bone marrow	Emergency administration of IV drug
Intraperitoneal catheter	Peritoneal cavity	Chemotherapy
Intraspinal catheter	Epidural or intrathecal	Pain management, chemotherapy
Intraventricular catheter	Lateral ventricle of brain	Chemotherapy, antifungal, antibacterial

Source: West VL. Alternate routes of administration. J Intraven Nurs. 1998;21(4):221–31.

on characteristics of the drug and drug concentration. It is imperative to calculate flow rates correctly to ensure that the medication is not delivered too quickly. Specific information needed to calculate flow rate includes:

➤ Desired rate of infusion (mL/min, mL/hr)
➤ Drug concentration (units/mL, mg/mL, g/mL)
➤ Volume of the bag containing the drug
➤ Set size (the set is the tubing the medication flows through that is connected to the catheter inserted in the patient. It has a roller clamp and drip chamber, which control drug delivery. Set sizes are defined as "drops/mL.")

An example calculation is as follows:

Medication Given IV

Desired Rate to be Infused = 30 mg/min
Drug Concentration Available = 15 mg/mL
Bag Size = 100 mL
Set Size = 20 drops/mL

Concentration and Rate

$$\left(\frac{1 \text{ mL}}{15 \text{ mg}}\right)\left(\frac{30 \text{ mg}}{1 \text{ min}}\right) = 2 \text{ mL/min}$$

IV Set Size

$$\left(\frac{20 \text{ drops}}{1 \text{ mL}}\right)\left(\frac{2 \text{ mL}}{1 \text{ min}}\right) = 40 \text{ drops/min}$$

Rate, Total Volume Available, and Total Running Time

$$\left(\frac{1 \text{ min}}{2 \text{ mL}}\right)(100 \text{ mL}) = 50 \text{ min}$$

The flow rate is the 2 mL/min or 40 drops/min, and the infusion will last 50 minutes.

Pumps or Infusion Controlled Devices

Parenteral infusion flow rates may be controlled by gravity or by an infusion-controlled device (pump).

➤ Gravity (without a controller)

• System based on hydrostatic pressure, controlled by clamps

Table 9-11 Characteristics of Various Infusion Control Devices or Pumps

Pump Type	Mechanism	Comments	Volume	Variance
Gravity Controller—Lifecare 75	Gravity driven	Electronically measures and compensates drip rate; good for nonviscous solutions	No volume limits	5–10%
Positive pressure Peristaltic	Tubing undergoes micropulses or constant massaging; linear or rotary pump	Inexpensive, use special sets to avoid tubing distortion	No volume limits	5–10%
Cassette—Piston Lifecare	Piston actuated	Dual piston available also; special tubing required	50–100 mL	2–5%

continued

Table 9-11 *Continued*

Pump Type	Mechanism	Comments	Volume	Variance
Cassette—Syringe Medifuse, Mini-Infusor	Mechanical or electric	Programmable; special tubing required	≤60 mL	2–5%
Syringe—AS50 Autosyringe	Electric	Programmable; good for slow flow rates, small volumes	≤60 mL	≤2%
Elastomeric—Homepump, Intermate	Nonelectric; constant elastic pressure; flow restricted rate	Limited pump volumes; small and portable; disposable	50–500 mL	10–20%
Vacuum pressure—prime CADI-120	Nonelectric; constant vacuum pressure; flow restricted rate	Specific flow rates; disposable	0.5–200 mL	Not available

Sources: Lindley CM, Deloatch KH. Infusion Technology Manual: A Self-Instructional Approach. Bethesda, MD: ASHP Special Project's Division; 1993;37–50, 82–91. Capes DF, Asiimwe D. Performance of selected flow-restricting infusion devises. AJHSP. 1998;55;351–9. Schleis TG, Tice AD. Selecting infusion devices for use in ambulatory care. Am J Health Syst Pharm. 1996;53:868–77.

- Used for peripheral sites only
- Requires frequent monitoring to check drip rate
- Example: ranitidine 50 mg/50 mL IV every 12 hours

➤ Infusion-controlled device

- Measured by various types of sensors
- Used for central or peripheral infusion
- Programmable, little monitoring
- Example: dopamine 400 mg/500 mL IV start at 2 mcg/kg/min

Multiple forms of infusion-controlled devices are currently available. Recent technology has developed smaller, more accurate devices. Table 9-11 explains in further detail characteristics of each type of device.

As technology continues to increase the availability of more convenient administration devices, the choices will broaden. It is imperative to maintain a working knowledge of this area of pharmacy to provide high quality care to the patient.

References

1. McPherson ML. Don't crush that tablet! Am Pharm. 1994;34:57–8.
2. Workman B. Safe injection techniques. Nurs Stand. 1999;13(39);47–53.
3. Turco SJ. Sterile Dosage Forms: Their Preparation and Clinical Applications. 4th ed. Philadelphia, PA: Lea & Febiger; 1994:7, 105.
4. Lindley CM, Deloatch KH. Infusion Technology Manual: A Self-Instructional Approach. Bethesda, MD: ASHP Special Project's Division; 1993:37–50, 82–91.
5. Burden M. A practical guide to insulin injections. Nurs Stand. 1994;8(29);25–9.
6. Phillips LD. Manual of I.V. Therapeutics. 2nd ed. Philadelphia, PA: FA Davis Company; 1997:199–204, 208–13, 398–420, 513.
7. LaRocca JC, Otto SF. Mosby's Pocket Guide to Intravenous Therapy. 3rd ed. St. Louis, MO: Mosby; 1997:42–60, 252.

8. West VL. Alternate routes of administration. J Intraven Nurs.1998;21(4);221–31.

9. Capes DF, Asiimwe D. Performance of selected flow-restricting infusion devices. AJHSP. 1998;55;351–9.

10. Schleis TG, Tice AD. Selecting infusion devices for use in ambulatory care. Am J Health Syst Pharm. 1996;53:868–77.

Chapter 10

Fluid and Electrolyte Therapy

Ronald L. Sorkness

Fluid and electrolyte therapy requires a careful assessment of a patient's current status and special needs to correct existing imbalances and to prevent new imbalances from developing. This chapter provides an overview of some basic concepts that are central to the design of intravenous (IV) fluid therapy, a review of the clinical assessment of fluid volume status, and the general approach to initiating fluid therapy.

DISTRIBUTION OF BODY WATER

A large portion of total body mass is due to water. The actual percentage is determined by the relative proportions of tissues with high water content (e.g., muscle and organs of the body) versus tissues with low water content (e.g., fat and bone). Figure 10-1 shows total body water as the percent of body weight for healthy males and females with average muscle and fat mass at various ages. Body water is located inside of cells (intracellular fluid [ICF]) and outside of cells (extracellular fluid [ECF]). ECF is divided further into a portion that is circulating in the blood vessels (plasma) and a portion that surrounds the cells outside the blood vessels (interstitial water). As shown in Figure 10-2, ICF comprises approximately two-thirds of total body water, and plasma accounts for approximately one-fourth of ECF, or only about one-twelfth of total body water. Water passes freely across most biologic membranes; thus, the water associated with the ICF, interstitial, and plasma compartments can equilibrate among the compartments. It is the *solute* residing in the various compartments that ultimately determines the distribution of body water among the compartments. Similarly, it is the solute contained in an intravenously administered fluid that determines how that fluid is distributed among the body compartments after equilibration.

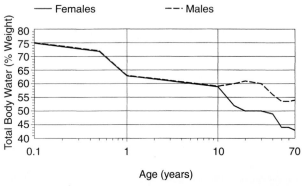

Figure 10-1. Average total body water as a percent of body weight by age and gender. Data from Parker HV et al. Colloquia on ageing. In: Ciba Foundation Colloquia on Ageing (vol. 4). Boston, MA: Little, Brown and Co.; 1958;4.

OSMOLALITY AND FREE WATER

Water and solute are intimately associated with one another by osmolar forces. Water will move across a semipermeable biologic membrane whenever an osmotic gradient exists, or whenever a larger number of particles is dissolved per unit of water on one side of the membrane compared with the other side. That is, if the membrane allows free passage of water but not solute, an osmotic gradient will

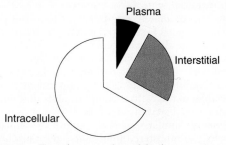

Figure 10-2. Distribution of total body water in an adult male.

cause water to pass toward the side with the greater number of dissolved particles. Eventually the shift of water will dilute the concentration of solute on one side and increase the concentration of solute on the other side of the membrane, so that the osmotic gradient no longer exists. This osmotic equilibration occurs constantly in the body, and osmotic gradients disappear as quickly as they develop. The fluids of all the body compartments, therefore, share a common *osmolality*.

Osmolality is defined as the number of particles dissolved per kilogram of solvent and is expressed as milliosmoles of dissolved particles per kilogram (or liter) of water (mOsm/kg). Note that the "kg" refers to *water* weight, not body weight, and that this unit of measure (i.e., kg) is preferred rather than *liters* of water to avoid confusion with *osmolarity*, which is defined as particles per liter of *solution*. Osmolality is approximately equal to molarity for dilute solutions of non-ionized molecules (e.g., glucose), and it is approximately twice the molarity for dilute solutions of strong monovalent electrolytes (such as sodium chloride). Osmolality can be measured using any of the colligative properties of solutions (osmotic pressure, water vapor pressure, freezing point depression, boiling point elevation). Clinically, osmolality is usually measured by using freezing point depression or vapor pressure. Body fluid osmolality also can be estimated mathematically if the concentrations of the major solutes are known. In plasma, nearly all the osmolality is accounted for by sodium salts, glucose, and urea; thus, if the measurements of serum sodium (in mmol/L), glucose (in mg/dL), and BUN (in mg/dL) are known, the osmolality can be estimated with the following formula:

$$\text{Serum Osmolality} = 2(\text{sodium}) + \text{glucose}/18 + \text{BUN}/2.8$$

Because body fluids are in osmotic equilibrium, the osmolality that is determined from serum should be identical to the osmolalities of interstitial and intracellular fluids at that point in time. The normal range for body fluid osmolality is approximately 280–295 mOsm/kg.

It is important to maintain body fluid osmolality within a narrow range to avoid large changes in cell volume. Because solute within the cells does not change quickly, fluctuations in osmolality result from fluctuations in intracellular water. Thus, cells are shrunken during elevated osmolalities and swollen during reduced osmolalities. Excessive changes in cell volume may alter cell functions or even destroy the cells. Thus, water balance is regulated carefully. Small increases in osmolality create a thirst sensation to encourage water intake and cause release of antidiuretic hormone to promote renal water reabsorption. In contrast, small decreases in osmolality inhibit release of antidiuretic hormone, allowing rapid water excretion into the urine.

These concepts also apply to the fluids used for IV therapy. Fluids that have an osmolality similar to that of body fluids and that have no effect on the volume of cells that are bathed in the fluids, are called *isotonic*. Although some of the commonly used IV fluids are isotonic, most have osmolalities well outside the physiologic range. Fluids having an osmolality of about 150–500 mOsm/kg, however, may be administered safely into peripheral veins. Solutions of even higher osmolalities may be infused into large central veins, due to the rapid dilution of the IV fluid by the volume of blood flowing through the veins. Table 10-1 shows some commonly used IV fluids, their solute content, and their calculated osmolalities. Dextrose (glucose) and sodium chloride are the solutes used for the basic solutions. Dextrose is metabolized quickly; therefore, it is a solute that can provide osmolality for the solution but it does not cause a net increase in body solute (i.e., administering 5% dextrose solution is physiologically equivalent to giving water without solute or *free water*). IV solutions can be thought of as combinations of isotonic fluid and free water, using combined sodium and potassium salts of 150 mEq/l as the definition of the isotonic portion of each. Table 10-1 also shows the free water equivalent volume for each of the solutions.

DISTRIBUTION OF BODY SOLUTE

In contrast to water, solutes (particularly ions and large molecules) do not pass through cell membranes readily, and concentration gradients for some ions are carefully regulated between ICF and ECF. Table 10-2 contrasts ICF and plasma concentrations for sodium, potassium, and

Table 10-1. Contents of Common IV Fluids

Solution	Osmolality (mOsm/kg, calculated)	Free Water (mL)	Dextrose (g)	Na$^+$ (mEq)	Cl$^-$ (mEq)	K$^+$ (mEq)	Ca^{++} (mEq)	Lactate$^-$ (mEq)
5% Dextrose	278	1000	50					
0.9% NaCl	308	0		154	154			
0.45% NaCl	154	487		77	77			
5% Dextrose/ 0.2%NaCl	355	773	50	34	34			
5% Dextrose/ 0.45%NaCl	432	487	50	77	77			
Lactated Ringer's	274	107		130	109	4	3	28

Table 10-2. Comparison of Ions in Intracellular Fluid and Plasma

Ion	Plasma (mEq/L)	Intracellular (mEq/L)
Sodium	142	12
Potassium	4.4	140
Chloride	104	4

chloride. Calcium, magnesium, and phosphate reside primarily in the intracellular environment, similar to potassium. However, sodium is the predominant cation of the ECF. Sodium is also the predominant factor in determining ECF volume. The kidneys regulate ECF volume by regulating sodium reabsorption, in part via the renin/angiotensin/aldosterone mechanism. Therapeutically, ECF volume can be altered by the amount of sodium that is included in the IV fluids. As mentioned previously, intracellular solute is relatively constant, so that intracellular volume is affected mainly by changes in osmolality. The following basic rule should be kept in mind: *ECF volume is regulated by sodium balance and ICF volume is regulated by free water balance.*

In ECF, differences between the interstitial and plasma (intravascular) components are more subtle. There is free equilibrium between plasma and interstitial fluid for not only water, but also all the ions and small molecules. Only large macromolecules (e.g., proteins) have restricted permeability across the capillary wall, and thus the principal difference in solute between plasma and interstitial fluid is a small protein concentration gradient. This gradient is important, however, in that it creates a small oncotic force that is responsible for preventing leakage of plasma out of the circulation and into the interstitial areas. Thus, plasma macromolecules help determine the equilibrium and distribution of ECF fluid between the intravascular and interstitial areas.

Figure 10-3 illustrates how the solute content of IV fluid determines its distribution in the body after administration. Free water (from 5% dextrose solution) distributes throughout the body in proportion to the pretreatment compartment volumes. In contrast, 0.9% NaCl, with no free water,

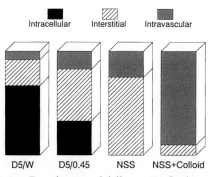

Figure 10-3. Distribution of different IV fluid types among intracellular, interstitial, and intravascular compartments. *D5/W*, 5% dextrose in water; *D5/0.45*, 5% dextrose and 0.45% NaCl; *NSS*, normal saline solution (0.9% NaCl).

stays entirely in ECF along with its sodium, distributing proportionally between plasma and interstitial compartments. Fluids with both free water and sodium distribute as predicted from their isotonic and free water components, and the addition of macromolecules (*colloid*) tips the ECF distribution toward the intravascular compartment.

CLINICAL ASSESSMENT OF FLUID STATUS

Most of the information that is useful for assessing a patient's fluid and electrolyte status, and for monitoring fluid therapy, can be obtained at the bedside and from a few routine laboratory tests. Because ICF and ECF compartments have different regulatory mechanisms and different pathology associated with fluid imbalances, one needs to evaluate each compartment. Additionally, when the extracellular compartment is considered, one needs to evaluate both the circulating (intravascular) and the extravascular (interstitial) portions. Box 10.1 summarizes physical findings and laboratory variables that are used for clinical assessment of fluid and electrolyte status.

Box 10.1   Clinical Assessment and Monitoring of Fluid
            Status

Total Body Water
  Body weight changes unrelated to changes in lean
    body mass
  Intake and output records

Extracellular Fluid Volume
  Extravascular ECF
    Signs of increased interstitial fluid:
      Peripheral or sacral edema
      Pulmonary congestion: crackles, radiograph,
        changes dyspnea, tachycardia, hypoxia
      Ascites or other sequestered (third space) fluid
    Signs of decreased interstitial fluid:
      Skin and mucous membranes: dry, decreased
        turgor
      Sunken eyes; depressed fontanelle in infants

  Intravascular volume
    Urine output: a sensitive indicator of intravascular
      volume if no organ failures are present
    Signs of renal hypoperfusion:
      Oliguria
      Urine chemistry: Na <15 mMol/l, specific grav-
        ity >1.015, osmolality >500 mOsm/kg
      Serum chemistry: increased BUN: creatinine ratio
        to >20
    Signs of peripheral hypoperfusion:
      Increased capillary refill time (e.g., in nailbeds)
      Temperature and color changes in extremities
      Decreased level of consciousness
    Orthostatic changes in pulse and blood pressure
    Signs of increased circulatory volume:
      S-3 heart sound
      Increased CVP, jugular venous distension, hepa-
        tojugular reflux

Box 10.1   *Continued*
___

Changes in blood hematocrit and hemoglobin with changes in intravascular water volume

Swan-Ganz catheter readings—CVP, occlusion pressure, cardiac output

Intracellular Volume
Serum osmolality
Thirst sensation
Mental status changes

TOTAL BODY WATER

Total body water is an indicator of the global balance of fluid. Daily changes in total body water are assessed with body weight and with intake and output (I&O) records. Body weight generally is the more accurate measure, although changes in lean body mass due to caloric imbalances need to be considered. I&O records should include all fluid intake, including food and IV medications, and all output, including urine, stool, and surgical drainage. It is difficult to estimate water content of food and stool, and I&O records do not quantify internal gains of water from metabolism (*water of oxidation*) or losses of water by evaporation (*insensible losses*). However, in acutely ill patients who are not eating solid food, who are not making significant stool, and who have a urinary catheter allowing accurate collection, the I&O records are extremely valuable for monitoring total body water balance.

Extravascular ECF

Extravascular ECF (interstitial fluid), the fluid that surrounds the capillaries and the individual cells of the tissues, normally makes up about 75% of the ECF volume. When total body fluid balance fluctuates (e.g., with dietary intake or with the menstrual cycle), most of the water volume changes occur in the extravascular ECF. Adults can increase this volume by about 2–3 liters before it becomes apparent; after that, edema begins to form at the parts of the body that are lowest with respect to gravity (e.g., ankles in an ambulatory person and at the sacrum of a person in a supine position). This is called *dependent* edema. Interstitial fluid also accumulates as sequestered fluid (third spacing) when the normal intravascular/interstitial equilibrium is upset (e.g., local edema associated with inflammatory conditions or the ascites associated with cirrhosis of the liver). When downward pressure is applied with a finger on the skin for a few seconds, the formation of a little pit in the surface indicates interstitial edema *(pitting edema)*. When interstitial fluid accumulates in the lungs, it may result in crackles that may be heard with a stethoscope. Fluid accumulation in the lungs also can be manifested as difficulty in breathing (dyspnea on exertion, orthopnea, shortness of breath reported by the patient), congestion appearing on a chest radiograph, or as compromised gas exchange in severe cases. Decreased interstitial fluid volume may cause dryness of the skin and mucous membranes and decreased skin turgor. Turgor is assessed by gently pinching a bit of skin between the fingers; instead of popping back normally on release, it exhibits *tenting* when turgor (or water content) is decreased. The eyes of a person with decreased interstitial fluid may appear sunken, and the tongue may be dry and furrowed. Severely fluid-depleted infants may exhibit a concavity over the fontanelle.

Intravascular Volume

Although plasma makes up less than 10% of total body water, it is critically important to maintaining circulation. Consequently, the assessment of intravascular volume receives highest priority in the evaluation of a patient's fluid status.

The kidney normally receives a generous proportion of cardiac output, and renal perfusion is a key factor in the regulation of ECF volume. When renal perfusion decreases, the kidney responds by reabsorbing more sodium, water, and urea from the filtrate. Conversely, when renal perfusion increases, filtrate volume increases, reabsorption mechanisms are blunted, and urine volume is increased. Renal perfusion is related to circulating volume and cardiac output. Thus, under normal circumstances, urine output and urine concentration are good indicators of circulating volume. Average urine output is approximately 1500 ml/day. Urine output <500 ml/day is called *oliguria*. When oliguria is caused by decreased renal perfusion, it is called *prerenal oliguria*. Prerenal oliguria is characterized by low urine output, concentrated urine (specific gravity >1.015 g/ml and osmolality >500 mOsm/kg), and a disproportional increase in plasma urea concentration (BUN:creatinine ratio >20 instead of the usual 10). Urine output, however, is not a good indicator of circulating volume in the presence of abnormal kidney function, heart failure (decreased cardiac output), or liver disease (redistribution of cardiac output).

Reduced circulating volume also may cause signs of hypoperfusion in other parts of the body. *Capillary refill time*, measured as the time necessary for a fingernail bed blanched by pressure to return to its pink color on release of the pressure, may increase from a typical time of <1 sec to ≥2 sec. The vasoconstrictive response to hypovolemia may decrease circulation of the extremities resulting in decreased surface temperature. When severe, the extremities may have a mottled or cyanotic coloring, and the skin surface may have evidence of piloerection and cold sweat. Hypoperfusion to the brain may result in mental status changes (e.g., confusion, agitation, coma).

Orthostatic changes in pulse and blood pressure may detect depletion of circulating volume in its early stages. The pulse and blood pressure of a normovolemic individual are not altered when the individual arises from a supine to a standing position. However, as circulating volume decreases, the pulse rate will increase on standing, and with further volume depletion the blood pressure will decrease as well. Patients with severely depleted circulating blood volume have elevated pulse and decreased BP even in the supine position.

An increase in circulating volume may be detected by pressure changes on the venous side of the circulation. The central venous pressure (CVP) can be measured directly with a catheter advanced into the right atrium of the heart. It can also be estimated from the level of the column of blood in the jugular veins in the neck (*jugular venous distension*). Increased venous blood volume may also be detected by eliciting jugular venous distension with manual compression of the liver (*hepatojugular reflux*). Increased blood volume also may make an S-3 heart sound become audible at the beginning of diastole.

The hematocrit (HCT) and hemoglobin (HGB) can reflect changes in plasma volume. For example, a loss of plasma volume resulting in a 20% reduction in total blood volume would cause a 20% increase in blood HGB concentration. The HCT and HGB values, however, are of limited usefulness if baseline values were not obtained before the patient's change in plasma volume or if the patient has experienced any blood loss.

The placement of a Swan-Ganz catheter into the pulmonary artery can provide valuable information when the circulating volume needs to be maintained within a narrow range. This catheter measures both CVP and pulmonary artery pressure. When the balloon at the tip is inflated, the catheter measures *wedge* or *occlusion* pressure, which is an approximation of the pressure that fills the left ventricle (*preload* pressure). In addition, the catheter has a temperature sensor that allows measurement of cardiac output by a thermodilution method.

Intracellular Volume

Intracellular volume cannot be measured with bedside techniques or routine clinical laboratory tests. However, as discussed previously, intracellular volume may change with fluctuations in osmolality due to a relatively constant amount of intracellular solute. Therefore, an increase of ICF volume can be assumed when the serum osmolality is low. In contrast, a high serum osmolality, and its associated sensation of thirst, generally indicate a decrease in ICF volume. Mental status changes may indicate that dangerous fluctuations in ICF are occurring, and might also reflect excessive swelling or shrinking of brain tissue within the rigid cranial structure.

GENERAL APPROACH TO IV FLUID THERAPY

IV fluid therapy is initiated based on estimates of the requirements of an individual patient and then adjusted as

---

Box 10.2   Design of Initial Fluid Therapy

---

(1)   Restore circulating volume if decreased
(2)   If severe imbalances are present, treat until out of danger range
(3)   Replace anticipated losses of water and electrolytes
(4)   Correct remaining imbalances gradually

---

necessary during the course of therapy. Adjustments are based on repeated assessments of the patient's fluid status. Box 10.2 summarizes the decision-making process used to design initial fluid therapy.

Circulating Volume

Circulating volume is a high priority of therapy, and hypovolemia with reduced tissue perfusion must be recognized and treated immediately. Solutions having little or no free water, such as 0.9% NaCl or Lactated Ringer's solution, are selected for this purpose, as they remain entirely in the ECF. In addition, red blood cells may be administered if the patient's HCT is less than approximately 30% and in some circumstances colloid solutions such as albumin or hetastarch may be administered to expand the intravascular volume more selectively.

Extreme Imbalances

Extreme imbalances in individual ions, osmolality, or acid-base may have profound physiologic and even life-threatening effects. Although such imbalances need to be addressed immediately, it is usually neither necessary nor desirable to correct them rapidly back to the normal range. The most prudent approach is to treat a severe imbalance immediately, but only to the extent necessary to move the imbalance out of the danger range. The remaining correction to the normal range may be accomplished gradually over 1–2 days. The reader is referred to the Suggested Readings for details regarding management of severe electrolyte, osmolar, and acid-base imbalances.

Replacement of Anticipated Losses

Replacement of anticipated losses of water and electrolytes is the central issue of fluid therapy after the urgent issues have been managed. In an adult patient with no preexisting imbalances, abnormal losses, or organ failures who is being supported on IV fluids for a few days, any regimen that provides some sodium, some potassium, and some free water is adequate. A commonly used fluid in this situation for an adult is 5% dextrose/0.2% NaCl with KCl 20 mEq/liter infused at 100 ml/hr. It is useful to keep this regimen in mind as a reference point from which adjustments may be made for deviations from this uncomplicated type of patient.

Adjustments to sodium intake are directed at the need for adjustments to ECF and intravascular fluid volumes. Losses of ECF volume via gastrointestinal losses, diuresis, excessive sweating, or wound drainage require replacement of both sodium and water if depletion of ECF volume is to be avoided. In contrast, sodium intake should be decreased when reduction of ECF volume is a therapeutic goal (e.g., edematous states such as congestive heart failure, liver disease, and nephrotic syndrome). A serum sodium concentration outside its normal range usually indicates an imbalance of *free water*, but by itself, the serum sodium concentration yields no information regarding sodium balance in the body. This is why ECF volume, and not the serum sodium concentration, is used as the guide for sodium balance.

Several common clinical conditions may increase daily potassium losses and require additional potassium replacement. Gastrointestinal fluids typically are potassium-rich compared with ECF; thus, gastrointestinal losses may tend to deplete potassium. Renal losses of potassium may occur with diuresis (drug-induced or osmotic), high-aldosterone conditions (congestive heart failure, liver disease), high doses of penicillin derivatives, alkaloses, and some renal tubular disorders. Potassium excretion by the kidneys is reduced in renal and adrenal insufficiencies. Drug therapy with potassium-sparing diuretics, angiotensin-converting enzyme inhibitors, trimethoprim, or heparin also can reduce potassium excretion. (Other than severe renal insufficiency, however, these factors usually do not necessitate reduction of potassium intake below normal maintenance.)

Free water losses are increased by conditions that enhance evaporative losses, such as a dry environment or a fever (about 13% increase in water losses for each degree Celsius increase in average body temperature). Diabetes insipidus, the failure of free water reabsorption by the kidneys due to lack of antidiuretic hormone or renal tubular defect, may result in massive free water losses that require careful replacement. Free water also is lost during diuresis or diarrhea involving osmotic substances (endogenous or ingested solutes). In general, losses due to these conditions may be replaced using fluids that are half free water (e.g., 5% dextrose/0.45% NaCl). In contrast, free water intake may need to be restricted for conditions in which renal free water excretion is limited by the presence of excess antidiuretic hormone (i.e., syndrome of inappropriate antidiuretic hormone).

Chloride also is an important ion for IV fluid therapy, and it is the usual salt used for sodium and potassium administration. Chloride replacement is particularly important in patients with losses of chloride-rich gastric secretions and in patients at risk for or having metabolic alkalosis. In contrast, nonchloride anions such as acetate, lactate, or bicarbonate may be substituted in conditions involving abnormal losses of bicarbonate (e.g., diarrhea, enterocutaneous fistulas, renal tubular acidosis).

Calcium, phosphate, and magnesium ions are usually not included in short-term IV replacement fluids, but need to be added to the regimen if IV therapy continues more than a few days. Phosphate and magnesium replacement may be necessary immediately if depletion of these ions is likely, as in malnourished or alcoholic patients or in patients with osmotic diuresis or diarrhea.

In summary, IV therapy consists of first attending to urgent imbalances of fluid compartment volumes and ion concentrations, and then designing a maintenance regimen that corrects remaining imbalances and replaces on-going losses. In a patient with normal daily turnover and healthy renal function, maintenance therapy need not be extensively individualized because the patient will keep everything in balance with normal physiologic homeostatic mechanisms. However, in patients with existing imbalances, organ failures, or abnormal losses that vary from hour to hour, IV therapy requires frequent reassessments and readjustments to achieve the therapeutic goal of optimal fluid and electrolyte balance. The concepts of body fluid chemistry and the methods of clinical assessment of fluid status that are outlined in this chapter should provide the clinician with the basic tools necessary to design fluid therapy for a patient.

Suggested Readings

Adrogue HJ, Madias NE. Management of life-threatening acid-base disorders. N Engl J Med. 1998;138:26–34,107–11.

Edelson GW, Kleerekoper M. Hypercalcemic crisis. Med Clin North Am. 1995;79:79–92.

Hellerstein S. Fluid and electrolytes: clinical aspects. Pediatr Rev. 1993;14:103–15.

Kitabchi AE, Wall BM. Diabetic ketoacidosis. Med Clin North Am. 1995;79:9–37.

Knochel JP. The pathophysiology and clinical characteristics of severe hypophosphatemia. Arch Intern Med. 1977;137:203–20.

Leier CV, Cas LD, Metra M. Clinical relevance and management of the major electrolyte abnormalities in congestive heart failure: hyponatremia, hypokalemia, and hypomagnesemia. Am Heart J. 1994;128:564–74.

Lorber D. Nonketotic hypertonicity in diabetes mellitus. Med Clin North Am. 1995;79:39–52.

McLean RM. Magnesium and its therapeutic uses: a review. Am J Med. 1994;96:63–76.

Oh MS, Kim H-J, Carroll HJ. Recommendations for treatment of symptomatic hyponatremia. Nephron. 1995;70:143–50.

Reber PM, Heath H. Hypocalcemic emergencies. Med Clin North Am. 1995;79:93–106.

Rose BD. Clinical Physiology of Acid-Base and Electrolyte Disorders. 4th ed. New York, NY: McGraw-Hill; 1994.

Saggar-Malik AK, Cappuccio FP. Potassium supplements and potassium-sparing diuretics. A review and guide to appropriate use. Drugs. 1993;46:986–1008.

Secki JR, Dunger DB. Diabetes insipidus. Current treatment recommendations. Drugs. 1992;44:216–24.

Sica DA, Gehr TWB. Diuretic combinations in refractory oedema states. Pharmacokinetic-pharmacodynamic relationships. Clin Pharmacokinet. 1996;30:229–49.

Chapter 11

Enteral Nutrition

Timothy D. Wolf

Enteral nutrition is a method of providing nutritional support to patients with normal gastrointestinal (GI) function who are unable to eat to meet metabolic demands. With the development of enteral formulas appropriate for a variety of disease states, nutrition delivery can be provided to the GI tract via artificial means. Clinical data studied after severe injury have shown that delivery of nutrition via the GI tract can reduce sepsis in critically injured patients.[1] As a means of nutritional support, enteral nutrition is preferred over parenteral nutrition because it is safe, effective, and economical for patients. It avoids the potential complications of parenteral therapy associated with central venous catheter insertion (e.g., catheter sepsis, pneumothorax, and catheter embolus). Administered by tube or by mouth, enteral products can serve as the sole source of nutritional support, as a dietary supplement to oral intake, or as an adjunct during transition from parenteral to oral feedings. For cases in which the enteral route for nutritional support is not viable, the reader is referred to Chapter 12, "Parenteral Nutrition." Calculations of adult nutritional requirements are presented in the that chapter.

The current chapter provides a basic understanding and appreciation of the various types of enteral products and pediatric formulas available. Approaches for administering and monitoring the products to ensure efficacy and minimize toxicity or interactions are highlighted. (See Chapter 12, "Parenteral Nutrition," for a detailed discussion of nutrition calculations.)

NUTRITIONAL TERMS

A wide variety of dietary terms are used to describe nutrition plans for patients. Some of the more common terms are listed below.

➤ *Clear Liquid Diet.* A clear liquid diet may be used before and after operative procedures, before many diagnostic tests, and during acute illness. It should only be used for a brief period in conditions requiring easily digestible, easily consumable nourishment. Clear liquid diets are low in irritants and contain foods that are liquid at room and body temperature.

➤ *General Diet.* A general diet provides various nutrients essential to the body for maintenance, repair, growth, and development. It is used for all patients not requiring restrictions, modifications, or special additions to their dietary regimen. A general diet includes milk and milk products, meat and meat substitutes, bread and cereal products, fruits and vegetables, saturated and unsaturated fats, and desserts.

➤ *High-Fiber Diet.* The high-fiber diet is designed to decrease transit time through the intestine, increase stool volume, and decrease intraluminal pressure. It may be prescribed for patients with constipation, hemorrhoids, diverticulosis, or irritable bowel syndrome. A high-fiber diet contains a minimum of 7 g crude fiber. Adequate fluid intake is critical to prevent constipation and bowel obstruction.

➤ *Low-Cholesterol Diet.* This diet limits the cholesterol intake to ≤300 mg/day; total fat should not represent more than 30% of the total daily caloric intake. It contains equal amounts of saturated, monounsaturated, and polyunsaturated fats. The calories provided are aimed at maintaining an ideal weight.

➤ *Low-Sodium Diet.* A low sodium diet is indicated in congestive heart failure (CHF), hypertension, liver cirrhosis, some renal diseases, and following the administration of sodium-retaining hormones or drugs (e.g., adrenocortical steroids). The various amounts of sodium per day that often are representative of a low-sodium diet are as follows: no added salt (NAS) (150–200 mEq); 90 mEq; 45 mEq; 22 mEq; and 11 mEq of salt per day.

➤ *ADA Diet.* This is a diet based on the American Diabetes Association (ADA) guidelines, which attempt to achieve control of blood glucose concentration and blood lipid levels. It provides adequate nutrition for growth and allows achievement and/or maintenance of reasonable weight to delay or prevent the complications associated with diabetes. Guidelines are available for insulin-dependent diabetes mellitus (IDDM), non–insulin-dependent diabetes mellitus (NIDDM), and diabetes during pregnancy.

➤ *Low-Carbohydrate, High-Protein, High-Fat Diet.* This diet is designed for patients recovering from a recent gastrectomy or who have developed a dumping syndrome. It is intended to prevent a hyperosmolar condition from developing in the proximal jejunum following gastrectomy. It is also used for patients who need to provide a gradual release of glucose into the bloodstream, (e.g., in the treatment of hypoglycemia).

➤ *Low- to Moderate-Protein Diets.* These diets minimize the accumulation of nitrogenous waste products (i.e., urea, uric acid, creatinine, organic acids, ammonia) when used in the treatment of hepatic disorders or in acute or chronic renal failure. Protein intake is approximately 0.4–1.2 g/kg ideal body weight (IBW) or a total of 20 to 60 g/day.

➤ *High-Protein Diets.* These diets are used during stress or trauma (e.g., surgery, burns, cirrhosis, infection, malnutrition, extreme heat or cold) or as replacement therapy for protein losses due to peritoneal dialysis or protein-losing enteropathy. These diets provide 1.5–2.0 g/kg IBW or 90–150 g/day of protein.

INDICATIONS/ CONTRAINDICATIONS FOR ENTERAL NUTRITION SUPPORT[2]

In general, enteral products are selected after a thorough and complete assessment of the patient's digestive/absorptive state and/or fluid and electrolyte demands. Beginning enteral feeds within 24–48 hours after severe injury has positive effects, whereas postponing it for 4–5 days may be too late to achieve reduced infectious complications. In addition, it is important to establish the delivery route (i.e., nasogastric [placed from the nose into the stomach], gastrostomy [stoma created from the abdominal wall into the stomach], or jejunostomy [stoma created from the abdominal wall into the jejunum for long-term postpyloric lateral feedings]), which is dependent on the patient's clinical condition. Nasogastric tubes are used in patients with a low risk of aspiration and a functional GI tract. The gastrostomy tube is preferred for long-term enteral access because of the ability to bolus their feedings and patient comfort. Needle catheter jejunostomy is attractive for short-term use of 3–4 weeks. These tubes are usually subject to a higher frequency of clogging and catheter kinking. A more permanent postpyloric access is the Witzel jejunostomy catheter. It is easier to administer both tube feedings and medications through these large-bore rubber tubes. Box 11.1 lists typi-

---

Box 11.1   Typical Indications and Contraindications of Enteral Nutrition

Indications	Contraindications
Carcinoma of the head and neck	Paralytic ileus
Radical surgery to the upper GI tract, oral pharynx, and upper respiratory tract	Failure to meet nutritional needs on a properly managed trial of enteral nutrition
Endotracheal intubation	Peritonitis
Esophageal stricture	Small bowel or gastric obstruction
Depressed mental status, anorexia nervosa	Abdominal distention
Swallowing difficulties/ dysphagia	Severe malabsorption
Paralysis	GI hemorrhage
Correction of malnutrition secondary to chronic disease (i.e., ulcerative colitis, Crohn's disease)	Enteral therapy associated with intractable diarrhea
When oral intake alone does not meet calorie protein needs	Intestinal ischemia
Hypermetabolic states, major body burns, and trauma	Pancreatitis
Chemotherapy	
Radiotherapy	
Geriatic patients	
Failure to thrive	

cal indications and contraindications for use of enteral nutrition.

PROFILE OF ENTERAL PRODUCTS

Commonly available enteral product formulas are described in Table 11.1. These products can further be categorized into the following groups according to ADA criteria:

➤ Standard oral supplements are most commonly used as tube feedings, are lactose-free, and are generally well tolerated by most patients. They contain 50–55% carbohydrates, 15–20% protein, and 30% fat. The caloric density is 1 cal/mL or greater, and the osmolality can be isotonic between 280 and 350 mOsm/L to hypertonic.

➤ Isotonic formulas are indicated for patients with normal gut function or when the GI tract has been at rest for more than 3 days. Fat calories are usually 50% of the formula as medium chain triglycerides, with the remaining percentage composed of corn and soy oils. The electrolyte composition of isotonic formulas is moderate to enhance flexibility of use, especially in patients with electrolyte imbalances.

➤ High-calorie/high-protein formulas are indicated for use in trauma, surgery, thermal injury, severe hypermetabolic states, multiple fractures, volume restrictions, and sensitivity. Like standard oral supplements, these formulations are lactose-free.

➤ Partially hydrolyzed peptide formulas are indicated for patients with protein or fat maldigestion/malabsorption (e.g., Crohn's disease, cystic fibrosis, fistulas, short-bowel syndrome) or during transition from parenteral to enteral feedings. The protein source is composed of essential amino acids that promote rapid and uniform nitrogen transport and absorption.

➤ High-nitrogen, partially hydrolyzed formulas are indicated for patients with extensive trauma, thermal injury, or hypercatabolic states when digestive and absorptive capacity may be marginal.

Table 11-1. Enteral Products Profile

Products	Na mmol/L (mg)	K mmol/L (mg)	Protein (g)	Fat (g)	Carbohydrate (g)	Water (mL)	Non-Protein Calorie: N ratio	Osmolality mOsm/kg (H$_2$O)	Calories (kcal/mL)
Standard Oral Supplements									
Ensure	36.8 (845)	40 (1564)	37.2	25.4	166	833	153:1	555	1.06
Boost	24 (550)	43 (1690)	43	17	171	840	125:1	590	1
Resource Liquid Nutrition	36.7 (845)	40 (1561)	37.2	37.2	145	823	153:1	430	1.06
Carnation Instant Breakfast	45.3	—	62.4	37.5	142	—	89:1	700	1.06
Attain	35	41	40	35	135	—	134:1	300	1
Isotonic Formulas									
Osmolite	27.6 (640)	26.1 (1020)	37.2	34.7	151.1	841	153:1	300	1.06
Isocal	23 (530)	34 (1320)	34	44	133	840	167:1	270	1.06
Nutren	27.1	32	40	38	127	860	134:1	300	1
High-Calorie/High-Protein Formulas									
Ensure Plus HN	51.3 (1180)	46.6 (1820)	62.6	50	200	769	125:1	650	1.5
Travasorb MCT Diet	15.2 (350)	26 (1000)	49.6	33	122.8	—	100:1	250	1
Boost Plus	37 (850)	38 (1480)	61	57	190	780	134:1	670	1.52
Reabilan HN Diet	(762)	(1250)	58	54	158	810	117:1	490	1.33
Partially Hydrolyzed peptide Formulas									
Travasorb HN Diet	40.1 (922)	30 (1171)	45	13.5	175	—	114:1	560	1
Vital HN	24.6 (566)	35.8 (1400)	41.7	10.8	185	867	125:1	500	1
Criticare HN	27 (630)	34 (1310)	38	5.3	220	850	149:1	650	1.06
Renal Failure									
Renalcal Nepro Diet	36.7 (845)	27.1 (1060)	70	95.6	222.3	699	154:1	665	2.0
			34	82	290	700	338:1	600	2.0
Amin-Aid	(<173)	—	19	46	365	740	800:1	700	2.0

Hepatic Failure									
Nutri Hep Diet	14 (319)	34 (1320)	40	21	290	760	209:1	690	1.5
Hepatic-Aid II	15 (<345)	6 (230)	44	36	168	740	148:1	560	1.2
High Nitrogen-Partially Hydrolyzed Formula									
Isotein IN	27 (620)	27.4 (1070)	67.8	33.9	156	652	86.1	300	1.2
Elemental Formula (Free Amino Acids)									
Tolerex	20.4 (468)	30 (1169)	20.6	1.4	231	860	284:1	550	1
Vivonex T.E.N.	20 (460)	20 (782)	38.2	2.8	206	845	149:1	630	1
Vivonex Plus	(610)	(1100)	45	6.7	190	850	115:1	650	1.0
Optimental	46 (1060)	45 (1760)	51.3	28.4	138.5	835	97:1	540	1.0
Trauma/Stress									
Impact	48 (1100)	36 (1400)	56	28	130	850	71:1	375	1.0
Immun-Aid	25 (575)	27 (1055)	80	22	120	820	53:1	460	1.0
Isotein HN (per 87 g packet)	(183)	(317)	20	10	46.7	—	86:1	300	1.2
Replete	38.1 (876)	38.5 (1500)	62.5	34	113	840	75:1	300	1.0
Traumacal	51 (1180)	36 (1390)	82	68	142	780	91:1	560	1.5
Promote	43.5 (1000)	50.6 (1980)	62.5	26.0	130	837	75:1	340	1.0
Perative	45.2 (1040)	44.2 (1730)	66.6	37.4	177.2	789	97:1	385	1.3
Protain XL	(920)	(1760)	57	30	129	830	—	340	1.0
Pulmonary Disease									
Nutrivent	51 (1170)	48 (1872)	67	94	100	780	116:1	330	1.5
Pulmocare	57 (1310)	44.2 (1730)	62	93	105	790	125:1	475	1.5
Respalor	55 (1270)	38 (1480)	76	71	148	770	102:1	580	1.52
Elemental Diet Formula									
Peptamen Diet	(560)	(1500)	40	39	127	850	131:1	270–380	1.0
Reabilan Diet	(700)	(1250)	31.5	40.5	131.5	850	175:1	350	1.0
Alitra Q	(1000)	(1200)	52.5	15.5	165	850	94:1	575	1.0
Sando Source Peptide	(1200)	(1600)	50	17	160	840	100:1	490	1.0

continued

Table 11-1. Continued

Products	Na mmol/L (mg)	K mmol/L (mg)	Protein (g)	Fat (g)	Carbohydrate (g)	Water (mL)	Non-Protein Calorie: N ratio	Osmolality mOsm/kg (H₂O)	Calories (kcal/mL)
Fiber Containing Formulas									
Jevity	40.4 (930)	40.3 (1570)	44.4	34.7	154.7	835	125:1	300	1.06
ProBalance Diet	(636)	(1300)	54	40	156	820	114:1	350–450	1.2
Ultracal	(877)	(1519)	44	45	123	850	128:1	310	1.06
Fiber Source	(917)	(1500)	43	41	170	820	151:1	390	1.2
High Fat, Low Carbohydrates Formula									
Pulmocare	57 (1310)	50.1 (1960)	62.6	92.1	106	785	125:1	475	1.5
Modular Components									
Polycose									23 kcal/tbsp
Medium Chain Triglyceride (MCT) Oil									7.7
Propac			1 pkt = 15 g						1 pkt = 78 kcal
Promod	0.6/6.6 kg	0.67/6.6 kg	5/6.6 g						28 kcal/6.6 g
Lipomul									6
Mirofipid									4.5
Moducal					0.95/g				3.8/kg
Low Calorie Formula Diets									
Medifast 70			70 g/500 cal						
Optifast 70			70 g/500 cal						

➤ Elemental formulas are indicated for maldigestion, mal-absorption, and protein restriction in patients with liver or renal disease. These products are low in fat; therefore, supplementation with purified unsaturated fatty acids (PUFA) is necessary for long-term use to prevent essential fatty acid (EFA) deficiency.

➤ Elemental diet formulas are indicated for maldigestion and malabsorption when protein restriction is unnecessary. These formulas have a high osmolarity and can cause diarrhea unless initiated slowly at a reduced concentration.

➤ Fiber-containing formulas are indicated for patients requiring tube feeding but not requiring a residue diet (i.e., unabsorbed dietary elements and total postdigestive luminal contents present following digestion, such as provided by fruits and vegetables). The fiber may help normalize whole gut transit time.

➤ High-fat/low-carbohydrate formulas are indicated for patients with compromised respiratory function and fluid restriction. These products provide concentrated nutrition and decrease carbon dioxide production and respiratory quotient.

➤ Modular components contain a single source of calories as carbohydrates, protein, or fat. Polycose is composed of a glucose polymer and has a negligible electrolyte content. Medium chain triglyceride (MCT) provides calories as fat for fat malabsorption states that accompany short-bowel syndrome and pancreatic insufficiency. Propac provides protein and is indicated for disease states with high protein requirements (e.g., burn/trauma, sepsis). Lipomul is a source of EFA and increases nonprotein calories without increasing the formula osmolality and carbohydrate load.

➤ Low-calorie formula diets are indicated for outpatient use as part of a specialized weight loss program under close medical supervision.

MONITORING THE TUBE-FED PATIENT

Once tube feedings are initiated, the patient must be monitored to ascertain efficacy of the nutritional support regimen and identify and correct intolerance problems, metabolic complications or other adverse effects. Patients should be weighed daily or as appropriate. The patient's input and output should be accurately recorded: the volume of tube feeding and volume of free water administered to the patient should be recorded separately. The frequency, consistency, and volume of stools must be recorded and monitored for any changes. Patients also should be observed for evidence of intolerance (e.g., abdominal distension or pain, nausea, emesis, diarrhea) and hydration status (e.g., edema, skin turgor, conditions of mucous membranes, rales). Patients who are alert and oriented should be asked to describe tolerance of therapy.

Laboratory tests should be monitored as follows to assess efficacy or toxicity of the regimen:

➤ Initially, a chemistry panel, electrolytes (serum), and hematology panel should be evaluated. The *chemistry panel* includes glucose, blood urea nitrogen (BUN), cholesterol, total bilirubin, alkaline phosphatase, gamma glutamyl transferase (GGT), aspartate aminotransferase (AST), lactate dehydrogenase (LD), creatinine, calcium, phosphorus, magnesium, uric acid, total protein, prealbumin, and albumin assessments. *Serum electrolytes* includes sodium (Na^+), potassium(K^+), chloride (Cl^-), and total carbon dioxide measurements. The *hematology panel* includes white blood cell (WBC) count, red blood cell (RBC) count, hemoglobin (Hgb), hematocrit (Hct), mean cell volume (MCV), and mean corpuscular hemoglobin concentration (MCHC) assessments.

➤ Follow-up laboratory tests includes electrolyte measurements daily for 5 days; chemistry, electrolytes, and hematology surveys weekly; and 24-hour total urea nitrogen as appropriate.

PROPER ADMINISTRATION OF TUBE FEEDINGS

The proper administration of tube feeding products is important to achieve and enhance patient tolerance. The following points should be considered when administering a particular product.

Continuous drip given over a 24-hour period is the preferred method for administration of tube feedings. Potential complications associated with tube feedings (e.g., hyperglycemia, pulmonary aspiration, and diarrhea) can be reduced by continuous feedings. Bolus feedings are not recommended and should not be given unless the feeding tube is in the stomach and previous feedings have been well tolerated.

To initiate a continuous tube feeding:

1. Depending on tube location, placement of the tube should be confirmed by irrigation with air or aspiration of stomach or small bowel contents. The pH of gastric fluid should be less than 4.0, unless the patient is receiving medications to control gastric acid, in which case the normal pH is 6.0 or less. If the pH is 6.0 or greater, the fluid may be intestinal or pulmonary. Normally, the pH of intestinal fluid is 7.5–8.0 and the pH of pulmonary fluid is approximately 7.6.

2. The product should be diluted to half strength, and administration started at 50 mL/hr (especially with high osmotic products).

3. If the feeding is tolerated (i.e., absence of glucosuria, hyperglycemia, diarrhea, abdominal discomfort, residuals <150 mL), the *rate* of feeding is increased by increments of 25 mL/hr each day until the desired rate of infusion is achieved.

4. Once the final rate (as determined by energy needs) is achieved, the *strength* of the product is increased from half to full strength (undiluted) in one-fourth increments every 24 hours, until full strength is achieved.

5. If diarrhea or abdominal discomfort is present after the advancement of the feeding, the previous rate or strength are returned to for another 24-hour period.

Before initiation of tube feedings, placement of the feeding tube is checked to make sure that the tube has been properly positioned. The patient is placed in an upright position with the head elevated to a 30° angle during feeding. Before subsequent feedings, gastric residuals are checked (i.e., amount of formula remaining in the stomach). If residuals are >150 mL, feedings should be held.

Adequate "free water" should be given to replace insensible water loss (500–1200 mL/day). Total fluid requirements should include insensible losses that range from 1–2 mL/kcal, with greater amounts for extrarenal losses (e.g., burns, fistulas, open wounds, fever) (see Chapter 10, "Fluid and Electrolyte Therapy," for a more detailed discussion). Adequate free water is especially important when administering high-protein formulas or >1 g/kg protein intake, because these products can produce a solute diuresis leading to dehydration. Input and output are recorded every 8 hours, with tube feeding volume recorded separately from water intake.

To minimize the risk of bacterial growth, commercial tube feeding products are refrigerated after opening. If the formula is not used within 24 hours, it should be discarded. No more than an 8-hour supply of feeding should be prepared and hung in the patient care area. The external tube and feeding bag are changed daily. The feeding tube is irrigated with 120 mL of water if the feeding is stopped for any reason and at least every 6–8 hours to prevent clogging.

Finally, if a tube feeding product is given orally, chilling improves palatability. If this is unacceptable, flavored products should be considered. Table 11.2 contains additional information on the complications of tube feeding.

Table 11-2. Tube Feeding Complications[3-5]

Type/Complication	Causes	Management
Gastrointestinal		
Diarrhea (most common)	Bacterial contamination of formula; improper administration; use of antibiotics; lactose intolerance; impaction; malnutrition; liquid drug formulations containing sorbitol; bowel infection from *C. difficile*	Discard tubing after 24 hr; use only 4–8 hr of feeding; use isotonic formula at tolerable rate by continuous delivery via pump; avoid or recognize drugs causing diarrhea; avoid lactose containing

Table 11-2.   *Continued*

Type/Complication	Causes	Management
	and pseudomembranous colitis	formulas; rule out impaction before treating diarrhea; use elemental formula or parenteral nutrition
Constipation	Low residue formula used in long-term, tube-fed patients	Provide additional fluids by mouth or tube feeding; increase ambulation or use a high-fiber, high-residue formula; administer bulking agents (psyllium)
Bloating	Presence of a mild ileus; intolerance to lipids in formula; swallowing excessive amounts of air (e.g., head and neck surgery)	Use elemental formulas requiring less digestion; increase ambulation; administer bisacodyl suppository
Inadequate gastric emptying	Gastric atony, prepyloric ulcers, bowel ileus; drugs such as theophylline, dopamine, anticholinergics calcium channel blockers, and meperidine which relax the lower esophageal sphincter	Verify tube placement; monitor stomach content residuals before bolus feedings or every 2–4 hr during continuous feedings

continues

Table 11-2. *Continued*

Type/Complication	Causes	Management
Vomiting	Psychological association with the illness; unpleasant odor of formulas containing free amino acids or the reinstilling of large amounts of aspirated gastric residuals	Reduce anxiety; use intact protein containing formulas or antiemetic when indicated; decrease the rate of delivery and feeding beyond the pylorus
Nausea	Delayed gastric emptying; gastric distention; formula too hot or too cold, or given too rapidly	Stop feedings and determine cause; check gastric residual to determine the progress of gastric emptying after 1–2 hr; restart feedings at slower rate and/or dilute
Gastrointestinal bleed (rare)	Some data suggest that enteral hyperalimentation may protect against GI bleeding while treating malnutrition	Discontinue enteral feeding and change to parenteral nutritional support
Mechanical		
Tube obstruction	Formula with a caloric density of 1.5–2.0 kcal/mL; inadequate crushing of medications or inadequate dilution/flushing of psyllium or antacids	Use feeding pumps for dense formulas and/or larger-bore feeding tubes; give medications as elixirs or mixed with water or formula; avoid mixing formulas with liquid medications with a pH 5;

Table 11-2. *Continued*

Type/Complication	Causes	Management
		instill a few mL of Coca-Cola or meat tenderizer to help unclog tubes; use cranberry juice for psyllium administration
Displacement	Vomiting; cough; incorrect tube placement; detached tape holding tube to nose	Check tube placement by x-ray; listen for air being injected through the tube into the stomach with a stethoscope, followed by aspiration of a small amount of gastric contents
Irritation	Esophageal reflux, peptic esophagitis; pressure necrosis of esophageal and tracheal wall at cuff inflation site	Provide nose and mouth care; change tape; increase salivation in the mouth by allowing chewing gum, hard candy, or ice chips
Rupture (rare)	Continuous tube feeding in a closed system	Periodic disconnection of feeding tube from the infusion apparatus; assess for abdominal distention; pain in upper left quadrant or epigastric area may be a sign of gastric rupture

continued

Table 11-2. *Continued*

Type/Complication	Causes	Management
Pneumonia	Gastric contents refluxing into bronchus secondary to delayed gastric emptying; improper placement of tube in tracheal or bronchus; incompetent lower esophageal sphincter	Place feeding tube beyond the pylorus; use small, soft feeding tube; keep maximum gastric content residuals to <150 mL
Metabolic Hyperglycemia	Common in patients who are diabetic, hypermetabolic, or receiving corticosteroids or glucagon	Check blood glucose and urine acetone frequently with advancing enteral feedings; administer insulin if needed; hydrate patient or change to a lower carbohydrate content formula **Note:** Hyperglycemic-hyperosmolar coma may occur if glucose is infused faster than 0.5 g/kg/hr, or if the patient is diabetic, a latent diabetic, or with hyperosmolar formulas causing intracellular dehydration
Tube feeding syndrome (develops 4–14 days after	*Signs and Symptoms:* Lethargy, cardiovascular instability, fever,	Monitor electrolytes, BUN, Hct, and fluid intake and

Table 11-2. *Continued*

Type/Complication	Causes	Management
feedings initiated)	confusion, and decreased level of consciousness *Results from:* Intake of excessive protein and inadequate fluids with subsequent dehydration, hypernatremia, hyperchloremia, and azotemia. Renal tubular dysfunction; primary water deficit; adrenal corticosteroid secretion producing sodium retention; advanced age and renal arteriosclerosis	output. Reduce protein content of formula and/or provide more free water
Hypernatremia	High sodium and low water intake	Monitor fluid intake and output, serum sodium, and BUN and rehydrate patient
Hyponatremia	Isotonic or hypotonic feedings; excessive antidiuretic hormone production; total body sodium deficiency or overhydration	Restrict fluids, administer diuretics, replace sodium losses
Hyperkalemia	Metabolic acidosis with or without renal insufficiency; anabolic metabolism; excessive potassium supplementation after tube feedings started	Monitor serum potassium and adjust formula

continued

Table 11-2. *Continued*

Type/Complication	Causes	Management
Hypokalemia	Diuretic use; GI losses; high doses of insulin; in combination with hypomagnesemia and hypophosphatemia in malnourished patients	Monitor serum potassium and adjust formula
Hyperphosphatemia	Renal insufficiency in tube-fed patients	Monitor serum phosphate and adjust formula
Hypophosphatemia	May occur in a malnourished patient placed on nutritional support who subsequently becomes anabolic	Monitor serum phosphate and adjust formula
Hypomagnesemia	Inadequate replacement of magnesium. May see: Increased reflexes, coarse tremors, muscle cramps, dysrhythmias, paresthesias, and positive Chvistek's and Trousseau's signs	Monitor serum magnesium and adjust formula
Hypozincemia	Sequestration of zinc in the liver resulting from systemic infection and decreased car decreased carrier protein levels in protein deficiencies.	Monitor serum zinc and adjust formula

PEDIATRIC ENTERAL NUTRITION

Indications and Goals

In infants, enteral nutrition is intended to provide adequate replacement for human breast milk. For those infants allergic or intolerant to various components of human breast milk or standard infant formulas, enteral nutrition should provide adequate substitute feeding.

Generally, caloric goals of pediatric enteral nutrition are calculated using the infant's weight:

➤ *Low-Birthweight Infants.* 120 kcal/kg/day.
➤ *6 Months.* 100–200 kcal/kg/day.
➤ *6 Months to 1 Year.* 100–105 kcal/kg/day.
➤ *>1 Year.* 80–100 kcal/kg/day.

Protein requirements for infants during the first year of life are 2–3 g/kg/day and should supply 7–16% of the total daily caloric intake. For low-birthweight infants, protein intake should be greater, at approximately 3.5–4 g/kg/day. The total daily caloric intake of carbohydrates and fats should be 35–to 65% and 30–55%, respectively.

Human Versus Cows' Milk Formulation

Normal infant formulas are formulated from cows' milk. Table 11.3 provides a comparison of the differences and similarities between whole cows' milk and human milk.

Methods of Altering Cows' Milk for Manufacture of Milk-Based Formulas[7]

A variety of approaches have been used to create milk-based formulas from cows' milk. First, the poorly absorbed butterfat is replaced by coconut and polyunsaturated vegetable oils to which vitamin E has been added to change the fat composition. For infants with pancreatic insufficiency (cystic fibrosis), bile acid deficiency, prematurity, or other malabsorption problems, MCT has been used. MCTs increase the absorption of calcium and phosphorus and may improve carbohydrate tolerance.

Next, the protein content is reduced by decreasing the total amount of calories from protein. In some instances, the lactalbumin:casein ratio is altered from 20:80 to 60:40 to more closely simulate breast milk. Soy protein formulas are promoted for use in infants allergic to milk protein. Others recommend that protein hydrolysate formulas be used. This recommendation is based on the concern that infants with severe allergy to cow's milk have intestinal mucosal damage sufficient to expose them to higher concentrations of foreign protein in soy protein formulas. These

Table 11-3. Comparison of Human Milk to Cows' Milk[7]

Component	Category	Cows' Milk	Human Milk
Fat	% of total calories	50%	55%
	Triglycerides	More difficult to absorb	More medium chain and monounsaturated fatty acids that are easier to absorb; contains lipoprotein lipase and bile salt stimulating pancreatic lipase
		Primarily short and long chain[a]	
		Primarily saturated	
Protein	% of total calories	20% (3 times that of breast milk)	7% (7–16% recommended)
	Lactalbumin: casein[b]	20:80	60:40
	Taurine[e] and cystine[d]	Almost none	High Levels
Carbohydrate[c]	% of total calories	30%	42 (35–65% recommended)
Form		Lactose	Lactose
Renal solute load		228 mOsm/L	79 mOsm/L
Sodium		2.2 mmol/100 mL	0.7 mmol/100 mL
Ca/PO$_4$ ratio		1.3:1	2–2.4:1

[a] Long chain triglycerides may form insoluble complexes with calcium.

[b] Casein is relatively insoluble and occurs in milk as a "tough curd," in contrast to lactalbumin which is highly soluble and occurs in milk as whey. The increased curd slows gastric emptying and may cause GI distress.

[c] Taurine is needed for maintenance of cellular structural and functional integrity.

[d] Increased cystine is needed because infants may not be able to convert methionine to cystine, which is necessary for somatic growth.

[e] Lactose is preferred as it increases the absorption of calcium and magnesium.

infants have demonstrated severe allergic manifestations when given soy protein formulas. However, life-threatening reactions to milk-based formulas have not been seen in most infants suspected of having milk-based adverse reactions, and they appear to tolerate soy protein formulas.[7] Likewise, protein hydrolysates may also be used in formulas for infants with food allergies or digestive disorders such as cystic fibrosis. Finally, the cystine content is sometimes increased to more closely simulate breast milk.

To more closely simulate human milk, the carbohydrate caloric source in milk-based formulas is increased to 40%. The added carbohydrate may be lactose, corn syrup, tapioca, sucrose, or dextrose. For infants allergic to or intolerant of lactose, lactose may be totally replaced.

The renal solute load in cows' milk is too high for routine infant feeding and can lead to dehydration. Milk-based formulas are formulated with a lower percentage of protein calories and a lower mineral content, which brings the renal solute load closer to that of human milk.

Finally, the mineral ratio of calcium to phosphorus in cows' milk may be altered to more closely resemble that of human breast milk.

Profile of Pediatric Formulas

Table 11.4 lists several examples of pediatric formulas. Product differences are described in Table 11.5.

Table 11-4. Pediatric Formulas Profile

Type	Product	Characteristics
Milk-based formulas	Enfamil	Lower sodium, 60:40 lactalbumin: casein ratio
	Similac	Similac with whey available
	SMA	Lowest sodium, 60:40 lactalbumin: casein ratio
Soy formulas	Prosobee	No sucrose
	Nursoy	Lower sodium
	Isomil	Isomil SF is available which is sucrose free
	RCF	Carbohydrate free, must supplement with fructose or glucose polymers (e.g., polycose)
Altered protein and/or fat	Nutramigen	Protein hydrolysate
	Pregestimil	Protein hydrolysate, MCT 40% of fat) and glucose polymers
	Portagen	Soy formulas with MCT (low essential fatty acids)
	Lofenalac	Low phenylalanine

continued

Table 11-4. Pediatric Formulas Profile

Type	Product	Characteristics
Low birthweight and premature infant formulas		Provide more calcium, protein, and sodium, an increased vitamin E to polyunsaturated fat ratio, altered carbohydrate consisting of lactose and corn syrup and part of the fat as MCT; some have increased zinc and/or folic acid
Renal formula	Similac PM 60/40	Low renal solute load with increased amounts of essential amino acids, low sodium, low phosphorus

ENTERAL FORMULAS AND DRUG COMPATIBILITY

Medication Administration

Medication dosage forms possess different characteristics that can affect how they are tolerated when administered through enteral feeding tubes. Capsules and tablets that are usually taken orally may be altered by crushing them to administer through a feeding tube.[9] When crushed, sublingual, buccal, time-released, or enteric-coated tablets or capsules may have an altered therapeutic effect and increased side effects or toxicity. Manually crushing these medications may result in small particles that, when administered, can adhere to the inside of the feeding tube and contribute to tube obstruction.[10]

Liquid dosage forms may have higher osmolality and a significant amount of sorbitol, which increase the

Table 11-5. Pediatric Formula Composition[6, 8]

Formula	Calories (kcal/30 mL)	Na (mmol/L)	K (mmol/L)	Cl (mmol/L)	Ca:P Ratio	Renal Solute Load	Protein (g/L)	Fat (g/L)	CHO[a] (g/L)
Standard Formulas									
Carnation Good Start	20	7	17	—	1.8:1	—	16	34	74
Kindercal	32	16	34	21	1:1	73	34	44	135
Mature human milk	22	7	14	12	1.6:1	99	11	45	68
Enfamil	20	9	18	12	1.5:1	108	15	37	73
Similac 20	20	11	20	15	1.3:1	90	15	36	72
SMA 20	20	6	14	10	1.5:1	199	15	36	72
Pediasure	29.6	16.5	33.5	28.5	1.2:1		30	49.7	109.7
Therapeutic Formulas									
Milk Allergy									
Alsoy	20	13	21	—	1.4:1	—	21	37	67
Gerber Soy Formula	20	10.4	21	—	1.3:1	—	20	36	68
Soyalac	20	13	21	12	1.7:1	129	21	37	67
Isomil	20	13	19	11	1.4:1	123	17	36	70
Nursoy	20	9	19	16	1.4:1	107	18	36	69
Nutramigen	20	14	19	16	1.5:1	128	19	34	74
Prosobee	20	11	21		1.3:1		20	36	69

continued

Table 11-5. Continued

Formula	Calories (kcal/30 mL)	Na (mmol/L)	K (mmol/L)	Cl (mmol/L)	Ca:P Ratio	Renal Solute Load	Protein (g/L)	Fat (g/L)	CHO[a] (g/L)
Fat/Carbohydrate Restriction									
Portagen	20	15.2	20	16	1.3:1	200	24	31	74
Pregestimil	20	14	19	16	1.5:1	125	19	38	69
RCF (Ross Carbohydrate Free)	12	13	19	15	1.4:1	126	20	36	0
High Protein or Calorie Requirements (LBW Infant Formulas)									
Enfamil Premature	24	14	23	19	2:1	152	24	41	89
Similac Special Care	24	15	27	21	2:1	156	22	44	86
Premie SMA	24	14	19	15	1.9:1	224	20	86	44
Sodium Restriction									
Lonalac	20	1.7	49	22	1.1:1	289	34	35	48
Lofenalac	20	14	18	13	1.3:1	133	22	26	88
Renal Insufficiency									
Similac PM 60/40	20	7	15	11	2:1	96	15.8	37.6	68.8
Elemental Diets									
Peptamen Junior Diet	30	20	33.8	30.4	1.25:1	—	30	38.5	137.5
Vivonex Pediatric	24	21.3	38.8	35	1.2:1	—	24	24	130

possibility of diarrhea. The osmolality of a liquid medication is the measurement of the number and size of particles per kilogram of solution. Many liquid medications have osmolalities greater than 1000 mOsm/kg. These medications can be diluted with water to minimize the occurrence of osmotic diarrhea according to the following formula:

Final volume = volume of liquid medication × mOsm of
liquid medication/desired mOsm
(300–500)

The volume of liquid medication is subtracted from the final volume to get the final diluent volume. Liquid medications should be diluted with at least 30 mL of water if this amount of water can be accommodated by the patient's fluid status.10

Drug-Nutrient Incompatibilities

Various medications can interact when administered concurrently with an enteral product (Tables 11.6–11.8). To avoid potential drug-nutrient incompatibilities, tube feedings should be discontinued and at least 15–30 mL of water instilled through the tube before and after drug administration. The most frequent compatibility problems involve strongly acidic or buffered syrups with pH values ≤4. Incompatibilities between formulas and drugs can cause immediate dumping, and the increased viscosity and particle size can clog feeding tubes.[11] At pH values ≤5, in vitro clotting has occurred with Pulmocare, Ensure Plus, Osmolite, Enrich, Ensure, and Resource.[12] Patients receiving warfarin may experience a reduced effect if the enteral products that contain vitamin K are not considered.

Pharmacokinetic Alterations[12, 13]

The pharmacologic actions of drugs which produce side effects such as nausea, vomiting, diarrhea, decreased appetite, and electrolyte and metabolic abnormalities may be similar to systemic effects that could be caused by enteral feedings. Likewise, medications' side effects must be con-

Table 11-6. Enteral Formulas and Drug Compatibility[13]

Product	Compatibilities		
	Osmolite HN	Vital	Osmolite
Aluminum hydroxide suspension (Amphojel)	C	C	I
Potassium gluconate (Kaon Liquid)	I	C	I
Potassium chloride powder (K-Lor)	C	C	C
Furosemide (Lasix)	C	C	C
Morphine sulfate	C	C	C
Magnesium and aluminum hydroxide with simethicone 20 mg (Mylanta)	C	C	C
Magnesium and aluminum hydroxide with simethicone 30 mg (Mylanta II)	I	C	I
Sodium phosphate (Phospho Soda)	I	C	I
Magaldrate (Riopan)	C	C	I
Cimetidine (Tagamet)	I	C	I

C, compatible; I, incompatible.

Table 11-7. Enteral Formulas and Drug Compatibility[14]

Product	Compatibilities	
	Enrich	Vivonex TEN
Cimetidine elixir	C	C
Prochlorperazine elixir (Compazine)	C	C
Docusate sodium elixir (Colace)	C	C
Diphenoxylate and atropine elixir (Lomotil)	C	C

Table 11-7. Enteral Formulas and Drug Compatibility[14]

Product	Compatibilities	
	Enrich	Vivonex TEN
Magnesium hydroxide (Milk of Magnesia)	C	C
Simethicone drops (Mylicon)	C	C
Metoclopramide syrup (Reglan)	I[a]	C
Diphenhydramine elixir (Benadryl)	C	C
Guaifenesin syrup (Robitussin)	I[b]	C
Pseudoephedrine (Sudafed)	I[c]	C
Acetaminophen elixir (Tylenol)	C	C
Ferrous sulfate elixir (Feosol)	I[d]	C
Potassium chloride elixir	C	C
Sodium phosphate (Fleets phosphosoda)	I[e]	C
Zinc sulfate capsules	I[f]	C
Amoxicillin suspension (Amoxil)	C	C
Nitrofurantoin suspension (Furadantin)	C	C
Cephalexin (Keflex)	C	C
Trimethoprim/sulfamethoxazole suspension (Septra)	C	C
Chlorpromazine concentrate	I[g]	C
Thioridazine concentrate	I[h]	C
Thiothixene (Navane)	C	C
Doxepin concentrate (Sinequan)	C	C
Phenobarbital elixir	C	C
Phenytoin suspension (Dilantin)	C	C
Digoxin elixir (Lanoxin)	C	C
Furosemide liquid	C	C

C, compatible; I, incompatible.
[a] Forms thin, granular formula.
[b] Separation particles.
[c] Thick, gelatinous mass.
[d] Large particles.
[e] Thin, granular
[f] Soft, gelatinous mass.
[g] Soft, thick.
[h] Thin, large particles.

Table 11-8. Interactions of Selected Formulas with Medications[15]

Product	Effect on Drug
Ensure	Theophylline: ↑ in osmolality Phenytoin susp: ↓ drug concentration[a] Methyldopa: ↓ drug concentration
Ensure Plus	Theophylline: ↑ in osmolality Phenytoin susp.: ↓ drug concentration[a] Methyldopa: ↓ drug concentration
Osmolite	Theophylline: ↑ in osmolality Phenytoin susp.: ↓ drug concentation[a] Methyldopa: ↓ drug concentration

[a] No significant drug concentration changes with injectable phenytoin.

sidered in patients receiving enteral formulas and not be solely attributed to formula intolerance. Further, drug bioavailability and metabolism can be altered by the concomitant use of enteral formulas. Factors that affect the absorption of drugs include the following: gastric emptying rate, composition of the formula or diet, GI pH, enteral feeding, and dissolution time for a solid dosage form (Table 11.8 and Box 11.2).[17]

Box 11.2 Drugs That Undergo Altered-Excretion and Absorption When Taken with Food[16]

Captopril	Nitrofurantoin
Carbamazepine	Penicillins
Dicumarol	Phenytoin suspension
Digoxin	Procainamide
Griseofulvin	Propranolol
Hydralazine	Rifampin
Hydrochlorothiazide	Tetracycline
Isoniazid	Theophylline
Metoprolol	

References

1. Moore FA, Moore EE. The benefits of enteric feeding. Adv Surg. 1997;30:141–54.

2. ASPEN Board of Directors. Guidelines for the use of parenteral and enteral nutrition in adult and pediatric patients. JPEN. 1993;17(4):1SA–52SA.

3. Breach CL, Saldanha LG. Tube feeding complications, part I: gastrointestinal. Nutr Support Serv. 1988;8(3):15–9.

4. Breach CL, Saldanha LG. Tube feeding complications, part II: mechanical. Nutr Support Serv. 1988;8(5):28–32.

5. Breach CL, Saldanha LG. Tube feeding complications, part III: metabolic. Nutr Support Serv. 1988;8(6):16–9.

6. Serrano Murphy VA, Bubica G. General pediatric therapy. In: Young LY, Koda-Kimble MA, eds. Applied Therapeutics: The Clinical Use of Drugs. 4th ed. Vancouver: Applied Therapeutics; 1988:1821.

7. Sagraves R, Kamper C, Doerr J. Infant formulas products. In: Covington TR, Berardi RR, Young LL eds. Handbook of Nonprescription Drugs. 11th ed. Washington, DC: American Pharmaceutical Association; 1996:393–422.

8. Benitz WE, Tatro DS. The Pediatric Drug Handbook. 3rd ed. St. Louis, MO: Mosby-Year Book, Inc.; 1995:330–5.

9. Mitchell JF. Oral dosage forms that should not be crushed: 1998 update. Hosp Pharm. 1998;33(4):399–415.

10. Guenter P, Jones S, Ericson M. Enteral nutrition therapy. Nurs Clin North Am. 1997;32(4):651–68.

11. Cutie AJ et al. Compatibility of enteral products with commonly employed drug additives. JPEN. 1983;7:186–91.

12. Marcuard SP, Perkins AM. Clogging of feeding tubes. JPEN. 1988;12(4):403–5.

13. Fagerman KE, Ballou AE. Drug compatibilities with enteral feeding solutions coadministered by tube. Nutr Support Serv. 1988;8(5):31–2.

14. Burns PE et al. Physical compatibility of enteral formulas with various common medications. J Am Diet Assoc. 1988;88(9):1094–6.

15. Holtz L et al. Compatibility of medications with enteral feedings. JPEN. 1987;11(2):183–6.

16. Egging P. Enteral nutrition from a pharmacist's perspective. Nutr Support Serv. 1987;7(4):17.

17. Varella L, Jones E, Meguid MM. Drug-nutrient interactions in enteral feeding: a primary care focus. Nurse Pract. 1997;22(6):98–104.

Chapter 12

Parenteral Nutrition

Joanne Whitney

Parenteral nutrition supplies require carbohydrate, protein, lipid, electrolytes, vitamins, and minerals intravenously to patients who are unable to assimilate nutrients via the gastrointestinal (GI) tract. It can maintain weight and metabolic integrity, replete malnourished patients with deficits in lean body mass accompanied by deficits in visceral and serum proteins, and restore hematologic and immune function integrity. Parenteral nutrition may be started and given in a hospital, a skilled nursing facility, or a patient's home. Because enteral nutrition is less costly, safer, and maintains absorptive and immunologic functions of the intestinal tract, the cardinal rule governing the prescribing of parenteral nutrition is that it should be used only when the gut is unavailable.

Peripheral parenteral nutrition is used when a patient requires intravenous nutritional support but does not have a central line. Peripheral parenteral nutrition requires good venous access and should be restricted to patients with mild to moderate stress who are not fluid-constrained. The concentration of dextrose used as an energy source should not exceed 10% for adults and 12.5% for children because the osmolality of higher dextrose concentrations can cause phlebitis of peripheral veins. Amino acid concentration should be limited to a maximum of 5% in adults and 3.5% in children. Lipid, which is isotonic, supplies a large percentage of the energy requirement and may be given separately or in the solution to minimize the development of phlebitis. Electrolytes, vitamins, and minerals are added. Peripheral parenteral nutrition is often used as a supplement to enteral feeding. Peripheral lines must be changed at least every 3 days in most institutions or when phlebitis occurs. Some add hydrocortisone, 5 mg/day, and heparin, 100–1000 units/day, to peripheral parenteral nutrition in an effort to reduce phlebitis.[1] The data are inadequate, however, and many institutions have discontinued the addition of hydrocortisone and heparin to peripheral parenteral nutrition solutions.

Total parenteral nutrition contains hypertonic concentrations (>300mOsm/L) of dextrose and amino acids and requires a catheter or port that empties into the superior or inferior vena cava. The term "total parenteral nutrition" is increasingly being replaced by the designation "parenteral nutrition." If lipid is added directly, the solution is a total nutrient admixture, also known as 3-in-1or All-in-One Parenteral Nutrition. Broviac, Hickman, and Groshong are commonly used central catheters. The Groshong catheter has a valve to prevent back flushing of blood, obviating the need for heparin flushes. The peripherally inserted central catheter (PICC line) can be placed by a nurse at the hospital bedside or at home. Placement into the vena cava must be verified by radiograph.

INDICATIONS FOR PARENTERAL NUTRITION

Every hospital should have institutional guidelines for the administration of parenteral nutrition. These guidelines often are developed by either a Nutrition Support Committee (a subcommittee of the Pharmacy and Therapeutics Committee) or by a committee consisting of physicians, pharmacists, nutritionists, and nurses. These committees may be primarily advisory bodies or committee members may direct the daily therapy of patients receiving nutritional support. Some Nutrition Support Committees issue guidelines for the administration of parenteral nutrition and initiate an order sheet that must be signed by the prescribing physician. Parenteral nutrition order sheets commonly contain abbreviated guidelines and information enabling physicians to devise patient-specific parenteral nutrition. Guidelines published by the American Society of Parenteral and Enteral Nutrition (ASPEN) are considered the gold standard for parenteral nutrition, and most institutional guidelines are based on them.[2] Representative guidelines for parenteral nutrition administration follow.

Cases in which parenteral nutrition is frequently used:

1. A patient with good nutritional reserves when it is anticipated that the GI tract will not be available for more than 7 days.

2. A patient who is severely malnourished or catabolic when it is anticipated that the GI tract will not be available for 5–7 days.
3. A patient with a nonfunctioning GI tract (e.g., severe malabsorption, short bowel syndrome, bowel resection, intestinal obstruction).
4. A patient who requires bowel rest (e. g., severe pancreatitis, enteric fistula, intractable diarrhea).

Cases in which parenteral nutrition may be helpful:

1. A patient under moderate stress (e.g., major surgery, trauma, burns) when it is anticipated the GI tract will not be available for 5 or more days.
2. A patient with inflammatory bowel disease not responding to medical therapy.
3. An immunocompromised patient with poor nutritional status and documented malabsorption who is receiving medical management and is not responding to enteral therapy.

Cases in which parenteral nutrition has little or no value:

1. A patient who has minimal stress or trauma when it is anticipated that the GI tract will be available within 5 days.
2. A pharmacy with good nutritional reserves when the use of parenteral nutrition would be for less than 7 days.
3. End-stage, terminally ill patients at comfort care level.

Specific adult diseases for which parenteral nutrition should be considered if guidelines are met:

➤ Short bowel syndrome; adequate absorption requires >40 cm, more in the elderly.
➤ Malabsorption syndromes (celiac disease, Crohn's disease).
➤ Motility disorders (ileus, intestinal pseudo-obstruction).
➤ Enterocutaneous fistulas.
➤ Radiation enteritis/chemotherapy.
➤ Severe pancreatitis without hyperlipidemia.
➤ Hyperemesis of pregnancy.
➤ Severe hypermetabolic states in which enteral feeding is contraindicated or inadequate (e.g., burns, sepsis with multi-organ failure, severe trauma, AIDS).
➤ Persistent vomiting secondary to obstruction, increased intracranial pressure, medication use, situations in which enteral feeding cannot be used.

➤ Severe malnutrition.
➤ Transplantation (bone marrow, liver, pancreas).

Specific pediatric conditions for which parenteral nutrition should be considered if guidelines are met:

➤ Extreme prematurity.
➤ Atresia of the GI tract and other GI anomalies.
➤ Treatment and prevention of necrotizing enterocolitis in premature and low-birthweight infants.
➤ Respiratory distress.
➤ Intractable diarrhea of infancy.
➤ Chronic renal or hepatic failure.
➤ Adverse effects of chemotherapy and radiation (radiation enteritis, vomiting, stomatitis).
➤ Abdominal wall defects and abdominal trauma to viscera.
➤ Cystic fibrosis.
➤ Inborn errors of metabolism.

NUTRITIONAL ASSESSMENT

Nutritional assessment consists of evaluations of diet, weight, medical and surgical histories, anthropomorphic and laboratory measurements, and a physical examination of the patient. Diet histories might uncover unusual patterns of eating, duration of anorexia, food allergies, and actual food intake. Weight loss (>5% in 1 month, >10% in 6 months) is significant in adults. Medical and surgical histories can reveal underlying pathology and risk factors for poor nutritional status. Anthropomorphic measurements of triceps and subscapular skinfold thickness estimate fat reserves, whereas mid-arm circumference predicts protein reserves. In pediatric patients, height/length ratios are compared to age-related percentiles to establish malnutrition. External head dimension is an additional parameter useful in evaluating the nutritional status of infants.

Low values of functional proteins (Table 12.1) may indicate deficient synthesis that could imply protein malnutrition. Serum albumin is most commonly used to assess protein nutritional status, but is of limited usefulness in determining acute nutritional changes because albumin has a long half-life. Proteins with shorter half-lives are used

Table 12-1. Serum Proteins Used to Ascertain Nutritional Status

Serum Protein	Normal Range	Half-Life (Days)
Albumin	3.5–5.0 g/dL	14–20
Fibronectin	1.66–1.98 g/dL	0.5–1.0
Prealbumin	10–40 mg/dL	2–3
Retinol binding protein	2.7–7.6 mg/dL	0.5
Somatomedin C (insulin-like GF 1)	0.55–1.4 U/mL	0.1–0.03
Transferrin	200–400 mg/dL	8–9

increasingly for monitoring improvements in protein malnutrition. Care should be taken in interpreting low or high concentrations of serum proteins, because their concentration in serum may be influenced by hydration state and by hepatic, renal, cardiac, or other underlying diseases. Measures of immunocompetence (e.g., T-cell counts, serum immunoglobulin concentration, complement levels, and leukocyte chemotaxis) have all been correlated with nutritional status. However, tests of delayed cutaneous hypersensitivity and total lymphocyte count are used more commonly in the clinical setting. Total lymphocyte count is normally 1800/mm^3 or greater. Leukocyte counts 800/mm^3 or less indicate severe malnutrition, but low counts may result from dehydration and underlying disease.

Micronutrient status should be assessed with the realization that disease processes also can affect micronutrient concentration. For example, alcoholism is associated with deficiencies in thiamine and folate. Zinc and ascorbic acid may be low in surgical patients. High doses of ascorbic acid, folate, and the B vitamins are often required in dialysis patients who are receiving parenteral nutrition. When laboratory tests are not available for the measurement of trace elements, clinical assessment of the patient can be used to predict the possibility of deficiencies. Baseline electrolytes, glucose, blood urea nitrogen (BUN), triglycerides, cholesterol, liver and renal function tests, complete blood cell count (CBC), and prothrombin time (PT) are necessary parts of the nutritional assessment of the patient who is to receive parenteral nutrition.

CALCULATING FLUID, KILOCALORIE, AND PROTEIN REQUIREMENTS

Fluid Requirements

A patient's fluid requirement can be increased by fever; losses from vomiting, diarrhea, nasogastric suction, and fistula drainage; underlying disease; and in infants by the use of radiant warmers and treatment with phototherapy (increases of 10–20%). For fever in adults, an additional 360 mL of fluid/day should be added for each degree Celsius above 37°. Losses other than from fever should be estimated as closely as possible and supplemental fluids given.

Adult fluid requirement:

➤ 100 mL/kg for first 10 kg
➤ 50 mL/kg for second 10 kg
➤ 20 mL/kg for kg above 20 kg

Case: D.D. is a 44-kg female with a temperature of 38.5° C. Calculate her daily fluid requirement.

$$\text{Maintenance fluid} = 1500 \text{ mL} + (24 \text{ kg} \times 20 \text{ mL})$$
$$+ 360 \text{ mL} (1.5) = 2520 \text{ mL}$$

Pediatric fluid requirement:

<10 kg = 100 mL/kg
$10\text{–}20$ kg = 1000 mL + 50 mL/kg for each kg > 10 kg
>20 kg = 1500 mL + 20 mL/kg for kg above 20 kg

Case: R.T. is a pediatric patient who weighs 7 kg.

$$\text{Maintenance Fluid} = 7 \text{ kg} \times 100 \text{ mL/kg} = 700 \text{ mL}$$

Energy Requirements

The kilocalories a patient needs daily are determined by basal metabolic rate, level of activity, and increased metabolism caused by the stress of trauma or disease. Basal metabolic rate varies with age, weight, height, gender, and disease state. True basal energy expenditure (BEE) can only be measured in a contained metabolic chamber. Resting energy expenditure (REE) can be determined by using formulas based on population studies or at a patient's bedside using indirect calorimetry with a metabolic measurement cart.[3] With indirect calorimetry, expired gases are analyzed to determine oxygen consumption (VO_2, in L/min) and carbon dioxide production (VCO_2, in L/min) from which REE can be calculated.

$$REE = [3.9 (VO_2) + 1.1 (VCO_2)] * 1440 \text{ min/day} = kcal/d$$

Case: D.R. is an 11-year-old, healthy girl who weighs 75 pounds. Her VO_2 = 0.125 L/min, VCO_2 = 0.110 L/min. Her REE can be calculated as follows:

$$REE = [3.9(0.125 \text{ L/min}) + 1.1 (0.110 \text{ L/min})]* \\ 1440 \text{ min/day} = kcal/day$$

$$REE = (0.49 + 0.12) * 1440 \text{ min/day} = kcal/day$$

$$REE = 0.61 * 1440 = 876 \text{ kcal/day}$$

In addition to energy expenditure, respiratory quotient (RQ = VCO_2/VO_2) can be calculated from the data and provides information on the preferential use of substrates. An RQ of 0.7 indicates primarily fat oxidation and an RQ of 1.0 indicates carbohydrate oxidation. Table 12.2 gives the energy source suggested by different RQs.

For patient DR (RQ = 110 mL/min/125 mL/min = 0.88), the RQ suggests a mixed dietary fuel source. Indirect

Table 12-2. Energy Source and Respiratory Quotient

Energy Source	Respiratory Quotient
Fat	0.7
Protein	0.8
Carbohydrate	0.95–1.0
Mixed fuel	0.85
Fat synthesis	>1.01
Hyperventilation	>1.10
Ketosis	<0.6

calorimetry is a useful tool but is expensive, and reproducible results require a skilled and experienced technician. In addition, underlying disease and trauma influence results. Indirect calorimetry cannot be used in patients on continuous airway pressure with chest tubes or when the fraction of inspired air is $\leq 50\%$. It has limited validity in infants and small children in whom a large amount of physiologic "dead space" is present.

CALCULATING ENERGY NEEDS FROM PUBLISHED FORMULAS

It has been estimated that there are 191 different published formulas derived from population studies to calculate REE. Because these formulas *are* derived from population studies, they are approximations, and the clinical response of the patient should be monitored to determine if the correct kilocalories are being supplied. When energy requirements are calculated, the patient's actual body weight (ABW) is customarily used. There are conditions, however, when ABW will not give an accurate estimation.

1. When a patient is edematous or overly hydrated but not obese, it is preferable to use the ideal body weight (IBW) as an estimate of dry body weight. It is not unusual for a patient to weigh up to 5 pounds more due to fluid overload.

Men: IBW (kg) = 50 kg (for first 5 feet)
$\qquad$ + (2.3 kg $\times$ # of inches > 5 feet)
Women: IBW (kg) = 45.5 kg (for first 5 feet)
$\qquad$ + (2.3 kg $\times$ # of inches > 5 feet)

Case: W.L., a 50-year-old man, 5'9", has congestive heart failure. ABW = 73 kg. What is his estimated dry body weight?

$$IBW = 50 \text{ kg} + (2.3 \text{ kg} \times 9'') = 70.7 \text{ kg}$$

2. For obese patients (>30% of IBW), metabolically active weight (MAW) should be used.

$$MAW \text{ (kg)} = IBW \text{ (kg)} + 0.25 \text{ (ABW} - IBW)$$

Case: U.J., a 59-year-old woman, 5'4", weight 84 kg. Calculate her MAW.

$$IBW = 45.5 + 2.3(4) = 54.7 \text{ kg}$$
$$MAW = 54.7 \text{ kg} + 0.25 (84 \text{ kg} - 54.7 \text{ kg}) = 62 \text{ kg}$$

3. If a patient is both obese and edematous, MAW is also used. In this case, some clinical judgment is needed to adjust ABW to dry body weight.

Case: E.K., a 58-year-old woman, 5'7", 92 kg, has experienced a 4-pound weight gain since the onset of pulmonary edema. Calculate her MAW. Since E.K. has gained 4 pounds, her ABW is subtracted by 4 pounds to give an estimated dry body weight. Convert pounds to kilograms.

$$IBW = 45.5 + 2.3(7) = 61.6$$
$$MAW = 61.6 + 0.25 \{(92 \text{ kg} - 4 \text{ lb}/2.2 \text{ kg}) - 61.6\} = 68.8 \text{ kg}$$

HARRIS-BENEDICT EQUATION[4] FOR REE

Men:

$$REE = 66.5 + \{13.75 \times \text{weight (kg)}\} + \{5 \times \text{height (cm)}\} - \{6.76 \times \text{age (years)}\}$$

Women:

$$REE = 655 \{9.56 \times \text{weight (kg)}\} + \{1.8 \times \text{height (cm)}\} - \{4.48 \times \text{age (years)}\}$$

Conversion factors: 2.2 lb. = 1 kg; 1 inch = 2.54 cm

Multiplying REE by activity and stress factors in Table 12.3 gives the approximate kilocalories needed. In practice, multiplying REE by 1.2–1.4 should supply sufficient kilo-

Table 12-3. Activity and Stress Factors for Harris-Benedict Equation

Activity Factors	Use	Stress Factors	Use
Confined to bed	1.2	Minor operation	1.2
Ambulatory	1.3	Skeletal trauma	1.3
Sepsis	1.6	Major burn	1.5–2.1

calories to account for activity and the stress of trauma and/or disease for most patients. Again, the degree of metabolic stress encountered by any one patient is based on clinical judgment unless actual calorimetric measurement has been made.

Case: R.Y., a 65-year-old man, 5'10", 72 kg, is on bowel rest secondary to Crohn's disease. Calculate his energy needs. R.Y. is neither obese nor edematous. ABW may be used.

$$REE = 66.5 + \{13.75 \times 72\} + \{5 \times 177.8 \text{ (cm)}\}$$
$$- \{6.76 \times 65\} = 1506 \text{ kcal}$$
$$1506 \times 1.2 = 1807 \text{ kcal}; 1506 \times 1.4 = 2109 \text{ kcal}$$

R.Y.'s energy needs are between 1808 and 2109 kcal. It is usual to choose somewhere in the middle of the range, so R.Y. would be given approximately 2000 kcal. However, if he were under greater stress, the higher value would be chosen.

Case: B.N., a 75-year-old woman, 5'2", 89 kg, has Stage III congestive heart failure. She gained 2.5 pounds in 2 days. Calculate her energy needs. The patient is edematous and obese. Subtract 1.1 kg from her measured weight and use MAW to calculate her REE as follows:

$$IBW = 45.5 + 2.3(2) = 50.1 \text{ kg; MAW} = 50.1$$
$$+ 0.25(87.9 - 50.1) = 59.6 \text{ kg} = 60 \text{ kg}$$
$$REE = 655 + \{(9.56 \times 60 \text{ kg}) + (1.8 \times 157.5 \text{ cm})$$
$$- (4.48 \times 75 \text{ years})\} = 1176 \text{ kcal}$$
$$1176 \text{ kg} \times 1.2 = 1411; 1176 \text{ kg} \times 1.4 = 1647 \text{ kcal}$$

Required energy needs are between 1400 and 1650 kcal/day

IRETON-JONES [5] FORMULAS FOR THE ILL OR INJURED PATIENT

These formulas were derived from indirect calorimetry studies of patients. Although not used as frequently as the Harris-Benedict equations, they are considered by many to predict REE more accurately and are applicable to patients on ventilators. The term estimated energy expenditure (EEE) is used to describe the kilocalories the patient requires daily.

$$EEE \text{ (ventilator)} = 1784 - 11(A) + 5(W) + 244(S)$$
$$+ 239(T) + 804(B)$$

$$EEE \text{ (spontaneous breathing)} = 629 - 11(A) + 25(W)$$
$$- 609(O)$$

EEE = kcal/day; A = age; W = Body Weight (kg); S = sex (male = 1; female = 0); T = Trauma, B = Burns, O = Obesity (if present = 1, absent = 0)

Case: R.Y. Consider that R.Y.'s Crohn's disease does not constitute major trauma. Calculate his EEE.

$$EEE = 629 - 11(65) + 25(72) = 1714 \text{ kcal/day}$$

R.Y.'s energy needs by Harris-Benedict were between 1808 and 2109 kcal, as shown in a previous equation.

Case: B.N., 87.9 kg as ABW.

$$EEE = 629 - 11(75) + 25(87.9) - 609 = 1392.5 \text{ kcal/day.}$$

B.N.'s energy needs by Harris-Benedict were between 1400 and 1650 kcal/day.

Alternately, a simple way to estimate REE is to multiply the patient's weight (with the appropriate adjustments) by a range of kcal/kg/day derived from population studies (Table 12.4). Although not as exact (neither age nor height is considered), these values are a useful approximation of energy needs. The range chosen depends on the degree of metabolic stress experienced by the patient. Whatever method is used, a clinician would monitor the patient and adjust kilocalories as dictated by monitoring. Patients rarely require >3000 kcal/day.

PEDIATRICS

Energy requirements for infants and children vary with age and growth rate. Caloric demands during growth stages are

Table 12-4. Ranges to Estimate Energy Requirements	
Maintenance	25–30 kcal/kg/day
Moderate stress	30–35 kcal/kg/day
Severe stress	35–40 kcal/kg/day

at least 5 kcal/g of weight gained. Normal growth proceeds at a rate of approximately 25–30 g/day for the first 6 months, 13–18 g/day for the next 6 months, and 5–7 g/day thereafter. Parenteral nutrition in infants which is aimed at inducing rapid "catch-up" growth can be hazardous and often results in hepatic steatosis, edema, and excessive fat deposition. Therefore, moderate gains are advised, particularly because children seem to be more at risk for hepatic complications associated with parenteral nutrition.

The recommended dietary allowance (RDA) is the main source of reference for the enteral caloric requirements of normal, active, growing children. The RDA can serve as a guideline for many children requiring parenteral nutrition (Table 12.5). For a premature infant, 90–110 kcal/kg are usually sufficient for growth. Inactivity, mechanical ventilation, a comatose state, and a warm environment (e.g., infants in an isolette) will decrease caloric requirements of infants and children. Basal calories will be increased by fever,

Table 12-5.   RDA Calorie Requirements for Children to Adolescents[a]

	Age	RDA: Enteral		TPN
		Energy (kcal/kg/day)	Protein (g/kg/day)	Protein (g/kg/day)
Infants	Premature	110–150	3.0–4.0	2.0–2.5
	0–6 mo	115	2.2	2.5–3.0
	6–12 mo	105	2.0	2.5–3.0
Children	1–3 yr	100	1.8	1.5–2.5
	4–6 yr	90–85	1.5	1.5–2.5
	7–10 yr	85–80	1.2	1.5–2.5
Males	11–14 yr	60	1.0	1.0–1.5
	15–18 yr	42	0.85	
	19+ yr[b]	40	0.80	
Females	11–14 yr	47	1.0	1.0–1.5
	15–18 yr	38	0.84	
	19+ yr[b]	35	0.80	

TPN, total parenteral nutrition.
[a] Reprinted with permission. Benitz WE, Tratos DS. Pediatric Handbook. 2nd ed., Chicago, IL: Mosby Yearbook Publishers, Inc.; 1988;339–47.
[b] Use adult energy assessments.

Table 12-6. Kilocalorie to Nitrogen Ratio by Patient Condition

Adult Patient Condition	Ratio of Nonprotein Calories to Gram of Nitrogen
Adult medical patient (stable)	125–150:1
Minor catabolic state	125–180:1
Severe catabolic state	80–100:1
No renal function	250–400:1

cardiac failure, major surgery, burns, severe sepsis, long-term growth failure, and protein calorie malnutrition (Table 12.6).

Protein Requirements

Amino acids are given to abate protein losses and provide essential amino acids. In the past, it was common to report total energy requirements as nonprotein kilocalories. The practice was based on the hypothesis that amino acids delivered would be spared to make protein and not be metabolized for energy. Because it is not really possible to determine if any individual amino acid is being used for protein synthesis or is being metabolized for energy, most authorities now use the amino acid contribution as part of the daily energy requirement.[6] Whether exogenous or endogenous amino acids are used for synthesizing new protein is difficult to determine, but the provision of exogenous amino acids does preserve visceral and serum proteins. Supplying the proper kilocalorie to nitrogen ratio allows for nitrogen calories to be used for anabolism rather than as an energy source, the so-called "protein sparing" effect. The kcal/nitrogen ratios listed in Table 12.6 can be used for various adult metabolic states. The optimal kcal/nitrogen ratio for children of various ages needs further study, but a ratio of 150–200:1 is considered optimal.[7] Daily protein requirements are based on the appropriate body weight estimation. If a patient's weight is less than the IBW, the ABW should be used. Giving more protein than is necessary stimulates urea production and increases the BUN concentration. If a patient is obese, MAW should be used, correcting for edema if necessary. If a patient is edematous, estimated dry weight should be used. Protein requirement is closely related to the proper functioning of the liver and kidney and must be adjusted accordingly. As with energy, protein requirements vary with degree of metabolic stress (Table 12.7). Patients who have renal failure must be given small amounts of protein, because they cannot clear large amounts of urea produced by protein catabolism. Some urea can be cleared by intermittent hemodialysis. If continuous ambulatory peritoneal dialysis (CAPD) or continuous arteriovenous hemodialysis (CAVHD) is instituted, even more urea can be cleared and more protein can be given.

A patient who has hepatic failure may have decreased branched chain amino acids, increased serum urea, and difficulty in clearing aromatic acids, and high serum ammonia. In the past, protein was restricted in such patients. The current thought is that the patient should not be denied protein because a critical goal of therapy is to maintain functional proteins. Consequently, clinicians usually begin at 0.8–1 g/kg and increase as tolerated up to a maximum of 2 g/kg. Patients who have hepatic failure and are encephalopathic are restricted to 0.6–0.8 g/kg of protein to avoid excess ammonia production. Essential amino acid composition of commercial amino acid formulations is not sufficient to supply enough essential amino acids if the daily amount of protein calculated falls below 40 g. The patient must be given additional essential amino acids.

Table 12-7. **Adult Protein Requirements**

Maintenance	0.8–1.0 g/kg/day
Moderately stressed	1.1–1.5 g/kg/day
Severely stressed	1.5–2.0 g/kg/day
Renal failure	
Nondialyzed	0.8–1.2 g/kg/day
Hemodialyzed	1.0–1.2 g/kg/day
CAPD, CAVHD	1.2–1.5 g/kg/day
Hepatic failure	1.0–2.0 g/kg/day
Hepatic failure with encephalopathy	0.6–0.8 g/kg/day

Newborn and premature infants have immature renal and hepatic enzyme systems and may be unable to tolerate full protein requirements. Initial intake of 1 g/kg/day protein with increases of 0.5 g/kg/day may improve tolerance.[8] Guidelines for protein administration for pediatric patients are shown in Table 12.5.

Case: D.E., a 45-year-old man, 5'8", 64 kg, is recovering after extensive bowel resection. His hepatic and kidney functions are normal. Calculate his daily protein requirement. D.E. is neither obese nor edematous. Use ABW although D.E. is slightly below IBW and under moderate stress because of the extensive bowel resection.

Protein requirement (g/day) = 1.3 g × 64 kg = 83.2 g/day

Protein requirement (g/day) = 1.5 g × 64 kg = 96 g/day

Protein requirement is between 83 and 96 g/day

Case: U.T., a 49-year-old man, 5'9", 50 kg, has a creatinine clearance of 25 mL/min. He is given parenteral nutrition because of severe pancreatitis. Calculate his daily protein requirement.

Protein requirement (g/day) = 50 kg × 0.8 g/kg = 40 g

If U.T.'s creatinine clearance had been normal, his weight would have been multiplied by a larger factor (1–2 g protein/kg) to supply more protein. However, clinicians should initiate protein replacement conservatively in patients with low creatinine clearances and increase it after monitoring BUN.

Case: One week later, U.T. undergoes hemodialysis. Calculate his protein requirement.

Protein requirement (g/day) = 50 kg × 1.0 g/kg = 50 g

Case: One month later, CAPD is instituted. Calculate U.T.'s protein requirement.

Protein requirement (g/day) = 50 kg × 1.3 g/kg = 65 g

Again, most clinicians would be cautious and use the patient's BUN to determine when and how much to increase protein.

NITROGEN BALANCE

Protein requirements may be monitored and modified by following nitrogen balance.[9] The goal of an optimum protein intake is to have a positive nitrogen balance of 2–4 g/day. To calculate nitrogen balance, it is necessary to have a complete 24-hour urine collection. The complete collection of urine is not easy to obtain, even in a hospital, because it is easy to lose a portion of voided urine and, thus, underestimate urinary nitrogen loss. Urine must be collected with great care and results must be carefully interpreted. Because of these problems, many institutions do not rely routinely on nitrogen balance tests, even though nitrogen balance is still the definitive method for estimating protein requirements.

$$N_{balance} = N_{in} - N_{out}$$

N_{out} = Urinary urea nitrogen (UUN) losses plus obligatory losses

Obligatory losses are those from stool, sweat, etc. and average 2–4 g/day

UUN is measured and reported as grams of nitrogen/day.

$$N_{balance} = \frac{\text{Protein in}}{6.25} - (UUN + 2)$$

One gram of nitrogen = 6.25 g protein. In this formula, 2 g has been chosen as the obligatory loss. If a patient has proteinuria, the loss of nitrogen from urinary protein must be factored into the equation.

$$\frac{\text{Urinary Protein}}{6.25} = \text{grams of nitrogen lost as protein in urine}$$

Case: Parenteral nutrition, 2000 mL, D25%, AA 4.25%, 250 ml of 20% lipids for 4 weeks has been ordered for a patient whose weight and functional proteins are unchanged from admission. Nitrogen balance study shows 2569 mL of urine and urinary urea nitrogen of 5.6 g/L. Calculate the nitrogen balance for this patient.

Protein/day = 0.0425 g/mL × 2000 mL = 85 g protein/day

UUN = 5.6 g/L × 2.6 L = 14.56 g nitrogen/day

$$N_{balance} = \frac{85}{6.25} - (14.56 + 2) = -2.96$$

This patient has a negative nitrogen balance, and additional protein should be added to the parenteral nutrition. By rearranging the formula and setting nitrogen balance to

+ 2, the number of grams of protein needed to achieve positive nitrogen balance of 2 can be calculated. Care should be exercised when using this number because of the inconsistencies related to estimation of nitrogen loss.

$$[(2 + UUN) + 2] \times 6.25 = X$$
$$[(2 + 14.56) + 2] \times 6.25 = 116$$
$$X = 116 \text{ g protein needed}$$

CALCULATING OTHER NUTRITIONAL REQUIREMENTS

Electrolytes

Standard concentrations of electrolytes in parenteral nutrition solutions vary with institutional guidelines. The concentrations shown in Table 12.8 are derived from healthy populations and are general guidelines. The electrolyte concentration of a parenteral nutrition solution should be based on the patient's chemistries and clinical condition. Patients may have significant deficits or excesses of serum electrolytes.

Calcium is often withheld from peripheral parenteral nutrition in infants and children because continuous infu-

Table 12-8. Guidelines for Amount of Electrolytes to be Added to Parenteral Nutrition Solutions

Electrolyte	Adults	Children
Sodium	0–140 mEq/L	2–4 mEq/kg (max:100–120 mEq/d)
Potassium	40–60 mEq/L (max: 100 mEq/L)	2–3 mEq/kg (max:100–120 mEq/d)
Chloride	0–140 mEq/L	3–5 mEq/kg
Phosphate	0–20 mmol/L	0.3–1mMol/kg
Calcium	4.5–9.0 mEq/L	0.5–1.0 mEq/kg
Magnesium	8–12 mEq/L	0.2–1 mEq/kg
Acetate	Varies	Varies

sion of calcium has been associated with extravasation and subsequent tissue necrosis. Calcium gluconate boluses can be used to maintain serum calcium. Attempts to correct significant electrolyte disparities with parenteral nutrition are ill advised. Parenteral nutrition solutions generally are infused over 24 hours, and electrolyte imbalances should be taken care of immediately. In addition, unusual loads of electrolytes in parenteral nutrition can lead to instability of the solution, and constant modification of electrolyte concentrations can result in wasting these very expensive solutions. Problems with severe electrolyte deficits should be corrected by giving oral supplements if possible or with intravenous fluids containing the appropriate electrolytes. Commercial amino acid solutions contain varying concentrations of sodium, chloride, potassium, phosphate, and other electrolytes as counter-ions to positively and negatively charged amino acids. The counter-ions in amino acid solutions should be included in calculations of electrolyte requirements. Acetate salts are included in parenteral nutrition to electrically balance these solutions. Under conditions of metabolic acidosis, it is common to increase to the maximum possible value (i.e., maximize) the concentration of acetate salts because acetate is converted metabolically to bicarbonate, which raises pH. The concentration of chloride salts, which lower pH, is minimized. It is not always possible to provide no chloride, because amino acid solutions contain chloride counter-ions. Conversely, under conditions of metabolic alkalosis, acetate is minimized to avoid raising pH and chloride maximized to lower pH. Again, eliminating acetate completely is not possible because there are acetate salts in amino acid solutions. Severe cases of metabolic acidosis or alkalosis should be resolved by fluids and electrolyte solutions and not by parenteral nutrition.

Early after parenteral nutrition is instituted, potassium, magnesium, and phosphate shift intracellularly because of increased synthesis of cells. As a result, serum concentrations of potassium, magnesium, and phosphate fall. This so-called "refeeding syndrome" should be anticipated and serum electrolytes monitored carefully during this period.

In contrast to the convention for adult patients in whom serum electrolytes are ordered as mEq/L or mmol/L, serum electrolyte concentrations for pediatric patients are ordered in mEq/kg or mmol/kg. The compounding form and final label put on pediatric parenteral nutrition solutions should use these units of measure. A not uncommon mistake in pharmacies is to enter units into compounding forms and final labels of pediatric electrolytes as mEq or mmol/liter. This can cause serious problems in a pediatric patient's serum electrolytes.

Case: A 65-day-old male, 2.7 kg, is receiving 288 mL of parenteral nutrition, 0.46% amino acids, 12.5% dextrose with 2.0 mEq/kg sodium, 1.0 mEq/kg potassium, and 0.3 mmol/kg phosphate. The parenteral nutrition should have contained 5.4 mEq sodium, 2.7 mEq potassium, and 2.7 mEq phosphate. The pharmacist, however, entered the electrolyte order into a computerized compounding system that used units/liter rather than per kilogram. As a result, the parenteral nutrition was compounded with 0.288 (the total volume) × 2.0 mEq sodium, 1.0 mEq potassium, and 1.0 mEq phosphorus giving 0.58 mEq of sodium, 0.29 mEq of potassium, and 0.29 mMol of phosphate. Mistakes of this kind can cause serious electrolyte disturbances and be life-threatening.

Vitamins

Vitamin requirements for adults and children are based on the recommended daily allowances and can be found in many standard textbooks on nutrition. The importance of multivitamins was made tragically clear when shortages occurred of commercially available adult and pediatric multivitamins. A fatality was reported to ASPEN which probably resulted from a thiamine deficiency in a patient receiving parenteral nutrition who did not receive multivitamins for 6 weeks. The compositions of the most used adult and pediatric preparations are shown in Table 12.9. Generally, 10 mL of MVI-12 is given for adults and children older than 11 years of age. Vitamin K (10 mg) may be given subcutaneously or may be placed in the parenteral nutrition once weekly. Additional vitamin K may be added depending on the patient's PT, but the dose should not exceed 10 mg/day.

For pediatric patients, 2 mL/kg/day to a maximum of 5 mL/day total of MVI-Pediatric is used. Individual vitamins may be added for patients with specific needs.

Table 12-9. Composition of Adult and Pediatric Multivitamin Solutions

Vitamins	MVI—Pediatric/5 mL	MVI-12—Adult/10 mL
A	2,300 IU (700 mcg RE)	3,300 IU (1mg RE)
D	400 IU (10 mcg)	200 IU (5 mcg)
C	80 mg	100 mg
Thiamine (B$_1$)	1.2 mg	3 mg
Pyridoxine (B$_6$)	1.0 mg	4 mg
Riboflavin	1.4 mg	3.6 mg
Niacin	17 mg	40 mg
Pantothenic acid	5 mg	15 mg
E	7 IU (7mg)	10 IU (10 mg)
Folic acid	140 mcg	400 mcg
B$_{12}$	1.0 mcg	5 mcg
K	200 mcg	—
Biotin	20 mcg	60 mcg

Trace Elements

Recommendations for normal requirements of trace elements may be found in standard nutrition textbooks. Obligate amounts of trace elements in premature infants, or in patients with specific clinical disorders, are not well defined. The serum concentrations of trace elements should be measured if available, and the patient should be monitored clinically for potential deficits of trace elements. Table 12.10 gives concentrations of trace elements in commonly

Table 12-10. Composition of Adult and Pediatric Trace Element Solutions

Trace Elements	Pediatric Solution (TES)/0.2 mL	Adult Solution (MTE)/5.0 mL
Zinc	100 mcg	5 mg
Manganese	6 mcg	0.5 mg
Copper	20 mcg	2 mg
Chromium	0.2 mcg	20 mcg
Selenium	—	100 mcg

used commercial preparations. Generally, adults are given 5.0 mL of the adult solution daily. Copper and manganese are eliminated primarily via the bile. For adult patients with cholestasis, trace elements are withheld and appropriate amounts of zinc, selenium, and copper are added to the parenteral nutrition separately. An additional 12 mg/L of zinc may be added to make up for excessive losses of small bowel fluids. Up to 17 mg/L may be used for losses in stool and ileostomy output. Preterm infants are given 0.2 mL of pediatric trace element/kg/day supplemented with 300 mcg/kg/day of zinc and 2 mcg/kg/day of selenium. Term infants and children <15 kg should receive 0.2 mL/kg/day of pediatric trace elements. Children 15 kg or greater should receive 0.3 mL of pediatric trace elements daily, and children older than 11 years of age should be given 5 mL of adult trace elements daily. If term infants, children <15 kg, and children 15 kg or greater are receiving parenteral nutrition for longer than 4 weeks, they should receive 0.2 mcg/kg/day of selenium. As in adults, trace elements are withheld from children with cholestatic liver failure, and zinc, chromium, and selenium are provided separately. Additional zinc may be required when small bowel fluid, stool, or ileostomy losses are significant. Serum zinc levels should be monitored. Selenium is excreted by the kidneys. When the patient has renal failure, selenium should be omitted from parenteral nutrition, and serum concentrations should be monitored. Iron may be required in patients receiving erythropoietin or after prolonged parenteral nutrition; however, the use of iron dextran in parenteral nutrition solutions is strongly discouraged. Patients receiving parenteral nutrition for long periods may develop deficiencies in trace elements due to inadequate intake or underlying diseases.[10]

ADDITIONS TO PARENTERAL NUTRITION SOLUTIONS

Many compounds can be added safely to parenteral nutrition and total nutrient admixtures although it is usually best to keep the solution as simple as possible. Additions to total nutrient admixtures should be very limited because of the ease of breaking the emulsion and the difficulty of viewing a precipitate. The addition of large amounts (>1 g) of ascorbic acid to parenteral nutrition should be avoided, because ascorbate is oxidized to oxalate which could precipitate calcium. To determine whether a compound is compatible, major references of intravenous stability and compatibility should be consulted. Manufacturers of parenteral nutrition stock solutions often have data on compatibility, but the practitioner should be careful in making sure that solutions reported are identical to those in use. If no data can be found, any requested addition should be considered incompatible.

Regular insulin is compatible with parenteral nutrition and total nutrient admixtures and is often included in the solution of diabetics. The addition of insulin controls mild glucose intolerance and allows higher concentrations of dextrose to be given. The recommended dose is 0.1 units of insulin/g of dextrose to maintain blood glucose at <200 mg/dL. If blood glucose is >200 mg/dL, insulin is increased by 0.05 units/g of dextrose. The minimum amount of insulin that should be placed into a parenteral nutrition solution is 10 units because lower amounts of insulin are adsorbed on the container and tubing. The maximum recommended concentration of insulin to be added to parenteral nutrition is 50 units/L. If a diabetic patient is receiving insulin in parenteral nutrition, he or she should be instructed to stop subcutaneous insulin unless counseled otherwise by the physician. H-2 blockers are commonly added to parenteral nutrition and total nutrient admixtures at manufacturers' suggested doses for intravenous use.

CHARACTERISTICS OF PARENTERAL NUTRITION CONSTITUENTS

A listing of all dextrose, amino acid, and lipid solutions that are commercially available is beyond the scope of this chapter. Detailed lists can be found in major drug information catalogs and in textbooks cited in the references. Before the advent of automatic compounding instrumentation, parenteral nutrition was compounded manually. Pharmacies would mix 500 mL bottles of 50% dextrose and 8.5% amino acids to produce 1000 mL of 25% dextrose and 4.25% amino acids. Even today, this is a common prescription sent to hospital pharmacies because prescribers are familiar with this formulation. Today, dextrose can be obtained in many concentrations and volumes. The most commonly used are 2000 mL bags of 50% and 70% dextrose-containing solutions for use in automated admixture compounders. Since dextrose is a monohydrate, each gram yields 3.4 kcal. At least 20% and 30% of kilocalories in parenteral nutrition are supplied as dextrose to provide energy and obligatory glucose for the brain. If the rate of glucose infusion exceeds the capacity of the body to oxidize glucose, glucose metabolism is directed to the production of fat. Most authorities consider that between 4 and 7 mg/kg/min (with 5 mg/kg/min being optimal) is a range that protects the patient from excessive CO_2 production and unwanted deposition of fat in the liver.[11] The metabolic condition of the body varies in different disease states and with burns and trauma. In such situations, the clinical condition should dictate the actual rate of dextrose administration. Because of their higher metabolic rate, the accepted rate of glucose infusion is higher in pediatric patients, with some authorities suggesting 20 mg/kg/min as the upper rate of glucose infusion

Case: B.G., a 58-year-old, 50-kg woman is hospitalized for a flare-up of Crohn's disease. Parenteral nutrition is 2100 mL of 15% D, 5% AA over 24 hours and 250 ml of 20% lipid over 8 hours. Is this dextrose rate within acceptable limits?

$$\begin{aligned} \text{Dextrose rate} &= \text{mg dextrose/kg/min} = 15 \text{ g/100 mL} \\ &\times 2100 \text{ mL} = 315 \text{ g/50 kg} \\ &= 6.3 \text{ g/kg/1440 min/day} \\ &= 4.38 \text{ mg/kg/hr (Acceptable)} \end{aligned}$$

Concentrations of L-amino acids most frequently used are 8.5%, 10%, and 15% in 1000-mL bottles. Fifteen percent solutions are very expensive and are held for situations in which high protein content and low fluid are necessary. Amino acids yield 4 kcal/g. The type and concentration of specific amino acids varies in commercial preparations. Some formulations have been devised for specialized conditions. Pediatric solutions contain significant amounts of cysteine, histidine, and tyrosine, amino acids that are considered semi-essential for infants. In addition, taurine is included because it has been reported to prevent cholestasis associated with parenteral nutrition in children. Formulations for patients with liver disease are rich in essential branched chain amino acids and low in aromatic amino acids. Branched chain amino acids are a major source of energy in muscle. Aromatic amino acids are a major source of ammonia, which can exacerbate encephalopathy. The ability of the aromatic amino acids, tyrosine, and tryptophan to cross the blood–brain barrier and form the false neurotransmitters proposed to be related to encephalopathy is competitively inhibited by branched-chained amino acids.[12] By providing a formulation rich in branched chain amino acids, muscle is supplied with a source of energy, protein synthesis is stimulated, and the possibility of encephalopathy is minimized.

Formulations used in renal failure are enriched in essential amino acids. By shifting the amino groups of essential amino acids to nonessential acids, urea production is reduced. The effectiveness of these formulations is intensely controversial, however, and they are used only in very special cases.

Lipids yield 9 kcal/g and are available as 10% and 20% emulsions of soybean or safflower oil fatty acids. The 10% emulsion provides 1.1 kcal/mL. The 20% emulsion provides 2.0 kcal/mL. Lipid emulsions are contraindicated in the following:

1. Patients with pathologic hyperlipidemia, triglyceride levels >400–500 mg/dL.
2. Patients with acute pancreatitis with hyperlipidemia.
3. Patients with lipoid nephrosis when accompanied by hyperlipidemia.
4. Neonates with hyperbilirubinemia since lipids displace bilirubin from albumin. If bilirubin is <10 mg/dL (direct <2 mg/dL) and free fatty acid to albumin ratio is 4, lipid may be given because displacement is unlikely.
5. Patients with egg allergy, because egg yolk phospholipids are used as emulsifiers.

Lipid is used to deliver calories and to prevent and treat essential fatty acid deficiency (EFAD). To prevent EFAD, at least 8% of the total kcal/day must be given as lipid emulsions. To treat EFAD, 15–20% of the total kcal/day must be provided by lipid emulsion. The usual proportion of fat kilocalories is 15–30% of total kcal/day. In adults who tolerate lipid emulsion (i.e., those whose serum triglycerides do not rise above 500 mg/dL), a greater proportion of fat calories (up to 40%) may provide a balanced nutrient solution. The percentage of total kcal/day contributed by lipid should not exceed 60%. Patients who may benefit from a higher percentage of calories as lipid include:

1. Fluid-restricted patients (fat provides a more concentrated form of calories).
2. Glucose-intolerant patients.
3. Patients with respiratory compromise (chronic obstructive pulmonary disease, adult respiratory distress syndrome).

If lipids are infused too quickly, triglycerides cannot be cleared fast enough and may deposit in the reticuloendothelial system, compromising immune function.[13] Authorities differ over the rate at which lipids should be infused. Values given are between 0.03 and 0.05 g/kg/hr, not to exceed 0.11 g/kg/hr. For home care patients who are receiving cycled parenteral nutrition, most authorities believe a rate of 0.15 g/kg/hr is acceptable. For infants and children, fat emulsions should be administered over as long a period as possible, preferably 20–24 hours. In premature and newborn infants in whom the enzyme systems are immature, the rate of 20% solutions should not exceed 0.8 mL/hr. In infants, 1.3 mL/hour is the limiting rate. Rates should be decreased when serum triglycerides are >200 mg/dL.

Case: Is B.G.'s rate of lipid infusion acceptable? Rate = Grams of lipid/kg/hr.

250 mL of 20% lipid contains 500 kcal and 55.55 g lipid
$$55.55 \text{ g}/50 \text{ kg}/8 \text{ hr} = 0.14 \text{ g/kg/hr}$$

This value is excessive for a hospitalized patient, and the time of infusion should be increased. If the time is increased to 12 hours, 55.55 g/50 kg/12 hr = 0.09 g/kg/hr, which (although high) is acceptable.

Use of an increased percentage of lipid in patients with respiratory diseases (50% of the nonprotein calories as fat) can lower the respiratory quotient, reduce ventilatory demands, and make it easier to wean patients off ventilators.

CALCULATING VOLUMES OF PARENT SOLUTIONS NEEDED TO COMPOUND PARENTERAL NUTRITION FORMULAS

Case: An order is for 2400 mL of D25%, AA5%. What volumes of dextrose and amino acid parent solutions are needed if D70% and AA10% are used?

$$25 \text{ g}/100 \text{ mL} = 0.25 \text{ g/mL} \times 2400 \text{ mL} = 600 \text{ g of}$$
$$\text{dextrose required}$$

$$D70 = 70 \text{ g dextrose}/100 \text{ mL} = 0.7 \text{ g/mL}$$

Divide grams of dextrose needed by g/mL of parent solution to obtain milliliters of parent solution needed.

$$\frac{600 \text{ g}}{0.7 \text{ g/mL}} = 857.14 \text{ mL}$$

$$2400 \text{ mL of 5\% AA} = 5 \text{ g}/100 \text{ mL} \times 2400 \text{ mL} = 120 \text{ g}$$
$$\text{required}$$

$$AA10 = 10 \text{ g amino acids}/100 \text{ mL}$$
$$= 0.1 \text{ g/mL}$$

Divide grams of amino acids needed by g/mL of parent solution to obtain milliliters of parent solution needed.

$$\frac{120 \text{ g}}{0.1 \text{ g/mL}} = 1200 \text{ mL}$$

857 mL of parent 70%D

$$\frac{1200 \text{ mL}}{2057 \text{ mL}} \text{ of parent 10\% AA}$$

Remaining fluid would be made up with sterile water for infusion.

TOTAL NUTRIENT ADMIXTURES

In many hospitals and home care companies, lipid is incorporated into parenteral nutrition as an additive much in the same way as multivitamins. That is, if a parenteral nutrition solution of D25, AA6, 2000 mL + 500 mL of 20% lipid is ordered, the pharmacist calculates the grams of dextrose and amino acids, and the milliequivalents or millimoles of electrolytes needed, on the basis of 2000 mL and adds 500 mL of 20% lipid. In other cases, the volume of lipid is intended to be included in the volume used to calculate the grams of dextrose and amino acids, and the milliequivalents or millimoles of electrolytes needed. Thus, orders for total nutrient admixtures must be written clearly and the prescriber's intentions clarified when necessary.

OVERFILL

The administration of a parenteral nutrition solution to a patient requires intravenous tubing (i.e., an administration set). Fluid must pass through the set and any extension sets on the patient's catheter. Some parenteral nutrition fluid may be lost in filling up the tubing and removing air bubbles (i.e., priming), while some will remain in the tubing after administration of the required volume. It is customary to provide an additional amount of fluid (overfill volume) to compensate for the fluid lost in these procedures. It is critical that when overfill is used, the amount of dextrose, amino acids, lipid (in a total nutrient admixture), electrolytes, and additives be calculated on the basis of the final volume, including overfill. In pediatric parenteral nutrition, particularly for low-birthweight infants, exact volume with no overfill is the rule.

CALCULATING SALTS NEEDED TO SUPPLY ELECTROLYTES AND BALANCING PARENTERAL NUTRITION SOLUTIONS

Commercially available stock solutions of the salts used to provide electrolytes in parenteral nutrition solutions are listed in Table 12.11.

Amino acid stock solutions used to make parenteral nutrition contain varying concentrations of positively and

Table 12-11.   Electrolyte Concentrations of Commercially Available Solutions

Solution	Concentrations
Sodium chloride	4.0 mEq/mL sodium and 4.0 mEq/mL chloride
Sodium acetate	2.0 mEq/mL sodium and 2.0 mEq/mL acetate
Sodium phosphate	4.0 mEq/mL sodium and 3.0 mmol/mL phosphate
Potassium chloride	2.0 mEq/mL potassium and 2.0 mEq/mL chloride
Potassium acetate	4.0 mEq/mL potassium and 4.0 mEq/mL acetate
Potassium phosphate	4.4 mEq/mL potassium and 3.0 mmol/mL phosphate
Calcium gluconate	0.48 mEq/mL calcium and 0.48 mEq/mL gluconate (1 g = 4.8 mEq Ca gluconate)
Magnesium sulfate	4.0 mEq/mL magnesium and 4.0 mEq/mL sulfate (1 g = 8 mEq MgSO$_4$)

negatively charged electrolytes, which serve as counter-ions to positively and negatively charged amino acids in order to maintain electrical neutrality. The pH and the counter-ions used to balance the charge of amino acid solutions differ depending on the formulation. These differences can be significant in different clinical settings. Table 12.12 gives the pH and counter-ion concentrations of three commercially available amino acid solutions. It is necessary to include the electrolytes used as counter-ions in the amino acid solution as a part of the electrolytes added to fulfill the electrolyte requirement of the parenteral nutrition solution.

Because electrolytes are charged ions and parenteral solutions need to be neutral, acetate or chloride salts are used to balance these solutions electrically. Although most pharmacies use computer programs to calculate the volumes of salts needed to provide ordered electrolytes and to balance parenteral nutrition solutions electrically, it is sometimes necessary to perform these calculations manually. Table

Table 12-12. Counter-Ion Concentrations in Amino Acid Solutions

	Travasol 10% (Clintec)	Aminosyn II 10 % (Abbott)	FreAmine III 10% (McGaw)
Electrolytes (mEq/L)			
Sodium		45.3	10
Chloride	40		<3
Acetate	87	71.8	~89
Phosphate			10 (mmol/L)
PH	5.86		6.68

12.13 demonstrates a worksheet that can be used to calculate the volume of each salt solution needed to supply the milliequivalents or millimoles of each electrolyte ordered. It also shows how to account for the electrolyte contribution from the amino acid solution and how to balance electrolytes so that the parenteral solution is neutral.

DIVALENT CALCIUM PHOSPHATE PRECIPITATION

The hazard of calcium phosphate precipitation in parenteral nutrition solutions cannot be overemphasized. Two deaths have been ascribed to the deposition of calcium phosphate crystals in pulmonary arterioles.[14] Although total nutrient admixtures must be compounded carefully because precipitates cannot be seen, any parenteral nutrition solution can form precipitates either during compounding, storage, or administration. Factors affecting the precipitation of calcium phosphorus are complex and include the following:

1. *Concentration of Calcium and Phosphate.* When the calcium phosphate solubility product is exceeded, a precipitate forms. Thus, it is important to consider the contribution of phosphate counter-ions from amino acid solutions.

Table 12-13. Worksheet for Balancing Electrolytes Using Acetate Salts

	Na	K	P	Cl	OAc	Ca	Mg
Total electrolyte (mEq, mmol) required in total parenteral nutrition (Multiply electrolytes/L by no. of liters required)	2.1 × 60 = 126	2.1 × 60 = 126	2.1 × 12 = 25.2	2.1 × 70 = 147		2.1 × 5 = 10.5	2.1 × 6 = 12.6
Electrolytes from AA solution (multiply the electrolytes in the AA solution by the no. of liters of AA solution required				40 × 1.05 = 42	88 × 1.05 = 92.4		

continued

Table 12-13. *Continued*

	Na	K	P	Cl	OAc	Ca	Mg
Electrolytes needed from additives (mEq, mmol) Where necessary, subtract electrolytes in AA solution from total electrolytes required	126	126	25.2	147 − 42 = 105		10.5	12.6
Concentration of Commercially Available Stock Electrolyte Solutions							
KPO_4 (3 mmol P/mL; 4.4 mEq K/mL)		36.9 mEq 8.4 mL	25.2 mmol 8.4 mL				
KCl (2 mEq/mL)		89.1 mEq 44.5 mL		89.1 mEq 44.5 mL			

	Na	K	Phos	Cl	OAc	Ca	Mg
NaCl (4 mEq/mL)	15.9 mEq / 4.0 mL			15.9 mEq / 4.0 mL			
NaOAc (4 mEq/mL)	110 mEq / 27.5 mL				110 mEq / 27.5 mL		
Ca gluconate (0.47 mEq/mL) (do not need to balance)						10.5 mEq / 22.3 mL	
Mg sulfate (4 mEq/mL) (do not need to balance)							12.6 mEq / 3.15 mL
Totals per liter (divide by no. of liters)	60 mEq	60 mEq	12.2 mmol	70 mEq	96.4 mEq	5 mEq	6 mEq

Rx: D25, AA5, 2. IL (includes overfill).

Electrolytes: Na 60 mEq/L; K 60 mEq/L; Cl 70 mEq/L; Phos 12 mMol/L; Ca 5 mEq/L; Mg 6 mEq/L.

Use Travasol 10% as amino acid stock solution containing Cl⁻ 40 mEq/L, OAc 88 mEq/L.

1. Row 1: Calculate the mEq or mmol of electrolytes needed (ordered amount × the liters of the parenteral nutrition solution).
2. Row 2: Calculate amount of electrolytes from amino acid solution (electrolytes/L of amino acid solution × liters of amino acid solution used).
3. Row 3: Subtract amount of electrolytes contributed by the amino acid solution from amount of electrolytes needed to find amount of electrolytes to be added.
4. Start balancing with potassium phosphate; 25.2 mmol phosphate required/ 3 mmol phosphate in potassium phosphate = 8.4 mL of potassium phosphate solution.
5. 8.4 mL of potassium phosphate × 4.4 mEq potassium/mL = 36.9 mEq of potassium.
6. Subtract contribution of potassium from potassium phosphate from total potassium needed = 89.1 mEq potassium still needed.
7. Use potassium chloride to supply remaining potassium. 89.1 mEq/2 mEq/mL potassium chloride = 44.6mL of potassium chloride solution and 89.1 mEq of chloride.
8. Subtract contribution of chloride from potassium chloride from total chloride needed = 15.9 mEq.
9. Supply remaining chloride with sodium chloride; 15.9 mEq chloride/4 mEq/ml sodium chloride = 4.0 mL sodium chloride and 15.9 mEq of sodium.
10. Subtract contribution of sodium from sodium chloride from total sodium needed = 110 mEq sodium still needed.
11. Complete the sodium requirement by using sodium acetate; 110 mEq/4 mEq/mL sodium acetate = 27.5 mL of sodium acetate and 110 mEq of acetate.
12. Calculate the volumes of calcium gluconate and magnesium sulfate needed to complete the calcium and magnesium requirements. Calcium and magnesium are balanced by their solution salts, gluconate and sulfate, which are not metabolized.
13. Check calculations.

Sum mEq or mmol for each electrolyte added. Divide by total volume of the parenteral nutrition solution.

The solution is balanced (i.e., electrically neutral). Their solution salts, gluconate and sulfate, balance calcium and magnesium. The 42 mEq of chloride and the 92.4 mEq of acetate contributed by the amino acid solution are balanced by counter-ion amino acids. For potassium, negative phosphate ions balance 36.9 mEq. This leaves 89.1 mEq positive charges from potassium and 126 mEq positive charges from sodium for a total of 215 mEq. Negative charges come from 89.1 mEq of chloride from potassium chloride, and 15.9 mEq of chloride from sodium chloride and 110 mEq of acetate from sodium acetate. Negative mEq add up to 215 mEq balancing positive mEq.

2. *Salt Form of Calcium.* Calcium gluconate is preferred because it is not as ionized as calcium chloride.
3. *Concentration of Amino Acids.* Table 12.14 gives the concentration of calcium and phosphate ions per liter that may be added in relation to the concentration of amino acids. Amino acids buffer parenteral nutrition solutions, keeping the pH in a range unfavorable for calcium phosphate precipitation. The low

Table 12-14. Maximum Allowable Calcium and Phosphate Concentration in Parenteral Nutrition in Relationship to Amino Acid Concentration

	Ca (mEq/L)	Phosphate (mmol/L)
2.1–3.0% amino acids	18	5
	15	6
	12	8
	10	10
	8	15
	5	40
3.1–4.0% amino acids	20	5
	15	8
	12	10
	10	15
	8	20
	6	30
	5	40
>4.0 % amino acids	25	5
	20	7
	15	9
	12	15
	10	20
	5	40

The data in this table apply to all dextrose concentrations. If the amount of calcium or phosphate to be added is between two numbers, the corresponding amount at the next lower level is chosen.

concentration of amino acids in pediatric parenteral nutrition coupled with low volume and the relatively high amounts of calcium and phosphorus needed for growth are particularly susceptible to these effects.

4. *pH of the Solution.* As the pH rises, the amount of divalent phosphate able to bind covalently with calcium increases. Commercially available amino acid solutions have different pHs. When changing from one to another, it is critical to judge the effect this may have on the amount of calcium and phosphorus that can be added safely to a parenteral nutrition solution.

5. *Temperature of the Solution.* More ionized calcium and divalent phosphate are available to react at higher temperatures. When the solution is being infused, ambient room temperature can increase the temperature of the solution and facilitate precipitation of calcium phosphate.

6. *Presence of Other Additives.* Strongly alkaline additives can increase pH, and divalent cations like magnesium can foster the precipitation of calcium phosphate. Lipids can increase the pH of solutions but rarely cause a problem because of the buffering capacity of the commonly used amino acid concentrations.

7. *Order of Mixing.* Phosphate salts should be added early in the preparation of parenteral nutrition. Calcium salts should be added later, near the time when the solution has reached its maximum dilution.

Because of the unpredictability of calcium phosphate precipitation, most institutions insert a 0.22 micron filter for parenteral nutrition solutions and a 1.2 micron filter for total nutrient admixtures in the path of the administration set in expectation of trapping calcium phosphate particles.

COMPOUNDING PARENTERAL NUTRITION UNDER SPECIAL CLINICAL CONDITIONS

Although many institutions now have automated, computerized compounding equipment, the pharmacist should understand and be able to prepare parenteral nutrition solutions without recourse to manufacturers' software.

Using Standard Parenteral Nutrition Solutions

Many hospitals and institutions, particularly those without computerized automated compounding equipment, use standard parenteral nutrition formulations, often with standard concentrations of electrolytes. Common parenteral nutrition formulations contain 20–25% dextrose with 5–6% amino acids and 10% or 20% fat emulsion. The amount of fat used in standardized total nutrient admixtures varies, but many institutions use 500 kcal from lipid.

Case: A 40-year-old woman, 5'3", 50 kg, is on bowel rest for 3 weeks. Needed: 1750 kcal/day, 60 g/day protein. Institution uses D25%, AA5% standard solution.

First, calculate milliliters of standard solution to supply 60 g of protein/day.

$$5\% \text{ Protein} = 0.05 \text{ g protein/mL of solution}$$

$$\frac{60 \text{ g}}{0.05 \text{ g/mL}} = 1200 \text{ mL of parenteral nutrition solution}$$

$$\text{Protein kcal} = 240 \text{ kcal}$$

Calculate kcal from 25% dextrose in 1200 mL of standard parenteral nutrition

$$\text{Dextrose kcal} = 1020 \text{ kcal}$$

1750 kcal desired − {240 kcal amino acids + 1020 kcal dextrose} = 490 kcal needed

Remaining kilocalories can be furnished from lipid, 20% 250 mL each day = 500 kcal/day. For a total nutrient admixture, the lipid would be added to the solution directly.

Minimizing Fluid in Parenteral Nutrition

Under certain clinical conditions when a patient is fluid-overloaded (e.g., congestive heart failure, chronic renal failure, hypoproteinemia, pulmonary edema), the fluid in parenteral nutrition must be minimized. Commercial amino acids are available as dilute (8.5%, 10%, and 15 %) solutions. Because of the low concentrations, amino acids stock solutions add considerable fluid to parenteral nutrition. Moreover, the maximum allowable amino acid concentration in parenteral nutrition is limited to 7%, further dictating that parenteral nutrition solutions are relatively dilute. The minimum amount of fluid that can be used, therefore, is circumscribed by the amount of fluid necessary to deliver the required amino acids.

Case: A 56-year-old woman, 5',5", 60 kg, has Stage III congestive heart failure complicated by edema and cardiac cachexia. She needs 1650 kcal/day and 75 g protein/day. For parenteral nutrition, 6% amino acid is reasonable for this patient. Determine the rate (mL/hr) of parenteral nutrition (delivered over 24 hours) using 6% as the final percentage of amino acids.

$$\frac{\text{Total g/protein/24 hr}}{\text{\% amino acids in parenteral nutrition}} = \begin{array}{l}\text{Rate of}\\\text{parenteral nutri-}\\\text{tion (mL/hr)}\end{array}$$

$$\frac{75 \text{ g/24 hr}}{0.06 \text{ g/mL}} = 52.08 \text{ mL/hr (52 mL/hr); kcal from amino}$$
acids = 300 kcal

Choose an amount of dextrose that will supply a significant number of calories for the parenteral nutrition. Twenty percent dextrose can be combined safely with 6% amino acids.

20% dextrose contains 0.2 g of dextrose/mL × 52 mL/hr × 24 hr = 250 g dextrose = 850 kcal from dextrose

Use 250 mL of 20% lipid (2 kcal/mL × 250 mL = 500 kcal to supply 500 kcal/day). Percentage of total kilocalories as lipid is 30%. For a total nutrient admixture, the 500 mL of lipid would be added directly to the admixture each day.

> 300 kcal (protein) + 850 kcal (dextrose) + 500 kcal
> (lipid) = 1650 kcal/day requirement.
>
> Total fluid = 52 mL/hr × 24 hr (amino acids and
> dextrose) = 1248 mL + 250 mL (lipid)
> = 1498 mL

Maintenance at ideal weight (57 kg) = 2240 mL, so there is a 742 mL saving of fluid that could be supplied by an additional infusion or held as required. Additional fluid could be saved if 25% dextrose was used and 250 mL of 20% lipid were given 4 times per week.

$$0.25 \text{ g/ml} \times 52 \text{ mL} \times 24 \text{ hr} = 312 \text{ g} \times 3.4 \text{ kcal/g} = 1060 \text{ kcal from dextrose}$$

$$1650 \text{ kcal (desired)} - \{300 \text{ kcal (amino acids)} + 1060 \text{ kcal (dextrose)}\} = 290 \text{ kcal}$$

It is not necessary to supply the exact amount of kcal/day.

Contribution from lipid can be averaged over a week (e.g., lipid given only on specific days of the week). If 250 mL 20% lipid is given 4 times per week, the yield is 2000 kcal/week (286 kcal/day), 17 % lipid.

$$\text{Fluid from lipid} = (250 \text{ mL (lipid)} \times 4 \text{ days} = 1000/7) = 143 \text{ mL/day}$$

$$\text{Total fluid} = 52 \text{ mL/hr} \times 24 \text{ hr} = 1248 \text{ mL} + 143 \text{ mL} = 1391 \text{ mL compared to } 1498 \text{ mL with } 20\% \text{ dextrose.}$$

For a total nutrient admixture, 145 mL of 20% lipid (2 kcal/mL) would be added directly to the admixture to provide 290 kcal from lipid.

Supplying Total Maintenance Fluid in Parenteral Nutrition

It is common to supply the daily total maintenance fluid required by a patient in parenteral nutrition. This is especially true in the home, where only one intravenous line may be available.

Case: A 60-year-old, 6', 75-kg man with short bowel syndrome needs 2600 mL/day, 2250 kcal/day, 95 g protein/day.

Use protein requirement to determine the percentage of amino acids in the final solution (maintenance fluid amount).

$$\frac{\text{Total g of amino acids}}{\text{Total daily fluid requirement (mL)}} = \% \text{ amino acids (g/100 mL)}$$

$$\frac{95 \text{ g amino acid}}{2600 \text{ mL}} \times 100 = 3.65\%; \text{ kcal from amino acids} = 380 \text{ kcal/day}$$

Calculate lipid to be used. Lipid is generally given as 20–40% of total calories, but it is not unusual to go as high as 60%.

If 20% is chosen; 2250 kcal/day $\times$ 0.2 = 450 kcal/day
from fat

Use 250 mL of 20% lipid (2 kcal/mL) to provide 500
kcal/day from fat = 22.2 % fat.

2250 kcal required $-$ {380 kcal (amino acids) + 500 kcal
(lipid)} = 1370 kcal

Calculate grams of dextrose needed to supply 1370 kcal.

3.4 kcal/g (caloric content of dextrose)

$$\frac{1370 \text{ kcal}}{3.4 \text{ kcal/g}} = 403 \text{ g dextrose}$$

$$\frac{403 \text{ g}}{2600 \text{ mL}} \times 100 = 15.5\% \text{ dextrose}$$

Final parenteral nutrition is 3.6% AA, 15.5% dextrose,
2600 mL + 250 mL of 20% lipid daily.

The 250 mL of lipid is probably inconsequential because
that amount can easily be handled by a patient with no fluid
problems. If an exact amount of fluid is required, the 250
mL of lipid can be subtracted from the total fluid requirement and the result used to calculate the percentages of dextrose and amino acids needed. For a total nutrient admixture, 250 ml of 20% lipid would be added to the parenteral
nutrition daily.

INITIATING PARENTERAL NUTRITION

Parenteral nutrition should be instituted at a slow rate (e.g.,
30–40 mL/hr), using the final concentration of dextrose,
amino acids, and lipids planned for therapy. The infusion
rate is increased by 30 mL/day as glucose tolerance permits
(i.e., serum glucose maintained at <200 mg/dL). Blood glucose monitoring via finger sticks every 6 hours (more frequently in patients in the intensive care unit) is indicated
until the infusion rate has stabilized. Alternatively, total
fluid may be infused to start, but a low concentration of
dextrose (e.g., 15%) may be run for 2–3 days. The concentration of dextrose would then be increased gradually to the
required concentration as tolerated by the patient.

If 24-hour parenteral nutrition must be discontinued, the rate of administration is gradually slowed to prevent rebound hypoglycemia. A typical approach is to reduce the hourly rate by 50% for 30 minutes, and then reduce that rate again by 50% for an additional 30 minutes before stopping the infusion. Alternately, the rate may be decreased to 50 mL/hr for the last hour before discontinuation. Some hospitals infuse 10% dextrose when parenteral nutrition is discontinued abruptly. Rebound hypoglycemia does not occur commonly in adults when parenteral nutrition is discontinued without tapering,[15] but parenteral nutrition should never be discontinued abruptly in infants or children.[16] Transition from parenteral nutrition to enteral or oral feeding is a gradual process. Parenteral nutrition is discontinued when enteral or oral intake achieves two-thirds of the patient's estimated needs.

CYCLING PARENTERAL NUTRITION

It is sometimes advantageous to supply parenteral nutrition over a shorter period of time than 24 hours. Generally, cycled infusions are given for 12 hours, but shorter or longer infusion times can be used depending on the patient's tolerance. Most infants and younger children cannot tolerate anything less than a 16-hour cycle. Twelve-hour infusion times are particularly useful in the home, giving the patient the freedom to perform tasks without having to carry around a bag and pump. Cycling is being used in hospitals increasingly. There is no evidence that parenteral nutrition is any less effective or that metabolic abnormalities occur more frequently when parenteral nutrition is cycled. Before beginning cycling, it must be assured that fluid requirements are met.

There are two approaches to cycling parenteral nutrition:

1. When patient is already receiving 24-hour parenteral nutrition. Several regimens can be used in this situation. A common regimen lowers the time of infusion on day 1 to 20 hours, on day 2 to 16 hours, and on day 3 to 12 hours. The infusion rate is adjusted accordingly. Depending on the patient's response, the cycling may be slower and the final duration of infusion may be longer.

2. When patient is initiated on parenteral nutrition with cycling. A common regimen begins parenteral nutrition at 30 mL/hr for 6 hours and the rate of infusion is increased by 20 mL/hour every 6 hours until the final rate is achieved.

The gradual discontinuation of parenteral infusion is affected by the rate of administration of the final solution. If the rate is >160 mL/hr, a two-step taper is often used. The first step is to decrease the rate of infusion by 50% for 1 hour, then to decrease the rate again by 50% for an additional hour, before discontinuation. If the rate of administration is <160 mL/hr, it is decreased by 50% for the last hour of the cycle and then discontinued. In the home, when electronic ambulatory pumps are used, rates of infusion may be decreased with a continuous ramping down for the last 1 or 2 hours of the infusion.

MONITORING OF PATIENTS RECEIVING PARENTERAL NUTRITION

Parenteral nutrition is an invasive therapy, and patients should be monitored carefully for metabolic abnormalities throughout the course of the therapy. The suggested regimen in Table 12.15 provides some guidelines for monitoring patients who require parenteral nutrition.

Monitoring of patients receiving parenteral nutrition should be individualized according to clinical status, chemical abnormalities, and severity of illness.

COMPLICATIONS OF PARENTERAL NUTRITION

Complications of parenteral nutrition can be categorized into mechanical, infectious, and metabolic. Mechanical complications include pneumothorax, air embolism, venous thrombosis, and catheter occlusion. Careful placement and radiographic evidence of catheter site can minimize the development of pneumothorax. Home care

Table 12-15. Clinical Monitoring of Patients Receiving
Parenteral Nutrition

Suggested Frequency	Monitoring Parameters
Baseline (within 72 hours hours before; 24 hours after therapy has begun)	Na, K, Cl, HCO_3, PO4, Mg, albumin, prealbumin, Ca, ALT, AST, Alk phos, T. bilirubin, creatinine, BUN, PT, blood glucose, TG, cholesterol, CBC, weight
Daily	Weight, finger stick glucose
Daily until stable (first 3–5 days, then 2–3 times per week)	Na, K, Cl, HCO_3, PO4, Mg, prealbumin, Ca, BUN, TG, intake and output, blood, glucose, urine glucose for neonates, children, weight
Weekly	For neonates: length/height, head circumference
Every 10–14 days	PT, ALT, AST, Alk phos, T. bilirubin, prealbumin
After 2 months and every 2 months thereafter	Selenium
Long-term pediatric patients	Triceps skinfold and mid-arm circumference may be used to assess progress in long-term patients

Additional chemistries that may be drawn include PTH, individual vitamins, minerals, trace elements, and visceral proteins (other than prealbumin).

patients, particularly, should be well educated in the care of their catheters to minimize problems with air emboli. If a catheter is occluded with fibrin from blood, one or two instillations of urokinase may dissolve the fibrin and restore flow to the catheter. In any case, nurses should never draw blood from, or give other medications through, a catheter dedicated to parenteral nutrition. Not only is the risk of occlusion enhanced, but also the potential for infection is increased. Fatty deposits from parenteral nutrition itself can

Table 12-16. Metabolic Complications, Causes, and Corrections of Parenteral Nutrition

Complications	Possible Cause(s)	Correction(s)
Hyperglycemia Glucosuria Hyperosmolar dehydration	Diabetes	Decrease dextrose concentration in parenteral nutrition
	Excessive glucose infusion rate	Reduce parenteral nutrition rate; adjust content to meet needs
	Hypoinsulinemia	Start insulin according to institution's guidelines
	Sepsis	
	Glucocorticoids	
	Potassium depletion	Ensure adequate potassium, phosphorus, chromium
Rebound hypoglycemia (<60 mg/dL after infusion)	Insulin secretion persists after abrupt discontinuation of concentrated glucose	Avoid sudden cessation of parenteral nutrition
		If parenteral nutrition is discontinued suddenly, start D10W infusion
		Discontinue insulin if added to solution
Hyperkalemia	Decreased renal function	Consider dialysis
	Excessive administration	Reduce/hold parenteral nutrition
	Low cardiac output	If severe, insulin or Kayexalate (by mouth or by enema
	Tissue necrosis and systemic sepsis	

continued

Table 12-16. Metabolic Complications, Causes, and Corrections of Parenteral Nutrition (*Continued*)

Complications	Possible Cause(s)	Correction(s)
Hypokalemia	Protein synthesis increases requirement (refeeding syndrome) Diuresis, GI losses Potassium wasting drugs	Increase K in parenteral nutrition Replace K by intravenous or oral route
Hyperphosphatemia	Excessive phosphate administration Renal insufficiency	Reduce phosphate in parenteral nutrition until normal achieved
Hypophosphatemia	Inadequate phosphate in parenteral nutrition Increased need due to anabolism	Increase phosphate in parenteral nutrition Replace phosphate by either intravenous or oral route
Hypervitaminosis/hypovitaminosis	Excessive or inadequate provision of vitamins	Adjust vitamins in parenteral nutrition
Hypermagnesemia	Excessive amount in parenteral nutrition Renal insufficiency	Reduce Mg in parenteral nutrition
Hypomagnesemia	Increased need due to anabolism	Increase Mg in parenteral nutrition Replace magnesium by either intravenous or oral route

Hypercalcemia	Excessive calcium in parenteral nutrition Excessive vitamin D Neoplasm	Reduce calcium in parenteral nutrition Give isotonic saline or other appropriate medical treat
Hypocalcemia	Increased requirement due to underlying medical problem	Increase Ca in parenteral nutrition as solubility of calcium phosphate allows
Hypertriglyceridemia	Intolerance due to underlying disease Inability to clear lipids	Reduce lipid to that needed to prevent essential fatty acid deficiency
Essential fatty acid deficiency	Inadeqaute lipid	Provide approximately 4–10% of daily calories as (250 mL of 20% lipid once or twice weekly)
Prerenal azotemia	Excessive amino acids in parenteral nutrition Insufficient nonprotein calories Inadequate hydration	Decrease amino acids in parenteral nutrition Provide adequate hydration
Hyperchloremic metabolic acidosis	Renal failure, diarrhea, pancreatic fistula, ileostomy, excessive chloride in total parenteral nutrition	Replace chloride salts with acetate salts in parenteral

continued

Table 12-16. Metabolic Complications, Causes, and Corrections of Parenteral Nutrition (*Continued*)

Complications	Possible Cause(s)	Correction(s)
Metabolic alkalosis	Diuretics, nasogastric suction, vomiting, hypokalemia, excessive acetate salts in parenteral nutrition	Replace acetate salts with chloride salts in parenteral
Zinc deficiency	Increased GI losses, wound healing	Increase Zn in parenteral nutrition
Copper deficiency	Failure to provide dose in parenteral nutrition	Provide minimum recommended dosage in parenteral
Hypercapnia	Excessive calories/carbohydrates	Decrease calories, then decrease dextrose
Hepatic/biliary dysfunction	Fatty liver	Avoid excessive dextrose
	Cholestasis	Overfeeding
		Provide adequate amino acids

occlude catheters. Careful instillation and removal of 0.1 N NaOH, 0.1 N HCl, cysteine HCl, or absolute ethanol can dissolve these precipitates.

Patients and nurses should observe scrupulous aseptic technique in dressing changes and care of catheters. Infections may appear as an erythematous, indurated area around the catheter site. In other instances, there may be only unexplained fever. It is often difficult to determine the exact source of a catheter-related fever. Cultures of the site or the catheter itself are frequently contaminated by the presence of skin bacteria so that identification of the infectious agent cannot be definitive. A course of antibiotics often resolves the problem. But care should be taken to minimize the use of vancomycin to avoid the emergence of resistant organisms. The last recourse is removal and replacement of the catheter.

The many metabolic problems that can be associated with parenteral nutrition as well as their possible causes and suggested corrections are given in Table 12.16. Clinicians caring for patients receiving parenteral nutrition should be experienced in the detection and resolution of these complications.

Acknowledgments

The author thanks the staff and the pharmacy students at the Drug Product Services Laboratory, Department of Clinical Pharmacy, University of California, San Francisco for their support.

References

1. Madan M et al. A randomized study of the effects of osmolality and heparin with hydrocortisone on thrombophlebitis in peripheral intravenous nutrition. Clin Nutr. 1991;10:309–14.

2. American Society of Parenteral and Enteral Nutrition, (ASPEN) Board of Directors. Guidelines for the Use of Parenteral and Enteral Nutrition in Adult and Pediatric Patients. JPEN. 1993;17(4):1SA–52SA.

3. Jequier E. Measurement of energy expenditure in clinical nutritional assessment. JPEN. 1987;11:86S–9S.

4. Roza AM, Shizgal HM. The Harris Benedict equation reevaluated: resting energy requirements and the body cell mass. Am J Clin Nutr. 1984;40:168–82.

5. Ireton-Jones CS. Energy expenditure assessment: predictive equations. Support Line. 1996;28(5):14–16.

6. Miles JM. Yes, protein should be included in calorie calculations for a TPN prescription. Nutr Clin Pract. 1996;11:204–5.

7. Easton LB et al. Parenteral nutrition in the newborn, a practical guide. Pediatr Clin North Am. 1982;29:1171.

8. Cochran EB et al. Therapy review: parenteral nutrition in pediatric patients. Clin Pharm. 1988;7:351.

9. Long C. Metabolic response to injury and illness: estimation of energy and protein needs from indirect calorimetry and nitrogen balance. JPEN. 1979;3:452.

10. Triplett WC. Clinical aspects of zinc, copper, manganese, chromium and selenium metabolism. Nutr Int. 1985;1(2):60.

11. Wolfe RR. Carbohydrate and requirements. In: Rombeau JL, Caldwell MD, eds. Clinical Nutrition: Parenteral Nutrition. 2nd ed. Philadelphia, PA: WB Saunders; 1975:113–31.

12. Fischer JE, Baldessarini RJ. False neurotransmitters and hepatic failure. Lancet. 1971;2:5–80.

13. Fischer JE et al. Diminished bacterial defenses with intralipid. Lancet.1980;2:819–20.

14. Hill SE et al. Fatal microvascular pulmonary emboli from precipitation of a total nutrient admixture solution. JPEN. 1996;20:81–7.

15. Krzywda EA et al. Glucose response to abrupt initiation and discontinuation of total parenteral nutrition. JPEN. 1993;17:64–7.

16. Bendorf K et al. Glucose response to discontinuation of parenteral nutrition in patients less than 3 years of age. JPEN. 1996;20:120–3.

Suggested Readings

Grant JP. Handbook of Total Parenteral Nutrition. 2nd ed. Philadelphia, PA: WB Saunders; 1992:368.

Holcomb BJ. Adult Parenteral Nutrition in Applied Therapeutics. 6th ed. Young LY, Koda-Kimble MA, eds. Vancouver, WA: Applied Therapeutics, Inc.; 1995:35-1–16.

Rombeau JL, Caldwell MD, eds. Clinical Nutrition: Parenteral Nutrition. 3rd ed. Philadelphia, PA: WB Saunders; 2000.

Wong AF. Pediatric Nutrition in Applied Therapeutics. 6th ed. Young LY, Koda-Kimble MA, eds. Vancouver, WA: Applied Therapeutics, Inc.; 1995:99-1–21.

Chapter 13

Common Calculations in Pharmacy Practice

Shelley L. Chambers

The practice of pharmacy requires the ability to perform calculations with the highest proficiency. Mastering this skill is achieved by training and practice. As students approach independent practice, they realize that patients will depend on their accuracy. Thus, students should double their efforts to perfect their calculation skills. This chapter reviews some of the more common and some of the much rarer but more complex calculations encountered in pharmacy practice. Students should take the time to look up those conversion factors, equations, or doses that they have not used often enough to remember well. Calculations that have not been performed before should be checked by another pharmacist.

CALCULATION FUNDAMENTALS

Proportions

Many of the calculations performed in pharmacy practice are **direct proportions**, that is, as one value increases, an associated value increases; or as one value decreases, an associated value decreases. An example of a direct proportion would be the calculation of doses based on weight. The recommended dose of amoxicillin is 7 mg/kg three times a day. The patient weighs 42 kg.

$$\frac{7 \text{ mg}}{1 \text{ kg}} = \frac{x \text{ mg}}{42 \text{ kg}}$$

In words, this equation states that the dose increases by the same proportion (factor) as the patient's weight increases. In the example, the related terms are in the same position in the fraction on either side of the equals sign. Solving for x:

$$(42 \text{ kg}) \frac{7 \text{ mg}}{1 \text{ kg}} = \frac{x \text{ mg}}{42 \text{ kg}} (42 \text{ kg})$$

$$x = (42 \text{ kg}) \frac{7 \text{ mg}}{1 \text{ kg}}$$

$$x = 294 \text{ mg}$$

As another example, how many milliliters of diltiazem injection, 5 mg/mL, should be drawn into a syringe to provide an 18-mg dose? Using the direct proportion method:

$$\frac{5 \text{ mg}}{1 \text{ mL}} = \frac{18 \text{ mg}}{y \text{ mL}}$$

Rearranging to solve for y:

$$(y \text{ mL}) \frac{5 \text{ mg}}{1 \text{ mL}} = \frac{18 \text{ mg}}{y \text{ mL}} (y \text{ mL})$$

$$(y \text{ mL}) \frac{5 \text{ mg}}{1 \text{ mL}} \frac{(1 \text{ mL})}{5 \text{ mg}} = \frac{18 \text{ mg} (1 \text{ mL})}{5 \text{ mg}}$$

$$(y \text{ mL}) = \frac{18 \text{ mg}}{5 \text{ mg}} (1 \text{ mL})$$

$$y = 3.6 \text{ mL}$$

The result of rearranging this direct proportion gives us the following relationship:

$$\text{volume} = \frac{\text{dose}}{\text{concentration}}$$

Inverse Proportions

The most common example of an **inverse proportion** is a dilution calculation. If 10 mL of a 5% solution is diluted to 100 mL, the concentrations are **inversely** related to the volumes:

$$\frac{10\ mL}{100\ mL} = \frac{x\%}{5\%} \qquad x = 0.5\%$$

When something is diluted, the volume goes up but the concentration goes down. In the case of an inverse proportion, the related values are in opposite positions in the fractions.

Conversion Factors and Conversion Between Systems of Measurement

There are two systems of measurement used in the United States: the avoir du pois system used by most of the lay public, and the metric system, which has been used by medicine and science for many years. The use of avoir du pois units still persists in medical charts and on prescriptions, so the pharmacist must know how to convert from avoir to metric units and when exact equivalents should be used for those conversions. Avoir units should be converted to metric units using exact equivalents (conversion factors with three significant figures) before compounding or dosage calculations are performed. For dispensing calculations, such as how much commercially available hydrocortisone cream to dispense when 1 oz (avoir) has been ordered, the pharmacist may use approximate equivalents. The relationship between the two systems is shown in Table 13.1.

USING CONVERSION FACTORS

Consider the following question: how many milligrams are contained in a 5-gr aspirin tablet? A conversion factor is a statement of equivalence, and this allows us to use

Table 13-1. Systems of Measurement

	Exact Equivalent	Approximate Equivalent
Units of length		
1 meter (m)	39.4 in	
1 inch (in)	2.54 cm	
Units of volume		
1 teaspoon (tsp)	5 mL	
1 tablespoon (tbs)	15 mL	
1 fluiddram (flz)	3.69 mL	
1 fluidounce (flZ)	29.6 mL	30 mL
1 pint (16 flz)	473 mL	480 mL
1 quart (32 flZ, 2 pts)	946 mL	1 L
1 gallon (4 qts)	3785 mL	
Units of weight		
1 kilogram (kg)	2.2 pounds (lb)	
1 gram (g)	15.4 grain (gr)	
1 grain (gr)	64.8 mg (65 mg)	60 mg
1 ounce (oz)	28.35 g	30 g
1 pound (lb)	454 g	

them as if they were fractions that equal one. The logic is as follows:

If 1 gr. = 65 mg then 1 gr./65 mg = 1 and 65 mg/1 gr. = 1

So the fraction may be inverted to suit the conversion desired:

$$5 \text{ gr. aspirin} \frac{(65 \text{ mg})}{1 \text{ gr.}} = 325 \text{ mg aspirin}$$

Note that the units, grains (gr), have canceled out, providing the answer in milligrams.

CONVERSION OF BODY WEIGHT

If the dose of fluconazole is 15 mg/kg and the patient weighs 35 lb, what is the appropriate dose?

$$1 \text{ kg} = 2.2 \text{ lb}$$

$$35 \text{ lb} \frac{(1 \text{ kg})}{2.2 \text{ lb}} = 15.9 \text{ kg}$$

Dose is $\dfrac{5 \text{ mg}}{\text{kg}}$ (15.9 kg) = 79.5 mg fluconazole

Dimension Analysis

Dimension analysis is a technique learned in physics or chemistry. The solution to a problem is determined by the units (dimensions) that the answer should have. It can be described as the use of a string of conversion factors, or appropriately related terms (see below), to provide an answer in the appropriate units. Many problems that can be solved with direct proportions can also be solved with dimension analysis. A particularly useful application of this technique is in the calculation of infusion rates. For example, consider an order for 10,000 units heparin sodium in 250 mL normal saline to be infused over 4 hours. The solution will be infused with an intravenous administration set that delivers 20 drops/mL. The nurse will set the flow rate once the infusion is connected to the patient by adjusting the number of drops/min delivered by the set. Thus, the pharmacist needs to type an infusion rate on the label using the units drops/min. This dimension analysis example begins with the related terms: 250 mL over 4 hours. Although this is not a conversion factor, the relationship of these terms is known because they are stated in the problem: 250 mL/4 hr. The other conversion factors or related terms need to be arranged so that the units mL/hr are cancelled out and the answer is in drops/min. The other related terms are 20 drops/mL and the well-known conversion factor of 60 min/hr. Starting with 250 mL/4hr, the dimension analysis setup is as follows:

$$\frac{(250 \text{ mL})}{4 \text{ hrs}} \frac{(20 \text{ drops})}{\text{mL}} \frac{(1 \text{ hr})}{60 \text{ min}} = \frac{20.8 \text{ drops}}{\text{min}}$$

Because a nurse cannot count 20.8 drops, this number is rounded up to the nearest whole number, 21 drops/min.

CALCULATIONS USED IN DISPENSING

Concentration Expressions and Labeling Conventions

An essential function of pharmacy practice is to ensure that the patient receives the right dose. This is often as simple as instructing the patient to take the appropriate number of tablets. In other cases, the right dose depends on the correct interpretation of a concentration expression. Table 13.2 presents the labeling conventions used in pharmacy practice to describe the strength/unit dose of manufactured dosage forms. Although these conventions are widely used, some are more easily understood than others.

Calculation Example

A patient has read that 12 mg β-carotene daily will provide protection from a variety of cancers. If 1 IU β-carotene is

Table 13-2. Labeling Conventions in Pharmacy

Dosage Form	Dose	Strength/Unit Dose	Dose to the Patient
Oral solids	g or mg	g or mg/tablet or capsule	Number of tablets or capsules
Oral liquids	g or mg	g or mg/5 mL or 15 mL	Teaspoons or tablespoons[a]
Topical products	inches or to cover	Percent w/w or w/v[b]	Inches or film to cover
Small volume parenterals	mg	mg/mL[c]	Number of mL
Large volume parenterals	g or mg	Weight (g or mg)/container	Volume per unit time
Ophthalmic or nasal liquids	Drops	Percent w/v[b]	Drops

continued

Table 13-2. *(continued)*

Dosage Form	Dose	Strength/Unit Dose	Dose to the Patient
Ophthalmic ointments	Inches	Percent w/w[b]	Inches
Suppositories	g or mg	g or mg/suppository	Number of suppositories
Inhalations	Inhalations	Weight/inhalation	Number of inhalations
Certain naturally derived drugs	International units[d]	International units/ unit dose	Number of mL, tablets
Certain electrolytes	mEq[c]	mEq/mL, tablets, tsp	Number of mL, tablets, tsp

[a] Doses of oral liquids for children often cannot be expressed conveniently in teaspoons, so milliliters are used in the instructions to the patient. It is important to double check the units in the sig because substitution of "teaspoons" for "milliliters" will produce a five-fold error in the dose.

[b] Percentage preparations are interpreted as follows: (1) for solids in solids, g/100 g; (2) for liquids in liquids, mL/100 mL; (3) for solids in liquids, g/100 mL.

[c] Occasionally, conventions other than mg/mL are used to expres the concentrations of injections. Some injectables are labeled in percent and should be interpreted as above (g/100, never mg/100). Ratio strength is an older convention used to express the concentration of dilute solutions such as epinephrine, 1:1000. The units of a ratio strength mixture are understood to be as follows: (1) for solids in solids, g/1000 g; (2) for liquids in liquids, mL/1000 mL; and (3) for solids in liquids, g/1000 mL.

[d] Units of potency are used to label insulin and a number of other natural products, an expression that describes the biological activity of a batch of natural drug rather than the weight. In some cases, units of potency may need to be converted to milligrams or micrograms of drug.

[e] The doses of various electrolytes are expressed as milliequivalents to account for the number of plus or minus charges contributed by the electrolyte. A milliequivalent can be defined as:

$$1 \text{ milliequivalent} = \frac{\text{weight of 1 millimole}}{\text{valence}}$$

For example,

$$1 \text{ milliequivalent of NaHCO}_3 = \frac{84 \text{ mg}}{1} = 84 \text{ mg}$$

and

$$1 \text{ milliequivalent of Na}_2\text{CO}_3 = \frac{106 \text{ mg}}{2} = 53 \text{ mg}$$

and

$$1 \text{ milliequivalent of CaCl}_2 \cdot 2\text{H}_2\text{O} = \frac{147 \text{ mg}}{2} = 73.5 \text{ mg}$$

equivalent to 0.485 mcg, how many milligrams of β-carotene are contained in a supplement with 25,000 IU?

$$25,000 \text{ IU} \frac{(0.485 \text{ mcg})}{1 \text{ IU}} \frac{(1 \text{ mg})}{1000 \text{ mcg}} = 12.1 \text{ mg beta carotene}$$

Calculation Example

A hospitalized patient has been receiving 3.6 g potassium chloride per day by continuous, intravenous infusion. How many Klorvess tablets (20 mEq KCl/tab) should this patient take daily to provide the equivalent dose of potassium (FW KCl 74.5)? By proportion:

$$\frac{74.5 \text{ mg KCl}}{1 \text{ mEq KCl}} = \frac{3600 \text{ mg KCl}}{x \text{ mEq KCl}} \qquad x = 48 \text{ mEq KCl}$$

$$\frac{20 \text{ mEq KCl}}{\text{tablet}} = \frac{48 \text{ mEq KCl}}{x \text{ tablets}} \qquad x = 2.4 \text{ tablets}$$

MILLIMOLES

The valence and therefore the number of equivalents of some ions (phosphate salts in particular) will vary with pH. Therefore, the concentration of this phosphate electrolyte is expressed as millimoles/milliliter (mmol/mL), and the dose may be expressed in millimoles. The source of phosphate for total parenteral nutrition (TPN) formulae is generally potassium phosphate injection that contains 236 mg of K_2HPO_4 and 224 mg of KH_2PO_4 per milliliter.

Calculation Example

How many millimoles of phosphate does the injection contain per milliliter? From a reference book:

1 millimole K_2HPO_4
  = 174 mg (which contains 1 mmole PO_4)
1 millimole KH_2PO_4
  = 136 mg (which also contains 1 mmole PO_4)

By dimension analysis, the answer in mmol/mL:

$$\frac{(236 \text{ mg K}_2\text{HPO}_4)}{\text{mL}} \frac{(1 \text{ mmole K}_2\text{HPO}_4)}{174 \text{ mg}}$$

$$= \frac{1.36 \text{ mmole K}_2\text{HPO}_4}{\text{mL}}$$

$$\frac{(224 \text{ mg KH}_2\text{PO}_4)}{\text{mL}} \frac{(1 \text{ mmole KH}_2\text{PO}_4)}{135 \text{ mg}}$$

$$= \frac{1.66 \text{ mmole KH}_2\text{PO}_4}{\text{mL}}$$

$$\begin{aligned}
&1.36 \text{ mmole PO}_4 \text{ as K}_2\text{HPO}_4 \\
+\ &\underline{1.66 \text{ mmole PO}_4 \text{ as KH}_2\text{PO}_4} \\
&3.02 \text{ mmole PO}_4/\text{mL}
\end{aligned}$$

Quantity to Dispense

A prescription will often not specify the quantity of drug to dispense, although the amount can be inferred from other information.

Calculation Example

Consider the following prescription:

Rx   Duricef 250/5cc
      Sig: 1 tsp q 12 h × 10 d.

This product is available as either a 50-mL or 100-mL container of powder for reconstitution. Because we know that 1 teaspoon = 5 mL and this dose will be administered twice a day, we can calculate:

$$\frac{(5 \text{ mL})}{\text{dose}} \frac{(2 \text{ doses})}{\text{day}} (10 \text{ days}) = 100 \text{ mL}$$

Calculation Example

Rx   Prednisone 20 mg tab
      Sig: Take 2 bid × 7 d, 1 bid × 7 d,
         1 qd × 7 d, 1 qod × 7 d.

The number of units to be dispensed can be calculated as follows:

$$
\begin{aligned}
2 \text{ bid} \times 7 \text{ d} &= 2 \times 2 \times 7 = 28 \\
1 \text{ bid} \times 7 \text{ d} &= 1 \times 2 \times 7 = 14 \\
1 \text{ qd} \times 7 \text{ d} &= 1 \times 7 \quad\;\; = \;\; 7 \\
1 \text{ qod} \times 7 \text{ d} &= \qquad\qquad = \;\; \underline{4} \\
&\qquad\qquad\quad\; 53 \text{ tablets}
\end{aligned}
$$

Duration of Therapy

Another calculation problem encountered in dispensing is that the amount of drug ordered or the shelf life of the preparation may not be adequate to provide for the intended duration of therapy.

Calculation Example

Rx Cephalexin 125/5 cc Disp. 100 mL
Sig: 3/4 tsp q 6 h × 10 d.

The patient will use $(0.75 \times 5 \text{ mL})$/dose × 4 doses/day = 15 mL/day

$$
\frac{100 \text{ mL}}{15 \text{ mL/day}} = 6.7 \text{ days supply}
$$

A larger amount than 100 mL will need to be dispensed to provide the patient with 10 days of treatment.

Calculation Example

Alternatively, the pharmacist may be interested in determining whether patients are using their medications as directed by calculating the expected number of days the medication should last. Consider the prescription below for an inhaler. The patient would like to pick up two canisters this month because she runs out before the end of the month.

Rx   Albuterol Inhaler Disp. 1
      Sig: 1–2 puffs qid.
      Refill prn.

The albuterol inhaler contains 200 actuations (puffs). Maximum usage is assumed. Using dimension analysis, the answer needs to be in days/container:

$$\frac{(200\ puffs)}{(container)}\frac{(1\ dose)}{(2\ puffs)}\frac{(1\ day)}{(4\ doses)} = \frac{25\ days}{container}$$

CALCULATIONS USED IN COMPOUNDING

Reducing and Enlarging Formulae with Factors

Many pharmacists who compound maintain formulation files that detail the amounts of ingredients required to make standard quantities of a preparation. On receipt of the prescription, the pharmacist then must reduce or enlarge the formula to make the amount specified in the prescription. This can be done easily using proportions. When using a series of calculations (e.g., increasing the size of a formula with many ingredients by some factor), it will be simpler to calculate the factor and apply it to each of the calculations. Consider the following formula for an oral suspending vehicle:

Sugar-Free Suspending Vehicle

Methylcellulose	1 g
Saccharin sodium	0.3 g
Benzoic acid	0.2 g
Water, q.s.	100 mL

It is desired to make 500 mL of the suspending vehicle to have on hand for dispensing oral liquids to patients who are unable to swallow tablets. The value of each ingredient in the formula must be increased by:

$$\frac{500 \text{ mL}}{100 \text{ mL}} = 5$$

methylcellulose	1 g × 5	=	5 g
saccharin sodium	0.3 g × 5	=	1.5 g
benzoic acid	0.2 g × 5	=	1.0 g
water, q.s.	100 mL × 5	=	500 mL

Admixture Calculations

Calculation Example

Box 13.1	Medication Orders
3/24/98 8 AM	Lidocaine 2 g, furosemide 800 mg in 1000 mL D5W Infuse at 25 mcg lidocaine/kg/min

The above admixture will be prepared with the 20% lidocaine injection and furosemide injection, 10 mg/mL. How many milliliters of the lidocaine injection and how many milliliters of furosemide injection are required to prepare the order? Using proportions:

Lidocaine $\dfrac{20 \text{ g}}{100 \text{ mL}} = \dfrac{2 \text{ g}}{y \text{ mL}}$ $y = 10 \text{ mL}$

Furosemide $\dfrac{10 \text{ mg}}{1 \text{ mL}} = \dfrac{800 \text{ mg}}{y \text{ mL}}$ $y = 80 \text{ mL}$

The pharmacist should add 10 mL of 20% lidocaine and 80 mL of 10 mg/mL furosemide to the admixture.

Calculation Example

Box 13.2	Medication Orders
3/25/98 6 AM	Potassium chloride 3g, enalaprilat 5 mg in 1000 mL D5W 1 liter per 24 hours

What volume of potassium chloride injection, 2 mEq/mL should be used to fill the order above? First convert the weight of KCl to milliequivalents:

$$\frac{74.5 \text{ mg KCl}}{1 \text{ mEq KCl}} = \frac{3000 \text{ mg KCl}}{x \text{ mEq KCl}} \qquad x = 40.3 \text{ mEq KCl}$$

Then calculate the volume of KCl injection to be used:

$$\frac{2 \text{ mEq}}{1 \text{ mL}} = \frac{40 \text{ mEq}}{y \text{ mL}} \qquad y = 20 \text{ mL}$$

Enalaprilat is available as 2-mL vials containing 1.25 mg/mL. How many vials are required to fill the order?

$$\frac{1.25 \text{ mg}}{1 \text{ mL}} = \frac{5 \text{ mg}}{y \text{ mL}} \qquad y = 4 \text{ mL}$$

Two vials are required to provide 4 mL.

INFUSION RATES

Large volume parenterals (e.g., the two orders above) are administered using two types of infusion devices: drip sets and infusion pumps. Infusion rates for drip sets are expressed in drops/min, and rates for infusion pumps are expressed in mL/hr.

Calculation Example

The order for potassium chloride and enalaprilat will be administered with a drip set that delivers 20 drops/mL. What infusion rate in drops/min should be used to administer the solution? The liter is intended to be delivered over 24 hours. The problem can be most conveniently solved using dimension analysis:

$$\frac{(1000 \text{ mL})}{(24 \text{ hours})} \frac{(20 \text{ drops})}{(\text{mL})} \frac{(1 \text{ hour})}{(60 \text{ min})} = \frac{13.9 \text{ drops}}{\text{min}} = \frac{14 \text{ drops}}{\text{min}}$$

Calculation Example

Assume that the first admixture for lidocaine and furosemide will be administered using an infusion pump to a patient who weighs 74.5 kg. What infusion rate should be typed on the label? The answer should be in mL/hr.

$$\frac{(1000\ mL)}{(2\ g)}\ \frac{(1\ g)}{(1000\ mg)}\ \frac{(1\ mg)}{(1000\ mcg)}\ \frac{(25\ mcg)}{(kg/min)}$$

$$\times\ (74.5\ kg)\ \frac{(60\ min)}{hour} = \frac{111{,}750}{2000} = \frac{56\ mL}{hour}$$

Dilutions

Dilution calculations are common in pharmacy practice and are among the most confusing to solve. Broadly, two types of dilution problems are encountered: those in which a more concentrated solution is diluted with a vehicle and those in which two concentrations of an ingredient are combined to achieve an intermediate concentration.

DILUTIONS WITH VEHICLE

When a more concentrated solution is diluted with a vehicle, the concentration of the product decreases and the volume increases. This category of problem can be conveniently solved as an inverse proportion:

$$\frac{Original\ concentration}{\textbf{Diluted concentration}} = \frac{\textbf{diluted volume}}{original\ volume}$$

The related terms (i.e., diluted concentration and diluted volume) are in *opposite* positions in the fractions on either side of the equation. When using this method, the concentrations should be expressed using the same convention [i.e., both in percent (w/v) or both in mg/mL], and ratio strength expressions should be converted to mg/mL or to percent.

Calculation Example

What volume of Zephiran chloride solution 17% should be used to prepare 1000 mL of a 0.1% solution? Using the inverse proportion method:

$$\frac{17\%}{0.1\%} = \frac{1000 \text{ mL}}{y \text{ mL}} \qquad y = 5.9 \text{ mL}$$

Calculation Example

How many milliliters of adult-strength amphotericin B, 5 mg/mL, and how many milliliters of sterile water for injection are required to make 10 mL of a neonatal concentration, 0.1 mg/mL? Using the inverse proportion method:

$$\frac{5 \text{ mg/mL}}{0.1 \text{ mg/mL}} = \frac{10 \text{ mL}}{y \text{ mL}} \qquad y = 0.2 \text{ mL amphotericin B}$$

$$\begin{array}{r} 10 \\ - \ \underline{0.2} \\ 9.8 \text{ mL SWI} \end{array}$$

Calculation Example

The instructions on the Domeboro tablets package states that two tablets in a pint of water make a modified Burow's solution equivalent to a 1:20 dilution. How should the patient be instructed to dilute the tablets to produce a 2.5% solution?

First convert the ratio strength expression to percent (w/v):

$$\frac{1 \text{ g}}{20 \text{ mL}} = \frac{x \text{ g}}{100 \text{ mL}} \qquad x = 5$$

Then solve the inverse proportion. From memory, Table 13.1, or a reference book, 1 pint = 473 mL.

$$\frac{5\%}{2.5\%} = \frac{x \text{ mL}}{473 \text{ mL}} \qquad x = 946 \text{ mL}$$

The patient should be advised to dilute the 2 tablets in 1 quart of water. Alternatively, the patient could dilute 1 tablet in 1 pint of water.

TWO CONCENTRATIONS OF AN INGREDIENT TO ACHIEVE AN INTERMEDIATE CONCENTRATION

When a calculation involves mixing two different strengths, a shorthand technique called alligation medial may be used. Alligation medial, which is used to determine the resulting concentration when two or more strengths are mixed, calculates a weighted average. Consider the following prescription for psoriasis:

Rx Alphaderm^R 30 g
Racet^R 30 g
Mix and dispense 60 g.
Sig: Apply to psoriatic lesions bid.

Alphaderm is a commercially available cream that contains 1% hydrocortisone and 10% urea. Racet contains 0.5% hydrocortisone and 3% iodochlorhydroxyquin. How should the product be labeled? In other words, what are the concentrations of hydrocortisone, iodochlorhydroxyquin, and urea in the final product? By alligation medial:

Percent hydrocortisone: the parts contributed by the hydrocortisone in each cream is calculated by multiplying the concentration by the weight of the cream:

Total parts		Ingredient parts
1×30	=	30
$0.5 \times \dfrac{30}{60}$	=	$\dfrac{15}{45}$

Divide ingredient parts by total parts:

$$\frac{45}{60} = 0.75\% \text{ hydrocortisone}$$

Percent iodochlorhydroxyquin:

Total parts		Ingredient parts
0×30	=	0
$3 \times \dfrac{30}{60}$	=	$\dfrac{90}{90}$

Divide ingredient parts by total parts:

$$\frac{90}{60} = 1.5\% \text{ iodochlorhydroxyquin}$$

Percent urea:

Total parts		Ingredient parts
10×30	$=$	300
$\dfrac{0 \times 30}{60}$	$=$	$\dfrac{0}{300}$

Divide ingredient parts by total parts:

$$\frac{300}{60} = 5\% \text{ urea}$$

Tonicity Calculations—E Value

Pharmacists occasionally prepare nasal, ophthalmic, or injectable solutions that must contain a total concentration of ionic and molecular solutes and must be approximately isoosmotic with body fluids. They usually strive to make such solutions equivalent to 0.9% sodium chloride which is considered isotonic, although the U.S.P. states that the eye can tolerate osmotic concentrations equivalent to 0.6–2.0% sodium chloride without significant discomfort.[1] The isotonicity of solutions for mucous membranes or injection may be adjusted using one of several approaches. The most versatile of these is the **E value method, which calculates the weight of sodium chloride equivalent to 1 g of drug or other solute.** In some cases, the E value of the drug has been tabulated,[2] and the amounts of water and isotonic vehicle to be added to prepare an isotonic product can be calculated using proportions.

Calculation Example

How much water and how much isotonic sodium chloride solution should be used to make 100 mL of a 4% cocaine hydrochloride solution isotonic? From a suitable reference,[2] the E value of cocaine hydrochloride is 0.16. An E value of 0.16 means that 1 g of cocaine hydrochloride is equivalent to 0.16 g NaCl in terms of the number of particles contributed to the solution. Use 4 g cocaine hydrochloride, suggesting the following proportion:

$$\frac{4 \text{ g drug}}{1 \text{ g drug}} = \frac{x \text{ g NaCl}}{0.16 \text{ g NaCl}} \qquad x = 0.64 \text{ g NaCl}$$

The 4 g cocaine hydrochloride is equivalent to 0.64 g NaCl. Because we know that 0.9% sodium chloride solutions are isotonic, we know that 0.9 g NaCl would make 100 mL isotonic solution. The proportion below calculates the amount of solution that can be made isotonic by adding water to 0.64 g of NaCl, the amount that is equivalent to our drug:

$$\frac{0.9 \text{ g NaCl}}{100 \text{ mL}} = \frac{0.64 \text{ g NaCl}}{y \text{ mL}} \qquad y = 71.1 \text{ mL}$$

The solution can be made from 4 g cocaine hydrochloride, 71.1 mL water, and $100 - 71.1 = 28.9$ mL isotonic saline.

CALCULATION OF E VALUE

Although many E values have been tabulated, the usefulness of this parameter lies in the fact that it can be calculated for any drug for which the molecular weight and empiric formula (or chemical structure) are known. Thus, the pharmacist confronted with the need to compound an isotonic product for a drug not previously tabulated can calculate an E value after consulting the appropriate reference books. The E value for a drug or other solute can be calculated from the following formula[3]:

$$\frac{x \text{ g NaCl}}{(58.5 \text{ g NaCl}/1.8)} = \frac{1 \text{ g drug}}{(\text{FW drug}/\text{MP})}$$

Where FW is the drug's formula weight in grams and MP is the number of moles of particles per mole of drug.

If the solute is a drug salt or a hydrate, the formula weight must include the weight of the counter-ion or waters of crystallization as well as the drug ion or molecule. The number of particles per mole of drug is based on the number of ions in the drug salt and can be determined from the formula or chemical structure. A nonelectrolyte drug will produce 1 mole of particles for each mole of drug. The approximations found in Table 13.3 for drug salts assume 80% dissociation of ions in solution.[3] Once the E value has been calculated, the pharmacist can calculate the amounts of water and isotonic vehicle or tonicity agent to be used to prepare an isotonic product.

Calculation Example

A physician has a patient with herpes keratitis and would like to use the acyclovir injectable to make a 2.5 % eyedrop. The injectable product is available as a 0.5-g vial of lyophilized powder. How much water and how much saline should be used to reconstitute the lyophilized powder to make 20 mL of an isotonic solution? From a reference book, the formula weight of acyclovir sodium is 247 and the formula is $C_8H_{11}N_5NaO_3$. Acyclovir is the monosodium salt and therefore would dissociate into 2 ions and

Table 13-3. Example Drug Solutes

Drug	Formula	Description	Moles of Particles Per Mole of Drug
Dextrose	$C_6H_{12}O_6$	Nonelectrolyte	1.0
Dipivefrin hydrochloride	$C_{19}H_{29}NO_5HCl$	Drug salt, 2 ions	1.8
Atropine sulfate	$(C_{17}H_{23}NO_3)_2H_2SO_4H_2O$	Drug salt, 3 ions	2.6
Ticarcillin disodium	$C_{15}H_{14}N_2Na_2O_6S_2$	Drug salt, 3 ions	2.6
Sodium citrate	$C_6H_5Na_3O_7$	Drug salt, 4 ions	3.4

(inferring from Table 13.3) would yield 1.8 moles of particles per mole (per 247 g) of the drug. Using the above formula:

$$\frac{x \text{ g NaCl}}{(58.5 \text{ g NaCl}/1.8)} = \frac{1 \text{ g acyclovir sodium}}{(247 \text{ g acyclovir sodium}/1.8)}$$

Rearranging and solving for x g NaCl:

$$x \text{ g NaCl} = \frac{1 \text{ g drug } (58.5 \text{ g NaCl}/1.8)}{(247 \text{ g}/1.8)}$$

$$x = 0.24$$

An E value of 0.24 means that 1 g of acyclovir sodium is equivalent to 0.24 g NaCl in terms of the number of particles contributed to the solution. Our vial contains 0.5 g acyclovir, suggesting the following proportion:

$$\frac{0.5 \text{ g drug}}{1 \text{ g drug}} = \frac{x \text{ g NaCl}}{0.24 \text{ g NaCl}} \qquad x = 0.12 \text{ g NaCl}$$

The 0.5-g drug contained in the vial is equivalent to 0.12 g NaCl. Because we know that 0.9% sodium chloride solutions are isotonic, we can set up the following proportion to calculate the number of milliliters of water and isotonic vehicle that should be added to make 20 mL solution.

$$\frac{0.9 \text{ g NaCl}}{100 \text{ mL}} = \frac{0.12 \text{ g NaCl}}{y \text{ mL}} \qquad y = 13.3 \text{ mL}$$

The eyedrop can be made from 0.5 g acyclovir sodium, 13.3 mL water, and 20 − 13.3 = 6.7 mL isotonic saline.

CALCULATION OF DOSES

As the understanding of drug kinetics has increased, so has the variety of ways to determine doses of drugs. These include dosing by age, by weight or lean body weight, by surface area, by creatinine clearance, by titration to a therapeutic endpoint, and by using pharmacokinetic parameters. Drug doses should be individualized whenever possible to elicit the desired therapeutic response with minimal side effects. The preferred method for determining a drug's dose depends on its margin of safety and the drug's kinetics.

Box 13.3 summarizes the equations used for the calculation of doses.

Box 13.3   Equations for the Calculation of Doses

---

1 kg = 2.2 lb

LBW (males) = 50 kg + 2.3 × no. of inches over 5 ft[4]

LBW (females) = 45.5 kg + 2.3 × no. of inches over 5 ft[4]

BSA (infants) = $M^{0.5378} \times H^{0.3964} \times 0.024265$[6]

BSA (children, adults) = $M^{0.425} \times H^{0.725} \times 0.007184$[7]

Jellife[8]:

$$Cl_{Cr} \text{ (males/1.73 m}^2) = \frac{98 - 0.8 \text{ (age} - 20)}{S_{cr}}$$

$$Cl_{Cr} \text{ (females/1.73 m}^2) = \frac{[98 - 0.8 \text{ (age} - 20)] \times 0.9}{S_{cr}}$$

Cockcroft and Gault[9]:

$$Cl_{Cr} \text{ (males)} = \frac{[140 - \text{age}] \times LBW}{72 \times S_{cr}}$$

$$Cl_{Cr} \text{ (females)} = \frac{[140 - \text{age}] \times LBW \times 0.85}{72 \times S_{cr}}$$

Age and Weight

The labeling of many drugs provides a dose or dosage range for adults, a second dose or dosage range for children, and a third for elderly patients. This is an adequate method for dosing drugs with a wide margin of safety and only requires calculations if, in addition to age, doses are described on a per unit weight basis.

A patient is 2.5 years of age and weighs 30 lb. He has a staphylococcal infection in the soft tissue of his right hand. The literature on cloxacillin sodium lists the dose for children under 20 kg as 50–100 mg/kg daily in 4 divided doses. How many milliliters of Tegopen (cloxacillin sodium) solution, 125 mg/5 mL, should the patient receive in each dose? Convert his weight:

$$(30 \text{ lb}) \frac{(1 \text{ kg})}{(2.2 \text{ lb})} = 13.6 \text{ kg}$$

Calculate the daily dose:

$$(13.6 \text{ kg}) \frac{(75 \text{ mg})}{(1 \text{ kg})} = 1020 \text{ mg/day}$$

Divide the daily dose into 4:

$$\frac{(1020 \text{ mg})}{(1 \text{ day})} \frac{(1 \text{ day})}{(4 \text{ doses})} = 255 \text{ mg/dose}$$

Calculate the volume he should receive:

$$\frac{(255 \text{ mg})}{(\text{dose})} \frac{(5 \text{ mL})}{(125 \text{ mg})} = 10.2 \text{ mL/dose or about 2 teaspoonsful}$$

Lean Body Weight

Because some drugs partition largely into body water or lean tissue and, to a much lesser extent, into adipose, an obese patient could receive more drug than required to produce therapeutic levels in the lean tissues if the dose was based on actual body weight. It is preferable, then, to calculate the patient's lean body weight and use this as the basis for calculating the dose of such drugs. The following equations can be used to calculate lean body weight[4]:

LBW (males) = 50 kg + 2.3 × # inches over 5 ft
LBW (females) = 45.5 kg + 2.3 × # inches over 5 ft

The digitalizing or loading dose of digoxin tablets is 10–15 mcg/kg. What is the appropriate dose for a 62-year-old woman who is 5 feet, 1 inch tall and weighs 188 pounds (85.5 kg)? Calculate lean body weight:

LBW (females) = 45.5 kg + 2.3 × 1
           = 47.8 kg

Calculate the digitalizing dose:

$$(47.8 \text{ kg}) \frac{(12.5 \text{ mcg})}{(1 \text{ kg})} = 597.5 \text{ mcg}$$

The patient should receive one 250-mcg tablet immediately and a second 250-mcg tablet in 6–8 hours.

Surface Area

Because body surface area (BSA) has a stronger relationship to renal clearance and to metabolic capacity than does body weight, BSA is preferred for calculating doses of drugs with narrower margins of safety. BSA may be conveniently taken from a nomogram.[5,6] Alternatively, body surface area may be calculated from the following equations[6,7]:

BSA (infants) = $M^{0.5378} \times H^{0.3964} \times 0.024265$
BSA (children, adults) = $M^{0.425} \times H^{0.725} \times 0.007184$

BSA is body surface area in m^2, M is mass in kg, and H is height in cm.

An adult patient is to receive cytarabine, 25 mg/m^2 × 1 dose, followed by cytarabine, 100 mg/m^2 every 24 hours × 7 doses. The patient is 6 feet, 1 inch tall and weighs 163 lb. How many milligrams of cytarabine should the patient receive in the first dose and how many in each subsequent dose? Convert his weight:

$$(163 \text{ lb}) \frac{(1 \text{ kg})}{(2.2 \text{ lb})} = 74 \text{ kg}$$

Convert his height:

$$(73 \text{ in}) \frac{(2.54 \text{ cm})}{(1 \text{ in})} = 185 \text{ cm}$$

Calculate his body surface area:

BSA = $74^{0.425}$ × $185^{0.725}$ × 0.007184
BSA = 6.23 × 44 × 0.007184
BSA = 1.97 m^2

Calculate the initial dose:

$$(1.97 \text{ m}^2) \frac{(25 \text{ mg})}{(\text{m}^2)} = 49 \text{ mg}$$

Calculate each subsequent dose:

$$(1.97 \text{ m}^2) \frac{(100 \text{ mg})}{(\text{m}^2)} = 197 \text{ mg}$$

Creatinine Clearance

Drugs that are primarily cleared from the body by the kidneys may accumulate to toxic levels in patients with renal dysfunction if either the dose or the frequency of administration is not modified. The literature on a number of drugs provides dosing tables for adjusting drug regimens based on the extent of renal dysfunction. A useful estimate of the degree of renal dysfunction is the creatinine clearance.[4] Creatinine is an endogenous substance that is filtered by the kidneys but not significantly reabsorbed or secreted. Thus, its clearance is an estimate of glomerular filtration rate. Serum creatinine levels can be measured easily and used to calculate creatinine clearance from one of the following formulae:

The **Method of Jellife** is adjusted for body surface area[8]:

$$Cl_{Cr} \text{ (males)} = \frac{98 - 0.8 \text{ (age} - 20)}{S_{cr}}$$

$$Cl_{Cr} \text{ (females)} = \frac{[98 - 0.8 \text{ (age} - 20)] \times 0.9}{S_{cr}}$$

Cl_{Cr} is creatinine clearance in mL/min/1.73 m^2, age is in years, and S_{cr} is in mg/dL. The units do not cancel out in this equation.

The following ranitidine regimens are suggested for patients with significant renal impairment[8]:

Cl_{Cr}	Regimen
50–100 mL/min	150 mg every 12 hours
<49 mL/min	150 mg every 24 hours

Which of the above regimens should be used for an 86-year-old woman who weighs 131 lb, is 60 inches tall, and has a serum creatinine of 1.9 mg/dL? Calculate her creatinine clearance:

$$Cl_{Cr} = \frac{[98 - 0.8 \ (86 - 20)] \times 0.9}{1.9}$$

$$= 21.4 \text{ mL/min}$$

Convert her weight:

$$(131 \text{ lb}) \frac{(1 \text{ kg})}{(2.2 \text{ lb})} = 60 \text{ kg}$$

Convert her height:

$$(60 \text{ in}) \frac{(2.54 \text{ cm})}{(1 \text{ in})} = 152 \text{ cm}$$

Calculate her body surface area:

$$BSA = 60^{0.425} \times 152^{0.725} \times 0.007184$$
$$BSA = 5.7 \times 38.2 \times 0.007184$$
$$BSA = 1.56 \text{ m}^2$$

Adjust the creatinine clearance by proportion:

$$\frac{(1.56 \text{ m}^2)}{(1.73 \text{ m}^2)} = \frac{x \text{ mL/min}}{21.4 \text{ mL/min}} \qquad x = 19.3 \text{ mL/min}$$

From the table, the patient should receive 150 mg ranitidine daily.

The **Method of Cockcroft and Gault** is adjusted for lean body weight[9]:

$$Cl_{Cr} \text{ (males)} = \frac{[140 - \text{age}] \times \text{LBW}}{72 \times S_{cr}}$$

$$Cl_{Cr} \text{ (females)} = \frac{[140 - \text{age}] \times \text{LBW} \times 0.85}{72 \times S_{cr}}$$

Cl_{Cr} is creatinine clearance in mL/min, age is in years, LBW is lean body weight in kg, and S_{cr} is in mg/dL. The units do not cancel out in this equation.

The following fluconazole regimens are suggested for patients with significant renal impairment[10]:

Cl_{Cr}	Regimen
50–100 mL/min	400 mg every 24 hours
20–49 mL/min	200 mg every 24 hours
10–19 mL/min	100 mg every 24 hours
< 10 mL/min	400 mg after each dialysis

Which of the above regimens should be used for a 70-year-old man who weighs 139 lb (LBW) and has a serum creatinine of 2.6 mg/dL?
Convert his weight:

$$(139 \text{ lb}) \frac{(1 \text{ kg})}{(2.2 \text{ lb})} = 63 \text{ kg}$$

Calculate his creatinine clearance:

$$Cl_{Cr} = \frac{[140 - 70] \times 63}{72 \times 2.6} = \frac{4410}{187.2}$$
$$= 23.6 \text{ mL/min}$$

From the table, the patient should receive 200 mg fluconazole daily.

PRACTICE PROBLEMS

1. A patient wants to refill the following prescription today.

   Rx: Lorcet 10/650 #60
   Sig: 1 tab po q 6 h prn pain.

   You note that the prescription was last filled 6 days

ago. How many tablets is the patient taking each day? Is the patient taking the prescription as directed? Lorcet tablets contain 10 mg hydrocodone and 650 mg acetaminophen. The maximum recommended daily dose of acetaminophen is 4 g. How many grams of acetaminophen is this patient taking each day?

2. The RDA of vitamin A for children between 4 and 6 years of age is 500 mcg retinol. A client would like to know if Bugs Bunny Complete Vitamins Plus Mineral Chewable Tablets with 5000 IU have the recommended amount of vitamin A (1 IU = 0.3 mcg retinol). How many mcg of retinol are contained in these tablets?

3. The following prescription needs to be filled:

Rx	Benadryl Cream 2%	30 g
	Zinc Oxide Ointment 20%	45 g

    Sig: Apply to chicken pox.

    You will mix a 30-g tube of 2% Benadryl Cream and a 45-g tube of 20% zinc oxide ointment to make the topical product prescribed above. What are the percent strengths of Benadryl and zinc oxide in the final product?

4. How many milliliters of ranitidine injection, 25 mg/mL, should be used to prepare 10 mL of a neonatal injection, 1 mg/mL?

5. If the neonatal dose of ranitidine is 1 mg/kg, how many milliliters of the above dilution should a 4 lb, 3 ounce neonate receive?

6. You have the prescription below for cefazolin eyedrops. Calculate the E value for cefazolin sodium, FW 477.5, $C_{14}H_{14}N_8NaO_4S_3$. How many milliliters of bacteriostatic water and how many milliliters of bacteriostatic saline should be used to make the eyedrop isotonic?

Rx Cefazolin sodium 50 mg/mL
disp. 20 mL

2 drops ou qid.

7. The infusion rate for intravenous insulin is 0.1 U/kg/hr until the glucose level drops below 250 mg/dL. If the insulin is prepared in 100 mL normal saline at a concentration of 1 U/mL, what infusion rate in mL/hr should be set for a 240-lb patient?

8. A mother has two children with chicken pox. You have recommended Benadryl syrup, 12.5 mg/5 mL for 2 days to reduce itching. She would like you to recommend a dose for each of the children. The older child weighs 40 lb and is 41 inches tall; the younger child weighs 18 lb and is 28 inches tall. The recommended dose is 150 mg/m^2 daily divided into 4 doses. How much syrup should each of the children receive in each dose?

9. You have a 83-year-old patient with renal dysfunction who is to receive ciprofloxacin for a urinary tract infection. She weighs 162 lb, is 5 feet, 6 inches tall, and her serum creatinine is 2.7. The labeling of ciprofloxacin specifies the following adjustments for patients with renal dysfunction:

Cl_{Cr}	Regimen
50–100 mL/min	750 mg every 12 hours
30–50 mL/min	250–500 mg every 12 hours
5–29 mL/min	250–500 mg every 18 hours

What dose of ciprofloxacin should the patient receive?

10. A patient is to receive 15 mEq magnesium gluconate (FW 414.6, $C_{12}H_{22}MgO_{14}$) twice daily by mouth for 2 weeks. How many 500-mg magnesium gluconate tablets should the patient receive in each dose? How many tablets will the patient need to complete the 2 weeks of therapy?

ANSWERS

1. The patient is taking 10 tablets/day, was directed to take 4 tablets/day, and is receiving 6.5 g acetaminophen/day.

2. 1500 mcg retinol.

3. 0.8% Benadryl and 12% zinc oxide.

4. 0.4 mL ranitidine injection and 9.6 mL water.

5. Neonate should receive 1.9 mL.

6. The E value for cefazolin sodium is 0.12. Use 13.3 mL bacteriostatic water and 6.7 mL bacteriostatic saline.

7. Infusion rate is 10.9 mL/hr.

8. The younger child is 0.386 m^2 and should receive 14.5 mg or 6 mL of the syrup per dose. The older child is 0.72 m^2 and should receive 27 mg or 11 mL of the syrup per dose.

9. By the Cockcroft and Gault formula, this patient's creatinine clearance is 14.8 mL/min. She should receive 250–500 mg every 18 hours.

10. The patient should receive 6 (6.2) tablets twice a day and will require 168 tablets to complete the 2 weeks of therapy.

References

1. The United States Pharmacopeia, XXIII, USP Convention, Inc., Rockvillle, MD; 1995.
2. Martin A, Swarbrick J, Cammarata A. Physical Pharmacy: Physical Chemical Principles in the Pharmaceutical Sciences. 3rd ed. Philadelphia, PA: Lea & Febiger; 1983.
3. Stoklosa MJ, Ansel HC. Pharmaceutical Calculations. 10th ed. Media, PA: Williams & Wilkins; 1996.
4. Shargel L, Yu ABC. Applied Biopharmaceutics and Pharmacokinetics. 3rd ed. Stamford, CT: Appleton and Lange; 1993.
5. Geigy Scientific Tables. 8th ed. Basel, Switzerland: Ciba-Geigy; 1981.
6. Haycock GB et al. Geometric method for measuring body

surface area: a height weight formula validated in infants, children and adults. J Pediatr. 1978;93:62–6.

7. DuBois D, DuBois EF. A formula to estimate the approximate surface area if height and weight are known. Arch Int Med. 1916;17:863.

8. Jellife RW. Creatinine clearance: bedside estimate. Ann Intern Med. 1973;79:604–5.

9. Cockcroft DW, Gault MH. Prediction of creatinine clearance from serum creatinine. Nephron. 1976;16:31–41.

10. Calvert JF, Hunter KA. Nomograms for dosing commonly used drugs by creatinine clearance. Hosp Pharm. 1993;28(11):1089–92.

Chapter 14

Clinical Pharmacokinetics

Y.W. Francis Lam and C.Y. Jennifer Chan

USE OF DRUG CONCENTRATIONS IN THERAPEUTIC DRUG MONITORING

The appropriate use of serum drug concentrations for optimization of drug therapy requires an understanding of the drug's pharmacokinetic and pharmacodynamic profiles. This chapter provides a general concept of clinical pharmacokinetics and its application in therapeutic drug monitoring. Important aspects of the pharmacokinetic profile and clinical insights on the use of drug concentrations are provided for each drug. Pharmacokinetic parameters for most commonly monitored drugs are provided in tables. However, specific dosing information for individual drugs is not covered, and readers are encouraged to consult other standard textbooks.

"Therapeutic Range" of Drug Concentrations

A therapeutic range represents a range of desirable drug concentrations, with upper and lower limits for which the *majority* of patients show effective therapeutic response with minimal drug-related side effects. In general, achievable drug concentrations that are below or above the usual therapeutic range are usually associated with decreased drug efficacy or increased drug toxicity, respectively. However, it is important to understand that the therapeutic range is essentially a probability concept and *not* an absolute entity. Attainment of drug concentration within the therapeutic range is associated with a high probability of therapeutic response and low probability of undesirable drug-related side effects. Individual patients can have good therapeutic response with "subtherapeutic" drug concentrations or can experience toxicity with "therapeutic" drug concentrations.

Many drugs (e.g., penicillin, cimetidine) possess a *wide therapeutic range* (i.e., the *toxic* drug concentrations are *much higher* than the *therapeutic* drug concentrations). Therefore, there is a wide margin of safety, and the dose can be adjusted based on the *clinical response* rather than drug concentration. On the other hand, some drugs (e.g., aminoglycosides, phenytoin, theophylline) have a narrow therapeutic range (i.e., the *toxic* drug concentrations are *close to* the *therapeutic* drug concentrations). In this case, interpatient and intrapatient variability in pharmacokinetic disposition of the drug may result in suboptimal therapeutic response if standard dosing regimens are used. For these drugs, monitoring of drug concentrations would be useful for optimal drug therapy.

Depending on the medical conditions being treated, the therapeutic range for a drug may not be the same. For example, higher concentrations of digoxin often are needed for rate control in atrial fibrillation than for the treatment of congestive heart failure. Similarly, higher concentrations of aminoglycosides are necessary for therapeutic management of pulmonary infections than for urinary tract infections. Therefore, when using drug concentrations to adjust the dosage regimen, it is important to know the clinical condition that is being treated.

In the pharmacokinetic literature, drug concentrations are usually referred to as either plasma drug concentrations or serum drug concentrations. Both plasma and serum samples refer to the aqueous component of the blood consisting of primarily water and other biologic substances such as albumin and globulin. However, clotting factors and fibrinogen are present in plasma and not in serum. Despite this difference in composition, the value of a drug concentration determined in plasma is the same as that determined in serum. For the purpose of discussion, unless otherwise mentioned, drug concentrations are serum drug concentrations.

Sampling Times

STEADY-STATE VERSUS NON–STEADY-STATE CONCENTRATIONS

The accepted therapeutic ranges of concentrations for different drugs refer to *steady-state* concentrations (i.e., when the rate of drug elimination in the patient equals the rate of drug administration). *Clinically*, steady-state concentrations are achieved after a time period equal to 3.3 × the elimination half-life of the drug, because 90% of steady-state concentrations are achieved by that time. If the drug's elimination half-life for the patient has not been previously characterized, the clinician can use literature values to estimate the approximate time required for achievement of steady-state.

Dosage regimen changes based on pre–steady-state drug concentrations could result in toxicity. Ideally, pre–steady-state drug concentrations should not be obtained. However, occasionally, a clinician may need to optimize the patient's dosage regimen before steady-state concentrations are achieved (e.g., in a life-threatening infection). In this case, pre–steady-state concentrations can be obtained to assist in the determination of a drug's volume of distribution and elimination half-life so that steady-state drug concentrations can be estimated, and dosage regimen adjusted, if necessary.

For any drug, administration of a loading dose to a patient can result in desirable therapeutic concentrations immediately but would not reduce the required time to reach steady-state concentrations. Likewise, if the patient has been receiving a drug for an extended period and a recent dose has been omitted, then it would also need a time-interval equal to at least 3.3 elimination half-lives to reach steady-state concentrations again. For drugs administered by continuous infusion, potential dose omission should be checked by reviewing nursing notes and even the volume of fluid left in the IV bag to ensure that drug administration has not been interrupted and that the rate of drug delivery has been recorded accurately in the chart.

SAMPLING OF PEAK VERSUS TROUGH CONCENTRATIONS

For drugs that are administered as an intermittent dosage regimen, either orally (e.g., theophylline, quinidine) or as short infusion (e.g., aminoglycosides, vancomycin), the steady-state drug concentration fluctuates between a maximum (peak) and a minimum (trough) concentration over the dosing interval. For the purpose of therapeutic drug monitoring, the trough concentration should be monitored for most drugs, especially those that are administered orally.

The trough concentration provides information on the minimum amount of drug present in the patient before the next dose administration. In addition, it is usually obtained at a defined time point within the dosing interval (i.e., right before the next dose). Since the rate of absorption varies significantly among different patients, it is usually difficult to determine the most appropriate blood sampling time for determination of a peak concentration. One rationale for obtaining a peak concentration is for evaluation of drug-related toxicity, since some drug-related side effects are related to concentration. However, when drug toxicity is suspected and it could be related to high concentration, then a blood sample should be obtained as soon as possible after the occurrence of the toxicity, regardless of whether it is a peak concentration or not. This is because that would be the concentration that should not be exceeded with subsequent dosage regimens.

There are drugs for which both the trough and the peak concentrations are monitored (e.g., aminoglycosides and vancomycin). This is to ensure optimal efficacy and minimal toxicity. In addition, both the peak and the trough concentrations are needed for clinicians to determine an elimination half-life and the volume of distribution, two pharmacokinetic parameters that vary significantly from one patient to another.

Most drugs follow at least a two-compartment pharmacokinetic profile, which means that soon after drug administration there is an initial rapid decrease in the drug concentration in the sampling compartment (i.e., plasma). During this "distribution phase," the drug is equilibrating between the intravascular and extravascular sites, and the drug concentration will better reflect the target site concentration *after* distribution is completed rather than *during distribution or before* completion of distribution. Therefore, when obtaining peak concentrations for assessment of drug therapy, it is important to obtain the blood sample after drug distribution is complete. This can vary from 30 minutes for aminoglycosides to 1 hour for vancomycin. If a blood sample for determination of peak drug concentration is obtained before distribution is complete, the value may be falsely elevated and dosage adjustments may be inappropriate. For drugs that are administered orally, the distribution phase is usually "hidden" during the absorption phase of the drug. In such cases, it is likely that distribution is completed before completion of the oral absorption process, which may takes up to 2–3 hours.

Indications for Therapeutic Drug Monitoring

Not all drugs require determination of drug concentrations for optimization of drug therapy. The following general criteria are considered appropriate indications for therapeutic drug monitoring:

1. The absence of a well-defined dose–response relationship, and there are no readily available therapeutic or toxic endpoints for outcome assessment.
2. Documented correlation between plasma or serum drug concentrations with pharmacologic and toxic effects.
3. Existence of a narrow therapeutic range of concentrations.
4. Existence of a significant variability in drug absorption, distribution, metabolism, and elimination among patients given the same standard dosage regimen.
5. Availability of drug assays for routine determination of serum or plasma concentrations.

In addition to serving as a guide for dosage adjustment, drug concentrations can occasionally be used to assess patient compliance.

The cost to determine the concentration of a drug in a patient ranges from approximately \$20–50; therefore, serum drug concentrations should not be obtained without due consideration for the cost. Although the majority of the criteria for therapeutic drug monitoring are present, blood sampling for determination of drug concentrations should occur at a time (e.g., steady-state peak and trough) that will yield the most desirable information. In addition, for appropriate interpretation of the measured drug concentrations and dosage regimen design, the following information should be either known or obtained:

1. The clinical condition being treated.
2. Whether adequate time has elapsed to ensure a steady-state condition. Is there any missing dose that

would affect the time required to reach steady-state concentrations?

3. The time the drug was administered and the time of completion of the drug administration process.

4. The time of sampling and the relationship of the previous dose to the sampling time.

5. Patient-specific factors that can influence drug disposition and, therefore, interpretation of the drug concentration.

Therapeutic Drug Monitoring Considerations for Pediatric Patients

Pediatric patients represent an unique population when providing therapeutic drug monitoring. Pharmacokinetic and pharmacodynamic variations are influenced by age, maturation process, and disease stage. In newborns and neonates, absorption of drugs from the gastrointestinal tract and intramuscular injection site is decreased and unpredictable.[1,2] On the other hand, percutaneous absorption of topically administered medications or chemicals is increased, resulting in potential risk of toxicity.[1,3,4] Total body water (predominantly extracellular water) is significantly larger in neonates, and the water component changes rapidly during the first year of life. Therefore, drugs that distribute to the extracellular water (e.g., aminoglycosides and neuromuscular blocking agents) will have larger volume of distribution than that reported in adults. Other factors that influence distribution of drugs in pediatric patients include rapidly changing fat composition; decreased protein binding due to lower albumin, glycoprotein, and globulin concentrations; and increased displacement by free fatty acid and unconjugated bilirubin.[1,5]

The maturation of the metabolic pathway during infancy is very complex. In general, neonates have 50–75% activity for Phase I metabolism. This function matures in 6 months and may exceed adult values during the first 2 years of life. Such changes in ability to handle hepatically eliminated drugs can result in a potential overdose in neonates or an underdose in infants and toddlers. For Phase II reactions, maturation occurs at a different rate. For example, conjugation by glucuronide reaches adult values at 2–4 years of age, whereas elimination by methylation is already functional in the fetus and neonate. Therefore, neonates and infants may eliminate a medication by a different metabolic pathway than adults.[1,2,5] Toxicities have been observed in pediatric patients due to elevated concentrations of carbamazepine 10, 11-epoxide, an active metabolite of carbamazepine.[6,7]

Renal function in full-term newborns is significantly decreased but rapidly improves, reaching the adult value by 2–5 months of age. It is important to remember that glomerular filtration rate (GFR) is correlated with postconceptual age. Therefore, a 4-week old infant born at 25 weeks gestational age will be less likely to be able to handle renally excreted medication when compared to a 4-week-old term infant. Interpretation of renal function using serum creatinine is more difficult in pediatric patients. At birth, serum creatinine reflects the mother's creatinine concentration. The serum concentration in the newborn will rapidly decrease and should be less than 0.5 mg/dL by the fifth day of life. A change of serum creatinine from 0.3 to 0.4 mg/dL represents a 30% increase in value, but this may simply reflect laboratory assay variability.[1,2,5]

The above differences in pharmacokinetic profiles contribute to the altered response to drugs. In addition, anatomic differences are also responsible for pharmacodynamic variation. For instance, newborns and neonates have an immature blood–brain barrier, immature neuromuscular transmission, and an incomplete sympathetic system. Certain diseases can also affect pharmacodynamics and pharmacokinetics of drugs. Patients with cystic fibrosis have altered oral absorption, increased volume of distribution, increased renal clearance, and increased hepatic metabolism for various medications.[8–11] In summary, understanding the maturation changes and the pharmacokinetic alterations in pediatric patients is important for providing optimal care.

DRUG MONOGRAPHS

Aminoglycosides

The aminoglycosides (gentamicin, tobramycin, amikacin, and netilmicin) are one of the primary antibiotics used for the treatment of serious gram-negative infections. These antibiotics are poorly absorbed from the gastrointestinal tract and, therefore, must be administered parenterally. Aminoglycosides are usually administered by intermittent short intravenous infusions over 30 minutes. The aminoglycosides distribute to a pharmacologic space similar to that of the extracellular fluid; hence, the volume of distribution can be affected by the pathophysiologic state of patients. Elimination of aminoglycosides is primarily dependent on the renal route; therefore, monitoring of renal function (usually in the form of serum creatinine or creatinine clearance) is an essential monitoring component to aminoglycoside therapy. Despite significant interpatient variability in distribution and elimination, the pharmacokinetic parameters (elimination half-life, volume of distribution, and clearance) of all aminoglycosides are the same. Therefore, the same pharmacokinetic equations can be used for dosage regimen design for all aminoglycosides.

Aminoglycosides	
Vd (should be adjusted for obesity and/or alterations in extracellular fluid status)	0.25 L/kg
Cl Normal renal function	Approximates Cl_{Cr}
Half-Life Normal renal function	2–3 hr

Therapeutic Range

The peak (obtained 30 minutes after the end of a 30-minute infusion) and trough concentrations for amikacin are usually 20–30 mg/L and 5–10 mg/L, respectively.[12] For the other three aminoglycosides, the respective ranges are 4–10 mg/L and 0.5–2 mg/L.[13-15] Because the pharmacokinetic parameters of all aminoglycosides are the same, the higher therapeutic peak and trough concentration ranges established for amikacin imply that the usual amikacin dosage regimen (15 mg/kg/day) for patients with normal distribution and elimination characteristics is usually about 3 to 4 times that of the other three aminoglycosides.

Therapeutic drug monitoring of the aminoglycosides provides a good example that the therapeutic range established for a specific drug can be different depending on the clinical condition of the patient. In general, higher drug concentrations of up to 10 mg/L are required for critically ill patients with sepsis or for treatment of deep-seeded infection such as pneumonia.[13] In contrast, relatively low concentrations (up to 5 mg/L) usually are sufficient for treatment of less serious infections such as simple urinary tract infection and cellulitis.[16] Abundant literature data documented that peak concentrations of less than 2–4 mg/L were less likely to result in successful therapeutic outcome.[14]

The risk of ototoxicity and nephrotoxicity remain major limiting factors associated with the use of aminoglycosides. Although controversy exists regarding the importance of peak and trough concentrations as contributing factors, exceeding the upper end of the peak and toxic concentration ranges has been associated with a higher incidence of toxicity. The risk is also higher in the presence of other risk factors such as prolonged therapy, concurrent nephrotoxic or ototoxic drugs, volume depletion, and preexisting renal function.[17–20]

Clinical Insights

1. Most of the published nomograms probably suffice for implementing the initial dosage regimen, especially for patients with normal fluid status and renal function. However, these nomograms normally incorporate fixed pharmacokinetic parameters or are designed to achieve fixed peak and trough concentrations. As a result, nomograms usually cannot account for the significant interpatient variability in aminoglycoside pharmacokinetic parameters and may result in subtherapeutic or toxic concentrations. Therefore, serum concentrations should be monitored early in therapy if aminoglycoside therapy is expected to be continued for more than a few days. These serum concentrations would enable the patient's pharmacokinetic parameters to be determined and the dosage regimen to be optimized for the treatment of his or her infection.

2. The significant interpatient variability of aminoglycosides dictates that in the presence of a significant change in extracellular fluid volume (e.g., congestive heart failure, dehydration) and/or renal function, the design of the initial dosage regimen should be able to take into consideration the anticipated changes in distribution volume and elimination half-life. This will allow therapy to be optimized as soon as possible. Follow-up concentration monitoring is especially important in patients with significant alteration in aminoglycoside pharmacokinetics.

3. Although the disposition of aminoglycosides is better described by a two-compartment pharmacokinetic model, literature data suggest no significant difference in predicted trough concentration using a one-compartment model versus a two-compartment model.[21] Therefore, for routine monitoring and dosage adjustment, the elimination half-life can still be calculated based on a one-compartment model and by using the peak and trough concentrations. Caution must be taken, however, to ensure that the peak concentration is obtained at least 30 minutes after the end of the infusion. Otherwise, the elimination half-life is underestimated.

4. Serum creatinine is usually used as a proxy measure for determining renal function; however, it usually lags behind the real change in patient's renal function by at least 24 hours. Therefore, urine output, if available, should be used in conjunction with the serum creatinine to monitor aminoglycoside therapy.

5. As with most laboratory parameters, it is more important to monitor for the trend of change in serum creatinine than for an individual value on a specific day. An increase in several serum creatinine determinations over several days (e.g., from 0.4 to 0.8 to 1.3 mg/dL) suggests a decline in renal function, even though all the measurements are within the normal range of serum creatinine reported by most clinical laboratories.

6. The decrease in lean body mass and decrease in creatinine production with aging dictate a more

cautious approach when estimating renal function in an elderly patient based on what appears to be a normal serum creatinine.

7. Nephrotoxicity induced by aminoglycosides is usually reversible on discontinuance of the drug. Although trough concentrations of greater than 2 mg/L (for gentamicin, tobramycin, and netilmicin) and 10 mg/L (for amikacin) have been associated with renal toxicity, the high trough concentrations may also be the result, and not the cause, of renal dysfunction. In fact, the use of elevated trough concentrations as an indication of early renal damage has been suggested by some researchers.[18,22]

8. The practice of administering the entire daily dose of aminoglycoside (5–7 mg/kg) every 24 hours has become more common.[23,24] As a result, peak serum concentrations would be much higher than would normally be considered "therapeutic." However, at this time, the desirable peak concentration to MIC ratio is not known for different microorganisms, for different types of infection, and for different aminoglycosides. In addition, the pharmacokinetics of gentamicin at high doses are different from that at the traditional doses.[24] Also, interpatient variability in distribution volume of the drug can affect the peak concentration significantly. The appropriate duration of high-dose aminoglycoside therapy is also not defined. Certain group of patients (pediatric patients, cystic fibrosis patients, and pregnant women) may not be good candidates for once-daily aminoglycoside dosing because of their unique aminoglycoside pharmacokinetics. In addition, experience in patients with endocarditis and immunocompromised patients is minimal. More clinical experience as well as dosing and concentration guidelines are needed before the practice can be applied to most patients.

Carbamazepine

Carbamazepine is primarily used clinically for the treatment of generalized seizures, simple and complex partial seizures, and trigeminal neuralgia. It is also used for management of bipolar depression in patients whose conditions do not respond to lithium. Carbamazepine is poorly water soluble, and absorption after oral administration of tablets is generally slow. Absorption is more rapid with the suspension formulation. Although the rectal route of administration is viable, absorption from this route is too slow for acute control of seizures.[25] Carbamazepine is eliminated primarily by the metabolic route, with one of the metabolites (10,11-epoxide) having some anticonvulsant activity and toxicity.[26]

Carbamazepine	
F	80%
Vd[a]	1–2 L/kg
Cl[a]	0.064 L/kg/hr
Half-life[b]	8–15 hr

[a] *The values for volume of distribution and clearance are approximations based upon oral administration data and an estimate of bioavailability.*
[b] *Half life is longer after single dose (no autoinduction).*

Therapeutic Range

The range of therapeutic serum concentrations for carbamazepine is 4–12 mg/L. In general, a lower range of 4–8 mg/L may suffice for patients who are receiving multiple anticonvulsants. For patients who are receiving carbamazepine monotherapy, a higher concentration range of 8–12 mg/L may be necessary. Although there is interpatient variability, most of the common central nervous system (CNS) adverse effects associated with carbamazepine (nystagmus, ataxia, blurred vision, and drowsiness) [12] occur more commonly when concentrations exceed 8–12 mg/L. There are a number of dermatologic and hematologic side effects that are not dose- and concentration-related, the most serious of which is the rare, but potentially fatal aplastic anemia.[26]

Clinical Insights

1. For monitoring of carbamazepine therapy, a baseline complete blood cell count (CBC) with differential,

platelet count, serum sodium, and liver function tests should be obtained before the initiation of therapy. If possible, a baseline evaluation of gait and nystagmus should be obtained for future comparisons.

2. Rare but potentially fatal blood dyscrasias (aplastic anemia, agranulocytosis, thrombocytopenia, and leukopenia) have been reported. Signs of bone marrow toxicity (e.g., fever, sore throat, easy bruising) should be monitored. On the other hand, frequent monitoring of the CBC after the patient's condition is stabilized with carbamazepine is unnecessary and unlikely to detect toxicity.

3. Most of the CNS side effects can be minimized by a slow titration of dose increases when therapy is initiated, or when the dose is increased so that patient tolerance to the effects can be developed over time. In addition, occurrence of CNS side effects with chronic therapy can be minimized with dosage reduction.

4. Autoinduction of carbamazepine metabolism occurs with each dose increase and usually takes about 4 weeks to complete. Therefore, determination of serum concentration before completion of autoinduction may result in overestimation of achievable concentration with a dosage regimen.

5. Polypharmacy is common in patients with epilepsy, and the potential of drug-drug interactions should always be considered when adding or deleting drug therapy. Concurrent drugs can induce or inhibit carbamazepine metabolism. In addition, carbamazepine is a potent enzyme inducer that can affect metabolism of concurrently administered drugs.

6. The suspension formulation achieves peak concentration quickly, and the total daily dose should be administered on a divided (e.g., four times a day) daily dose schedule using smaller doses to minimize fluctuations in peak to trough concentrations. The incidence of side effects or breakthrough seizures should be decreased with this method of administration of carbamazepine suspensions.

Digoxin

Digoxin is primarily used as an inotropic agent in the treatment of congestive heart failure and for slowing ventricular rate in supraventricular tachyarrhythmias such as atrial fibrillation. The extent of bioavailability after oral administration varies with different dosage forms. Despite a large distribution volume, it has low affinity to fatty tissue; therefore, dosing should be based on ideal body weight. Between 60 and 80% of an absorbed dose is eliminated by the kidneys. Patients with significant renal insufficiency often have a decreased Vd (4.5–5 L/kg) and a decreased capacity to eliminate the drug. These patients require a smaller loading dose and less frequent or smaller maintenance doses. This is also important for the elderly, who in general have a physiologic decrease in kidney function with advancing age and reduced muscle mass.

Digoxin	
F	
Tablet	0.7
Elixir	0.8
Gelatin capsule	1.0
Vd (after distribution complete)	7.3 L/kg
Cl[a]	57 mL/min + 1.02 Cl_{Cr}
Half-Life	2 days

[a] *Altered by congestive heart failure.*

Therapeutic Range

The relationship between digoxin concentrations and pharmacologic effects is more clearly defined for its positive inotropic effects in management of congestive heart failure than for its negative chronotropic effects to slow ventricular rate in atrial fibrillation. Although there is considerable variation among patients, serum concentrations of approximately 0.8–2 µg/L (ng/mL) are generally considered to be therapeutic for digoxin inotropic effects.[27,28] Higher concentrations of 1.5–2.5 ng/ml are necessary for rate control in most patients.[29] Considerable variation also exists in the relationship between digoxin concentrations and toxic effects.[28] Therefore, ECG monitoring, clinical observation, and laboratory evaluations are as important as digoxin concentrations for monitoring of digoxin therapy.

Clinical Insights

1. Interpretation of serum digoxin concentrations for optimal dosing design should ideally be made after steady-state is attained, that is, approximately 6–8 days after initiation of maintenance regimen in patients with normal renal function, and up to 20–22 days in patients with renal impairment.

2. Blood sampling for determination of any digoxin serum concentrations must take into account its prolonged distribution phase. High concentrations obtained during the distribution phase are not correlated with its clinical effect. The clinician should wait at least 6 hours after an intravenous dose and 8 hours after an oral dose to obtain the blood sample. Therefore, a standard collection time (preferably as a trough concentration before administration of the patient's daily dose) should be instituted.

3. For rapid control of ventricular rate in the acute management of atrial fibrillation, digoxin loading doses generally are divided into 3 or 4 doses (e.g., one-half, one-quarter, one-quarter given every 6 hours) to assess the clinical effect of each dose before administration of the next. In this clinical setting, determination of digoxin concentration in between dosing is likely of minimal benefit and is not cost-effective. The need for further dosing can be guided by the patient's clinical response and ECG results. In addition, there is a high possibility that the blood sample obtained during the loading dose phase primarily reflects the distribution phase of the previous dose. Even if that can be avoided, clinical decisions about further dosing in the acute setting probably cannot await the laboratory assay determination and subsequent reporting of the results.

4. Determination of digoxin concentrations is appropriate for patients with significant renal impairment, for patients with clinical deterioration after initial good response, when toxicity or drug interaction (e.g., with quinidine) is suspected, and for evaluating noncompliance and/or the need for continued therapy.

5. Some medical conditions (e.g., hypokalemia, hyperthyroidism, and hypothyroidism) can change the

sensitivity of the patient to pharmacologic effects of digoxin independent of any change in concentration. Therefore, in addition to renal function and concurrent therapy, electrolytes (especially potassium) and thyroid status should be assessed.

6. The most common assay for determination of digoxin concentrations is radioimmunoassay (RIA). Although RIA is very sensitive, it has the drawback of low specificity. It can cross-react with digoxin-like immunoreactive substances (DLIS). DLIS can account for as much as 50% of the total digoxin concentration determined by RIA and are present in patients with renal failure, in patients with hepatic failure, and in pregnant women during the third trimester.

Ethosuximide

Ethosuximide has been used primarily for the treatment of absence seizures. It is rapidly absorbed, with peak concentrations generally achieved within 7 hours. Similar to carbamazepine, the lack of an intravenous formulation precludes the determination of absolute bioavailability, although it generally is assumed to be complete. It is eliminated by metabolism to an inactive metabolite that is excreted in the urine as glucuronide. Approximately 20% of the unchanged drug is excreted in the urine.

Ethosuximide	
F	100%
Vd	0.7 L/kg
Cl	0.23–0.39 L/kg/day
Half-Life	30–50 hr

Therapeutic Range

The therapeutic concentration range for ethosuximide (measured just before the next dose) is 40–100 mg/L. Most patients with concentrations in this range respond with a significant or complete reduction in seizure activity; whereas those with concentrations below 40 mg/L are less likely to have their conditions well-controlled.[30–33] The incidence of adverse effects associated with ethosuximide therapy is relatively low and does not correlate well with drug concentrations. Many patients with concentrations in excess of 100 mg/L experience no side effects.[34] Drug concentrations are, therefore, primarily used to evaluate a patient's potential for clinical response and compliance.

Clinical Insights

Nonlinear kinetics have been described in the literature for ethosuximide, primarily with higher concentrations.[35,36] Therefore, caution needs to be exercised with dosage increments at the upper end of the therapeutic range.

Lidocaine

Lidocaine is commonly administered intravenously for the acute treatment of severe ventricular arrhythmias. It has very low oral bioavailability, and absorption from the intramuscular route is slow and variable. After intravenous administration, its pharmacokinetic profile follows a two-compartment model, with rapid distribution (distribution half-life of about 8 minutes) to well-perfused tissues such as the brain and the heart. Therefore, lidocaine serum concentrations can decrease to below that of the therapeutic range despite administration of a loading dose and initiation of maintenance infusion. To maintain lidocaine concentration within the therapeutic range, it is necessary to administer "mini" bolus doses (one-half of original loading dose) every 8–10 minutes. Lidocaine primarily binds to α-1-acid glycoprotein (AAG) in the plasma (approximately 70%). Lidocaine is almost exclusively metabolized by the liver to two pharmacologically active metabolites: monoethylglycinexylidide (MEGX) and glycine xylidide (GX). The kidney is a minor excretion route for lidocaine.

Lidocaine	
Vd	0.9–2.3 L/kg
Half-Life	100–300 min
Cl	4–10 mL/min/kg

Therapeutic Range

Lidocaine concentrations of 2–5 mg/L are usually associated with therapeutic control of ventricular arrhythmias,[23–25] although concentrations higher than 5 mg/L may be needed in patients with life-threatening ventricular arrhythmias. Lidocaine has a narrow therapeutic range, and toxic effects are generally dose-dependent or concentration-dependent. There is considerable interpatient variability in the concentration-effect relationship. Minor CNS side effects (e.g., dizziness, mental confusion, and blurred vision) can be observed in patients with concentrations as low as 3–5 mg/L. Seizures are usually associated with concentrations exceeding 9 mg/L.[37–40]

Clinical Insights

1. Concurrent medical conditions such as congestive heart failure and liver disease can decrease the clearance of lidocaine and the expected therapeutic responses with the usual doses. Therefore, a reduction of dose by as much as 40% may be necessary for these patients.

2. MEGX is primarily eliminated by the liver, and GX is eliminated by both the liver and the kidney. Therefore, in patients with liver and/or renal disease, accumulation of the metabolites may contribute to CNS toxicity.

3. AAG is an acute phase reactant; as such, its concentration can increase with stress or pathophysiologic conditions such as acute myocardial infarction (especially during the first week after infarction). An increase in the serum concentration of AAG decreases the free fraction of lidocaine temporarily due to enhanced protein binding. The increase and subsequent decrease in AAG concentration can further complicate interpretation of lidocaine kinetics and effects in patients. Careful concentration and clinical monitoring are required .

4. Because lidocaine is rapidly distributed to the brain and the heart, intravenous bolus doses should be administered at a rate not faster than 50 mg/min, so that the patient is not exposed to transient but toxic concentrations of lidocaine, especially in the brain.

Seizures and arrhythmias may occur and may not always be preceded by other toxic signs (e.g., confusion, dizziness).

5. The clearance of lidocaine decreases with continuous dosing.[41,42] Therefore, infusions lasting longer than 24 hours require diligent monitoring of concentrations and of clinical responses. If necessary, doses should be reduced.

Lithium

Lithium is primarily used to treat patients with bipolar depression. Absorption of lithium after oral administration is fastest with the liquid formulations. However, the bioavailability is comparable among the liquid preparations, tablets, and capsules. Lithium absorption can be delayed significantly with meals. Lithium is not bound to plasma proteins and is distributed extensively in the intracellular compartment. The primary elimination route is via the kidney, with clearance directly proportional to glomerular filtration rate. In addition to renal function, lithium elimination can also be affected significantly by sodium loading or sodium depletion.

Lithium	
F	100%
Vd	0.5–1.2 L/kg
Cl	10–40 mL/min
Half-Life	18–29 hr

Therapeutic Range

The usual range of therapeutic concentrations for lithium is reported to be 0.4–1.5 mEq/L, but this range can be further refined depending on the stage of therapy. In patients receiving chronic therapy, most respond with concentrations that range from 0.6–1.2 mEq/L. Occasionally, in patients with acute mania, higher concentrations of 0.8–1.5 mEq/L may be necessary; however, chronic therapy at these higher concentrations is not usually the goal.[43–45] In general, the lowest lithium concentration that controls the manic state is the desired endpoint. Lithium carbonate salt contains 8.12 mEq of lithium per 300 mg tablet or capsule. Lithium is also available as 300 mg (8.12 mEq) or 450 mg (12.18 mEq) extended-release capsules and as an oral solution that contains 8 mEq/5 mL.

The most common side effects associated with lithium therapy are nausea, vomiting, anorexia, epigastric bloating, and abdominal pain. These adverse effects seem to occur after administration of large doses of rapidly absorbed dosage forms and may be due to high gastrointestinal concentrations or high plasma concentrations. Many of these effects subside with continued therapy, but they occasionally persist. CNS side effects (e.g., lethargy, fatigue, muscle weakness, and tremor) are usually associated with plasma concentrations exceeding 1.5 mEq/L.[44,45]

Clinical Insights

1. Administering lithium preparations with meals will decrease both the rate of absorption and the achievable peak concentration. Meals, therefore, may help minimize the incidence of some of the adverse effects (e.g., tremor and polyuria). Side effects may also be minimized in some patients by use of the slow-release lithium dosage formulations.

2. The daily dose of lithium should be divided into two or more doses, and trough concentrations should be obtained 12 hours after the last dose.

3. Lithium reabsorption follows sodium reabsorption in the proximal tubule. Therefore, patients with precipitous changes in fluid balance or electrolytes due to drug therapy (e.g., thiazide diuretics) that result in increased sodium (and lithium) reabsorption are at increased risk of toxicity.

Phenobarbital

Phenobarbital, a long-acting barbiturate, is used in the treatment of seizure disorders (including status epilepticus not adequately controlled by phenytoin or benzodiazepine). Absorption after oral and intramuscular dosing is rapid and complete. Phenobarbital distributes to all body tissues, including fat. It is primarily eliminated by the liver and the kidney, and the renal excretion capacity can be increased by forced diuresis and/or alkalization of urine.

Phenobarbital	
F	Approximately 1
Vd	0.6–0.7 L/kg
Cl[a]	0.1 L/kg/d
Half-Life	3–5 days

Therapeutic Range

The usual reported therapeutic range of phenobarbital concentrations is from 15–40 mg/L. In most patients, 10–30 mg/L are sufficient for seizure control,[46] and concentrations higher than 40 mg/L usually produced side effects (such as depression and ataxia)[47] with no additional therapeutic benefit.

Clinical Insights

1. Phenobarbital has an average half-life of 5 days; and steady-state concentrations are achieved 2 or 3 weeks after the initiation of a maintenance regimen. Therefore, when therapeutic concentrations of 20 mg/L are required immediately for treatment of status epilepticus, a loading dose of 15 mg/kg can be administered intravenously, usually in 3 divided doses of 5 mg/kg.

2. Because phenobarbital distributes to fatty tissue, loading doses for morbidly obese patients should be based on total body weight.[48]

3. Due to phenobarbital's long elimination half-life, blood samples for determinations of concentrations can be obtained at any time during the dosing interval.

4. With an average clearance value of 0.1 L/kg/day, steady-state phenobarbital concentrations can be estimated by multiplying the daily dose in mg/kg (usually 2 mg/kg/d) by a factor of 10.

Phenytoin

Phenytoin is primarily used in patients for control of seizures. Although the bioavailability of phenytoin is generally assumed to be complete, the rate and extent of oral absorption are dose-dependent. The usual oral maintenance dose is 200–400 mg/day, and doses exceeding 400 mg (e.g., 15 mg/kg as oral loading dose) would need to be administered as several 400-mg doses separated by 4 hours. The rate of absorption also varies among different formulations, and caution needs to be exercised when switching brands or using different generic products. Intramuscular administration should be avoided because of slow and erratic absorption. Approximately 90% of phenytoin is bound to albumin. This provides a challenge in the interpretation of phenytoin concentration in patients with altered protein binding (e.g., patients with renal failure or hypoalbuminemia, and patients with concurrent drugs that displace phenytoin from the binding sites). In addition, the metabolism of phenytoin is saturable. Therefore, modest changes in the maintenance dose can result in disproportionate changes in steady-state plasma concentrations. Less than 5% of a dose of phenytoin is excreted unchanged via the kidneys.

Phenytoin	
F	1.0
Vd	0.65 L/kg
Cl	Concentration dependent
Vm	7 mg/kg/day
Km	4 mg/L
Half-Life	Concentration dependent

Therapeutic Range

Total concentrations of 10–20 mg/L are generally accepted as therapeutic for phenytoin in most patients.[49–51] Concentrations in the range of 5–10 mg/L can be therapeutic for some patients, but concentrations below 5 mg/L are unlikely to be effective.[52] For patients with these low concentrations and no improvement or deterioration in clinical condition, the need for continued therapy should be reevaluated. About 90% of phenytoin is normally bound to albumin. Therefore, the therapeutic range of unbound concentrations is 1–2 mg/L (Fig. 14-1, Column A). Several phenytoin side effects (e.g., gingival hyperplasia,

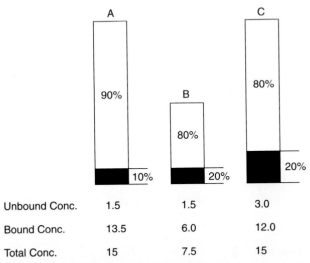

Figure 14-1. Relationship between the extent of phenytoin protein binding and its concentrations (total, unbound, and bound).

folate deficiency, and peripheral neuropathy) are not related to concentrations. On the other hand, most of the CNS side effects are dependent on concentration. Far-lateral nystagmus, the most common CNS side effect, usually occurs in patients with phenytoin concentrations greater than 20 mg/L. Other CNS symptoms such as ataxia and diminished mental capacity are frequently observed in patients with concentrations exceeding 30 mg/L and 40 mg/L, respectively.[50]

Clinical Insights

1. Oral bioavailability of phenytoin can be reduced significantly by concomitant oral nutrition supplements (e.g., Osmolite) administered as nasogastric feedings. These can necessitate the use of very large doses ranging from 800–1000 mg 3 times a day. The most practical way of circumventing this problem is to administer phenytoin intravenously. If

that is not possible, then consistent implementation of the following procedure can help minimize the problems. Nasogastric feeding is stopped 2 hours before dose administration. The nasogastric tube is flushed with 60 mL of water after dose administration. Another 2 hours should pass before nasogastric feeding is resumed.

2. Only Dilantin capsules should be dosed once daily. As with other sustained-release formulations, the capsules should not be crushed.

3. The capsule and intravenous formulations are available in the form of phenytoin sodium, which is 92% of phenytoin acid. Although this may not be important at the low end of the therapeutic range, the 8% difference in phenytoin content between the sodium salt preparations and that of chewable tablets and suspension (100% phenytoin) can become significant when an individual patient's metabolic capacity is close to the saturation point. Because the metabolic saturation point in individual patients is difficult to predict, the difference in the phenytoin acid content among the different formulations should always be considered when switching phenytoin formulations.

4. Hypotension can occur with intravenous administration due to the propylene glycol diluent.[49] Therefore, the rate of phenytoin infusion should not be greater than 50 mg/min. Fosphenytoin, a prodrug of phenytoin, is available for parenteral use. The addition of a phosphate group to the chemical structure of phenytoin results in a more soluble chemical entity; therefore, there is no need for the propylene glycol as a diluent for fosphenytoin.

5. Fosphenytoin dosing should be based on phenytoin equivalent (the molecular weight of fosphenytoin is 1.5 times that of phenytoin). Phenytoin concentration should be determined no sooner than 2 hours after intravenous administration and no sooner than 4 hours after intramuscular administration. By these times, cleavage of phosphate group from phenytoin via the activity of phosphatases is complete.

6. As a result of capacity-limited metabolism, half-life and clearance of phenytoin are dose-dependent, and the time to achieve steady-state concentrations is not simply a function of 4 to 5 times the elimination half-life.

7. The clinical significance of drug interactions with phenytoin as a result of protein binding displacement is usually overstated. Although the displacement of phenytoin from albumin binding sites can result in an increase in the unbound phenytoin concentration, the increase is only transient. The increased unbound concentration is available for distribution *and* elimination. Therefore, unless elimination of the unbound drug is *also* impaired, the unbound concentration will eventually return to the predisplacement value once the steady-state condition is established. Since the pharmacologic effect is related to unbound concentration, dosage adjustment is not necessary in patients with binding displacement but no change in elimination of unbound concentrations.

8. The issue of protein binding displacement is important, however, for appropriate interpretation of phenytoin concentration[53] in patients with altered protein binding (e.g., as a result of hypoalbuminemia, resulting in an unbound fraction of 0.2). The total concentration of phenytoin would be lower once a new steady-state condition is established. However, because the unbound concentration remains the same (Fig. 14-1, Column B), dosage adjustment is again not necessary in patients with an altered degree of binding but no change in elimination of unbound concentrations. If a decision is made to double the dose because the total concentration is lower, the unbound concentration would double and results in toxicity (Fig. 14-1, Column C).

9. Equations to "equate" the measured total phenytoin concentration to that which would be observed under normal binding conditions should be used so that inappropriate dosage adjustments can be avoided.[54] These equations differ somewhat depending on whether patients have one or more sources of altered binding (renal failure, concurrent displacing drug, hypoalbuminemia).[55]

Procainamide

Procainamide is primarily used for the treatment of supraventricular and ventricular tachyarrhythmias. Its absorption is relatively rapid, with about 70–95% of a dose absorbed after oral administration of a rapid-release formulation (concentrations peak 1–2 hours after administration) and sustained-release products (concentrations peak 3 hours after administration). A 25% reduction in the distribution volume of procainamide occurs in patients with congestive heart failure, and dosage reduction is necessary. Procainamide is eliminated unchanged by the kidney (about 50%) and is metabolized (via phase II acetylation) to N-acetyl procainamide (NAPA). Compared to procainamide, elimination of NAPA is dependent on renal function to a greater extent (approximately 87% of a dose is excreted unchanged by the kidney).

Procainamide	
F	0.85
S (HCl salt)	0.87
Vd	1.5–2 L/kg
Half-Life	2–5 hr

Therapeutic Range

Based on early investigations, procainamide concentrations of 4–8 mg/L are usually considered therapeutic.[56,57] However, recent data suggest that concentrations up to 14 mg/L may be appropriate in some patients with severe arrhythmias that were unresponsive to other antiarrhythmic agents.[58–60] Minor toxicities such as gastrointestinal disturbances, weakness, mild hypotension, and ECG changes (10–30% prolongation of the PR, QT, or QRS intervals) usually do not occur at concentrations less than 8 mg/L. On the other hand, early investigation suggested that toxicities may develop in as many as 30% of patients when concentrations exceed 12–13 mg/L.[57] Since NAPA also possess antiarrhythmic activity and toxicity, the concentration-effect relationship of procainamide is complicated. Care should be taken to evaluate carefully the risk versus benefit of high-dose therapy in any patient with concentrations above the therapeutic range of 4–8 mg/L.

Clinical Insights

1. Hypotension may occur if intravenous procainamide is administered too quickly. The rate of infusion should not be faster than 25 mg/min.

2. The short plasma half-life of procainamide requires the use of 3- to 4-hour dosing intervals for the rapid-release products and every-6-hours intervals for the sustained-release formulations. This is in contrast to the usual longer dosing intervals with sustained-release formulations of other drugs.

3. Wax matrix carcasses or "skeletons" of the sustained-release tablets may come through intact in the stool. This is not a concern because the drug is absorbed despite the recovery of the wax matrix.

4. N-acetylation of procainamide to NAPA is polymorphic. In general, patients receiving procainamide can be divided into two groups: slow acetylators and rapid acetylators. In general, slow acetylators have drug concentrations of PA greater than NAPA; rapid acetylators have concentrations of NAPA greater than PA.

5. Most clinical laboratories report the concentrations of both procainamide and NAPA. The electrophysiologic activity of NAPA is different from that of procainamide, and monitoring of NAPA concentration is not necessary to evaluate efficacy. However, assessment of NAPA concentrations may be appropriate in some patients[61] (e.g., those with diminished renal function), because NAPA is primarily eliminated by the kidneys and accumulates to a much greater extent than procainamide.

6. In addition to concentration monitoring, a baseline QT interval should be obtained, if possible, before initiation of therapy or before dosage increase. Prolongation of QT interval >25–50% of the baseline value necessitates at least the consideration of dosage reduction.

Quinidine

Quinidine is used in the management of atrial fibrillation and ventricular arrhythmias. It is available for oral administration as the sulfate, gluconate, or polygalacturonate salts, with the sulfate salt having the highest bioavailability. Peak concentration occurs faster with the sulfate salt (within 1 hour) compared with the gluconate and polygalacturonate salt formulations (within 3–6 hours). Quinidine has a high degree of plasma protein binding (about 90%), primarily to AAG.[62–65] The distribution volume is decreased up to 50% in patients with congestive heart failure. Quinidine is primarily eliminated by the liver to several metabolites, one of which (3-hydroxy-quinidine) may possess some antiarrhythmic activity. Approximately 20% of quinidine elimination is by the renal route.

Quinidine			
	Vd	Cl	t½
	1.8–3.0 L/kg	3–5 mL/min/kg	7 hr
	S	F	
Quinidine sulfate	0.82	0.73	
Quinidine gluconate	0.62	0.70	
Quinidine polygalacturonate	0.62	?	

Therapeutic Range

A number of quinidine assays of varying specificity for the parent drug are available.[66,67] Each assay is associated with a different therapeutic range of concentrations. It would be prudent to check on the specificity of the assay used by the clinical laboratory for determination of quinidine concentration within an individual hospital.[66] Nonspecific assays (such as the protein precipitation assay and benzene double extraction assay) measure various amounts of metabolites and therefore have a higher therapeutic range of concentration. Based on specific assays, such as enzyme immunoassay and fluorescence polarization immunoassay, quinidine concentrations of 1–4 mg/L are considered to be within the therapeutic range.[68,69] Of the different gastrointestinal side effects reported in patients receiving quinidine, diarrhea is the most common, with as much as 30% of patients affected, some of whom may require discontinuance of the drug. The gastrointestinal side effects occur after both oral and intravenous administration and are not related to drug concentrations.

Clinical Insights

1. The various salt forms contain different amounts of quinidine base: sulfate salt (83% of quinidine base), gluconate salt (62%), and polygalacturonate salt (60%). This difference needs to be taken into consideration when switching quinidine formulations.

2. Quinidine can be administered intravenously using the gluconate salt; however, most clinicians are reluctant to administer quinidine by the parenteral route because life-threatening hypotension has occurred. If the intravenous route of administration is desirable or necessary, the risk of hypotension may be minimized by slow infusion (e.g., at a rate of not greater than 0.2–0.3 mg/kg/min).

3. Aluminum hydroxide gel can be used to counteract quinidine-induced diarrhea without affecting its absorption.[70] Patients may develop tolerance to the gastrointestinal side effects if the dosage is slowly titrated to therapeutic concentrations over 1 week. In addition, sustained-release products are claimed to produce less gastrointestinal side effects.

4. The plasma protein binding of quinidine can be reduced (e.g., in patients with chronic liver disease) [69,71] or increased (e.g., following acute stress such as surgery).[63] Alterations in protein binding only affect transiently the unbound fraction and the unbound quinidine concentrations. Altered quinidine binding may complicate interpretation of the relationship between the measured quinidine concentration (which represents both the bound and unbound drug) and

clinical response (especially immediately after any change in the degree of protein binding). Therefore, a patient with an unexpected high quinidine concentration should be evaluated for the presence of clinical factors known to alter quinidine binding. More importantly, the clinical response (e.g., changes in PR, QRS, or QT intervals on ECG) of the patient should be assessed carefully to ensure that it is consistent with any change in drug concentration.

5. Similar to procainamide, quinidine can prolong the QT interval. Therefore, a baseline QT interval should be obtained, if possible, before initiation of therapy or before dosage increase. Prolongation of QT interval >25–50% of the baseline value necessitates at least the consideration of dosage reduction.

Theophylline

Theophylline is a bronchial smooth muscle relaxant that is widely used in the treatment of bronchial asthma and other respiratory diseases such as chronic obstructive pulmonary disease. Numerous oral formulations of theophylline, aminophylline, and other theophylline salts are available, most of which have bioavailability close to 100%. Theophylline is poorly soluble in water and can only be administered intravenously as the more soluble ethylenediamine salt of theophylline, aminophylline, which contains 80% of theophylline. Theophylline distributes to body water. The Vd in most patients is relatively constant, ranging from 0.45–0.5 L/kg. Metabolism of theophylline in the liver accounts for the majority of drug elimination.

Theophylline	
F	100%
Vd[a]	0.45–0.5 L/kg
Cl[b]	0.035–0.04 L/hr/kg
Half-Life	8.3 hr

[a] *The use of total body versus ideal body weight in obese patients is uncertain*
[b] *Clearance highly variable amont patients.*

Therapeutic Range

The usual therapeutic concentration for theophylline is 10–20 mg/L[72–74]; however, improvement in pulmonary function can be observed with concentrations as low as 5 mg/L.[72] In addition, the bronchodilating effects of theophylline are proportional to the log of the theophylline concentration. Therefore, as the theophylline concentration increases, there will be a less-than-proportional increase in bronchodilation.[75] This concentration-effect relationship and clinical experience suggest that concentrations exceeding 15 mg/L are likely to produce more side effects without significant increase in pharmacologic effect. Nausea and vomiting can occur at concentrations as low as 13–15 mg/L.[74,76] However, these less severe side effects are not always observed and cannot be used as reliable indicators of the more severe side effects (e.g., cardiac arrhythmias,[75,77] seizures[75,78]) that are associated with higher drug concentrations ($\geq$40–50 mg/L). In eight patients with theophylline-induced seizures, only one patient had "warning" toxicity signs such as nausea, vomiting, tachycardia, or nervousness.[78] Seizures have been reported in patients with theophylline concentrations less than 30 mg/L.[78,79]

Clinical Insights

1. In most adult patients requiring theophylline, the use of sustained-release preparations (such as Theo-Dur) on a twice-daily regimen at a dosage that is based on pharmacokinetic considerations would result in relatively constant therapeutic concentrations for a major portion of a dosing interval.

2. Food has a variable effect on the extent of absorption of different theophylline sustained-release formulations. High-fat foods have been reported to cause "dose dumping" of some extended-release products such as Theo-24, in which a major portion of the drug is absorbed during the first 4 hours rather than evenly over the entire 24-hour period.[80]

3. Children metabolize theophylline rapidly and may require every-8-hours dosing of sustained-release products.

4. Theophylline is extensively metabolized via cytochrome P450 enzymes: CYP1A2 and CYP3A4.

Therefore, its elimination can be increased with smoking (affecting CYP1A2) and enzyme inhibition (affecting CYP1A2 and CYP3A4).

5. Although saturable metabolism of theophylline occurs in some patients, theophylline clearance is generally linear within the therapeutic range. Nonlinearity generally occurs with concentrations exceeding 20 mg/L. The average reduction in clearance is approximately 20%.

Valproic Acid

Valproic acid is currently used in the treatment of various generalized seizure disorders with the exception of absence seizures. It is rapidly absorbed after oral administration, with peak concentrations achieved within 1–3 hours for the syrup and gelatin capsule formulations. The rate of absorption is slower for the enteric-coated tablet and the sprinkle preparations. Bioavailability of all oral preparations is close to 100%. Valproic acid is highly bound (90–95%) to albumin. The extent of binding is concentration-dependent, ranging from 10% at 50 µg/mL to 30% at 80 µg/mL. With concentrations exceeding 100 mg/L, the unbound fraction has been reported to be close to 20%.[81] It is extensively metabolized by the liver, with less than 10% of the drug excreted unchanged via the kidney.

Valproic acid	
F	100%
Vd	0.1–0.5 L/kg
Cl	8–13 mL/hr/kg
Half-Life	6–12 hr

Therapeutic Range

The therapeutic range for valproic acid is 50–100 mg/L[82–84]; however, concentrations exceeding 100 mg/mL do not appear to be associated with obvious signs of toxicity. Concentrations as high as 150 mg/L have been advocated. However, these concentrations may not be achievable in some patients as a result of dose-limiting gastrointestinal side effects such as nausea, vomiting, diarrhea, and abdominal cramps. Sedation and drowsiness are relatively uncommon side effects that may, in part, be due to the interaction between valproic acid and other concurrent antiepileptic drugs. Other infrequent side effects include alopecia, a benign essential tremor, thrombocytopenia, and hepatotoxicity. Although not clearly established, high concentrations of valproic acid have been associated with hepatotoxicity.[82,85,86]

Clinical Insights

1. Although the rate of absorption from the use of enteric-coated tablets may be slower, this formulation can be used to minimize gastrointestinal side effects.

2. Diurnal variation in valproic acid clearance has been reported, and the concentrations of valproic acid in the afternoon or evening are lower than in the morning. Therefore, it is important to standardize consistent blood sampling times (e.g., morning trough concentration) for therapeutic drug monitoring.

3. Valproic acid can inhibit the metabolism of a number of other drugs such as phenobarbital. In addition, valproic acid can displace highly protein-bound drugs such as phenytoin from their albumin binding sites. Therefore, similar to other antiepileptic drugs, the potential of drug-drug interactions should be considered when adding or deleting drugs to a patient's regimen.

4. Although valproic-acid–induced hepatotoxicity is rare, it is a serious complication of therapy and should be considered in any patient with elevated liver enzymes.[85,86] Unfortunately, the predictive value of laboratory monitoring for occurrence of hepatotoxicity induced by valproic acid is low.

Vancomycin

Vancomycin is a bactericidal antibiotic with a gram-positive spectrum of activity that includes methicillin-resistant *Staphylococcus aureus*. It is also an alternative to penicillin in patients who have a history of serious penicillin allergy.[87–90] It is poorly absorbed orally and must be administered intravenously for treatment of systemic infection. After administration, vancomycin pharmacokinetics follow a multicompartment model, with a distribution half-life as long as 90 minutes. Elimination of vancomycin is primarily via the kidney by glomerular filtration.

Vancomycin	
Vd	0.5–1 L/kg
Cl	$[0.65][Cl_{Cr}]$
Half-life	8–10 hr

Therapeutic Range

The desirable peak concentrations (obtained 1 hour after the end of an 1-hour infusion) range from 20–40 mg/L, and the desirable trough concentrations range from 5–15 mg/L.[87,88,91–93] However, 20–30 mg/L are generally sufficient for treatment of most infections. Peak concentrations greater than 50–80 mg/L have been associated with ototoxicity.[87,89,94] The minimum inhibitory concentration for most strains of staphylococci is less than 5 mg/L; therefore, vancomycin trough concentrations should be maintained above 5 mg/L. Although some clinicians recommend maintaining trough concentrations between 10 and 15 mg/L for enhanced efficacy in patients with endocarditis,[91,93] there are reports of increased nephrotoxicity with trough concentrations >10 mg/L.[95] Other major side effects, such as the red man syndrome, are not correlated with drug concentrations.

Clinical Insights

1. Red man syndrome (characterized by flushing, tachycardia, and hypotension) is associated with histamine release. Its incidence is higher with rapid infusion rates. To minimize its occurrence, vancomycin should be infused slowly (e.g., 1 g over at least 60 minutes). Even at this rate of infusion, some patients will experience flushing and tachycardia.[96] The syndrome may also be managed by premedication with an antihistamine.

2. Although nephrotoxicity was originally associated with vancomycin use, this was probably due to an impurity present in the original formulation; there have been no recent reports of nephrotoxicity caused by vancomycin alone.[87,97] A much greater risk factor for nephrotoxicity is the presence of concomitant aminoglycoside[95] or the use of an aminoglycoside within the previous 6 weeks.

3. Some high-flux dialysis membrane (e.g., polysulfone) can eliminate vancomycin more rapidly in patients undergoing hemodialysis than previously reported.[98] Similar to aminoglycoside, a postdialysis rebound in concentration occurs. It is probably advisable to wait at least 1–2 hours after dialysis before serum concentration is obtained.

4. Given the normal elimination half-life of vancomycin in patients with normal renal function, pharmacokinetic calculations based on bolus administration rather than infusion administration should be sufficient for estimation of individual pharmacokinetic parameters and subsequent dosage regimen modification.

References

1. Stewart CF, Hampton EM. Effects of maturation on drug disposition in pediatric patients. Clin Pharm. 1987;6:548–64.

2. Besunder JB, Reed MD, Blumer JL. Principles of drug biodisposition in the neonate. A critical evaluation of the pharmacokinetic-pharmacodynamic interface (part I). Clin Pharmacokinet. 1988;14:189–216.

3. Rutter N. Drug absorption through the skin: a mixed blessing. Arch Dis Child. 1987;62:220–1

4. Ginsburg Cm, Lowry WL. Absorption of gamma benzeo hexachloride following application of Kwell shampoo. Pediatr Dermatol. 1983;1:74–6.

5. Besunder JB, Reed MD, Blumer JL. Principles of drug biodisposition in the neonate. A critical evaluation of the pharmacokinetic-pharmacodynamic interface (part II). Clin Pharmacokinet. 1988;14:261–86.

6. So EL et al. Seizure exacerbation and status epilepticus related to carbamazepine-10,11 epoxide. Ann Neurol. 1994;35:743–6

7. Rane A, Hojer B, Wilson JT. Kinetics of carbamazepine and its 10.11-epoxide metabolite in children. Clin Pharmacol Ther. 1976;19:276–83.

8. Christensson BA et al. Increased oral bioavailability of ciprofloxacin in cystic fibrosis patients. Antimicrob Agents Chemother. 1992;36:2512–7.

9. Dove AM et al. Altered prednisolone pharmacokinetics in patients with cystic fibrosis. J Pediatr. 1992;120:789–94.

10. Kearns GL. Hepatic drug metabolism in cystic fibrosis: recent developments and future directions. Ann Pharmacother. 1993;27:74–9.

11. Spino M. Pharmacokinetics of drugs in cystic fibrosis. Clin Rev Allergy. 1991;9:169–210.

12. Pechere JC, Dugal R. Clinical pharmacokinetics of aminoglycoside antibiotics. Clin Pharmacokinet. 1979;4:170.

13. Noone P et al. Experience in monitoring gentamicin therapy during treatment of serious gram-negative sepsis. Br Med J. 1974;1:477.

14. Jackson GG, Riff LF. Pseudomonas bacteremia: pharmacologic and other basis for failure of treatment with gentamicin. J Infect Dis. 1971;124(suppl):185.

15. Klastersky J et al. Antibacterial activity in serum and urine as a therapeutic guide in bacterial infections. J Infect Dis. 1974;129:187.

16. Cox CE. Gentamicin: a new aminoglycoside antibiotic: clinical and laboratory studies in urinary tract infections. J Infect Dis. 1969;119:486.

17. Jackson GG, Arcieri G. Ototoxicity of gentamicin in man: a survey and controlled analysis of clinical experience in the United States. J Infect Dis. 1971;124(suppl):130.

18. Schentag JJ et al. Clinical and pharmacokinetic characteristics of aminoglycoside nephrotoxicity in 201 critically ill patients. Antimicrob Agents Chemother. 1982;5:721.

19. Wilfret JN et al. Renal insufficiency associated with gentamicin therapy. J Infect Dis. 1971;124(suppl):148.

20. Federspil P et al. Pharmacokinetics and ototoxicity of gentamicin, tobramycin, and amikacin. J Infect Dis. 1976;134(suppl):200.

21. Hatton RC, Massey KL, Russell WL. Comparison of the predictions of one- and two-compartment microcomputer programs for long-term tobramycin therapy. Ther Drug Monit. 1984;6:432–7.

22. Goodman EL et al. Prospective comparative study of variable dosage and variable frequency regimens for administrations of gentamicin. Antimicrob Agents Chemother. 1975;8:434.

23. Nicolau DP et al. Experience with a once-daily aminoglycoside program administered to 2,184 adult patients. Antimicrob Agents Chemother.1995;39:650.

24. DeMczar DJ et al. Pharmacokinetics of gentamicin at traditional versus high doses: Implications for once-daily aminoglycoside dosing. Antimicrob Agents Chemother. 1997;41:1115.

25. Graves NM, Kriel RL. Rectal administration of antiepileptic drugs in children. Pediatr Neurol. 1987;3:321–6.

26. Bertilsson L. Clinical pharmacokinetics of carbamazepine. Clin Pharmacokinet. 1978;3:128.

27. Smith TW. Digitalis toxicity: epidemiology and clinical use of serum concentration measurements. Am J Med. 1975;58:470.

28. Smith TW, Harber E. Digoxin intoxication: the relationship of clinical presentation to serum digoxin concentration. J Clin Invest. 1970;49:2377.

29. Aronson JK, Hardman M. ABC of monitoring drug therapy: digoxin. Br J Med. 1992;305:1149–52.

30. Browne TR et al. Ethosuximide in the treatment of absence seizures. Neurology. 1975;25:515.

31. Sherwin AL et al. Improved control of epilepsy by monitoring plasma ethosuximide. Arch Neurol. 1973;27:178.

32. Penry JK et al. Ethosuximide: relation of plasma levels to clinical control. In: Woodbury DM, Penry JK, Schmidt RP, eds. Anti-epileptic Drugs. New York, NY: Raven Press; 1972:431–41.

33. Sherwin AL, Robb JP. Ethosuximide: relation of plasma levels to clinical control. In: Woodbury DM, Penry JK, Schmidt RP, eds. Anti-epileptic Drugs. New York, NY: Raven Press; 1972:443–8.

34. Sherwin AL et al. Plasma ethosuximide levels: a new aid in the management of epilepsy. Ann Royal Coll Surg Can. 1971;14:48.

35. Bauer LA et al. Ethosuximide kinetics: possible interactions with valproic acid. Clin Pharmacol Ther. 1982;31:741–5.

36. Smith GA et al. Factors influencing plasma concentrations of ethosuximide. Clin Pharmacokinet.1979;4:38–52.

37. Gianelly R et al. Effect of lidocaine on ventricular arrhythmias in patients with coronary heart disease. N Engl J Med. 1967;277:1215.

38. Jewett DE et al. Lidocaine in the management of arrhythmias after acute myocardial infarction. Lancet. 1968;1:266.

39. Seldon R, Sasahara AA. Central nervous system toxicity induced by lidocaine. JAMA. 1967;202:908.

40. Thompson PD. Lidocaine pharmacokinetics in advanced heart failure, liver disease, and renal failure in humans. Ann Intern Med. 1973;78:499.

41. LeLorier J et al. Pharmacokinetics of lidocaine after prolonged intravenous administrations in uncomplicated myocardial infarction. Ann Intern Med. 1977;87:700–2.

42. Davidson R, Parker M, Atkinson A. Excessive serum lidocaine levels during maintenance infusions: mechanisms and prevention. Am Heart J. 1982;104:203–8.

43. Elizur A et al. Intra:extracellular lithium ratios and clinical course in affective states. Clin Pharm Ther. 1972;13:947.

44. Salem RB. A pharmacist's guide to monitoring lithium drug-drug interactions. Drug Intell Clin Pharm. 1982;16:745.

45. Amdisen A. Lithium. In: Evans WE, Schentag JJ, Jusko WJ, eds. Applied Pharmacokinetics: Principles of Therapeutic Drug Monitoring. 2nd ed. Vancouver: Applied Therapeutics; 1986:978–1002.

46. Buchthal F et al. Relation of EEG and seizures to phenobarbital in serum. Arch Neurol. 1968;19:567.

47. Plass GL, Hine CH. Hydantoin and barbiturate blood levels observed in epileptics. Arch Int Pharmacodyn Ther. 1960;128:375.

48. Wilkes L, Danziger LH, Rodvold KA. Phenobarbital pharmacokinetics in obesity: a case report. Clin Pharmacokinet. 1992;22:481–4.

49. Louis S et al. The cardiocirculatory changes caused by intravenous dilantin and its solvent. Am Heart J. 1967;74:523.

50. Kutt H et al. Diphenylhydantoin metabolism, blood levels and toxicity. Arch Neurol. 1964;11:642.

51. Lund L. Effects of phenytoin in patients with epilepsy in relation to its concentration in plasma. In: David DS, Prichard NBC, eds. Biological Effects of Drugs in Relation to Their Concentration in Plasma. Baltimore, MD: University Park Press; 1972;227.

52. Lascelles PT et al. The distribution of plasma phenytoin levels in epileptic patients. J Neurol Neurosurg Psychiatry. 1970;33:501.

53. Reidenberg MM. The binding of drugs to plasma proteins and the interpretation of measurements of plasma concentrations of drugs in patients with poor renal function. Am J Med. 1977;62:466.

54. Winter M. Basic Clinical Pharmacokinetics. 3rd ed. Vancouver: Applied Therapeutics; 1994:312–6.

55. Liponi DL et al. Renal function and therapeutic concentrations of phenytoin. Neurology. 1984;34:395.

56. Koch-Weser J. Pharmacokinetics of procainamide in man. Ann N Y Acad Sci. 1971;169:370.

57. Koch-Weser J, Klein SW. Procainamide dosage schedules, plasma concentrations and clinical effects. JAMA. 1971;215:1454.

58. Engel TR et al. Modification of ventricular tachycardia by procainamide in patients with coronary artery disease. Am J Cardiol. 1980;46:1033.

59. Giardina EV et al. Efficacy, plasma concentrations and adverse effects of a new sustained release procainamide preparation. Am J Cardiol. 1980;46:855.

60. Greenspan AM et al. Large dose procainamide therapy for ventricular tachyarrhythmia. Am J Cardiol. 1980;46:453.

61. Vlasses PH et al. Lethal accumulations of procainamide metabolite in renal insufficiency [abstract]. Drug Intell Clin Pharm. 1984;18:493.

62. Chow MS et al. Pharmacokinetic data and drug monitoring: antibiotics and antiarrhythmics. J Clin Pharmacol. 1975;15:405.

63. Fremstad D et al. Increased plasma binding of quinidine after surgery. A preliminary report. Eur J Clin Pharmacol. 1976;10:441.

64. Piafsky KM. Disease-induced changes in the plasma binding of basic drugs. Clin Pharmacokinet. 1980;5:246.

65. Kessler KM. Blood collection techniques; heparin, and quinidine protein binding. Clin Pharmacol Ther. 1979;23:204.

66. Guentert TW et al. Divergence in pharmacokinetic parameters of quinidine obtained by specific and non-specific assay methods. J Pharmacokinet Biopharm. 1979;7:303.

67. Hartel G, Harjanne A. Comparisons of two methods for quinidine determination and chromatographic analysis of the difference. Clin Chem Acta. 1969;23:124.

68. Powers J, Sadee W. Determination of quinidine by high-performance liquid chromatography. Clin Chem. 1978;24:299.

69. Conrad KA et al. Pharmacokinetic studies of quinidine in patients with arrhythmias. Circulation. 1977;55:1.

70. Romankiewicz JA et al. The non-interference of aluminum hydroxide gel with quinidine sulfate absorption: an approach to control quinidine-induced diarrhea. Am Heart J. 1978;96:518–20.

71. Kessler KM et al. Quinidine pharmacokinetics in patients with cirrhosis, or receiving propranolol. Am Heart J. 1978;96:627.

72. Mitenko PA, Ogilvie RI. Rational intravenous doses of theophylline. N Engl J Med. 1973;289:600.

73. Bierman CW et al. Acute and chronic therapy in exercise induced bronchospasm. Pediatrics. 1977;60:845.

74. Jenne JW. Pharmacokinetics of theophylline: application to adjustment of the clinical dose of aminophylline. Clin Pharmacol Ther. 1972;13:349.

75. Piafsky KM, Ogilvie RI. Dosage of theophylline in bronchial asthma. N Engl J Med. 1975;292:1218.

76. Jacobs MH et al. Clinical experience with theophylline: relationships between dosage, serum concentration and toxicity. JAMA. 1976;235:1983.

77. Ogilvie R et al. Cardiovascular response to increasing theophylline concentrations. Eur Clin Pharmacol. 1977;12:409.

78. Zillich CW et al. Theophylline-induced seizures in adults. Ann Intern Med. 1975;82:784.

79. Yarnell PR, Chu NS. Focal seizures and aminophylline. Neurology. 1975;25:819.

80. Hendeles L et al. Food induced "dose-dumping" from a once-daily theophylline as a cause of theophylline toxicity. Chest. 1985;87:758–65.

81. Kodama Y et al. Binding parameters of valproic acid to serum protein in healthy adults at steady-state. Ther Drug Monit. 1992;14:55–60.

82. Pinder RM et al. Sodium valproate: a review of its pharmacological properties in therapeutic efficacy in epilepsy. Drugs. 1977;13:81.

83. Graham L et al. Sodium valproate, serum level, and critical effect in epilepsy: a controlled study. Epilepsia. 1979;20:303.

84. Sherard ES et al. Treatment of childhood epilepsy with valproic acid: result of the first 100 patients in a 6-month trial. Neurology. 1980:30:31.

85. Suchy FJ et al. Acute hepatic failure associated with the use of sodium valproate. N Engl J Med. 1979;300:962.

86. Donalt JT et al. Valproic acid and fatal hepatitis. Neurology. 1979;29:273.

87. Alexander MB. A review of vancomycin. Drug Intell Clin Pharm. 1974;8:520.

88. Kirby WMM et al. Treatment of staphylococcal septicemia with vancomycin. N Engl J Med. 1960;262:49.

89. Banner WN Jr, Ray CG. Vancomycin in perspective. Am J Dis Child. 1984;183:14.
90. Cunha BA, Ristuccia AM. Clinical usefulness of vancomycin. Clin Pharm. 1982;2:417.
91. Rotschafer JC et al. Pharmacokinetics of vancomycin: observations in 28 patients and dosage recommendations. Antimicrob Agents Chemother. 1982;22:391.
92. Blouin RA et al. Vancomycin pharmacokinetics in normal and morbidly obese subjects. Antimicrob Agents Chemother. 1982;21:575.
93. Mollering RC et al. Vancomycin therapy in patients with impaired renal function; a nomogram for dosage. Ann Intern Med. 1981;94:343.
94. Farber BF, Mollering RC Jr. Retrospective study of the toxicity of preparations of vancomycin from 1974 to 1981. Antimicrob Agents Chemother. 1983;23:138.
95. Ryback MJ et al. Nephrotoxicity of vancomycin, alone and with an aminoglycoside. J Antimicrob Chemother. 1990;25:679–87.
96. Newfield P, Roizen MF. Hazards of rapid administration of vancomycin. Ann Intern Med. 1979;91:581.
97. Cook FV, Farrar WE. Vancomycin revisited. Ann Intern Med. 1978;88:813.
98. Lanese DM et al. Markedly increased clearance of vancomycin during hemodialysis using polysulfone dialyzers. Kidney Int. 1989;35:1409.

Chapter 15

Clinical Drug Monitoring

Teresa A. O'Sullivan and Ann K. Wittkowsky

Clinical drug monitoring is the most basic element of pharmaceutical care.[1] All the therapeutic knowledge the pharmacy student possesses is useless unless it can be applied in a structured and consistent manner to detect and solve patients' problems. This structured process is clinical drug monitoring. It includes each of the following activities[2]:

➤ Gathering objective and subjective patient information.
➤ Analyzing that information to determine medical and drug-related problems.
➤ Setting therapeutic goals for each medical and drug-related problem.
➤ Developing and enacting a treatment plan to reach the therapeutic goals.
➤ Developing and enacting a monitoring plan to see if the treatment works or causes any harm.
➤ Documenting all of the above (subjective and objective information, analysis, and plan) in a coherent and systematic manner so that the next care provider can continue the process.

All the above steps are necessary components of clinical drug monitoring. No step can be skipped, or good patient care will be sacrificed.

The following sections provide clinical drug monitoring guidelines for the pharmacy student to follow when dealing with patients.

Determining Patient Discussion Issues

The clinician must talk to the patient. The discussion will be more comfortable and productive if the clinician first scans the patient's chart or profile to determine some discussion issues. The following should be considered:

➤ The current medication list (patient profile or most recent medication administration record [MAR]). What medications has the patient been prescribed? What likely disease states are present?

➤ Patient compliance/adherence (patient profile or most recent MAR). How often does the patient get his or her medications for chronic conditions refilled? In an institutional setting, the pharmacist will want to check the MAR to see if the patient has been receiving or refusing his or her medications.

➤ Disease state control (recent progress notes). Monitoring notes written by other health care providers will be useful in an institutional or clinic ambulatory setting. (In a community pharmacy setting, however, the pharmacist may not have extensive documentation of previous disease state control.) The pharmacist should look for disease state monitoring data obtained through interview, physical examination, and laboratory values. Well-written progress notes will include this information. In the absence of well-written progress notes, information from previous visits or admissions, an admission summary (for hospitals or long-term care settings), or current laboratory data can be reviewed to gain an idea of the patient's medical problems. In this situation, an interview with the patient or their caregiver will provide invaluable information to determine disease state control.

➤ Cost (patient profile will contain costs; most recent MAR will not). Are any chronic medications high-cost? Is there any indication that lower-cost agents have not worked? Physicians distributing drug samples often facilitates the initiation of high-cost, brand name products without initial trials of low-cost agents.

➤ Adverse drug effects (recent progress notes), including drug allergy information. Are there any medications that may have been prescribed to treat side effects from other medications? When thinking about adverse drug reactions, the "as needed" or "prn" portion of the MAR is useful because prn medications are often given to combat side effects from routinely scheduled medications. For instance, if the patient begins asking for a laxative shortly after beginning opiate therapy for pain, opiate-induced constipation can be suspected.

To summarize, before interviewing the patient, the pharmacist should look at the patient's medication list in the chart or profile in any setting, the MAR in an institutional setting, and any previous care notes that would indicate how well the patient's disease states are controlled.

It should be remembered that the first step is to identify discussion questions quickly, *not* to read the patient's chart from beginning to end. This is because the most important source of information regarding patients' problems are the patients themselves, not their charts. For a pharmacy student who has not seen many patient charts, it will be easy to spend hours (literally) reading the chart, aimlessly writing everything down, and not identifying what information is important and what is not. Only after the patient interview can the chart information be used efficiently.

Interviewing the Patient

Obtaining subjective information from the patient is the most important step in the database-building process. The pharmacist must make it a priority to interview every patient to whom he or she is assigned, unless the patient is intubated or comatose.

Before beginning the interview, pharmacists should introduce themselves and explain their role on the health care team (which is to optimize the patient's drug therapy). The pharmacist should ask if this is a good time for the patient to be asked some questions about his or her medication use. (A pharmacist's first few interviews will probably take at least 10 minutes if a patient's drug regimen is simple and longer if the regimen is complicated. This time will decrease as the pharmacist gains more experience.) If it is not a good time for the interview (e.g., the patient is in a hurry, has visitors, or is going for a diagnostic test), another time should be scheduled.

Many experienced clinicians use the Standard Organization for Patient History and Physical Database (the "H and P"; Box 15.1) as a mental "nudge" for directing an interview. This helps to ensure that the proper information is gathered completely and consistently. Individual pharmacists may choose to design their own data collection forms. However, regardless of the data collection method selected, the pharmaceutical care database must include detailed information about medication use, including prescription medications, nonprescription agents, disease states, drug allergies and adverse drug reactions, the patient's level of understanding the disease state, the patient's overall attitude about medications and disease states, and the patient's height and weight.

Box 15.1   Standard Organization of Patient History and
            Physical Data

ID (identifying information): patient age, gender, race.

CC (chief complaint): a one-phrase description of the patient's reason(s) for seeking medical and/or pharmaceutical care. Identification of the probable diagnosis is sometimes given as a chief complaint but is not strictly correct.

HPI (history of the present illness): summarize the events that led to the patient's decision to seek care. Organize chronologically if possible.

PMH (past medical history):

➤ Brief summary of medical problems not presented in the HPI.

➤ Organized by problem in order of most important to the least important. This may be a different order than the physician uses. The pharmacist's definition of importance is based on the need for drug therapy monitoring. Numbering or bulleting each medical problem will enhance organization.

➤ An indication of the date of onset or duration of each problem, and the current status of the problem, are useful.

DH (drug history): some data may be obtained from the chart, but the majority will be obtained by interviewing the patient. The drug history includes:

a. Name, dose, frequency, reason for use, duration of use, efficacy, toxicity, and indication of all prescription, OTC, and herbal medications that the patient has taken during the past month.

   • All drug indications should be reflected in the past medical history.
   • Identify name/telephone number of pharmacy and medication management issues.

b. Medications previously used for the medical condition and reasons why they were discontinued.

Box 15.1   *Continued*

c.   Recreational drug use. This includes history and current use of tobacco, ethanol, and illicit drugs.

d.   Allergies or contraindications for drug use. Allergy history should include a description of the allergic reaction.

e.   Compliance/adherence. Assess the patient's comprehension of drug therapy, knowledge of side effects/toxicity, compliance to drug regimen (including reliability), compliance aids, and needs for further intervention. Note any language or disease state barriers to compliance.

FH (family history): genetic predisposition or occurrence of *relevant* diseases in other family members.

SH (social history): includes information regarding living situation, support systems, lifestyle, employment, and work environment (risks/chemical exposure) *that may affect drug therapy*.

ROS (review of systems): this is a *subjective* review of bodily systems as voiced by the patient during the interview.

PE (physical examination): this is an *objective* review of bodily systems obtained during the examination of the patient. At the very least, this should include vital signs (heart rate, blood pressure, respiratory rate, temperature), weight, and height.

Both the ROS and the PE begin with general statements about the patient (subjective for ROS and objective for PE) and then move on to specific findings starting at the patient's head and moving down the body to the feet ("head to toe"). Students should always obtain clarification of data from PE or ROS that they do not understand. When presenting this information to the preceptor or other health professional, students should *only present data pertinent to the case*. If findings are normal, state as such and do not elaborate.

Labs (laboratory data): obtain all laboratory data pertinent to the problem list. At a minimum, report the baseline seven laboratory values (Na, K, Cl, CO_2, glu-

continued

Box 15.1 *Continued*

---

cose, BUN, and Cr), CBC (WBC/diff, Hct, and platelets), liver function tests (AST, ALT, alk phos, and total bili; albumin and PT/INR are reasonable indicators of metabolic capacity). If the patient is febrile and/or an infection is suspected, report Gram stain and C&S findings.

Other relevant diagnostic tests: (CXR), EKG, CT, EEG, etc.

PRESCRIPTION MEDICATIONS

All prescription medications that the patient is currently taking should be reviewed. For each drug, the following should be noted:

➤ Drug, dose, route, frequency, indication (this is the *patient's* version of the indication).
➤ Efficacy ("Tell me how you know that this medication is working for you.").
➤ Toxicity ("Are there any problems that you are having that you think may be caused by this medication?"). If the patient says "No," the pharmacist should probe with a few of the most common side effects.
➤ Compliance ("How often do you actually take this medication?" or "Tell me what interferes with your ability to take the medication regularly."). What does the patient do if a dose is missed? The pharmacist should try to verify if cost, dosing frequency, adverse effects, or personal beliefs may be an obstacle to compliance. If the patient is able to state clearly how he or she ensures that all drugs and doses are taken on time and as prescribed, then the pharmacist will feel more comfortable trusting their compliance self-assessment.
➤ Medication management issues. How does the patient store his or her medications? Is the patient able to administer the medication easily (e.g., tablet size can sometimes be a problem)? How many physicians does the patient see? What is the name and telephone number of the pharmacy(ies) at which the patient gets his or her prescriptions filled? How does the patient remind himself or herself to obtain refills? Is transportation to the physician or pharmacy a problem? The pharmacist should inquire about

technique and maintenance of devices (such as spacers, peak flow meters, blood pressure monitors, or blood glucose monitors) used to facilitate drug delivery or monitor drug therapy. The patient should demonstrate inhaler use technique to the pharmacist and use of any other devices if the pharmacist suspects suboptimal technique.

NONPRESCRIPTION AGENTS

These include over-the-counter (OTC) medications, herbal and other natural remedies, vitamins and minerals, and nondrug therapy. The following "head to toe" review of systems approach should be used to inquire about nonprescription agents used by the patient. In addition to gaining valuable information about nonprescription agents the patient uses routinely or infrequently, it will also often identify disease states that may not have been identified through the prescription medication portion of the interview.

➤ Head, eyes, ears, nose, and throat (HEENT): nose, ear, or eye drops; nasal inhalers; analgesics used for headache or sinus pain; dental products.
➤ Respiratory tract: antihistamines, decongestants, OTC inhalers.
➤ Gastrointestinal: antacids, antiflatulents, antidiarrheals, laxatives, hemorrhoidal preparations.
➤ Genitourinary: urinary antibacterials; vaginal antiinfectives; usual amount of fluid consumed daily; what kind of fluid (e.g., soda versus water versus lite beer).
➤ Musculoskeletal: aspirin, antiinflammatory agents, acetaminophen, or combination pain medications.
➤ Hematologic: iron, B_{12}, folate.
➤ Dermatologic: psoriatic, seborrheic, antiinfective, or analgesic topical preparations; corn/callus pads or other foot care.
➤ Neurologic: medications for insomnia, motion sickness, anxiety, lethargy.
➤ Overall/system-wide: vitamins; naturopathic, homeopathic, or other alternative health care products. Tobacco and alcohol use, noting favored product, quantity, frequency, and duration of use. Nonprescribed (illicit) drugs for recreational purposes (patients are more likely to be honest if asked questions about illicit drug use in a matter-of-fact manner).

If the patient uses nonprescription products for a particular medical problem, the pharmacist should establish how often the medical problem occurs, if the nonprescription therapy works, and if the therapy causes any side effects. Patients should be asked where they usually buy nonprescription products and how they obtain answers to questions about the products (i.e., is there a pharmacist or other health care professional available to answer their questions).

DISEASE STATES

The list of disease states that the patient appears to have should be reviewed with the patient. The pharmacist should also ask if there are other disease states or medical problems that are not included on the list.

DRUG ALLERGIES AND ADVERSE DRUG REACTIONS

If a patient states that he or she is allergic to a certain drug or has had an adverse reaction to a certain drug, as much of the following information as possible should be obtained. This information should be obtained for every drug that the patient notes.

➤ Name of the drug to which the reaction occurred. Were there occurrences of similar reactions when drugs in same class were taken? How many times was the drug used without adverse sequelae before the reaction occurred? These two questions will help to discern between adverse reactions and drug allergies, and also an adverse reaction that may be a one-time event (e.g., ibuprofen was once associated with nausea but it had been taken many times previously without sequelae; a label of "allergic" in this case may be incorrect).

➤ Reason the patient took the drug. Likelihood of viral infection preceding drug use, if the reaction was a rash.

➤ Complete description of physical symptoms of the reaction. A physical assessment should be conducted if the adverse drug reaction is currently in progress. If the patient reports a rash, hives versus a maculopapular rash should be differentiated.

➤ Timing of reaction versus administration of the drug ("How soon after you took the drug did this reaction happen?" "How many days or doses into therapy were you when this reaction occurred?"). Any information about other medications administered around the same time that the reaction occurred may also be useful.

➤ Other allergies or intolerances (e.g., food, nickel, latex). Drug vehicles or inert ingredients may contain something to which the patient will react.

If it is determined that a patient is incorrectly labeled as "allergic" to a drug or other substance, the preceptor should be consulted about the possibility of removing the allergy label and flag from the patient's chart or profile.

LEVEL OF UNDERSTANDING THE DISEASE STATE

Patients should be asked to describe their disease (e.g., "Just to give me an idea of your understanding of congestive heart failure, please describe what is happening."). The pharmacist should probe for understanding of the effects of overtreatment, undertreatment, or sporadic treatment of the disease (e.g., "Tell me what long-term complications you may avoid if your blood pressure is lowered."). The patient should also be asked about therapies used *previously* for each disease state. Drug names, doses, frequencies, duration of use, efficacy, toxicity, and compliance should be noted for each medication previously used.

OVERALL ATTITUDE ABOUT MEDICATIONS AND DISEASE STATES

Some questions can provide important information about a patient's cultural and personal beliefs that might affect current or future drug therapy ("Tell me how you feel about medication use, in general." "How do you feel your medications impact your quality of life?")

PATIENT HEIGHT AND WEIGHT

A patient can be asked his or her height and weight if it is not possible for the pharmacist to measure the patient or if there is no access to recent height and weight measurements made by other health care professionals.

Objective Data Collection

➤ Any physical examination necessary to test a hypothesis about drug-related problems should be conducted (see

Chapter 20, "Approaches to Evaluating Drug-Related Problems").

➤ Current and past laboratory data should be checked. It should be discerned if there have been any changes that might support drug efficacy or toxicity.

➤ Diagnostic test results should be reviewed to determine if they support drug efficacy or toxicity. These will also provide an estimation of the severity of the medical problems.

➤ The patient's pharmacy should be contacted if there are any questions about current prescription drug doses. Questions regarding refill patterns can be asked to confirm compliance. A patient's family members, caregivers, or physician can be contacted if they can provide valuable information regarding the patient's response to therapy. The preceptor should be consulted before any calls are made.

If a pharmacy student wishes to obtain information from an objective parameter that has not been previously ordered, he or she must be able to explain to the preceptor why the information will be helpful and cost-justified in confirming the tentative pharmaceutical diagnoses. The student should also be able to justify which tests or procedures must be done immediately and which ones can be delayed until the most emergent problem(s) is/are addressed.

Definition of Current Medical Problems

After the subjective and objective data have been collected, a list of all the patient's current medical problems—problems that the patient is experiencing or being treated for at this time—needs to be made. These medical problems should be numbered and placed in order of importance, starting with the medical problems needing the most immediate attention (the student will need to justify to the preceptor *why* they need immediate attention) and ending with the problems that can be addressed later.

Determining the Goals of Therapy for Each Medical Problem

The pharmacy student must determine a goal for each medical problem for which the patient will receive drug or non-drug therapy. Trying to solve a problem without first setting a therapeutic goal is similar to getting into a car and starting to drive before the destination is decided. The four primary goals for therapy include the following:

➤ Cure a disease (e.g., infection).
➤ Eliminate or reduce a patient's symptoms (e.g., pain control, congestive heart failure).
➤ Arrest or slow a disease process (e.g., diabetes, cholesterol reduction to reduce the risk of coronary heart disease).
➤ Prevent a disease or other unwanted condition (e.g., immunization, contraception).

There are other secondary goals that the clinician and the patient will have. Attaining these secondary goals will maximize the ability to attain the patient's primary goals. Secondary goals include the following:

➤ Avoidance of adverse effects.
➤ Convenience.
➤ Cost-effectiveness.
➤ Patient education.

A measurable, patient-specific endpoint is determined for each goal. The endpoint can be objective (e.g., blood pressure measurement in a patient with hypertension) or subjective (e.g., patient self-rating of cancer pain using a pain scale). To ensure comparability of measurements, the same method of endpoint measurement must be used every time. In addition, the goal must be reasonable for a particular patient. For example, it is not reasonable to set a goal of "no pain" for a patient with severe rheumatoid arthritis. Instead, decreasing the pain to a level at which the patient can perform most of the necessary activities of daily living is more practical.

Analyzing Subjective and Objective Data to Determine Drug-Related Problems

Box 15.2 contains a list of drug-related problems (DRPs) that may occur in individual patients. To help identify whether a patient has any actual or potential DRPs, the pharmacist should ask the following questions about each of the medications the patient is taking:

➤ Are there any medical problems (diagnoses) identified by the prescriber or pharmacist for which no drug therapy has been prescribed? If the answer is "Yes," it may

Box 15.2   Drug-Related Problems

Drug needed
➤ Drug indicated but not prescribed. A medical problem has been diagnosed, but there is no indication that treatment has been prescribed (although treatment may not be needed)
➤ Correct drug prescribed but not taken (noncompliance)

Wrong drug
➤ Inappropriate drug prescribed (no apparent medical problem justifying the use of the drug, not indicated for the medical problem for which it has been prescribed, medical problem no longer exists, duplication of therapy, less expensive alternative available, drug not covered by formulary, drug not available for other reasons)
➤ Failure to account for pregnancy status, age of patient, other contraindications
➤ Incorrect nonprescription agent self-prescribed by the patient
➤ Harmful recreational drug use

Wrong dose
➤ Prescribed dose too high (requires adjustments for kidney and liver function, age, body size)
➤ Correct prescribed dose but overuse by patient (overcompliance)
➤ Prescribed dose too low (requires adjustments for age, body size)
➤ Correct prescribed dose but underuse by patient (undercompliance)
➤ Incorrect, inconvenient, or less than optimal dosing interval (consider use of sustained-release dosage forms)

Adverse drug reaction
➤ Side effects
➤ Allergy

> **Box 15.2**   *Continued*

➤ Drug-induced medical problem
➤ Drug-induced laboratory change

Drug interaction
➤ Drug-drug interaction
➤ Drug-disease interaction
➤ Drug-nutrient interaction
➤ Drug-laboratory test interaction

be appropriate for no medication to be given (e.g., a patient with Type II diabetes who has been able to achieve acceptable blood glucose control with diet alone). On the other hand, perhaps the pharmacist failed to identify a drug that was prescribed for the patient, the pharmacist misunderstood the indications for a drug that he or she thought was being used for something else, or the prescriber inadvertently forgot to order something for the patient. These situations should be investigated, and a plan for any necessary interventions made.

➤ Are there any drugs prescribed for the patient with no apparent indication? If the answer is "Yes," the pharmacist has failed to identify one of the patient's medical problems, overlooked an unusual use of a drug specific to the patient, or identified a possible inappropriately prescribed drug. These situations should be investigated, and necessary steps should be taken.

➤ Is the patient taking the medications as prescribed? Is there evidence of noncompliance, overuse, or underuse by the refill patterns? If "Yes," the reason should be discerned (a confusing regimen, high cost, side effects, personal or cultural beliefs about the medication or disease states, or presence of interacting drugs are all possibilities).

➤ Is the regimen cost-effective? Is there any medication that the patient is taking for which there is a lower-cost alternative? If so, has that alternative been tried? If the alternative has been previously used, was the dose maximized? Are all medications covered by the patient's insurance company? Is there any evidence of therapeutic duplication? Could more than one of the patient's medical problems be treated with one drug?

➤ Is the treatment working? If the answer is "No," there could be several explanations such as undercompliance, drug ineffectiveness, a dose that is too low, or a drug interaction that has led to a lower than desired serum drug concentration.

➤ Are the doses correct? The patient's age (especially pediatric and geriatric patients), weight, renal and hepatic functions, dosing schedule, and dosage form (regimen convenience, possible need for sustained-release products, cost-effectiveness) should all be considered.

➤ Is the treatment causing toxicity? Could any of the medical problems be drug-induced? Are any abnormal laboratory values drug-induced?

➤ Are there any contraindications to be considered? If the profile indicates prior allergies, the current regimen should be screened for possible cross-reacting drugs. If the patient is receiving a potential cross-reacting drug without deleterious effect, this needs to be noted for future therapeutic consideration. The possibility of pregnancy should be considered and inquired about in women of child-bearing age who are not using oral contraceptives and who are to receive a medication that could adversely affect a fetus.

A list of DRPs is constructed using the answers to the above questions. Each DRP should correspond to one of the medical problems. It is helpful to write the lists alongside each other.

In addition to determining DRPs, justification for each must also be determined. There must be a sound defense for each DRP detected.

Identifying Reasonable Therapeutic Alternatives for Each DRP

Various drug classes and nondrug therapies should be considered in the process of solving DRPs. For each therapeutic option, the following should be determined:

➤ The evidence for efficacy.
➤ The likelihood and severity of adverse medication effects.
➤ The number of daily doses.

➤ The effects (either positive or negative) of the option on the patient's other diseases.
➤ The cost relative to the other agents.

The pharmacy student will have learned much of this information in his or her therapeutics series, but some of the information may have been forgotten. Therefore, the student should be prepared for re-reading during the clerkship. Additionally, the student should make it a practice to search the primary literature regularly to determine the most effective treatments. The ability to clearly summarize the most recent evidence supporting (or disputing) each treatment option will facilitate providing the best possible care. The preceptor will query students extensively about therapeutic alternatives, so this important step should not be neglected.

Choosing and Individualizing the Best Therapeutic Option

If a thorough and complete job has been done collecting and evaluating the benefits and hazards of each of the therapeutic options, then choosing the most reasonable therapeutic option should be easy. The option must then be individualized to fit the characteristics of the patient. This is where knowledge about height and weight (for pharmacokinetic dose considerations), concomitant diseases and medications (for drug-disease and drug-drug interactions), and compliance history (to determine frequency of doses) will be vital. If the plan includes drug therapy, then drug, dose, route, frequency, and duration of therapy need to be specified. All drug and nondrug plans should include some degree of patient education.

Designing a Monitoring Plan for Efficacy and Toxicity

After choosing a therapeutic regimen, a monitoring plan needs to be designed. The monitoring plan should be specific: exactly *what* will be measured, *who* will do the measuring, *how often* will it be done, *when* will it be time to change or discontinue the therapy, and *what* is the backup plan. The student must be able to defend all of the above measures. This will be easy if the monitoring parameters are cheap, quick, and noninvasive, but more difficult if they are expensive, lengthy, or invasive.

Documenting the Decision-Making Process

It is professionally unacceptable and legally dangerous to provide care for a patient and not record the care decisions and the reasoning behind those decisions. Clerkship experiences are valuable because they provide the student with the time to gain the practice necessary to produce a brief yet informative note in a short amount of time.

All documentation notes should begin with the date and time that the information is recorded and include a header identifying the type of information provided (e.g., "pharmacy progress note," "pharmacy compliance assessment"). Good notes will also include a brief one-phrase overview of the reason for the note. This one-phrase overview should identify patient age, gender, and primary issue (e.g., "67 yo male presenting with uncontrolled hypertension," "82 yo female with probable adverse drug reaction").

SOAP FORMAT

The most commonly used documentation format is referred to by the mnemonic, "SOAP," which stands for *s*ubjective information, *o*bjective information, *a*ssessment, and *p*lan. Other health care providers (e.g., nurses, physicians) use this format and will recognize and feel comfortable reading a SOAP note.

The content of a SOAP note written by a pharmacist will be subtly different from that written by another type of health care provider, primarily in the assessment section. Whereas a physician's assessment will produce a disease state diagnosis and a nursing assessment will evaluate the patient's psychosocial and physical health care needs, a pharmacist's SOAP note assessment will primarily identify DRPs.

Before a SOAP note is begun, the following must be defined clearly:

➤ What are the patient's most important DRPs that need to be addressed *now*?

➤ What is the evidence that each problem exists?

➤ What are the therapeutic goals for each problem?
➤ What are the therapeutic options for each problem?

The answers to each of these questions will form the content of the assessment section of the SOAP note. Therefore, the assessment is "written" mentally before the actual SOAP note is begun. After the problems are defined, subjective and objective information needed to justify why those problems exist should be written down.

The first paragraph should be preceded with an "**S:**" and will contain subjective information, which is patient information obtained through interview. The information source should be identified (e.g., patient or caregiver). Examples of subjective information include patient-provided information about disease symptoms, OTC medications used, drug allergy descriptions, and compliance. All information included in the subjective section *must* directly support either the assessment or plan. Information that does not support the assessment or plan is extraneous and should be omitted.

The second paragraph will be preceded by an "**O:**" and will contain objective information (i.e., information obtained by verifiable means). Objective information is obtained by physically examining the patient, viewing laboratory data, checking prescription records for doses and refill patterns, and locating medication costs from a printed or on-line formulary. All information included in the objective section *must* directly support either the assessment or plan. Information that does not support the assessment or plan is extraneous and should be omitted.

Some information can be either subjective or objective, depending on how it is obtained. For example, weight and blood pressure would be subjective if reported by the patient, but objective if measured by a health care provider. A list of prescribed medications would be listed as subjective information if provided verbally by the patient, but objective if obtained from a pharmacy profile. The most important thing to remember when composing the subjective and objective portions of notes is that *only information pertaining directly to the assessment should be included*. Any subjective and objective information extraneous to the assessment of the patient's drug-related problem should be omitted. This will keep the note brief and focused.

The third paragraph will be preceded by an "**A:**" and will contain the pharmacist's assessment of the patient's medical and drug-related problem(s). It must include the explanation of why the pharmacist thinks the problem exists. If the subjective and objective paragraphs are written well, the problem should be obvious to the reader by the time he or she arrives at the assessment paragraph. Nevertheless, a succinct summary justifying each problem is crucial to establishing credibility and demonstrating a logical thought process. Reliance on innuendo is to be avoided at all costs.

Other information included in the assessment paragraph are the therapeutic goals and a brief discussion of the therapeutic alternatives. Each therapeutic alternative should include a brief phrase that describes why the option is either beneficial or not optimal. If this is done well, the reader will know exactly what the recommendation will be before he or she begins to read the proposed plan in the next paragraph.

The fourth paragraph should begin with either a "**P:**" or "**R:**" and will detail either a plan (P), or recommendation (R), whichever is most appropriate for the situation. In a prescribing situation (such as with prescriptive authority or nondrug or OTC primary care), the plan should be phrased as an order. In a nonprescribing drug therapy work-up, the plan may be documented as a recommendation for a change or concurrence with current drug therapy. In all cases, the plan should include individualized dosing instructions (drug, dose, route, frequency, and, when applicable, duration of therapy). All recommended medications should be referred to by their generic names. Dosing instructions must be specific. Ranges should not be used. The exact dose and frequency should be identified.

After the drug or nondrug therapy is delineated, the monitoring plan must be detailed. This will include specifically what (e.g., laboratory test, symptom) should be measured, who should measure it (patient, caregiver, or pharmacist), when and how frequently the measuring should occur, and at what point changing therapy will be considered. A backup plan for use in the event of therapeutic failure should also be noted here.

ALTERNATIVE FORMATS

Other formats advocated for written communication of pharmaceutical care, such as FARM (*f*indings, *a*ssessment, resolution, and *m*onitoring) and CORE (*c*ondition, *o*utcome desired, *R*x regimen, *e*valuation parameters) have been described in detail elsewhere.[3] Close examination of these other formats reveal that they are all variations on the same theme found in SOAP notes: problem identification (including data to justify existence of problem), proposed or implemented solution, and method for evaluating whether the solution works.

Written communication can also use preprinted check-off forms, such as care pathways or protocols, or dictation (i.e., transcription of taped information to written form). Because pharmaceutical care activities such as unexpected DRPs cannot be recorded completely using a preprinted form, these activities should be documented by adding a written addendum to the progress notes. If dictation is used to document pharmaceutical care, the same format and style should be followed as that for a written note.

DOCUMENTATION NOTE STYLE TIPS

Length. In general, physicians like brief notes and lawyers like detailed notes. The trick lies in choosing words carefully to maintain a balance between the two. This can be most easily accomplished through careful use of phrases, rather than sentences, and by including *only* the information needed to support the assessment and plan and nothing more. As a general rule, notes should not exceed one page.

Format. The subjective and objective portions of notes lend themselves well to the use of bullets followed by words or terse phrases. These phrases can be placed in a horizontal list with each separate piece of information separated by commas or can be listed vertically.

Some preceptors will ask students to address each different medical problem or DRP in a separate SOAP note. Other preceptors will allow students to address more than one problem in a SOAP note as long the note is organized coherently. To facilitate organization of such an assessment, each separate problem should be numbered. For each problem, the student should identify the problem and justify its existence, describe the therapeutic goal, and outline the reasonable therapeutic alternatives.

Recommendation statements should be concise. Brief phrases should be used. Recommendations should not begin with, "I recommend . . . " or any other leading statements. Recommendations are not justified in this section; all justification occurs in the assessment. If more than one problem is addressed in the assessment and each problem has been numbered there, then the recommendations should be numbered similarly (e.g., recommendation 1 corresponds to problem 1, recommendation 2 to problem 2, etc.) If only one problem is addressed in the assessment, then the drug/nondrug therapies and monitoring plans can be listed using bullets.

Abbreviations. Abbreviations should be avoided whenever possible. It may be safe to abbreviate common laboratory values, the four main vital signs, height and weight (although specify units), and common diagnostic tests (e.g., CXR, XRAY, CT, MRI, FEV_1, FVC), but abbreviation of anything else may result in miscommunication among health care providers, leading to suboptimal care. Drug names are never abbreviated. Many institutions have an approved abbreviations list; the pharmacy student should obtain a copy of this list on the first day at a new site. Pharmacists working in different settings or sites in the same geographic area should consider assembling a list of approved abbreviations to be used by all. The old adage of "When in doubt, spell it out" cannot be overemphasized.

THE FIVE MOST COMMON DOCUMENTATION MISTAKES

Inclusion of Extraneous Information. It takes much practice to get to the point at which a note contains no excess information. The student may be tempted to list all of a patient's medications and medical problems in a note, rather than just those that pertain to the problem assessed. Excess information will confuse the reader, drawing his or her attention away from the main point of the note. This can be avoided by mentally "writing" the assessment portion of a note first. All data included in the subjective and objective portions should support the assessment or plan directly. Only those facts necessary to convince the reader of the accuracy of the conclusions should be included.

Exclusion of Important Information. Another common error is the omission of subjective and objective data crucial to the support of the assessment or plan. For example, if a note states that a patient's hypertension is not responding to therapy because the patient is being noncompliant but does not provide compliance data in the subjective or objective portions of the note, the reader will at best be confused and at worst may discredit the writer's conclusions and ignore the recommendations. Again, mentally writing the assessment portion first will provide the opportunity to include supportive facts in the subjective and objective portions of the note.

This rule presupposes that all necessary data have been gathered. Obviously, important information will be excluded in a note if such data are not obtained. The only way this can be avoided is through the use of a complete and consistent information-gathering process.

Information in the Wrong Place. Information that is misplaced will lend a disorganized feel to a note and be confusing for the reader. It is common for SOAP writers to place subjective information in the objective section and vice versa. Some pharmacists avoid this misplacement by using a combined S/O heading, rather than having a separate heading for each. Another common misplacement occurs when new subjective or objective information is placed in the assessment or plan portion of the note. This is extremely distracting for the reader. Extra room should be left at the end of the subjective and objective portions of the note, so that if important data have been omitted while writing the assessment or plan, they can be put in the proper places.

Vague or Unclear Information. There are two areas of the SOAP note in which vague or unclear words or phrases are most likely to be used. The first area is the presentation of subjective information in a nonquantifiable fashion. For instance, the vague phrase, "History of kidney problems," could mean anything from mild dysuria to dialysis. Use of nonspecific measurement descriptions such as "decreased," "increased," "recent," "history," "symptoms," "problems," and "changes" should be avoided. Whenever possible, patient parameters should be quantified at baseline and after changes have occurred. For example, it is better to write, "BP 160/95 (2 readings); 145–150/85--90 over last calendar year." This gives the reader more useful information than just noting "BP increased."

The monitoring plan is the second common location of unclear information. It is tempting to use vague words or phrases such as "monitor renal function," but this does not tell the reader what specifically should be measured or examined, how often that measuring should occur, who will perform the measuring, and when a therapeutic alteration will be considered. The use of vague words such as "follow," "assess," "explain," "monitor," "review," "provide," "consult," and "educate" should be avoided in the monitoring plan. "Measure," "observe," "ask," or "tell," should be used instead. In addition, the writer should specify exactly what should be measured, observed, asked, or told.

Lack of Clear Reasoning Supporting Problem Existence or Choice of Recommendation. The most ubiquitous documentation error is the lack of logical reasoning behind problem identification and therapeutic recommendation. Lack of this supportive reasoning may lead a reader to question the credibility of the note and discount or disregard the pharmacist's advice. In the assessment section, it should be stated clearly *why* the pharmacist thinks a problem exists and *why* the proposed treatment seems to be the most optimal therapeutic option.

Objective critique of SOAP notes is an excellent way of improving clarity. Figure 15-1 shows an evaluation instrument that can be used for self-evaluation or for the evaluation of other's SOAP notes.

EXAMPLE

The following is a complete patient work-up including history and physical examination, medical problems with goals and endpoints, drug-related problems with justification, treatment alternatives, recommendations and monitoring plans, and a SOAP note summarizing the important issues.

The scenario is as follows. It is the first day of the clinical clerkship at a community pharmacy. Mr. Smith, a 68 year-old man who has been a patient at this pharmacy for several years, presents a prescription for "Coumadin 2 mg #30, i po qd" to the pharmacy student. The information

Element	Comments
Heading	
-Date, time?	
-Identification of pharmacy note?	
-One phrase overview of reason for note?	
Subjective/Objective Information	
-Enough information to support assessment statements?	
-Only information directly pertaining to assessment is included (i.e., no extraneous information)?	
Assessment	
-Clear identification of problem?	
-Logical reasoning supporting existence/importance of problem?	
-Identification of reasonable goals for therapy?	
-List of reasonable therapeutic alternatives, with benefits and/or hazards of each?	
Recommendation	
-One recommendation clearly stated?	

Figure 15-1. Documentation note evaluation (continues).

-Therapeutic recommendation complete/detailed (i.e., drug, dose, route, frequency, duration of therapy)?				
-Detail of patient education content and comprehension?				
-Plan for monitoring complete for both efficacy and toxicity (what will be monitored, who will monitor, how often monitoring will occur, when therapeutic improvement or goals should be reached)?				
-Justification for expensive/involved medication plan?				
-Brief identification of back-up therapeutic recommendation if primary plan fails?				
Closing				
-Closing statement, if appropriate?				
-*Legible* signature, printed ID (e.g., RPh, PharmD, pharmacist), contact information if appropriate?				

Figure 15-1. Continued.

sources available to the student are Mr. Smith, his pharmacy profile, and a log of his laboratory values, which the pharmacist has asked him to bring every time he comes to the pharmacy. The following information is the patient history and physical data, the student's assessment of Mr. Smith's situation, and the chart note.

Patient History and Physical Database

ID: A 68-year-old man.

CC: Needs an increase in warfarin dose due to decreased efficacy of past dose.

HPI: The patient takes warfarin daily for deep venous thrombosis (DVT) prevention. INR today was 1.5, and the physician has decided to increase the warfarin dose from 5 mg by mouth daily to 7 mg by mouth daily. The patient has been instructed to take one 5-mg tablet and one 2-mg tablet daily and to return for reassessment in 2 weeks.

PMH:

➤ DVT, 2 months ago.

➤ Hip replacement surgery, 3 months ago.

➤ Atrial fibrillation, single episode 4 years ago; no symptoms are currently reported.

➤ Congestive heart failure (CHF), diagnosed 7 years ago.

➤ Chronic obstructive pulmonary disease (COPD), diagnosed 5 years ago.

➤ Anterior myocardial infarction (MI), 14 years ago indicating coronary artery disease (CAD); no current chest pain.

DH:

Prescription medications:

➤ Warfarin 5 mg by mouth every day for 2 months (DVT; same dose since discharge from hospital 2 months ago).

➤ Digoxin 0.25 mg by mouth every day for 7 years (CHF).

➤ Ipratropium 2 puffs four times a day for 5 years (COPD).

➤ Albuterol 2 puffs four times a day for 5 years (COPD).

Nonprescription medications:

➤ Multivitamin with iron and minerals, one by mouth daily for 7 months.

➤ Psyllium 1 scoop in a glass of water for constipation daily for 4 years.

➤ Bismuth salicylate 4 tablespoonfuls as needed for diarrhea (took 1 dose twice in the past year for stomach flu).
➤ Alfalfa tablets 2–3 every day for health; friend recommended this to him about 1 month ago.

Compliance information:

➤ Medication refill records indicate that the patient obtains refills on time.
➤ The patient obtains all prescription and OTC medications from this pharmacy.
➤ The patient bought alfalfa tablets at a health food store.

Recreational drug use:

➤ 40-pack year smoking history: quit 2 years ago.
➤ Occasional alcohol use: 1–2 drinks/week; no recent change in this amount.

Allergies: denies history of medication or environmental allergies.

FH: Father died of acute MI at age 54.

SH: Retired; lives with spouse who assists with medication management at home; denies any changes in ingestion of vitamin-K–containing foods.

ROS: No current complaints.

Lungs: Clear sputum, no spells of coughing recently; denies shortness of breath (SOB), dyspnea on exertion (DOE), and paroxysmal nocturnal dyspnea (PND); sleeps with one pillow; is comfortable walking short distances (no change from 3 months ago).

CV: Denies chest pain.

Skin: Denies bleeding or bruising.

GI: Stools are dark brown.

GU: Urine is clear, yellow; no blood.

PE: 5'10", 80 kg today (usual weight).

HR: 85 beats/min, regular rhythm; blood pressure: 135/82 mm Hg; respiratory rate (RR): 20 breaths/min; temperature 37.2°.

No bruising found on arms, legs, or face.

Labs:

INR:

1.5   Today
1.9   2 weeks ago
2.4   4 weeks ago
2.6   6 weeks ago
2.3   At discharge, 8 weeks ago

Albumin:

4.5 g/dL   5 months ago

Current Medical Problems	Goal of Therapy	Measurable Endpoint
Recent DVT	Prevent recurrent thromboembolism	Therapeutic INR
CAD	Prevent angina and MI	No anginal episodes
CHF	Symptom control	No episodes SOB, edema, PND
COPD	Symptom control	No DOE, SOB, PND

Current Drug-Related Problems	Justification	Therapeutic Alternatives
Underanticoagulation (wrong dose? drug interaction?)	Subtherapeutic INR Possible causes: Diet (no recent change) Ethanol (patient denies) Underlying disease state change (no evidence to support) Drug interaction (recent addition of natural product that contains varying amounts of vitamin K) Compliance (no evidence of noncompliance)	Increase warfarin dose (problematic considering inconsistent amount of vitamin K in alfalfa tablets) Discontinue (D/C) alfalfa. In this case, patient would need additional anticoagulant effect until a therapeutic INR is achieved. Low-molecular-weight heparin can be used on an outpatient basis; unfractionated heparin requires hospitalization *continued*

Pharmacy Practice Manual

Continued

Current Drug-Related Problems	Justification	Therapeutic Alternatives
Inadequate MI prophylaxis (needs drug?)	Current AHCPR guidelines recommend aspirin and beta-blocker for all patients after MI unless contraindicated	ASA 325 mg po qd ASA 81 mg po qd (lower dose will minimize risk of bleeding with concomitant warfarin) Beta-blocker (contraindicated wih COPD)
Inadequate CHF and post-MI mortality benefit (needs drug?)	Current ACC/AHA guidelines recommend ACEI for all patients with CHF; SAVE, AIRE, and TRACE trials support use after MI to reduce mortality	Angiotensin-converting enzyme (ACE) inhibitor Angiotensin receptor antagonist
COPD overmedicated (wrong drug?)	1995 study conducted in The Netherlands showed increased costs and no additional benefit of two bronchodilators over one alone	D/C albuterol (preferred due to CHF) D/C ipratropium

Recommendation	Monitoring Plan

Anticoagulation
  D/C alfalfa tablets
  Start enoxaparin 80 mg (1 mg/kg) SQ q 12 hr. D/C when INR ≥2.0
  Continue warfarin at current dose; instruct patient to self-administer SQ medication
	Return for INR check in 5 days
	Patient to self-monitor for signs/symptoms (S/S) of DVT: calf warmth, tenderness or pain
	Patient to call provider immediately if experiences chest pain or SOB

Continued	
Recommendation	Monitoring Plan
	Patient to self-monitor for S/S of minor, moderate, and major bleeding: visual check for gum, urine, stool, skin bruising, epistaxis
MI prophylaxis ASA 81mg po qd	Patient to self-check for bleeding as noted above; stool guaiac in 3 months
CHF/post-MI mortality benefit	Check BP in 1 week (goal systolic BP 100–120)
Lisinopril 5 mg po qd; first dose at bedtime; titrate dose upward weekly to maximal doses (20 mg po q 12 hr) as tolerated per BP and serum creatinine (SCr)	Check SCr now for baseline and again in 1 week Patient to self-monitor for and report dizziness/lightheadedness and any increase in coughing frequency
COPD D/C albuterol	Patient to self-monitor and report any increased incidence of SOB, DOE, or PND

Today's date and time

Pharmacy note regarding anticoagulation and other drug therapy for 68-year-old white man.

S:

➤ Pertinent medical history: DVT 2 months ago; CHF for 7 years; COPD for 5 years; anterior MI 14 years ago.

➤ ROS: denies coughing, SOB, DOE, PND, chest pain, bleeding or bruising, blood in stool or urine; pain, tenderness, or swelling of the lower extremities.

➤ Occasional alcohol use: 1–2 drinks/week; no recent change in this amount.

➤ Denies any changes in ingestion of vitamin-K–containing foods; has taken alfalfa 2–3 tablets (for general

health) every day for approximately 1 month per
friend's advice.

O:

➤ 5'10", 80 kg today (usual weight). HR: 85 beats/min,
regular rhythm. BP: 135/82 mm Hg. RR: 20 breaths/
min.

➤ No bruising found on arms, legs, or face.

➤ INR: 1.5 today; 1.9 2 weeks ago; 2.4 4 weeks ago; 2.6 6
weeks ago; 2.3 at discharge 8 weeks ago.

➤ Pertinent prescription medications: warfarin 5 mg po qd
(same dose for the past 2 months), ipratropium 2 puffs
QID, albuterol 2 puffs QID.

A:

1. INR ≤2.0 associated with increased risk of recurrent
   DVT. Addition of alfalfa coincides with decreased
   INR. D/C of alfalfa preferable to increasing warfarin
   dose, because varying vitamin K content of tablets
   confounds dose titration. Patient has been
   underanticoagulated for at least 2 weeks but shows no
   signs/symptoms of acute DVT. Addition of outpatient
   enoxaparin for a few days until INR is in therapeutic
   range is necessary and would be more cost-effective
   than admission to the hospital for treatment with
   unfractionated heparin.

2. Suboptimal CHF and post-MI mortality benefit. Use
   of aspirin for CAD and ACE inhibitor for CHF and
   post-MI is associated with decreased mortality. Low
   dose aspirin is necessary to avoid increased risk of
   major bleeding complications associated with
   concomitant warfarin therapy. Beta-blocker use also
   associated with decreased risk of subsequent MI but is
   relatively contraindicated in this patient because of
   COPD.

3. Use of two bronchodilator inhalers is not superior to
   one for COPD (Am J Respir Crit Care Med
   1995;151:975). Ipratropium preferred over albuterol
   in this patient due to potential for beta-
   agonist–induced CHF exacerbation.

R:

1. D/C alfalfa tablets. Start enoxaparin 80 mg SQ q 12
   hr. D/C when INR ≥2.0. Continue warfarin at

current dose. Instruct patient to self-administer SQ medication. Return for INR check in 5 days. Instruct patient to self-monitor and report calf warmth, tenderness, or pain; chest pain or SOB; excessive blood in gums, urine, stool, nose, dermis.

2. Start: ASA 81 mg po qd; lisinopril 5 mg po qd; first dose at bedtime; titrate dose up by 5 mg every week to maximum 20 mg po qd as tolerated per BP (check in 1 week; goal: systolic BP 100–120) and SCr (check today and in 1 week). Patient to report any dizziness or increased coughing.

3. D/C albuterol. Patient to report any increase in SOB, DOE, or PND.

Pharmacist signature

CONCLUSION

In summary, whether with a patient in the hospital, in the clinic, or at the pharmacy counter, the student should perform the following steps:

➤ Quickly scan the chart or profile to identify issues that need to be discussed with the patient.
➤ Obtain subjective data by interviewing the patient.
➤ Gather objective data by physical examination and review of pertinent laboratory parameters, MAR or patient fill records, and diagnostic tests and consultations.
➤ Summarize the patient's medical problems and drug-related problems and set goals for the therapy of those problems that need to be addressed immediately.
➤ Consider the potential benefits and hazards of all reasonable therapeutic alternatives. Select the alternative that has the highest likelihood of efficacy, a minimum of toxicity, and seems the most cost-effective.
➤ Determine the optimal dose, route, frequency, and duration for the patient's pharmacokinetic, concomitant drug and disease state, economic, and compliance needs.
➤ Design and implement a monitoring plan to determine if the recommendation works or causes unreasonable toxicity.
➤ Document the decision-making process.

At first, this process will seem long and cumbersome, but with practice it will become quick and effortless. By taking the responsibility for clinical drug monitoring, the student will become a practitioner that patients and health care colleagues will respect and trust.

References

1. Hepler CD, Strand LM. Opportunities and responsibilities in pharmaceutical care. Am J Hosp Pharm. 1990;47:533–43.
2. Strand LM, Cipolle RJ, Morley PC. Documenting the clinical pharmacist's activities: back to basics. DICP. 1988;22:63–6.
3. Canaday BR, Yarborough PC. Documenting pharmaceutical care: creating a standard. Ann Pharmacother. 1994;28(11):1292–6.

Chapter 16

Documentation in Pharmacy Practice: A Pharmacist-Lawyer's Perspective

Kenneth R. Baker

DOCUMENTATION IN A CHANGING PROFESSION

Pharmacists oversee the distribution of dangerous drugs in the United States and in most industrialized countries in the world. In the United States, state and federal laws restrict the sale of dangerous drugs to pharmacies and a few other channels. The federal and state governments have mandated a mass of records that must be maintained to show that restrictions on these drugs are observed.

Even before the development of laws requiring precise documentation, the pharmacist was a record-keeper. From the very beginning, formulations for compounded prescriptions were recorded—not just the drugs used, but the formulas and methods of mixing. The role of the pharmacist required that knowledge be preserved so procedures could be repeated with consistency. Such information was too important to be left to memory.

Pharmacists today have taken on new roles and duties. By necessity, this has forced a reorganization of many of the tasks associated with the pharmacist's traditional roles. The pharmacist has left many of the mechanical, nonjudgmental jobs to para-professionals. Those roles are now being transferred to the pharmacy technician and increasingly to machines. It is the pharmacist, however, who is still legally responsible for seeing that each step is performed correctly and is documented properly.

As the role of the pharmacist expands and changes, the amount, and in some cases the importance, of documentation becomes greater. This chapter explores the role of the pharmacist as documenter and record-keeper. The need and desirability of documentation in the pharmacist's roles as manager of drug distribution and as patient risk manager are discussed. In addition, as the role of the pharmacist continues to expand, the need to document what was done and why it was done will also expand. The reasons, purposes, and manner of documentation are discussed as are the legal uses of documentation.

This chapter is not designed to provide the pharmacist with a complete list of all laws and rules requiring documentation and record-keeping. Rather, this chapter serves to remind pharmacists that these requirements exist and of the importance of this documentation.

THE PHARMACIST'S CHANGING ROLE

The role of the pharmacist can be described as two-fold. The newest of these roles has evolved over the past two decades. This role has been called pharmaceutical care, but by whatever name, the role is as protector, or risk manager, of the patient. With all drugs there are risks and benefits of taking the medication. The prescriber performs a risk–benefit analysis and prescribes a drug to treat the patient. The order is then taken to a pharmacist, whose job it is to assist the patient in managing the potential risks of taking the drug.

Even today, pharmacy continues to evolve and an even broader role of the pharmacist is beginning to emerge—that of risk assessor. Until recent years this has been the role of the physician or prescriber. In many states, pharmacists have been granted limited prescribing functions, usually by protocol, or collaborative agreement, developed between the pharmacist and a physician. Under these arrangements, it may be the pharmacist who initiates changes in the medication or directions for its use according to the protocol. In this case the pharmacist performs a part of the risk–benefit analysis, which may include triage diagnosis.

COURT DECISIONS REFLECT CHANGING DUTIES

Through the 1980s it could generally be said that the pharmacist who filled a prescription correctly, with the correct drug, in the correct strength, and with the directions as written by the physician was safe from lawsuits. These mechanical functions were generally seen by the courts as the extent of the pharmacist's duties. This is no longer the rule. Beginning in 1990, the courts have recognized additional duties and responsibilities for pharmacists, allowing lawsuits against pharmacists even when the prescription is filled correctly. The evolution of these duties can be seen in court decisions over the past two decades. Reviewing a few of these cases also illustrates the need for the pharmacist to develop documentation skills in new areas.

In 1985, the Indiana Appellate Court rejected the concept of a legal duty on the pharmacist's part to warn a patient of common side effects of a prescribed drug. The Court said, "The duty to warn of hazards associated with prescription drugs is part and parcel of the physician-patient relationship."[1] The Court added:

> The injection of a third-party in the form of a pharmacist into the physician-patient relationship could undercut the effectiveness of the ongoing medical treatment. We perceive the better rule to be one which places the duty to warn of the hazards of the drug on the prescribing physician and requires of the pharmacist only that he include those warnings found in the prescription.[2]

The patient in this case, Ronald Ingram, was prescribed Valium, which was filled by the defendant pharmacy. After taking several doses of the prescription, he fell and subsequently sued the pharmacy, Hooks Drugs, Inc., for failing to warn him the drug could cause drowsiness. The Court rejected Ingram's claim holding, as a matter of law, that the pharmacist could not be held to have such a duty. The Indiana Court concluded:

> Ingrams' position would require a pharmacist filling a prescription for Valium to give the entire list of side effects and cautionary statements. Such a voluminous warning would only confuse the normal customer and be of dubious value. This matter is better handled by a treating physician.[2]

At the time of this ruling, this was the general standard. According to the Indiana Court in 1985, the pharmacist's only duty was to fill the prescription correctly. Discussing medication with the patient was the exclusive role of the physician. With this limited duty, little documentation beyond that required by law for the dispensing function was necessary.

This limited legal view of a pharmacist's duty began to change. In 1990 the Tennessee Court of Appeals heard *Dooley v. Everett*,[3] a more involved case against a pharmacist in which the Court was asked to find that the pharmacist had a duty to review a physician's prescription and intervene. Brandon Dooley was a minor child who was taking theophylline for his asthma. The child's physician later prescribed erythromycin, which was filled at the same pharmacy as the earlier theophylline prescription. The child suffered cerebral seizures that the parents alleged were the result of toxic levels of theophylline in his blood caused by the erythromycin. The physician and the pharmacy were sued.

The trial court had dismissed the case against the pharmacy based on the principle that the pharmacist had no duty to warn or intervene. The Court of Appeals overruled the trial court and reinstated the case against the pharmacist. In part, the Court said:

> The pharmacist is a professional who has a duty to his customer to exercise the standard of care required by the pharmacy profession in the same or similar communities as the community in which he practices his profession.

> There is a disputed issue of fact in the record regarding whether the duty to discover and warn customers of potential drug interactions is included within the general scope of the duties a Tennessee pharmacist owes to its customers.[3]

The Tennessee Court looked at the case as a question of professional standard of care. To determine the minimum professional standard of care to be applied to the practice of pharmacy, the Court reviewed the testimony of an expert witness—a practicing pharmacist. The Court quoted the expert's testimony:

> "Pharmacy is a profession that requires considerable knowledge about drugs and how they affect the human

body;" that "pharmacists recognize that there exists a standard of care applicable to the practice of pharmacy in [Tennessee];" that "there are certain duties and responsibilities generally accepted by the members of the pharmacy community;" that the "accepted standard of care of professional practice for the profession of pharmacy as they existed in Lawrenceburg, Tennessee, and similar communities in 1987" included that "pharmacies maintain a patient profile system" and that "the patient profile should be reviewed by the pharmacist prior to filling a new prescription for *several* purposes" including a determination of whether the new drug prescribed for the patient and presented for filling to the pharmacist interacts with any other drug currently ordered for the patient.

He further testified: [T]he standard of care also required the pharmacist alerted to the interaction to call the Erythromycin prescriber, alert him or her to the potential interaction, and/or advise the patient or patient's representative of the potential interaction and encourage him or her to (1) have his or her serum Theophylline levels monitored and/or (2) be alert for side effects of Theophylline toxicity . . . . [T]he pharmacist is required to alert the patient or patient's representative to the potential interaction.[3]

Based partly on the expert's opinion, the Court found the pharmacist may have a duty to review the prescriptions and warn the physician and/or the patient of potential interactions. The Court held it was for the jury to determine the extent of the pharmacist's duty and whether the pharmacy met the minimum standard of care in this case.

The *Dooley* case was not alone in finding a pharmacist may be liable for failing to review and warn a patient of potential adverse drug reactions. A Louisiana Court held that a hospital pharmacist had a limited duty to inquire or verify a drug order when a prescribing physician made a clear error or mistake in prescribing. When a physician ordered Vibramycin to be given intramuscularly rather than intravenously, the pharmacist could not merely fill the order but was required to at least check with the physician.[4]

The pharmacist may also have a duty to monitor the patient's use of a drug. In *Lasley v. Shrakes Country Club Pharmacy*[5] a patient sued his physician and pharmacy for injuries and pain and suffering caused by his addiction after 10 years of prescriptions for glutethimide and codeine. The trial court had dismissed the pharmacist and pharmacy from the case because, the court said, a pharmacist had no duty to warn Lasley or his physician of the potentially addictive nature of drugs legitimately prescribed for Lasley.[6] The Arizona Court of Appeals disagreed and reinstated the case, finding a jury could find such a duty and could find the pharmacist had failed to meet his minimum standard of care.

This concept of minimum standard of care is important to the pharmacist in deciding what is necessary to document. Every profession has a minimum standard that each member of the profession must meet. Any professional who is found to have performed his or her duties below that minimum is negligent. In a malpractice case a pharmacist may be required to show what actions were taken and why other actions were not taken. Pharmacists must understand what is required of them and how and when to make notations that can be used later to show that they performed to the standard of the profession. Courts do not set these standards, rather they are set by the profession itself and may be set by the laws and regulations that govern the profession. To understand fully what is expected of pharmacists in both duty and documentation, pharmacists must be familiar with the laws governing their profession.

STATUTES AND REGULATIONS AND THEIR EFFECTS ON DUTY AND DOCUMENTATION

Pharmacy has been called "the most regulated profession." This may or may not be true, but the amount of documentation required of pharmacists can seem staggering. Both state and federal governments require pharmacists to maintain records. As the legal overseer of drug distribution in the United States, the pharmacist is constantly under surveillance and has statutory record-keeping requirements. This documentation is necessary to ensure the proper management of drug distribution in the United States.

Federal and state laws require records be kept to ensure compliance with the regulations and statutes passed to safeguard the public. The first level of such laws and regulations is the state pharmacy practice act. The regulations of the states vary, but many of the state pharmacy acts are based on the National Association of Boards of Pharmacy "Model Practice Act." The Model Practice Act was written by representatives of several state boards of pharmacy through their national association to provide a guide for individual state boards and to provide some uniformity of laws among the states. This model act illustrates the documentation requirements pharmacists face in their states. It is useful to use the NABP Model Practice Act as a guide to documentation. Each pharmacist should be familiar with the pharmacy law and regulations in the state in which he or she practices, because they vary from state to state.

The Model Practice Act, and most state acts, declares that the primary purpose of the law is to protect the public, not the pharmacist. This is an important concept the pharmacist should recognize. The Model Practice Act states:

> It is the purpose of this Act to promote, preserve, and protect the public health, safety, and welfare by and through the effective control and regulation of the Practice of Pharmacy; the licensure of Pharmacists; the registration of technicians; the licensure, control, and regulation of all sites or Persons, in or out of this State that Distribute, Manufacture, or sell Drugs (or Devices used in the Dispensing and Administration of Drugs), within this State, and the regulation and control of such other materials as may be used in the diagnosis, treatment, and prevention of injury, illness, and disease of a patient or other individual.

Section 103. Statement of Purpose.

Because the purpose of pharmacy rules and regulation is for the protection of the public, documentation required under these acts flows from this purpose. Most pharmacists are aware of the record-keeping requirements and that if the records are not kept as mandated, discipline can be applied. Such documentation serves to protect the public, but it may also protect the pharmacist by providing proof that the pharmacist complied with the law.

State boards of pharmacy require documentation of each prescription drug dispensed. Typical requirements include a prescription or drug order containing the name and address of the patient, the name and address of the prescriber, the date prescribed and the date dispensed, directions for use, a prescription or order number, the name and strength of the drug, and identification of the pharmacist dispensing (e.g., see Oklahoma Statutes[7]). Such information is required to be retained for a specified amount of time, typically 5–7 years. Pharmacists do not think of these requirements as documentation, but they are exactly that.

Federal law also mandates documentation connected to the pharmacist's duties of drug dispensing. This is particularly true when dealing with controlled substances. A record of all controlled substances received and dispensed and an inventory of such drugs must be maintained. The federal government provides the forms to be used and maintained for these purposes. Most pharmacists are familiar with the daily controlled drug printouts required by federal and state law. Failure to maintain these records can result in civil fines and criminal and administrative penalties.

Court cases, laws, rules, and regulations help to define what is expected of pharmacists. They help establish the minimum expected under professional standards of practice. When considering documentation, pharmacists need to consider what is required as part of those professional standards. Pharmacists can expect that they may be required to show, through proper documentation, that at a minimum they fulfilled the following duties:

1. To dispense the drug as prescribed.
2. To correctly interpret and communicate to the patient the directions for use.
3. To maintain all required records.
4. To perform a prospective drug review before dispensing a prescription or drug order.
5. To inquire of the patient and/or physician when there is an apparent error in the prescription or drug order until, in the pharmacist's professional judgment, the error has been corrected or the question resolved to the extent that the physician made a risk assessment decision.

6. To monitor drug use for abuse and overuse and to warn the patient and/or physician of use.

7. To warn the patient and/or the physician of those items that, in the pharmacist's judgment, are necessary.

8. To perform those items of pharmaceutical care mandated by law.

THE PATIENT RISK MANAGEMENT ROLE: PHARMACEUTICAL CARE

The newer roles of the pharmacist also require documentation. Unlike those necessary for the dispensing function, they are generally not required, with some exceptions. Because these are not required, the pharmacist may consider them less important. This could be a mistake. The purpose of documentation should first be to protect and serve the patient. The patient's chart exists primarily to allow caregivers to view a history of treatment and experience. So it must be with pharmacist documentation.

With the introduction of new duties, the pharmacist must now learn to document beyond the requirements of the law. The pharmacist must document to the extent required for the patient's well-being. The old role of the pharmacist was as dispenser of medication upon the order of a physician. The new role of the pharmacist is as patient risk manager. This is not a completely new duty—it is a logical extension of the old duties. However, the old duties are not gone, they have simply been expanded. Pharmacists have not exchanged one set of required documentation for another. The pharmacist's role of record-keeper has grown.

Pharmacists are entering into a new role that takes them to a new level of documentation. No longer is the pharmacist's role exclusively that of overseer of drug distribution; now, the pharmacist is the primary professional responsible for pharmaceutical care of the patient. Increasingly, the pharmacist is becoming more responsible for drug therapy outcomes. Many state boards of pharmacy have adopted this as a mandatory charge for a pharmacist in professional practice. In the NABP Model Practice Act, the pharmacist in charge has the duty of:

> Developing quality assurance programs for pharmacy services designed to objectively and systematically monitor and evaluate the quality and appropriateness of patient care, pursue opportunities to improve patient care, and resolve identified problems. Quality assurance programs shall be designed to prevent and detect drug diversion.

> *Model Rules for Pharmaceutical Care, § (2) (a)*

These are not novel concepts, but as they become codified, they present new areas in which pharmacists may be required to demonstrate at a future date that they performed these tasks at least to a minimum level of competency. For a given patient, the pharmacist will be unable to recall in detail what actions were taken. This is the task of documentation.

Previously, the documentation required of the pharmacist involved *what* mechanically was done. The new roles of the pharmacist involve *why* something was done as well. Just as the physician can be held responsible for assessing the risk to the patient and choosing a particular drug to treat a condition, and may thus be called on to later prove that he or she made such decisions in a reasonable manner, the pharmacist may be held responsible for managing the risk to the patient of the selected drug therapy, and may be called on to later prove his or her judgments and decisions were reasonable. It becomes important to record actions, judgments, and decisions made and to track them so others, including the pharmacist, can track the patient's care.

DOCUMENTATION IN CIVIL LAW: PROOF OF WHAT AND WHY

The primary use of documentation is to protect and treat the patient, but documentation can protect the pharmacist as well. Documentation may be introduced as proof in a civil lawsuit or in an administrative hearing, such as before a board of pharmacy, of what the pharmacist knew at the time, what decision he or she made, and why that decision was made. Without such proof, the court or board may be left to speculate, and the pharmacist may have to rely on his or her imperfect memory.

In civil law, the question usually is, "Did the pharmacist act reasonably?" The judgment of what is reasonable is determined by the facts and what the pharmacist knew, or should have known, at the time of the event. The standard applied is an objective one and assures the same standard will be applied to everyone. The standard is not applied with retrospective "20/20 vision," but from the view of the apparent risk and under the circumstances existing at the time. The test is, "What would the reasonable, prudent pharmacist with the same or similar knowledge, acting under the same or similar circumstances, have done at the time?"[8] Only if the pharmacist can demonstrate what knowledge he or she had at the time and what circumstances existed at the time, can the pharmacist be judged properly.

Use of Documentation

The facts in a 1996 Michigan case serve as an illustration of the potential use of documentation in the pharmacist's role of patient risk manager.[a] The pharmacist in *Baker v. Arbor Drugs*[9] received a prescription for Robert Baker for Tavist-D, a cold product containing a decongestant. The same pharmacy had in recent days also filled Mr. Baker's prescription for Parnate, a monoamine oxidase (MAO) inhibitor. The patient eventually suffered a stroke and later committed suicide. The computer apparently detected the potential interaction, but, according to the pharmacist, the technician overrode the message. The computer documented the interaction detection by printing an "I" on the printout, which was later introduced as evidence. The pharmacist testified that had she known the patient was taking Parnate, she would not have filled the Tavist-D prescription.

---

[a] This case is useful here for illustration only. The case was decided not on pharmacist duty, but on a related theory of advertising law. (The pharmacy had a duty because it advertised it had taken on the duty of screening for interactions.) Because the pharmacist was not made aware of the previous prescription of Parnate, no documentation of the type discussed here was made. See *Baker v. Arbor Drugs*, 544 N.W.2d 727 (Mich. Ct. App. 1996)

If able to reverse time to the moment of the pharmacist checking the prescription, and presuming the pharmacist had a duty to, and did, perform a prospective drug review on this prescription, there are two possible scenarios, both requiring documentation. In each scenario, it should be presumed the pharmacist discovered the potential interaction. Either the pharmacist would have filled the prescription for Tavist-D or would have refused to fill it. Either decision could have been called into question at a later date. What facts would need to be preserved to judge properly the reasonableness of the pharmacist's action?

SCENARIO ONE

The pharmacist notes the interaction and fills the second prescription. In this hypothetical situation, the pharmacist notes the following facts:

> I called the doctor and told him of the interaction and its severity. I cited the page in the PDR. The doctor said that he is aware of the interaction but believes the patient stopped taking Parnate 2 weeks ago. He believes this is a safe time. I told the doctor that the patient had refilled the Parnate 15 days ago. He asked me to check with the patient. I talked to the patient, informed him of the potential serious interaction, and asked when he last took the Parnate. He said he has not taken one since the day he had it filled last. I decided the doctor's decision of proper time interval was reasonable and filled the Rx. Dated: _____ Signed _____

Even if it is later discovered that the patient did not tell the truth about when he last took the Parnate and if the physician's notes do not indicate a conversation, and even if the pharmacist can no longer recall the exact events, the documentation can be used to show the facts and reasonableness of the pharmacist's judgment.

SCENARIO TWO

The pharmacist refuses to fill the Tavist-D prescription. Although she explains her reasons to both the physician's office and the patient, both make charges that she is interfering with the physician-patient relationship and with the physician's right to prescribe. The physician's records show no telephone call from the pharmacy. The patient did not fill the prescription at any other pharmacy because, according to the patient's later testimony, "The pharmacist intimidated me." In this hypothetical situation, the pharmacist notes the following facts:

> I called the doctor's office but could not get through to the physician. The receptionist, Sally, said he could not be disturbed. I told Sally of the interaction and its severity and cited the page in the PDR. Sally said, "OK," and promised that she would inform the doctor and he would call me if he wanted to discuss it. I talked to the patient, informed him of the potential serious interaction, and asked when he last took the Parnate. He said he is still taking it. I told him I could not fill the prescription and advised him not to fill it elsewhere. The patient seemed upset. Dated: _____
> Signed _____

These scenarios illustrate not perfect, but adequate, documentation. In each case the facts as understood by the pharmacist at the time of the event are preserved and can be used to test the reasonableness of the pharmacist's actions. Because of the drugs involved and the severity of the interaction, the pharmacist may have been able to defend herself without the notes. Documentation, however, provides dramatic evidence from the time of the events and has an air of accuracy that would be missing if the pharmacist testified just from memory.

LEGAL RULES REGARDING DOCUMENTATION

The best use of documentation is to provide a recording that can be used later to better treat the patient. Every pharmacist knows, however, that documentation can, and often is, used by lawyers in court. Although there are rules of evidence that provide detailed guidelines governing the introduction and use of documentation, and although these rules can often be subject to debate among lawyers, in a general sense, the rules covering the use of documentation in trial are relatively simple.

A trial is a search for ultimate truth through an adversarial process. Each side in a trial believes it is correct. To convince an impartial third party, a judge or a jury, of its version of truth and thus win a decision in its favor, each side presents evidence proving its version of the truth. Documentation is a part of that evidence.

Evidence can be anything tending to prove something relevant to the case. This may be the testimony of a witness to an event. For example, a nurse may testify that she recalls seeing the pharmacist talking to the patient's physician and heard the pharmacist tell the physician an interaction was possible if a particular drug was given to the patient. The testimony may help or hurt either side of the case. It may concern a central element of the case or it may involve a very small fact.

Another type of evidence may be a writing made at or near the time the event which the writing documents. This writing is called documentation. Not all writings and not all testimony, however, will be allowed as evidence in court. If the nurse in the above example did not hear the pharmacist's conversation, but instead was told about the conversation by someone who was there, the testimony may be ruled hearsay and not allowed. Hearsay is an out-of-court statement introduced in court to prove the truth of the matter stated. With a few exceptions, hearsay is not allowed to be used as proof.

There are several reasons for not allowing hearsay as evidence in court. If another person is allowed to testify as to what he or she heard someone else say, then the person who actually spoke the words would not be under oath, and the court could not be certain the words spoken were true. Another reason is that small details of the conversation, including what the persons were doing at the time, the exact words used, and the intent of the speaker may be significant; therefore, the search for truth must allow cross-examination of the person who actually heard the words spoken. A second-hand report by a person who only heard what a witness to the conversation stated could only be used to prove that the original witness gave an account of what was heard.

The same is true of an out-of-court written statement. If it is important that the written words be accepted as true, then the person who wrote the words would generally have to be present in court, be placed under oath, and be subject to cross-examination. The witness could then testify to his or her knowledge of when the words were written and exactly what the words meant at the time. There are exceptions to this rule, but generally the best evidence is the testimony of the witness who wrote the document, not the writing itself. An often-heard objection in a court of law is, "I object to the introduction of the document, it is hearsay. I can't cross-examine a piece of paper." There are many appropriate responses to this objection, but the attorney making the objection is correct in that he or she cannot cross-examine the document, only the person who wrote the document can be cross-examined.

These are several ways in which documentation can be used in court. Some regularly kept business records are admissible as an exception to the general rule against hearsay. Such records must be original entries made in the routine of the business by someone who had personal knowledge of the event. In addition, the entry must have been made at or near the time of the event. Because the person who made the entries would be the best evidence of the truthfulness of the recorded event, that person must be shown to be unavailable to testify at trial.[10] Many records made in pharmacy practice would meet these requirements.

Documents may also be used in court if they show a prior inconsistent statement of the witness. It is therefore important for a pharmacist who is called as a witness to review all documentation entries he or she made regarding the event prior to testifying. If there are prior inconsistent statements, the pharmacist witness should be ready to explain the differences. Prior documents should *never* be destroyed, no matter what they say or how inconsistent they may seem.

Statements for the purpose of medical treatment or diagnosis may be admissible under court rules as an exception to the hearsay rule. In addition, description of medical history or symptoms, if they form the basis of treatment or diagnosis, are usually admissible, even if hearsay. It is generally viewed that such statements tend to be truthful because of the patient's strong motivation to be truthful at such times.[10]

From the pharmacist's point of view, the best use of documentation is to refresh memory. By the time a court is involved in a dispute, 2 or 3 years may have elapsed from the time the event took place. All human memory fades with time. A writing made at or near the time of the event can refresh the pharmacist's recollection of the events. The experience of a Midwestern community pharmacist provides a good example of the use of contemporaneous notes to refresh memory.

Almost six months after partially filling two controlled substance prescriptions for a patient, the pharmacist received a visit from a board of pharmacy inspector who informed the pharmacist that the prescriptions were forgeries. The board inspector questioned the pharmacist's reasons for partially filling the prescriptions, with an underlying suspicion that the pharmacist knew something was wrong with the prescriptions at the time of filling. The pharmacist made no notes on the prescriptions or in the computer at the time of filling. The pharmacist was left with only faint memory that there was something unusual at the time and confessed to the inspector, "I must have had some question in my mind about the prescriptions when I filled them." The pharmacist was charged with a professional violation because if he questioned them, he had a corresponding duty to go further and verify the prescriptions. Only after the pharmacist was officially reprimanded did the truth emerge. The reason for the partial fill was the customer only had enough money for half of each prescription. The pharmacist did not know, and had no reason to believe, there was any problem with the prescription. Had the pharmacist been able to refer to notes made at the time of filling, the inspector's questioning would have pointed toward the pharmacist's innocence. Such documentation can be used in a court of law in the same manner, to refresh recollection.

At times, documentation does not sufficiently refresh the writer's recollection of the events. However, it does allow the writer to recognize the writing as one prepared by himself or herself and to testify that the notes made at the time were true. Many months or years after an event, the pharmacist may have no knowledge of the event, even when shown his or her own notes. In such a case, a judge may allow the notes themselves to come into evidence. There are legal requirements for the use of the notes, however. The witness offering the notes in evidence must have had firsthand knowledge of the event; the writing must have been made at a time sufficiently near the time of the event when the witness did have a clear and accurate memory of it; and the witness, while having no present recollection, must be able to testify that the notes were accurate at the time.[11]

Some general knowledge of the legal uses of documentation is useful to pharmacists. This knowledge may forewarn pharmacists as to what type of items should be documented and what items need not be documented. Pharmacists should remember, however, that either side in a legal case can use documentation. This fact should not prevent documentation, because the truthful notation of facts may be among the best ways to arrive at the ultimate goal of judicial proceedings—the search for truth.

WHAT TO DOCUMENT AND WHEN

Having reviewed the pharmacy and legal uses of documentation and the need for documentation, the pharmacist should consider the manner of documenting. With the pharmacist's new duties and responsibilities added to the time-honored ones, the pharmacist's time is becoming a valuable asset. A pharmacist must learn to be judicious in what is documented. The examples used here provide insight into the purpose and usefulness of documentation, but if every routine decision were completely documented, the pharmacist would have little time to practice pharmacy. Perfect documentation may have to yield to practical considerations. A few simple rules provide at least minimal levels of documentation.

When to Document

1. When the law requires a record (e.g., prescription records, controlled substance records, etc.).
2. When the law requires a pharmacist to perform certain acts that the pharmacist may later be called on to prove (e.g., in the Model Act, the pharmacist in charge must develop a quality assurance

program).[b] When routine duty requirements are necessary to show a duty performed (e.g., OBRA '90 type requirements [drug review, counseling, patient records]. Note: A system should be used to allow routine documentation to be accomplished quickly with as little time as possible).

3. When there are nonroutine events (i.e., those that are unusual or out of the ordinary), such as in the hypothetical scenarios discussed in the *Baker v. Arbor Drugs* example.

4. When there are therapeutic notations and drug use notes that may affect future treatment decisions.

5. When there are extraordinary measures taken for or on behalf of the patient (e.g., extra time spent training or retraining the patient in oral inhaler use).

6. When relatively routine matters can be documented quickly (e.g., a note in the computer [or on the back of a prescription] such as, "Part fill, not enough money" or "Part fill to see if patient can tolerate side effects").

7. When there are procedures that may need to be replicated (e.g., method of compounding or intravenous preparation).

8. When nursing home or hospital medication notes (e.g., "Patient taking anticoagulant—monitor regularly and note results. No aspirin.") necessary for physicians, nurses, or other caregivers are made.

9. When there are potential or foreseeable future problems that may need a special alert (e.g., anticoagulants; MAO inhibitors; "Patient history may show potential for abuse—monitor refills").

10. Whenever the pharmacist questions a prescription or feels it necessary to contact the prescriber.

---

[b] NABP Model Pharmacy Act., *Model Rules for Pharmaceutical Care*, § (2) (a). "Developing quality assurance programs for pharmacy services designed to objectively and systematically monitor and evaluate the quality and appropriateness of patient care, pursue opportunities to improve patient care, and resolve identified problems. Quality assurance programs shall be designed to prevent and detect drug diversion."

11. Whenever the pharmacist warns a patient of a potential interaction, allergy, or especially dangerous side effects.

12. When there is any other situation in which professional judgment suggests that future proof of facts known or reasons for judgment may be required.

Documentation of Nonroutine Events

As the professional goes about the routine of daily business life, events occasionally occur that are out of the ordinary. In some ways these events are the easiest to document, because they are unusual. The patient who is particularly trying or whose medication is unusual, cries out, "Better make a note." The wise pharmacist listens to such instincts.

The more unusual the situation, the more likely it is that the pharmacist may be called on to recall in some detail the events and the reasons for decisions. Patients involved in unusual medical situations may be more likely to face a recurrence of the events. Thus, it may be more likely that future caregivers treating the patient need to understand prior decisions and the reasons for them. This may allow for a better future response for that patient.

Documentation of Legally Mandated Acts

As discussed previously, state regulations require the pharmacist or the pharmacist in charge to perform certain duties. When such duties become a part of the law, the state has the right to inspect and demand proof that the pharmacist performed these duties. In some cases, the documentation itself may not be required by the law; however, the burden of proof may be on the pharmacist. The NABP Model Act, for example, mandates that the pharmacist in charge "develop a quality assurance program." If this language were adopted by a particular state, an inspector may demand evidence. Documentation of the steps taken, conversations held, and plans implemented will be more persuasive than the pharmacist verbal assurance, "I did that."

Such documentation not only protects the pharmacist, it also provides continuity and an assurance that the plan will work. Pharmacists must acquaint themselves with the regulations in their state. The same may be said for hospital or institutional rules. In addition to administrative reasons, such rules or regulations may be used in court to show the pharmacist did, or did not, perform up to institutional requirements.

Documentation of Medical Notations

Several of the items in the "What to Document" section refer to information regarding a patient's pharmaceutical use or needs. Pharmacists in long-term care facilities review medications of each resident monthly and record their findings. Depending on the information, the physician, the director, or the nurse may have to respond to these findings. This form of documentation is medically required.

The pharmacist's professional duty is to care for the patient. This was earlier characterized as the duty of patient risk manager. Just as physicians, hospitals, nursing homes, and nurses find it necessary to chart the patient's medical progress, the pharmacist should note the patient's pharmaceutical progress. What items should be covered are determined by the pharmacist's judgment in a particular case. Generally, this can be expressed as what information will be needed to make future medical or pharmaceutical decisions.

Documentation can be a history of what was done, a notation regarding thoughts on future needs to change medications, notes concerning how a patient is progressing while taking a particular drug, notations concerning side effects or reactions that can be expected, or proposals of what course of action to follow if the current drug regimen fails.

Documentation of Routine Duties

The most difficult items to document habitually are the routine duties of the pharmacist. To expect a pharmacist to document each time a patient is counseled, or each time he or she performs a routine drug review, seems to be an exercise in futility. In actuality, however, pharmacists do document matters just as routine, and do it consistently. A pharmacist records in great detail each drug order sent to the floor for each patient. Years later, records reveal what drug was dispensed, in what quantity, for what charge, and on what day. This type of documentation was performed even before computers were used. Aside from the regulatory requirements, all pharmacists recognize that if they could not show at any future time what medication was given, they may be at the mercy of a patient who later charged that the pharmacist must have dispensed the wrong drug, because the medication did not work in the way it was expected.

In today's world of pharmacy, it may be as necessary for the pharmacist to prove the patient was counseled, was asked what other medication were being taken, was asked about allergies, and in each case what the answers were. A number of claims are brought each year against ambulatory pharmacists who have dispensed a prescription with a non-safety cap. Although in many of these cases the patient requested no safety cap, the burden falls on the pharmacist to prove the request. After a child has been injured by a parent's or grandparent's prescription medication, the parents or grandparents say (and many times believe) that they were not asked and did not request "no safety cap."

In most cases, documentation is required for the patient's benefit. Routine, duty-related requirements are just as often for the benefit of the pharmacist. The problem with documentation of routine duties is that the vast majority of the documentation is not necessary. The majority of the time, no claims or accusations will ever be made. Once in a while, however, an incident will occur that requires looking for prior documentation. If the documentation is not done each time, it may not be available when the pharmacist needs it. Routine documentation need not be time-consuming or elaborate. An example is documentation of a routine telephone prescription in an ambulatory pharmacy.

By their nature, telephone prescriptions rely on oral communication. The words can be misunderstood or the speaker can be confused. If the pharmacist receives a prescription over the telephone which is later found to be incorrect, it will be perceived that the pharmacist made the mistake. If a physician or nurse misstates the name of the drug during a telephone prescription, the pharmacist, who first becomes aware of the error months or years later, will have no memory of what was said or know whose error it was. Simple documentation, however, can preserve the actual events.

A telephone prescription documentation and risk management technique is called "Echo, Verify, and Document." When any prescription is received by telephone, the pharmacist should always "echo" back the entire prescription before ending the conversation by saying, "Let me make sure I got that right." As each part (patient name, drug name, dosage, directions) of the prescription is echoed, the pharmacist places a checkmark on that part. The pharmacist then asks for verification, "Is that correct?" When the nurse or physician indicates what the pharmacist echoed was correct, the pharmacist places a "V" (for verified) on the prescription face and places his or her initials next to the "V" and the date. If the pharmacist rewrites the prescription, these notes should be attached to the telephone prescription to be filed as a "hard copy." The Echo, Verify, and Document prescription will look like the one in Figure 16-1.

Very seldom will the proof of what was said be necessary, but when it is, the proof will be available. Six months or even years later a pharmacist can state that although he or she does not remember the events, he or she can testify what the markings on the prescription indicate. The pharmacist

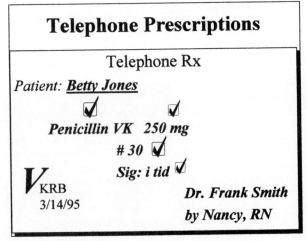

Figure 16-1. Echo, verify, and document.

can say, "The check marks mean I repeated each section of the prescription. The 'V' indicates that the person calling verified that what I said was correct." Simple documentation, such as that shown in Figure 16-1, can be effective.

The secret of documenting routine duties is in making the documentation part of the routine, just as a pharmacist does when recording a drug used and the prescription number issued. If documentation is too complicated or too time-consuming, it will not be done. Again, some compromise between completeness and ease may be necessary.

Documentation of Special Alerts

In *Hooks-SuperX v. McLaughlin*[12] the Indiana Supreme Court ruled, for the first time in that state, that pharmacists could be tried in a civil court for damages resulting from the pharmacists' failure to monitor a patient's abuse of a controlled substance. The Court opinion does not reveal that shortly after the ruling, the case was settled out of court for little more than nuisance value because the pharmacy's documentation showed repeated calls to the physician alerting him to the patient's use. The documentation showed the pharmacists had monitored the patient's use. They had performed their duty.

In today's harried practice of high-volume prescription filling, it is less likely than ever that pharmacists will know which patients to monitor. Documentation in such cases not only is useful in protecting the pharmacists, but it is necessary to protect the patient. A note in the computer can warn all pharmacists to review this patient's frequency and allow the patient to be warned of the dangers before a problem begins. The documentation permitted in most computer programs also allows entry of a short note to warn all pharmacists of special situations, such as a patient receiving anticoagulation therapy or special patient needs (e.g., "Speak loudly, patient is hard of hearing").

WHERE TO DOCUMENT

The choice of where to document is often dictated by the use of the documentation. Pharmacist's comments used as a history, as precautionary notes to alert the pharmacist or other health care providers of patient needs, and as an aid in future treatment must be made where they will be found by the one who needs the information. A nursing home patient who is taking an MAO inhibitor will require that all nurses and prescribers be knowledgeable of the drug use and its importance. If the nursing home rules allow pharmacists to add notations to the patient chart, the pharmacist may choose this as the place for documentation. In addition, notes of dietary restrictions may be noted on a special kitchen dietary guide, if one exists. The pharmacist familiar with the rules and routine following in nursing homes must make the decision based on the questions, "Where will the note be read?" and "Who needs to know?"

If the patient chart is not available to the pharmacist, the nurse's notes or physician's notes may be appropriate. A pharmacist may have to create a special pharmacist medication chart and work with the nurses and administration to mandate its review at the beginning of each shift. Remembering that the primary purpose of such documentation is to protect the patient, the pharmacist may have to become inventive in documentation.

In the hospital and in ambulatory pharmacies, the computer may provide the best place for documentation. Some information mandates the use of the computer for documentation. Information that can be accessed by the computer database when new medication for the patient is added can provide drug review information at the time of entering a new order. Allergy databases, drug databases, and disease state databases all make use of the computer's ability to store and retrieve large amounts of information quickly.

Some information is documented only to refresh memory later because of an unusual event. For example, if a patient refuses to listen to information the pharmacist believes is critical to the patient's use of the medication, such as how to use an inhaler properly, documentation may provide later proof of the pharmacist's attempt to counsel the patient. A special documentation portion of the computer may be a good place to note this experience. The pharmacist should also realize, however, that this information may be necessary during refills of the prescription and should be retrievable at that time. If a "pharmacist notes" portion of the computer is used in a pharmacy, each pharmacist should also be instructed to review this section for each patient.

Some notes are important at the time of the event and for later proof, but will not be needed routinely for the patient. In a community or ambulatory pharmacy, this type of information may best be documented on the back of the new prescription. The back of the prescription has the advantage that it is likely to be found if a complaint regarding the prescription is later made, because the new prescription is usually available. The disadvantage of the back of the prescription is the information is unlikely to be seen with each refill. Once again, this depends on the use of the information. If a pharmacist calls a physician to inquire if the physician knew that the drug prescribed may cause an adverse event when taken with another drug the patient is taking, the physician's answer should be documented. Because the primary purpose of this documentation may be to prove later that the pharmacist warned the physician, and thus the pharmacist did his or her duty, noting the conversation on the back of the prescription may be all that is necessary.

There may be times when none of the places discussed are available or are the most convenient place to put notes. For those times, a pharmacist may start a documentation journal. A pharmacist documentation journal is usually in chronologic order of events and is solely for the purpose of later proof of the event. This is usually documentation to protect the pharmacist, not for the patient, because the entry will usually only be viewed when a complaint regarding a particular instance is made.

Incident or Peer Review Report Documentation

One final place for documentation should be distinguished. Regardless of the care a pharmacist uses and regardless of the professional nature and efficiency of a pharmacy operation, errors will occur. When an error does happen and the pharmacist becomes aware of it, an entry must be made. In most hospitals and most retail pharmacies, this entry is on an incident report, or a peer review report. There are two purposes of these entries. The first is as a potential claims report. If an error reaches a patient, administration and/or management personnel must be made aware of it so steps can be taken to minimize the effects of the error on the patient and the institution. Usually called an incident report, this documentation can be necessary to resolve a potential claim.

The second use of such documentation is as a peer review report. Pharmacists in both hospital and retail practice are becoming increasingly aware of the need of instituting a quality assurance program to reduce errors. Every error reported becomes an opportunity to improve.

A WORD OF CAUTION

As a general rule, documentation should be of facts that will be needed in the future by pharmacists or other health care providers to make a decision or a judgment. Opinions of a personal nature, unless necessary for future or present treatment, are generally not warranted. Opinions without a factual basis are also not wise, nor are comments regarding another's decisions, unless the documentation is necessary for treatment.

Certain words are opinion words and should be avoided unless their use is judged as absolutely necessary and the writer knows all surrounding facts. Words such as "sloppy," "poor," "aberrant," "defective," "faulty," and "substandard" denote a judgment and require significant investigation. Words such as "inadequate," "undesirable," "inappropriate," and "unsatisfactory" state an opinion that may be appropriate in some instances. These words are usually used in documentation as merely showing frustration and a difference of opinion. If such words are judged necessary, they should not be used in a chart or patient records, but in a place and at a time calculated to change a course of treatment after careful consideration.

No professional appreciates being labeled as careless or negligent, particularly if the label is applied in a place where others will be privy to the accusation. A pharmacist is not likely to convince a prescriber to change a course of treatment if the physician sees the choice ridiculed in the patient's record. Words of blame such as "erroneous," "regretful," "foolish," "terrible," "unfortunate," and "wrong" should be avoided. The temptation to make a legal opinion by using words such as "negligent," "mix-up," "mistake," "fault," and "inadvertent" should also be overcome.

Professional documentation should be truthful, factual, and serve the purpose of assisting the patient. A patient chart is not an appropriate place for a war of words and accusations between two otherwise professional persons. Documentation should be complete but it must also be concise.

CONCLUSION

Documentation is valuable in the professional practice of pharmacy for both the protection of the patient and the protection of the pharmacist, who may be unfairly charged with a negligent or unprofessional act. Most people, including pharmacists, are not good documenters. In the day-to-day pressure to accomplish their professional tasks, pharmacists tend to focus their energies on performing their duties to the patient. Extra time taken during the performance of these duties, or after the duties are finished, to make notations of what happened or the basis of judgments made may seem unnecessary. Pharmacists need to train themselves to think of necessary documentation as a part of the job, rather than as an inconvenience.

To train themselves to recognize documentation as a part of the job, it is valuable for pharmacists to understand the uses of documentation. The most important reasons are professional. Pharmaceutical care is usually a continuing process of judgments and decisions, making it important for future caregivers to know the reasons and facts surrounding past treatment.

The primary reason to document is not for use in court. However, pharmacists should understand that documentation can and will be used in court and that, in court, documentation is often a double-edged sword. It may help and it may hurt.

Professional pharmacists need to become good documenters. The emphasis, however, must be on "professional." The mark of a professional is a reputation for truthfulness. All entries must be truthful and should be for a legitimate pharmacy purpose. If the pharmacist feels that what he or she is about to document could be embarrassing and the pharmacist would feel uncomfortable having to show the documentation to others, then the pharmacist should probably not perform the act in the first place. Perhaps the most important rule in documenting is, "Think first, then do, then write."

References

1. *Ingram v. Hooks*, 476 N.E.2d 881, 886 (Ind. App. 1985).
2. *Ingram v. Hooks*, 476 N.E.2d 881, 887 (Ind. App. 1985).
3. *Dooley v. Everett*, 805 S.W.2d 380 (Tenn. App 1990).
4. *Gassen v. East Jefferson General Hospital*, 628 So.2d 256 (La. App. 1993).
5. *Lasley v. Shrakes Country Club Pharmacy*, 880 P.2d 1129 (Ariz. Ct. App. 1994).
6. *Lasley v. Shrakes Country Club Pharmacy*, 880 P.2d 1132 (Ariz. Ct. App. 1994).
7. Oklahoma Statutes, Title 59, Chapter 8, § 355, et seq.
8. W. Page Keeton et al, Prosser and Keeton on the Law of Torts § 32 (5th ed. 1984).
9. *Baker v. Arbor Drugs*, 544 N.W.2d 727 (Mich. Ct. App. 1996).
10. *USC Fed. Rules of Evidence*, Art. VIII, Rule 803 with annotations.
11. *United States v. Kelly*, 349 F.2d 720, 770–71 (2nd Cir. 1965).
12. *Hooks SuperX v. McLaughlin*, 642 N.E.2d 514 (Ind. 1994).

Chapter 17

Over-the-Counter Drug Therapy

William R. Garnett

INTRODUCTION

The pharmacy profession has adopted pharmaceutical care as the philosophy that is guiding its educational and practice development. The basic premise of pharmaceutical care is that the pharmacist will take responsibility for and be accountable for the outcomes of drug therapy. The use of over-the-counter (OTC) drugs provides the pharmacist with an excellent opportunity to practice pharmaceutical care. There is a growing demand for OTC drugs and an increasing number of potent drugs being converted from prescription to OTC status. The pharmacist has complete access to the patient when selecting an OTC drug and can individualize the treatment plan. Patients benefit from pharmacists' counseling about OTC drugs through more appropriate use of these drugs, which helps to reduce health care costs. Pharmacists need to promote the contributions that they can make in maximizing the use of OTC drugs.

SELF-CARE ENVIRONMENT

The focus of health care has shifted. For many years health care was paternalistic, with health care providers deciding what they thought was best for the patient and then telling the patient what to do. In the past 25 years, however, patients have demanded a greater role in deciding the course of their therapy. Patients now expect to know why the drug is being used, what the name of the drug is, how they are going to respond to the drug, and what the side effects of the drug are. Patients are often asked to make choices about the benefits and risks of treatment options. Patients view OTC drugs as a means of increasing their autonomy and as a way of reducing their health care costs.

A recent survey (Self-Medication in the 90's: Practices and Prescriptions. Washington, DC: Nonprescription Drug Manufacturers Association, 1992;9–13) illustrated these opinions with the following findings:

- ➤ 70% of consumers prefer to endure the symptoms of a disease without medication if possible.
- ➤ 85% of consumers believe that they should have access to OTC drugs to relieve minor medical problems.
- ➤ 94% of consumers believe that care should be taken when using an OTC drug.
- ➤ 94% of consumers would take the same OTC medication again if similar symptoms returned.
- ➤ 54% of the participants believe that they have saved time and money by using OTC drugs.
- ➤ 66% of consumers favor more OTC switches.
- ➤ 81% of consumers believe that pharmacists are a good source of OTC drug information.

It has been estimated that 57% of all health problems can be treated with an OTC drug. Therefore, it is not surprising that the use of OTC drugs is increasing. The trust placed in pharmacists by patients provides an excellent opportunity for increased involvement in OTC drug therapy selection and monitoring.

THE OTC DRUG MARKET

The use of OTC drugs is increasing. The sales volume of OTC drugs exceeds $30 billion and is expected to exceed $36 billion by the year 2002. Approximately 60% of all dosage units consumed (prescription and nonprescription) are OTC drugs. The per capita expenditure for OTC drugs is approximately $90 per year and is increasing. Persons older than 65 years of age comprise approximately 14% of the population but take approximately 25% of prescription and 33% of all OTC drugs. This segment of the population is rapidly increasing. There are over 400 medical disorders that are treatable with one or more nonprescription drugs. Of approximately 3–5 billion health problems treated anually in the United States, about 2 billion or 57% are treated with a nonprescription drug. Managed care plans have identified that management of many health problems with OTC medications reduces the utilization of expensive health care resources and is very cost-effective. (Covington Timothy R. "Self-Care and Nonprescription Pharmacotherapy." The Handbook of Nonprescription Drugs. 12th ed. Washington, DC: American Pharmaceutical Association; 2000:3–14.)

As has often been stated, the pharmacist is the most accessible health care provider. Consumers view the pharmacist as a good source of drug information. However, the number of OTC drugs obtained in a pharmacy is decreasing. The percentage of OTC drugs bought in a pharmacy has dropped from approximately 70% to less than 40%. This clearly decreases revenue for the pharmacy. Also, if consumers purchase OTC drugs without consulting with a pharmacist, they are potentially at risk if they fail to understand completely how to use OTC drugs or if the OTC drugs are used inappropriately. Inappropriate use of OTC drugs will increase the cost of health care. Therefore, pharmacists should encourage patients to consult with them about the appropriate use of OTC drugs.

OTC DRUGS ARE DRUGS

Many patients and some health care providers view OTC drugs as little more than placebos. Some people still refer to "patent medicines" and have the philosophy that the dose is "one for a man and two for a horse." These views may emanate from the traveling medicine men days and an earlier process for OTC drug approval. However, it is important to realize that the drugs available OTC are potent compounds and should be treated with the same respect as prescription drugs.

Many years ago, drugs could be marketed OTC without rigorous testing. However, a few years ago the FDA conducted a thorough review of all of the OTC drugs and set standards for the pharmacologic activity if the label claimed a specific action. Now there is a formal procedure for approval of drugs for OTC status. The procedure is similar to approval of prescription drugs. There must be efficacy trials, and the label must be reviewed and approved by the FDA. Under this new process, there have been some very potent compounds (e.g., the nonsteroidal antiinflammatory drugs [NSAIDs] and the histamine II antagonists [H_2RAs] that have achieved OTC status). Many other drugs are being considered for a switch to OTC status.

OTC drugs have pharmacologic activity and have the potential to relieve or cure patient complaints. However, because they are potent compounds, they also have the potential to cause patient problems.

POTENTIAL PROBLEMS WITH OTC DRUG USE

The FDA does not have authority over OTC drug advertising. The advertising of OTC drugs is regulated by the Federal Trade Commission. Because OTC drugs (e.g. H_2RAs, oral analgesics) are widely advertised, it is possible for consumers to become confused or misinformed. This can lead to inappropriate OTC drug use.

Many patients may be confused about the appropriate use of an OTC drug. For example, a patient with daily episodes of heartburn may continue to take OTC drugs that are approved for heartburn for up to 14 days when a prescription drug is more appropriate for chronic use. Also, patients may not differentiate symptoms. For example, a patient may have point tenderness between the sternum and the umbilicus that occurs in the early morning hours and is often relieved by food. This is a classic presentation of duodenal ulcer disease. However, the patient may not recognize this and inappropriately treat the condition with OTC drugs such as antacids or H_2RAs when they are not indicated for this condition. Another example of inappropriate OTC drug use is the patient who uses OTC analgesics for inflammatory disorders. The doses of the NSAIDs that are approved for OTC use are analgesic doses and are not antiinflammatory doses. In these conditions, the patient may obtain some relief but not receive adequate treatment for curing the disease or completely relieving the symptoms. Therefore, inappropriate OTC drug use many prolong the disease by causing a delay in seeking appropriate care. Consultation with a pharmacist could help maximize the use of OTC drugs for appropriate indications and duration of therapy.

Also, many patients do not consider OTC drugs as medications. When they are providing a medication history, many patients only mention prescription medicines until they are prompted to remember OTC drugs by questions such as "Do you take anything for a headache?" or "Do you take anything for an upset stomach?" Many patients clearly take the use of OTC drugs more casually than prescription drugs.

OTC drugs are drugs, and they can cause side effects and interact with other drugs. If these side effects and interactions are not suspected and detected, they can cause significant medical problems. Although the OTC label is required to list the most common side effects and interactions, patients may not read the label or understand the nature of the problem. For example, the label may warn of an interaction between cimetidine and warfarin. However, the patient knows that he or she is taking Coumadin and does not make the connection that Coumadin is warfarin. Side effects may also occur. The patient may take an OTC antihistamine to relieve the symptoms of allergic rhinitis and become sleepy. Without consultation, patients may not realize that they should use caution when driving if they are taking OTC antihistamines. Because patients often do not include OTC drugs in their medication history, OTC-induced drug interactions and side effects may go undetected when the patient sees a physician. Pharmacists should encourage patients to record and report all medications, including OTC drugs, that they are taking when giving a medication history.

As more drugs are switched from prescription to OTC status, problems may occur because patients know the names of the drugs but do not know the OTC dose. When drugs achieve OTC status, they may keep their prescription trade name because of name recognition. However, the OTC dose is usually lower than the prescription dose. This is clearly stated on the label. However, a patient may have taken Zantac (ranitidine) 300 mg per day for a peptic ulcer and not realize that the OTC dose for heartburn is 75 mg twice a day. The patient may increase the dosage units to take the dose that he or she is familiar with.

> ## PHARMACISTS' ROLE IN MAXIMIZING THE USE OF OTC DRUGS

Be Familiar with OTC Drugs and Drug Labels

It is important to know what OTC drugs are available in a given pharmacy. It is estimated that there are more than 300,000 individual OTC drug products currently being marketed. However, they contain only about 700 distinct active ingredients. There are many OTC products with different names but with the same active ingredients. For example, there is a plethora of analgesics but they all contain acetaminophen, aspirin, nonacetylated salicylates, and other NSAIDs. Thus, with all the OTC analgesics advertised, there are only eight drugs that are analgesics.

Mylanta provides an example of drugs with the same trade name but different active ingredients. Mylanta liquid is an antacid containing a mixture of aluminum hydroxide and magnesium hydroxide. Mylanta capsules contain famotidine, which is an H_2RA.

The active ingredients in OTC drugs may change without a change in the trade name. For example, the formulations of many of the analgesics changed when phenacetin was removed from the OTC market, but the trade names remained the same.

In addition, patients may take the same drug with different trade names and not realize that they are taking more of the drug than is recommended.

There are some OTC drugs that are marketed regionally and may be very popular with consumers in a given area. These drugs may not get national exposure through advertising, but it is important for the pharmacist to know the availability, ingredients, and usefulness of these regional products.

Specific information is required by the FDA to be on the label of an OTC drug. The information required consists of the product name and ingredients, product indications and claims, package contents, directions for use, contraindications, warnings, adverse reactions, indications for seeking medical attention, expiration date, batch code, and label flags. This information is directed at the consumer, not the health professional. The pharmacist should read these labels to ensure that patients can understand the information and to determine where additional information is necessary. Patients should be encouraged to read the label and to ask any questions that they might have about the information on the label. Some OTC drugs provide additional patient information materials. Pharmacists should review this information to determine suitability for patients.

Obtain Additional Information About OTC Drugs

Although the package insert may provide valuable information, pharmacists may need additional information to counsel patients adequately about OTC drug use. There are books (e.g., "The Handbook of Nonprescription Drugs") devoted to OTC therapy. It is harder to obtain comparative and evaluative information on herbal medicines and dietary supplements. Some textbooks and journal articles are provided in the Suggested Readings section. The Internet provides a means of rapid retrieval of data. Data searches of specific topics can be performed in a short period of time. When performing data searches, pharmacists should be cautious about information found on web sites. Journal articles have been through a peer review process; web sites may only provide opinions or be overly biased in support of a given therapy.

Develop an Action Plan

Patients will come to the pharmacy and request a specific OTC drug product or will seek help form the pharmacist in selecting an OTC drug for a specific complaint. The pharmacist must ensure that it is appropriate to use an OTC product and then individualize the OTC drug selection. In some cases, the pharmacist must convince the patients that the medication they requested is not the best one for their condition. After making an OTC drug product selection, the pharmacist should monitor the patient's response through patient follow-up. Figure 17-1 provides an algorithm for implementing pharmaceutical care with OTC drugs.

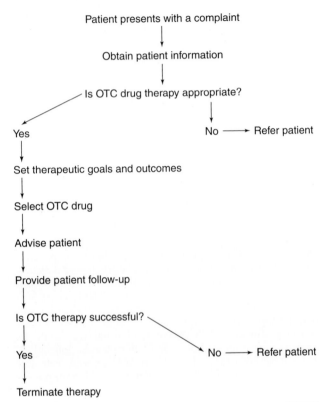

Figure 17-1. Algorithm for pharmacist management of OTC drug therapy.

When Patient Has a Specific Complaint

DETERMINE IF OTC DRUG THERAPY IS APPROPRIATE

Pharmacists must ensure that OTC drugs are used appropriately. OTC drugs are intended for short-term treatment of uncomplicated disease states that can easily be recognized (Box 17.1). OTC drugs should never be used to mask the symptoms of a more serious disease that requires careful diagnostic evaluation and prescription drug treatment. If there is a doubt about the appropriateness of OTC drug therapy, the patient should be referred for a medical evaluation. To do this pharmacists must assess the patient's condition by interview, observation, and inspection. Initially the pharmacist should identify if the person to whom he or she is talking is the person that has the complaint and will use the OTC drug. The pharmacist should ask a series of questions (Box 17.2) to identify specific patient symptoms, chronicity of disease, severity of disease, and patient risk factors. The pharmacist should observe and inspect the patient also. Increasingly, the observation and inspection of the patient involves physical examination. This process will differentiate self-treatable conditions from conditions requiring medical intervention. For example, if the patient wants something for a rash, the pharmacist should look at the rash. The pharmacist should consider that the rash could be a drug-induced rash from another drug that the patient is taking. Also, the patient may call a reaction a skin rash when it is a more severe eruption, e.g., a Stevens-Johnson reaction. After the pharmacist determines that the rash is related to contact dermatitis (e.g., poison ivy) and involves a modest area of the body, an OTC therapy may be recommended.

Additionally, the pharmacist should obtain a history that is more thorough than a simple complaint. For example, a patient may request something for a cough. A description of

647

Box 17.2   Questions for the Patient Interview

Who is the patient?
How old is the patient?
Is the patient male or female?
Does the patient have any other medical problems?
Is the complaint a chronic disease?
Does the patient have any allergies?
Can you describe the problem?
When did the problem start?
How long does it last? Does it come and go, or is it
    continuous?
Does the problem limit daily activities?
Is this a new problem or a recurrence?
Are there other problems that occur concurrently?
Does any food, drug, or activity make the problem
    worse?
Does anything relieve the problem? What has helped in
    the past?
What has been done to treat the problem?
Is the patient eating a special diet?
Is the patient taking any prescription, nonprescription,
    or social drugs?
Has the patient experienced adverse reactions in the
    past?

the cough should be explored. Although it may be appropriate to recommend a cough medicine to someone with a
mild cold, the pharmacist might make the wrong recommendation if he or she does not ask additional questions. If
the patient has a cough but also describes night sweats and
a history of blood in the sputum, the pharmacist should suspect tuberculosis and refer the patient for medical evaluation. The frequency of symptoms obtained by patient history may also indicate that the patient needs a referral. For
example, mild and infrequent heartburn symptoms may be
treated or prevented with OTC H_2RAs. However, if the
pharmacist determines that the patient has a classic picture
of heartburn but the symptoms are occurring daily or several times per week, OTC therapy would be inappropriate
and the patient should be referred to a physician.

Pharmacists should not recommend OTC therapy when it is not indicated or would mask the symptoms of a severe disease. For example, a patient may have a complaint of abdominal pain that is suggestive of duodenal ulcer. Although an OTC H_2RA or antacid may provide short-term symptom relief, this is inappropriate therapy. Patients with duodenal ulcers should undergo endoscopy and be evaluated for the presence of *Helicobacter pylori*.

Pharmacists provide a valuable service by screening patients to determine if OTC therapy is indicated. Physician referral should occur when the symptoms are too severe and require a definitive diagnosis, when the symptoms are minor but have persisted with no identifiable cause, the symptoms have returned repeatedly for no identifiable cause, or the pharmacist is in doubt about the patient's medical condition. A referral to a physician is a valuable contribution to the patient's health care.

SET THERAPEUTIC GOALS

All therapy should be directed toward accomplishing some definable objective. For example, if a patient has a headache and it has been determined that there is no cerebrovascular accident in progress and there is no other significant neurologic problem, an OTC analgesic is appropriate. The goal of therapy would be to stop the headache. The goals of some therapy may be to prevent symptoms from occurring. For example, H_2RAs may be used to prevent heartburn when the patient knows that he or she will be exposed to factors that precipitate symptoms. Therapeutic goals help define therapeutic outcomes, which are quantifiable and measurable.

SELECT THE OTC DRUG

After determining that OTC drug therapy is appropriate and defining the goals of therapy, pharmacists should individualize therapy by helping the patient select the most appropriate OTC drug. This individualization of therapy will depend on the information obtained during the patient interview. For example, a patient requests a recommendation on an analgesic. If the patient is female and needs something for menstrual cramps, an NSAID is most appropriate. If the patient is taking warfarin, acetaminophen may be a better choice. If the patient has a history of ulcers, NSAIDs and aspirin should be avoided. Therefore, pharmacists can individualize OTC therapy by avoiding drug interactions, anticipating side effects, and defining what OTC drugs work better in special populations.

ADVISE THE PATIENT

After helping the patient select an OTC drug for self-therapy, the pharmacist should advise the patient on its use. The areas for advisement are similar to the those used in consultation for prescription drugs. The pharmacists should ensure that the patient understands the reasons, goals, and outcomes of self-treatment. The pharmacist should provide a description of the drug, instruct the patient on how to administer the drug, and inform the patient about the treatment guidelines. The patient should also understand how to evaluate a positive response to therapy and how to detect side effects when they occur. The pharmacist should be available to patients if they have any questions about their OTC therapy.

SET THERAPEUTIC END POINTS

There should be a limit to the duration of OTC therapy—either the condition is resolved or the patient needs medical referral. By helping the patient set specific therapeutic goals at the initiation of OTC drug therapy, pharmacists can help patients set limits on the use of OTC drugs. For example, if a headache persists or is reduced in severity but persists for 2 or 3 days while taking an OTC analgesic, the patient should be referred to a physician. The OTC drug label will provide guidelines for the maximum duration of self-therapy. By adhering to these guidelines, the use of OTC drugs can be maximized. Extending the use of OTC drug therapy beyond the approved time limits may delay the time for effective therapy. For example, extended use of H_2RAs may delay the diagnosis of gastroesophageal reflux disease and effective treatment.

PROVIDE PATIENT FOLLOW-UP

Although many pharmacists provide OTC drug recommendations, not many provide adequate patient follow-up. However, the only way to determine if the recommendation was appropriate is to monitor the patient. The basic premise of pharmaceutical care is to take responsibility for therapeutic outcomes. Patient follow-up is essential for OTC drug recommendations for which the pharmacist helps to select the drug. Patient follow-up would also reinforce in patients' minds that pharmacists are concerned about their well-being and response. The patient follow-up could be brief. Pharmacist extenders could obtain basic information and put the patient in contact with the pharmacist if there are questions or problems. This could be done by telephone. During the telephone call, it could be determined if the patient had a desirable response or a negative response. The call could determine if the need for OTC drug therapy has been met and the patient has discontinued the OTC therapy, or if the patient continues to need OTC therapy. Need for OTC therapy after the maximum duration of recommended therapy would be a reason to refer the patient for additional evaluation. For example, a patient may obtain an OTC H_2RA for heartburn. The symptoms may be minimized or even abolished with OTC therapy. However, if the symptoms continue or return when the patient discontinues the OTC H_2RA, the patient should be referred for additional evaluation. This referral is an integral part of taking responsibility for therapeutic outcomes and pharmaceutical care.

DOCUMENT ACTIVITIES

It is becoming increasingly important for pharmacists to document their activities in patient care. There is the obvious legal advantage of documenting evaluations and recommendations. There is also the need to document activities to demonstrate effectiveness for reimbursement. Although there are simulation studies that suggest that OTC drug therapy is cost-effective, pharmacists may find it difficult to be reimbursed for OTC recommendations. Third-party payers will reimburse for services that they perceive to be cost-effective. Therefore, pharmacists need to show the value of their services in an attempt to obtain reimbursement.

When Patient Requests a Specific Drug

If the patient requests a specific drug, the pharmacist must determine if the use is appropriate and if that is the best drug for that patient. This process begins by determining what condition the patient intends to treat. This process is similar to the one described above. Again, it may be appropriate to refer the patient to a physician. If self-therapy is appropriate, the pharmacist must decide if the patient's choice is the best choice. The pharmacist should determine why the patient wants that drug. The pharmacist should ask how the patient heard about the drug. Did a physician recommend it? Does the patient have a prescription for that drug? If the pharmacist does not believe that this is the best choice for a given patient, the pharmacist should explain why another selection is better. As described above, the pharmacist needs to monitor the patient and provide patient follow-up.

BENEFITS OF OTC DRUG COUNSELING TO PHARMACISTS

There are clear professional benefits to the pharmacist for being involved in OTC drug therapy selection. It is an excellent opportunity to practice pharmaceutical care. With OTC recommendations, the pharmacist can interview, observe, and inspect the patient. The amount of information available to the pharmacist is limited only by the thoroughness with which he or she reviews the patient. There are no data in a patient's chart that the pharmacist does not have access to. The pharmacist can help determine the appropriateness of self-therapy. With OTC recommendations, the pharmacist helps the patient make the most appropriate choice of drugs. The pharmacist does not have to contact another health care provider to discuss the choice of therapy. By providing follow-up, the pharmacist can evaluate the success of the recommendations and let patients know of his or her concern for their welfare.

In addition to the professional benefits, there are economic benefits also. The number of OTC drugs obtained in a pharmacy is decreasing. If the patient does not receive counseling and help from the pharmacist in selecting OTC drugs, then it does not matter where the patient obtains the OTC drugs. If there is no value to the patient in obtaining OTC drugs in a pharmacy, then pharmacists should not complain if patients obtain OTC drugs at more convenient locations.

BENEFITS OF OTC DRUG COUNSELING TO PATIENTS

Clearly, many patients can benefit from pharmacists' recommendations for OTC drug therapy. Pharmacists can help identify patients who are good candidates for self-therapy. Pharmacists can provide patient education and direct patients to additional sources of information. Pharmacists can individualize OTC drug therapy and avoid drug interactions. Appropriate use of OTCs have been shown to reduce health care costs. Finally, by being better informed, patients are empowered to take a more active role in their own therapy.

SUMMARY

The availability of OTC drugs allows patients to manage many problems rapidly, economically, and conveniently. However, inappropriate use and misuse of OTC drugs can increase the risk of drug misadventures that result in increased health care costs and a more seriously ill patient. Pharmacists can improve the usefulness of OTC drug therapy by helping select patients appropriate for self-therapy and referring patients who need medical evaluation. Pharmacists can individualize OTC drug therapy to improve drug selection. By providing patient monitoring and follow-up, pharmacists can maximize therapeutic outcomes. Pharmacists should promote to patients their value in selecting OTC therapy.

Suggested Readings

American Pharmaceutical Association. Handbook of Nonprescription Drugs. Washington, DC: 2000.

Anderson RA et al. Quick Access Professional Guide to Conditions, Herbs, & Supplements. Newton, MA: Integrative Medicine Communications; 2000.

Astin JA et al. A review of the incorporation of complementary and alternative medicine by mainstream physicians. Arch Intern Med. 1998;23(158):2303–10.

Ausman LM. Criteria and recommendations for vitamin C intake. Nutr Rev. 1999;57:222–4.

Blumenthal M et al. Complete German Commission E Monographs: Therapeutic Guide to Herbal Medicines Developed by a Special Expert Committee of the German Federal Institute for Drugs and Medical Devices. Newton, MA: Integrative Medicine Communications; 1998.

Blumental M, Goldberg A. Herbal Medicine: Expanded Commission E Monographs. Newton, MA: Integrative Medicine Communications; 2000.

Chan TY. Monitoring the safety of herbal medicines. Drug Saf. 1997;17:209–15.

Cohen MH. Complementary & Alternative Medicine: Legal Boundaries and Regulatory Perspectives. Baltimore, MD: Johns Hopkins University Press; 1998.

Gardiner P, Kemper KJ. Herbs in pediatric and adolescent medicine. Pediatr Rev. 2000;21:44–57.

Hardy ML. Herbs of special interest to women. J Am Pharm Assoc. 2000;40:234–42.

Kayser-Jones J et al. A prospective study of the use of liquid oral dietary supplements in nursing homes. J Am Geriatr Soc. 1998;46:1378–86.

Lewis DP et al. Drug and environmental factors associated with adverse pregnancy outcomes. Part II: improvement with folic acid. Ann Pharmacother. 1998;32:947–61.

Mannion M. The Pharmacist's Guide to OTC & Natural Remedies. NY: Penguin Putman, Inc.; 1999.

Mar C, Bent S. An evidence-based review of the 10 most commonly used herbs. West J Med. 1999;171:168–71.

Marrone CM. Safety issues with herbal products. Ann Pharmacother. 1999;33:1359–62.

Medical Economics Staff. 1999 PDR for Nonprescription Drugs & Dietary Supplements. Montvale, NJ: Medical Economics Co.; 1999.

Newton GD et al. New OTC drugs and devices 1999: a selective review. J Am Pharm Assoc. 2000;40:222–33.

Nonprescription Drug Therapy. St. Louis, MO: Facts & Comparisons; 1999.

Parents need help with children's doses of nonprescription drugs, study suggests (news). Am J Heath Syst Pharm. 1997;54:2288–9.

PDR for Herbal Medicines. Montvale, NJ: Medical Economics Co.; 1998.

Physician's Desk Reference for Nonprescription Drugs and Dietary Supplements. Montvale, NJ: Medical Economics Co.; 1999.

Porter JA. Increasing the use of nonprescription drugs in a group-model HMO. Am J Health Syst Pharm. 1998;55:1357–1358, 1361.

Pray WS. Nonprescription Product Therapeutics. Philadelphia, PA: Lippincott Williams & Wilkins; 1999.

The Review of Natural Products. St. Louis, MO: Facts & Comparisons; 1996.

Scannell KM, Marriott BM, Costello RB. The role of dietary supplements for physically active people (762 citations). U.S. Dept. of Health and Human Services, Public Health Service, National Institutes of Health, National Library of Medicine, shipping list no: 99-0003-M. Available at: http://www.nlm.nih.gov/pubs/cbm/dietsup.html.

Seibel MM. The role of nutrition and nutritional supplements in women's health. Fertil Steril. 1999;72:579–91.

Smolinske SC. Dietary supplement - drug interactions. J Am Med Wom Assoc. 1999;54:191–192, 195.

Soller RW. Evolution of self care with over-the-counter medications. Clin Ther. 1998;20(suppl C):134–40.

Tyler L. Understanding Alternative Medicine: New Health Paths in America. New York, NY: Haworth Herbal Press; 2000.

Winslow LC, Kroll DJ. Herbs as medicines. Arch Intern Med. 1998;158:2192–9.

Chapter 18

Patient Consultation in the Cycle of Patient Care

Marie Gardner

A 55-year-old woman states that she does not need her psychotropic medications despite clear symptoms. An 18-year-old deaf student has a new prescription to be filled. A 60-year-old man asks about side effects of his blood pressure medications. These scenarios illustrate the types of patients and communication challenges faced by both pharmacy students during clerkships and practicing pharmacists. To be effective during patient consultations, the pharmacist must have some sense of the patient as an ill person, be knowledgeable about diseases and medications, and use certain verbal and nonverbal skills relating to consultative techniques.

In today's climate of pharmaceutical care, patient consultation is one of the cornerstones on which good pharmacy practice is built. Pharmacist-patient consultation encompasses a broad range of activities, including medication counseling, symptom and disease assessment, compliance assessment, and clinical interviewing to obtain a medication history. During clerkships, students consult with patients in a variety of settings under the guidance of the preceptors. The first part of this chapter provides an overview of medication counseling, one aspect of patient consultation, throughout the cycle of patient care. Later in the chapter, specific communication skills for optimal medication counseling are reviewed.

THE CYCLE FROM BEGINNING TO END

Experienced practitioners know that every meeting between the pharmacist and the patient presents an opportunity for consultation. Once the patient enters the cycle of care, unique relationships begin to be formed and continue throughout the patient's involvement in the health care system. In contrast to the past, when patients formed solid, long-lasting relationships with their pharmacist and physician, today patients transition between various care settings frequently, from hospital to home to nursing home to clinic and back to the hospital. It is important for students and practitioners to keep in mind that the first encounter with a patient is most likely not the patient's first encounter with the health care system. Most patients have already been counseled by other health care practitioners. They will have firsthand knowledge and experience with illnesses, medications, and the health care system. These experiences factor into every subsequent encounter. It is important that students understand this, for they must work from where the patient is, from what the patient knows and thinks about his or her medications. This is the first important concept— to know the patient. Keeping this broad perspective will help the student plan some of the elements of patient consultation.

AT HOSPITAL ADMISSION

Case History

SCENARIO ONE

Mr. K. is a 78-year-old white man who was admitted to the hospital for treatment of acute stroke. His history includes hypertension treated with various medications, lastly oral clonidine and HCTZ, and BPH, S/P TURP. Noncompliance is noted in the admission notes. The patient is been treated with physical therapy, HCTZ at the usual dose, and a clonidine patch to be changed weekly. Pharmacist A reviews the chart and visits Mr. K. on his last hospital day. After proper introduction, the pharmacist informs Mr. K that once at home, his doctor wants him to continue taking HCTZ once a day. The patient is also informed that his clonidine pill has been changed. He will now be taking it in a patch, as he has been during his hospital stay. The pharmacist informs him that it must be put on once a week, on the same day of the week. The patient is shown how to apply the patch medication. Because of the noncompliance note on the problem list, the pharmacist asks how the patient took medications before admission and recommends a 7-day pill box to help compliance. The pharmacist concludes by asking whether the patient has any questions. Mr. K., who has so far responded with only one- or two-word answers, states that he has no questions.

SCENARIO TWO

Once again, Mr. K is the patient. In this scenario, however, discharge counseling is planned from the beginning of the hospital stay. Pharmacist B met the patient at admission and has followed his progress. Because the pharmacist was aware that stroke could affect mentation, open-ended questions such as, "What is the name of your new medicine?" were used. It was noted that the patient had poor recall of information from one day to the next. The pharmacist probed with questions regarding past medication use and discovered an incontinence problem due to diuretic use. This may have contributed to poor compliance. The pharmacist followed Mr. K's course of rehabilitation and is aware of a right-sided weakness that may affect the patient's ability to apply the patch medication. Pharmacist B also recommended a 7-day pill box but planned to counsel the caregiver of the patient and provide written supplemental information.

A COMPARISON

What made Pharmacist B's consultation so different? First, knowing the patient. Second, appreciating the interrelationships between disease state, medication, and compliance. The pharmacist continually made observations about the patient's mental and physical state that could affect compliance. Through interview techniques and demonstration of skill, the pharmacist uncovered deficits in the patient's abilities to self-medicate. Pharmacist A was not aware of these but could have been if proper counseling technique had been used. Failure to ask open-ended questions resulted in the false assumption that the patient knew how to take his medication. Failure to ask the patient to demonstrate how to apply the patch was also a mistake.

In addition to using good technique throughout, Pharmacist B applied the knowledge of stroke complications involving mental and physical deficits. The open-ended questions used for consultation are especially important when one suspects cognitive problems or a physical limitation affecting medication usage. The second pharmacist also considered the effects of the diuretic on the existing urinary tract problem. Many patients who have incontinence due to diuretics cease taking them or alter their schedule to avoid incontinence interfering with their daily lives.

Pharmacist B was familiar with Mr. K throughout the hospital stay. This provided a more thorough foundation for performing discharge medication counseling. This case reinforces the second important concept—that discharge counseling on medications should be planned from the time of the patient's admission. For example, instead of thinking about just insulin dosages, blood sugars, and electrolytes in a patient admitted with diabetic coma, the pharmacist should also think about compliance issues and drug use patterns that might have led to the admission. The bottom line is to think beyond the *acute* problem to the *chronic* care issues as well, right from the start.

As can be seen in Figure 18-1, hospitalization provides an opportunity to consider many factors affecting medication use by the patient. Daily follow-up visits provide additional clues to tailor counseling to the patient's needs. Discharge medication counseling then becomes a time to review and emphasize important aspects of medication use, following which the community pharmacy takes over the continuing education and monitoring of the patient's progress. Each of these areas will be discussed in more depth in the following sections. Relevant communications skills needed for medication counseling are also discussed.

When patients are admitted to the hospital, students are expected to review the patient's chart and assess the regimen for drug-related problems. The student may be expected to visit the patient either as part of the medical team or with the preceptor. The "REAP" mnemonic (Box 18.1) can be used to help plan medication counseling. The reason for admission should be considered; noncompliance could be the cause. The drug regimen should be evaluated. The pharmacist must consider how many and what kinds of diseases the patient has as well as how many and what medications are prescribed. The patient's physical, emotional, and mental states should be assessed in light of the patient history. All potential drug-related problems should be

On Hospital Admission

Is non-compliance the reason for admission?
Does patient take many medications?
Does patient have asymptomatic diseases?
What drug-related problems are present?
How is patient currently managing medications?
How is patient coping with his illnesses?

↓

On Daily Follow-up

Have I established good rapport?
What medications are being changed?
Any new diagnoses?
What is patient's emotional, mental and physical state?
Is patient accepting need for treatment?

↓

At Discharge

Has regimen been simplified?
Does patient agree with prescribed treatments?
Have I verified patient's understanding of medications?
Have I reviewed a plan for assuring compliance?

↓

During Community Follow-up

Have I established rapport with patient?
Have I verified patient's understanding of
prescribed medications?
Have I checked for and addressed compliance barriers?
Have I assessed disease control?
Have I assessed complications from disease and treatment?

Figure 18-1. Medication counseling in the cycle of care.

Box 18.1 **Plan for Discharge Medication Counseling
with REAP**

*R*eason for admission (is it due to a drug-related problem or noncompliance?)
*E*valuate current medication regimen for drug-related problems, including noncompliance
*A*ssess the patient's knowledge base and skills to self-medicate; assess compliance-promoting strategies
*P*lan to avoid drug-related problems after discharge

listed, and anything that needs correction during the hospital stay should be determined. Thus, the patient's medication management will be improved after discharge.

The patient's knowledge of medications and their self-medication skills should be assessed. Interviewing the patient is helpful in this regard. The pharmacist should begin with an introduction, stating that he or she is helping to assure that the patient gets the best effects from the medications being taken. Questioning should begin with the most important medications and those that relate to the primary problem, such as insulin use in a patient who has diabetes. The focus should also be on those drugs with multiple daily dosings and those with special administration techniques, such as inhalers. This is a good opportunity to obtain as much information as possible regarding medication use to delineate problems that can be addressed during the hospital stay. Chapter 15 provides a good overview of the necessary skills involved. It also has a sample form suitable for conducting the medication history, which includes items relating to compliance, functional limitations, and others affecting medication usage. During the interview, the pharmacist should consider the patient's level of cognition and affective state. Any physical deficits that might affect medication-taking behavior should also be noted and considered when prescribing medication. For example, it may be too difficult for a patient who has had a stroke or who has rheumatoid arthritis to use an eye drop medication.

After all data have been collected and reviewed, the risk factors for poor compliance or drug-related problems can be assessed. These should be addressed during the patient's stay, and planning should begin regarding the aspects of drug therapy or compliance strategies that will be reviewed at the time of discharge.

The patient's overall state (disposition, knowledge of disease state or medication, communication skills) is an important factor. During the hospital stay, the pharmacist can form an impression of the patient as both a person and a clinical entity. This will allow a better evaluation of what will be important to include in daily follow-up care and in discharge planning.

It is critical to recognize that the patient also has a treatment plan in mind. In addition, patients may not be totally honest with health care providers. They may minimize or exaggerate their needs for medication, especially analgesics. Their agenda may be to obtain a medication they have seen on television or heard about through a friend. Patients who are frequent users of health services have underlying needs of long-standing duration. Some do not really want to get well. Students are often naïve and think that the patient is in agreement about care. If this were so, there would be no compliance problems. Although most patients are cooperative and establish a trusting relationship with their providers, some do not. In addition, managing medications can still be a problem even among those who have good rapport with their providers. This reinforces the first important concept—get to know the patient.

DAILY FOLLOW-UP

As the hospital stay progresses, much important information can be gathered during daily visits to the patient (daily rounds). The physician's discharge plan is comprehensive and inclusive of all therapies. The pharmacist's discharge plan focuses on optimizing drug use by the patient. To this end, daily or every-other-day visits can reveal potential barriers to successful medication management in the outpatient setting.

One common problem is that the medication regimen changes during hospitalization. New medications and changes in currently prescribed medications need to be noted to help plan discharge counseling. These should ideally be reviewed with the patient every day. It is not necessary to review medications that will be used in the short term; the focus should be on those likely to be continued during outpatient care. Changes in the medication regimen are often confusing to the patient, who is sometimes not even aware that new medications have been prescribed.

When new clinical conditions are diagnosed, the patient is forced to confront yet another change. If the news is negative, patients may experience a sense of loss relating to their health and begin to go through Kübler-Ross stages of grief.[1] These include shock and denial followed by anger, depression, bargaining, and acceptance. If a patient is in denial (the first stage), then discussion of proper medications use at that point is often fruitless. The patient must have accepted the presence of an illness as warranting treatment. The patient should be allowed to discuss the issue openly. The pharmacist should use empathic listening and try to discern when the patient moves to a point of readiness to learn. For example, a patient newly diagnosed with diabetes might be aware of treatment with insulin and begin to ask about using it. This is the opportune moment to address issues regarding newly prescribed medications. The pharmacist should be careful to avoid overwhelming the patient with too much information, and offer his or her availability for further assistance.

During daily follow-up visits, the patient's mood, mental state, and physical state should be observed to discern how well the patient is coping with changes in health status. If the patient states, "It's not really worth it anymore," this is a sign of hopelessness and that future compliance will be unlikely. Conversely, the patient may see the illness as something that can be beaten with the help of medication. Obviously, counseling needs differ from case to case. A supportive climate, nonjudgmental attitude, and empathic responding are more important than information in the first case. Health care providers sometimes believe that if patients are provided with enough information, they will comply with therapy. Health care professionals often feel a sense of failure when a patient who has been counseled many times shows up again and again with exacerbations of illness related to noncompliance. Nevertheless, a health care provider cannot make a patient comply with a therapy. Managing a chronic illness requires a commitment in time and energy and the acceptance that there is a problem that needs treatment. Many patients are just not ready to commit to being an active partner in their care, which is what compliance requires.

Practitioners often feel frustrated when patients do not follow through with instructions. This can lead to anger and resentment toward the patient. To prevent this, there should be realistic expectations about what the patient can handle. The pharmacist should listen closely to what the patient says for clues like those mentioned above and match the counseling to the patient's level of need.

Problems with cognition are also common and not readily identified during hospitalization. One study showed that cognitive problems were present in approximately 35% of hospitalized adults but went unrecognized by medical caregivers.[2] During daily rounds, the pharmacist should provide a few specifics about current medications such as dosages or serum levels. The patient should be asked to repeat the information during the next day's visit. This can help to discern the patient's ability to retain information. Improvements or declines in mental status should be assessed over time. When memory impairment seems likely, the pharmacist should plan to counsel the caregiver and provide written supplemental information.

Patients may also have physical impairments that might affect the ability to self-medicate, such as the patient with arthritis who is prescribed an inhaled medication. During discharge counseling, the pharmacist should take the time to have the patient demonstrate the proper use of medication equipment or delivery vehicles whenever possible. Other more subtle limitations include weakness, such as patients who have had strokes or those with musculoskeletal illnesses, which may affect the patient's ability to manipulate medication containers. These barriers are sometimes hard to detect, but proficiency is gained with experience.

PATIENT DISCHARGE

Applying the above strategies during the patient's hospital stay will result in several important outcomes: (1) establishment of the pharmacist-patient relationship, (2) identification of drug-related problems, and (3) recommendations for specific strategies to enhance proper medication management after discharge. By the time of discharge, the pharmacist should know the patient quite well and have developed a trusting relationship. Because of daily intervention, the patient is aware of new medications and changes in existing therapies. The pharmacist will know how adept the patient is at managing medications and if the patient has any special concerns regarding medications. Perhaps recommendations have been made to streamline the drug regimen to enhance compliance or to improve medication management, such as suggesting a compliance aid. When discharge counseling is approached in this manner, the actual discharge consultation can be quite brief and to the point.

A typical discharge counseling session includes review of each prescribed medication in terms of indication, dosage, administration, and self-monitoring, including any necessary follow-up laboratory tests or appointments. Any concerns the patient has about medication usage should be queried for and resolved. Most importantly, compliance expectations and measures implemented to meet them are established. Written supplements should be given as needed. The specific verbal communication skills applied to medication counseling and compliance assessment are described in the following sections.

MEDICATION COUNSELING TECHNIQUES

Today's pharmacists have shifted from the traditional method of patient counseling, which involved talking at the patient, to an interactive dialogue with the patient. With the former method, the pharmacist provided information and then asked, "Do you have any questions?" This style of counseling does not allow the pharmacist to assess the patient's experience or knowledge from prior use of the medication. The pharmacist-patient consultation program (PPCP) techniques developed by the Indian Health Service 3 decades ago, and further refined in collaboration with colleagues from across the United States, teach an interactive method of consultation, one that seeks to *verify* what the patient knows about the medication and *"fill in the gaps"* with only the most basic information when needed.[3] Research shows that people forget 90% of what is heard within 60 minutes of hearing it.[4] Imagine how much more difficult it is for the patient who is in pain or cognitively impaired to retain technical information during counseling. By making the patient an *active* participant in the process, increased learning will occur. Active patient participation in the consultation is accomplished through the use of specific, open-ended questions to uncover the patient's current knowledge about the medication. Between questions, the pharmacist can provide information to enhance patient understanding. These specific techniques are linked to consultation outcomes. Assuring the patient has proper knowledge to self-medicate, addressing compliance issues, and assessing clinical problems are contained within the framework of the consultation skills outlined below.

THE PRIME QUESTIONS AND SHOW AND TELL TECHNIQUE

The basic PPCP consultation techniques involve two sets of questions, one for new prescriptions (Prime Questions) and the other for refill medications (Show and Tell Questions), shown in Box 18.2. Medication counseling using these

---

Box 18.2   The Pharmacist-Patient Consultation Program (PPCP) Medication Counseling Skills[3]

THE PRIME QUESTIONS FOR NEW PRESCRIPTIONS

(1)   What did the doctor tell you (were you told) the medication is for?
      What problem or symptom is it supposed to help?
      What is it supposed to do?

(2)   How did your doctor tell you (were you told) to take the medication?
      How often? How much? How long?
      What does X times a day mean to you?
      What did your doctor say to do if you miss a dose?

(3)   What did the doctor tell you (were you told) to expect?
      What good effects? Bad effects? Precautions to take?
      What should you do if a bad reaction occurs?

SHOW-AND-TELL QUESTIONS FOR REFILL PRESCRIPTIONS

(1)   What do you take this medication for?
(2)   How have you been taking it?
(3)   What kinds of problems are you having with it?

questions not only makes the patient an active participant in the learning process, but also provides an organized approach to reviewing medication information. A structured approach has been associated with improved recall of prescription instructions.[5] The pharmacist can praise the patient for knowing correct information, clarify misunderstandings, and add new information as needed. In terms of consultation outcomes, the technique assures proper knowledge by the patient and identifies new clinical problems or compliance issues. The PPCP techniques are commonly used in community pharmacy practice but are applicable to any practice in which patients are counseled. The steps in the consultation process are described below.

Begin Medication Counseling

Whether in the hospital at discharge or in the community pharmacy, counseling should begin by the establishment of a rapport between pharmacist and patient. The pharmacist should introduce himself or herself and state the purpose of the consultation. If the patient is not familiar to the pharmacist, identification should be verified by either asking for identification or simply asking, "And you are . . . ?" If the patient cannot hear well or has a language barrier, it will be evident at this point. In such cases, the caregiver should be counseled. A private space should be found for cases in which sensitive information is to be discussed. Examples include consultations on vaginal products or in cases of medications for a sexually transmitted disease. Before discussing the medications, it should be assured that the patient is comfortable and has sufficient time to be counseled. The pharmacist should face the patient and maintain the appropriate interpersonal distance (1.5–2 feet) during the consultation.[6]

Conduct the Medication Counseling

If the patient has a new prescription, the Prime Questions are used. Otherwise, the Show and Tell questions are used. It is not necessary to provide additional information if the patient provides correct answers to the questions. After asking the second Prime or Show and Tell Question, it may be important to ask the additional questions shown in Box 18.2 that probe exactly how a medication is to be taken. For example, the patient is asked at what times would he or she take an antibiotic prescribed three times a day. Additional information should be provided if the patient lacks appropriate knowledge in these areas. The second Prime Question is also when special administration of medications should be addressed. The patient should demonstrate how to apply a patch or use an inhaler. Repeated review is often necessary to assure proper technique and optimal benefit from the medication. Other questions to include under the second Prime Question are how long to take the medication, what to do when a dose is missed, and how to store the medication. Intersperse "telling" the patient information with open-ended questions that will keep the patient an active participant in the consultation. The counseling session should be a means to verify what the patient knows rather than a time to overload the patient with information. Keep information brief and to the point.

The third Prime Question relates to expected beneficial and adverse effects. Many issues can be discussed within this third question. With respect to beneficial effects, patients often do not know what to expect from taking the medication. Although they might relate pain relief with a newly prescribed analgesic, it is more difficult for patients to understand how digoxin might help atrial fibrillation. This is the time to explain that it regulates the heart beat. It is even more difficult for patients to understand how taking a medication will help an asymptomatic condition or prevent a disease. Providing explanations on drug effects may take more time in these cases but the benefits may be significant in the long run. It is usually necessary to relate the drug to a complication of disease such as stroke from the asymptomatic hypertensive disease.

Patients have often been told nothing about adverse effects. Research shows that patients want information about their medications, especially adverse effects, and that providing such information does not lead to the development of those reactions in most cases.[7,8] In fact, patients worry more about the bad effects from medications than dosage or even indication. If the patient is unaware about adverse effects, counsel him or her on the most common ones, those that are life-threatening, or those that are most serious and advise what to do if an adverse reaction is suspected.

When counseling on a new medication, it is helpful to raise compliance concerns. A universal statement is a useful opener. An example is, "Mr. K., a lot of patients have trouble fitting taking medication into their daily schedule. What's been your experience?" It is important to link medication-taking to a daily activity to help promote compliance. Pill boxes and calendars are also helpful, especially when placed where the patient can see them easily. A partnership approach should be used. Additional compliance-enhancing skills are discussed later in this chapter.

End the Medication Counseling

The *final verification* is a summary technique that assures the patient has sufficient knowledge to self-medicate correctly. The pharmacist should say to the patient, "Just to make sure I didn't leave anything out, please go over with me how you are going to use the medication." Avoid putting the patient on the defensive by saying things such as, "Just to make sure *you* know . . . " At the final verification, the patient should describe correct use of the medication. Any errors should be corrected, and additional information can be given. Means to obtain help if needed should be provided, such as the pharmacy's telephone number or a business card. Written supplements should be given as indicated.

For refill prescriptions, Show and Tell questions are used. This is especially useful in community practice in which patients are seen regularly between physician visits. Consultation on refill medications is mandated in some states. The medication should be shown to the patient (i.e., by opening the bottle and displaying the contents), and the pharmacist should check to make sure the correct medication is in the bottle. The pharmacist then asks the questions, usually in the order shown in Box 18.2. If the patient answers incorrectly to the second question, the patient may be noncompliant or the physician may have changed the dosage. The pharmacist will need to discern the reason for the discrepancy. As with the second Prime Question for new medications, the second Show and Tell question allows the patient to demonstrate proper use of an inhaler or other medication requiring special administration.

The Show and Tell Questions are commonly used in community practice when counseling on refill medications. However, they are essentially the same as questions used to take a medication history and are applicable to institutional settings or any time when chronic medication use is reviewed with a patient.

HANDLING DIFFICULTIES DURING COUNSELING

In addition to using good verbal and nonverbal skills in consultation, practitioners must apply specific techniques to overcome difficulties complicating the consultation. Some common barriers and the skills to manage them are listed in Table 18.1. These relate to functional and/or emotional issues. Functional barriers have specific strategies for management, whereas emotional barriers require the use of active listening skills.

Dealing with emotional barriers is difficult for some practitioners and requires active listening and reflecting responses. The terms "active listening," "empathic listen-

Table 18-1. Common Barriers Affecting Consultation

Barrier	Helpful Techniques
Language barrier	Identify barrier with open-ended questions
	Use pictures; contact translator
Counseling a third party	Be careful regarding confidentiality; ask for identification; provide written supplements; ask patient to call
Hearing-impaired	Use print material; move to a quiet space; speak more loudly
	Use final verification technique
Vision-impaired	Use interactive dialogue, final verification
	Provide large-print material
Patient has mental disorder	Identify problem early with open-ended questions
	Counsel caregiver; repeat information and use final verification
	Provide written supplements

ing," and "reflective responding" are often used inter-changeably. The common thread is the use of specific verbal responses that indicate a heightened awareness and interpretation of the patient's thoughts and feelings. These are called "reflecting responses." When pharmacists respond with a reflection of what the patient is saying, thinking, or feeling, they are letting the patient know that they are truly listening. This provides the patient with the opportunity to admit feelings, clarify thoughts, and bring forth additional information. Reflecting responses are especially called for when the patient is demonstrating emotions. Angry looks, averted eye contact, and head drooping are examples of nonverbal signs that convey certain emotional states. Remarks such as, "Well, I *guess* I could try that medicine," suggest concerns that need to be gently brought to light.

To make a reflecting response, the emotion the patient seems to be exhibiting must be identified by observing their verbal and nonverbal signs. The pharmacist can think of the emotion as being mad, sad, glad, or scared. Each has a range, such as being concerned about a side effect to being profoundly frightened by a previous serious drug reaction. The second step is to put the word describing the feeling state into a sentence structure. Examples include, "Sounds like you're (frustrated, mad, happy) about your visit with the doctor," or "I can see that this is (frustrating, worrisome) for you." The pharmacist should avoid saying things such as, "I know what you're going through," or "I understand how you feel," unless he or she has had the same experience.

Setting limits with patients is also troublesome for most practitioners. Setting limits controls availability for consultation and unnecessary interruptions. It is also needed when differences of opinion cannot be resolved or when the patient is overly talkative. Table 18.2 illustrates some examples of how pharmacists can balance meeting the patient's needs with their own. Students are often eager to meet the patient's every expectation. This can trap the student in a dependency relationship with a difficult patient. Dealing with difficult patients can be frustrating, and the student must learn to use limit-setting to maintain a healthy perspective on providing care. Other reviews dealing with patient-related barriers can be found elsewhere.[6,9]

Table 18-2. Setting Limits in the Encounter

Example	Useful Skills for the Pharmacist
Patient is overly talkative	Take control by piggybacking onto one of the patient's comments (e.g., "I know you don't like hospitals so let's talk about how your medicines can keep you out of here")
	Interrupt the patient as gently as possible
	Use patient's name to register attention
Patient consistently wants lengthy encounters	Realize patient's need for attention
	State clear limits on consultation (e.g., "I can only discuss this medication now with you...")
Patient interrupts your daily routine	Realize patient's need for attention
	Set time period for your availability (e.g., "I can meet with you for no more than 5 minutes after lunch")
Patient continues to discuss issues that cannot be resolved	Realize patient is frustrated, wants attention, or desires control
	Acknowledge the differences (e.g., "We disagree on whether you should keep taking this medication")
	Use diverting tactics, switch to discussing something else
	State need to move on to next task

ENHANCING COMPLIANCE

The problem of noncompliance continues to plague the best efforts toward maximizing the use of many therapies. Although compliance with therapy for *acute* problems is necessary for good outcomes, compliance with treatment for many *chronic* medical conditions is vitally important to manage them. As mentioned previously, the *patient's acceptance* that a problem exists and his or her acceptance of the value of treatment form the essential foundation for compliance.

Students and practitioners trained in the treatment of diseases often feel they are in control of the patient's problems. Except for those few patients in institutional settings, the *patient* controls the outcome of his or her disease by taking or not taking prescribed medications. The practitioner's role is to facilitate the patient using medications to the best benefit. A partnership approach is therefore necessary. Patient satisfaction, compliance, and improved outcomes are linked to a partnership style of the provider-patient relationship.[10–12]

Applying the concept of a partnership approach involves shared expectations about care, including compliance, and helping patients meet these expectations. During the first consultation, it may be necessary for the pharmacist to ask questions about the patient's perceptions about medication. The pharmacist might ask, "How do you feel about taking this medication?" The patient's answers may reveal his or her awareness of a disease process and acceptance of treatment. At other times, the patient may feel ambiguous about the value of treatment. If so, the pharmacist should provide valid information and offer an opinion. The patient should have time to consider the information. The pharmacist should determine what the patient's expectations are about treatment, given good compliance. During Prime Question consultation, questions such as, "If you take this medication, how do you think it will help?" can be asked. Again, valid information that will help the patient decide to comply should be provided. After determining that pharmacist and patient expectations are similar, expectations about compliance can be set.

Previously, techniques for medication counseling on new and refill prescriptions were reviewed. Facilitating the patient's compliance with medications begins with using the PPCP skills to verify that the patient has the appropriate *knowledge* base for medication management, checking *skills* required to administer medications (e.g., by having the patient demonstrate inhaler technique), and asking about *compliance strategies* to maximize benefit from the medications.

Students and practitioners often overwhelm the patient with information and explanations about medication effects. It is best to start small and focus on verifying that the patient simply know what the medication is for and how to take it correctly. Also, the patient should know the main adverse effects and how to monitor if the medication is working. Specific information should be provided in small amounts. For example, for the patient with a new prescription for warfarin, a basic medication counseling session should review the indication as well as instructions to take the drug at the same time every day to enhance compliance, to take what actions if the dose is missed, to watch for bleeding, to keep appointments for blood work, and to not take any nonprescription medications without checking with the pharmacist first. A written supplement is a good addition to this consultation to cover specific drug interactions and monitor parameters regarding bleeding.

After using the PPCP consultation questions, it should be stressed that compliance is very important to successful outcomes. The pharmacist should state that it is sometimes difficult to adopt the habit of taking medication every day, but that the pharmacist will help the patient do this successfully. The patient should be asked if there is something that would aid him or her in remembering to take the medication. A medication box may be needed. The patient should be aware that questions about compliance will be asked at forthcoming visits. In using these strategies, the patient and pharmacist come to an agreement on the fact that treatment is needed and what methods will aid in compliance. This basic approach is repeated any time the medication regimen changes. It sets up conditions to optimize compliance but does not guarantee it. Other skills are needed to probe for potential compliance problems during return visits.

MONITORING COMPLIANCE IN COMMUNITY PRACTICE

Community pharmacy practice presents a unique opportunity to follow the patient's progress over time. This involves the ongoing monitoring for specific outcomes related to disease control, disease and treatment complications, and medication compliance. Good medication compliance is often necessary for disease control, and drug complications such as side effects can be a barrier to compliance. Before discussing compliance assessment, the assessment of disease control and complications during the consultation needs to be considered.

While using the Show and Tell technique, the pharmacist should listen for symptomatic complaints that reveal poorly controlled diseases or disease complications. Alternatively, resolution of symptoms might suggest benefit from drug therapy. Any *new* symptom requires evaluation. The patient should be asked when the symptom started, how long it has been present, any treatment for it, what it is like, what makes it better or worse, and what other symptoms are present. Thorough probing will help differentiate between symptoms related to a disease versus a drug. For example, a patient who was recently prescribed carbamazepine for a seizure disorder complains of dizziness possibly due to the medication. During the interview, the patient states that her dizziness had been present off and on for several years, suggesting that the problem was not due to the medication.

Disease-specific symptom questions should be used. For example, a patient refilling furosemide and an angiotensin-converting enzyme inhibitor for newly diagnosed congestive heart failure might be asked about breathing and endurance. Objective information can also be evaluated, such as a blood glucose level in a patient with diabetes or at least asking about recent glucose values. One way to conduct the consultation is to ask all three Show and Tell questions and then follow with, "Now I want to ask about how your diabetes is doing. What have your blood glucose readings been this week?"

Additional follow-up questions are needed to assess *complications* due to drug effects. Proper probing for this requires knowledge of the signs and symptoms from adverse drug reactions. When the patient is queried with the third Show and Tell question, "What kinds of problems have you had?" the patient may again reveal a specific symptom that requires evaluation. A few simple, specific questions targeting disease progression and medication effects will greatly enhance the consultation and provide a global assessment of the patient's condition.

Practitioners tend to assume that when a patient is doing well and has no complaints it must be because the medication is working and not causing problems. It is assumed that the patient is compliant with therapy. Assumptions should never be made. The patient may feel well and be noncompliant. Perhaps the patient tried the medication and had a reaction that prompted him or her to stop taking it. Research indicates that medication compliance is a continuing problem. One study found that one-third of patients do not get their original prescription filled, another one-third take it incorrectly, and the final one-third take it as prescribed.[13] Being aware of the frequency with which patients have compliance problems should raise the index of suspicion, so that every patient is a potential noncomplier until proven otherwise. Furthermore, the onus is on the professional to recognize and correct compliance-related problems. In the following section, a specific communication model that is built on PPCP techniques and addresses compliance is reviewed.

The Recognize, Identify, and Manage Model

The Recognize, Identify, and Manage (RIM) Model is a process used by pharmacists to enhance patient compliance.[13] In the *recognize* step, specific communication skills are used to explore subjective and objective findings to detect potential compliance problems. Following this, other specific probes are used to *identify* and categorize the type of compliance problem. Finally, strategies to *manage* the compliance problem are reviewed.

Subjective findings are statements made by the patient. Objective findings are based on hard data, such as that in the drug profile. In the recognize step, the patient's drug profile is reviewed for evidence of potential compliance problems *before* the patient is counseled on the medication. Items to look for include lateness on refills, the most common objective finding, and times when the patient requests refills on some but not all chronic medications. Findings suggestive of noncompliance require further exploration before a definite compliance problem can be ascertained, because there can be rational explanations for the objective findings. Gaps in refills may be due to patients getting refills at another location, or the physician may have told the patient to change the dosage schedule or to stop the drug altogether.

When the profile indicates potential noncompliance, medication counseling should begin with the Show and Tell questions for the refill. The pharmacist should listen carefully to the patient's answers for any clues hinting at noncompliance, especially to the second Show and Tell question. Patients will sometimes give expected answers, "That's my blood pressure pill and I take it every day. I have no problems with it." If the refill record indicates that the patient is overdue for medication, the pharmacist should probe the compliance issue in a nonthreatening manner. To do this, a *supportive compliance probe* should be used. This is structured using "I" language and reflects the pharmacist's concerns. The "I noticed/I'm concerned" formula should be used. For example, "Mr. K, I noticed this clonidine patch prescription was due to be refilled 3 weeks ago. I'm a little concerned about that." The patient may volunteer that the physician has changed the medication regimen or that it was obtained elsewhere.

Another useful communication tool is the *universal statement* (e.g., "Many patients have trouble remembering when to take this medication, especially since it's only changed once a week. What's been your experience?") Suggesting that the patient is not the only one who has a problem managing medications allows him or her to discuss the situation without fear of criticism.

The communication skills listed above are useful to address objective signs suggesting noncompliance. In addition, the patient may provide the pharmacist with clues to compliance problems by certain types of verbal remarks. Some may be quite obvious, such as when the patient asks, "Why do I have to keep taking this medicine?" This can be thought of as a "red flag" because it is obvious that the patient wishes not to take the prescription. More commonly, however, the comments are more subtle. Examples of these vague clues, called "pink flags" include the following: "My doctor *says* I should take it . . . ," "My doctor *wants* me to . . . ," or "I'm *supposed* to be taking." These are usually picked up when the first two Show and Tell questions are asked. Another pink flag is a long pause during the patient's reply, which may indicate potential problems.

It is likely that patients use pink flags because they want to appear to be in agreement and avoid conflict, or because they want to keep peace or please another person. Patients know that compliance is expected of them, and they do not wish to disappoint, displease, or anger the health care practitioners taking care of them. They would rather have the practitioners believe that they are compliant. Pink flags should be thought of as the patient "testing" how the health care provider will respond to noncompliance. If the provider is sensitive to the potential problem and makes the appropriate response, the patient will respond by discussing the truth. Reflecting responses are an ideal way to facilitate this. As an example, there is a patient refilling a prescription for theophylline three times a day for a respiratory condition. When asked, "How are you taking the medication?" the patient hesitates and then says, "I'm supposed to take it three times a day." Pharmacists who miss the pink flag, *supposed to*, will usually say "That's right. The doctor wants you to take three a day." It would be better to say, "Sounds like you feel that three a day isn't right for you," and then discern how much the patient is actually taking.

Using reflecting responses, even if not exactly on target, tells the patient that the hesitation has been recognized and that the pharmacist wants to talk about it. It is nonthreatening and allows the conversation to unfold naturally.

Patients may openly ask, "Does this medicine have any side effects?" or "Is this anything like (specific drug)?" There are two options to respond. One is to simply answer the question, and the other is to ask for more information before answering the question. These questions should be considered as possible pink flags as well. Suggested follow-up responses include "Why do you ask?" or a reflecting response such as "Sounds like you have some concerns about this medication." As mentioned in the beginning of this chapter, patients often have knowledge about medications, either through direct experience or through a family member's medication use, or they may have heard or read about a medication's effects. Do not discount the patient's views. Patients who believe their concerns were not addressed may not trust future advice and will certainly be unwilling to directly confront future medication issues. The patient's concerns should be identified before an alternate viewpoint is provided.

The above verbal techniques address the *recognize* phase for assessing compliance. Using them may confirm the presence of a compliance problem, following which the use of other probing questions can identify the type of compliance problem (*knowledge deficits, practical limitations,* and *atti-*

tudinal barriers). In the case of knowledge deficits, patients have insufficient information, insufficient skills, or misinformation that prevents compliance. In a recent case, a patient was refilling nitroglycerin ointment much more often than expected. When asked to demonstrate the 0.5-inch application, the patient applied a 0.5-inch deep layer onto the paper rather than 0.5 inches in length. The Show and Tell technique uncovered the problem, and the pharmacist was able to provide education to fix the compliance barrier.

The second category involves practical limitations or barriers. These range from not having transportation to obtain medication to multiple daily doses to vision and hearing difficulties that complicate consultation. Again, the Show and Tell questions can reveal deficits in hearing or vision, as when the patient cannot read the prescription label. Confusion about dosing will be apparent with the second Show and Tell question, and the third question may reveal the presence of adverse drug effects that are contributing to or causing noncompliance.

The third category is attitudinal barriers. These are pervasive, difficult to detect, and even more difficult to manage. As mentioned previously, a patient not accepting the presence of a disease process is a barrier to compliance with medications and other treatments. However, even when the disease is acknowledged, the value of treatment may be questioned. This is especially an issue in this era of increased interest in herbal and nontraditional therapies. As outlined by the health belief model, perceived severity of risk compared with perceived benefit of treatment plays a large role in determining patient compliance.[14] Other factors, such as patients' desire to be in control and patients' belief that they can successfully implement the recommended treatment, also strongly influence compliance.[15] There are also pervasive patient ideas (such as, "I can develop immunity to a medication's effects," "If one pill helps, then two must be twice as good," and "If I feel good, then I don't need medication") that are barriers to compliance. These theories are difficult to replace with scientific-based reasoning, perhaps because they originate in the patient's experience, which can be a powerful reinforcer.[16]

It may take a while in consultation to identify which barriers to compliance are present and are most important. Patients may have several barriers operating at once. The pharmacist should focus on one strategy at a time, being patient and assessing the patient's progress consistently over time at follow-up visits. Once the cause for the noncompliance has been categorized, then a specific strategy to *manage* that problem can be implemented. Most knowledge and skill deficiencies can be corrected successfully with education and training. Providing a video or written supplement that visually shows good inhaler technique is one example. Practical barriers respond to specific measures such as simplifying drug regimens, using easy-to-open containers, and enlisting the aid of a spouse or caregiver. Some practical barriers, such as lack of transportation to the pharmacy or lack of funds to purchase medications, are not as easily solved.

Attitudinal issues tend to be the most complex and difficult to resolve. It takes patience, practice, careful listening, a supportive climate, and repeated conversations with the patient before the patient will acknowledge one of these barriers. A patient will only do so when he or she feels that the pharmacist will not be critical or argumentative. Using all the communication skills mentioned above will provide the optimum environment for ongoing discussion of disparate views. Repeated efforts to enlighten may, over time, change the patient's views of disease and the value of treatment.

WHAT NOT TO DO

When dealing with patients, the pharmacy student must remember to do many things. The following list contains some things that the student must remember not to do:

➤ Do not expect the perfect patient. Patients may take medications in ways different than the textbook indicates. They may take medications that are ineffective. It is the pharmacist's duty to discover if current therapies are helping and then your judgments about the drug regimen. The patient should be counseled accordingly.

➤ Do not expect to know everything. A pharmacist must read, research, and ask for help when needed.

➤ Do not be afraid to make mistakes—just learn from them.

➤ Do not second-guess the prescriber in front of the patient. Comments such as, "I'm not sure why you're getting this drug when we usually use (another therapy)," should be avoided. This creates confusion and doubt in the patient's mind and can lead to conflict between medical and pharmacy staff. If the pharmacist has doubts about a prescribed drug or therapy, the physician should be consulted in a private and professional manner for clarification.

➤ Do not leave the patient without hope. Pharmacists will counsel patients whose diseases are progressing despite maximal therapeutic efforts. These patients may be looking for answers that are not there. Statements such as, "You're getting all the prescribed medications available for X condition," are not helpful and should be avoided. What patients need is support. Pharmacists should use reflecting responses such as, "It must be very frustrating to feel like you're not getting any better."

➤ Do not judge the noncompliant patient. Examples include patients who abuse certain substances or the patient with lung cancer who still smokes. Dealing with such patients can be frustrating to the health care provider because of the provider's *unrealistic expectations* about the patient's participation in care. Health care providers expect patients to share the same views about the need for treatment. Nevertheless, a health care practitioner should never "give up" on a patient. An open, honest, and sincere presence should be maintained, and information should ne provided that is appropriate to the patient's level of readiness to accept responsibility for his or her health care.

CONCLUSION

The techniques and issues discussed in this chapter contribute to good rapport with patients and success in helping patients manage chronic illnesses.

Students should seek out model practitioners, observe their skills and techniques, and then practice these skills and techniques during the clerkship. The strategies discussed in this chapter will also be helpful. Clerkships are designed to provide experience under the guidance of others with more wisdom. Such opportunities should be taken advantage of because experience is the best teacher.

References

1. Kübler-Ross E, Wessler S, Avioli LV. On death and dying. JAMA. 1972;221:174–9.
2. Gallo JJ, Reichel W, Andersen L. Handbook of Geriatric Assessment. 1st ed. Rockville, MD: Aspen Publishers Inc.; 1988.
3. Boyce RW, Herrier RN, Gardner ME. Pharmacist-Patient Consultation Program, Unit 1: An Interactive Approach to Verify Patient Understanding. New York, NY: Pfizer Inc.; 1991.
4. Bolton R. People Skills. New York, NY: Simon & Schuster Inc.; 1979.
5. Gardner ME, Hurd PD, Slack MK. Effect of information organization on recall of medication instructions. J Clin Pharm Ther. 1989;14:1–7.
6. Pharmacist-Patient Consultation Program, Unit 2: Counseling Patients in Challenging Situations. New York, NY: Pfizer Inc.; 1993.
7. Lamb GC. Can physicians warn patients of potential side effects without fear of causing those side effects? Arch Intern Med. 1994;154:2753–6.
8. Gardner ME et al. A study of perceived importance of medication information provided in a health maintenance organization setting. Drug Intell Clin Pharm. 1988;22:596–8.
9. Groves JE. Taking care of the hateful patient. New Engl J Med. 1978;298:883–7.
10. Roter D, Hall J. Doctors Talking with Patients, Patients Talking with Doctors. New York, NY: Auburn House; 1992.
11. Anderson LA, Zimmerman MA. Patient and physician perceptions of their relationship and patient satisfaction: a study in chronic disease management. Patient Educ Counsel. 1993;20:27–36.
12. DiMatteo MR. The physician-patient relationship: effects on quality of health care. Clin Obstet Gynecol. 1994;37:149–61.
13. Pharmacist-Patient Consultation Program, Unit 3: Counseling to Enhance Compliance. New York, NY: Pfizer Inc.; 1995.
14. Eraker SA, Kirscht JP, Becker MH. Understanding and improving patient compliance. Ann Intern Med. 1984;100:258–68.

15. Viinamaki H. The patient-doctor relationship and metabolic control in patients with Type 1 (insulin-dependent) diabetes mellitus. Int J Psychiatry Med. 1993;23:265–74.
16. Leventhal H. The role of theory in the study of adherence to treatment and doctor-patient interactions. Med Care. 1985;23:556–63.

Chapter 19

Public Health Practices

Bernard Sorofman and Connie Kraus

INTRODUCTION

Health, as defined by the World Health Organization, is complete physical, mental, and social well-being. To achieve and maintain complete health, society must undertake activities that can be defined broadly as "public health." These are activities intended to optimize individual health through healthy lifestyles and an environment that contributes to health in a positive manner. Health professional practice conditions that contribute to public health are defined by the Institute of Medicine as (1) the assessment of the health of populations, and (2) the assurance that interventions are in place to maintain the health of individuals. These two, along with the construction of public policy to achieve them, are the basic elements of public health in society. They are built on a foundation of scientific knowledge and grounded in the notion that the burdens and benefits of membership in society are distributed fairly.

Public health activities operate on two levels simultaneously. Common are those that are "one-on-one" with patients—individual-level care to optimize a patient's health. However, the health professional can and should also be involved in community-level care. Public health activities that assure clean water, sanitation, proper housing, and clean air all contribute to the prevention of disease on a population level.

WHY IS PUBLIC HEALTH IMPORTANT TO PHARMACY?

Pharmacists are challenged today with a new role, pharmaceutical care, that increases their obligations as a health provider. Pharmacists are personally responsible for achieving long-term health outcomes for patients. This results in a demand for continuous care to assure positive, long-term patient outcomes. Therefore, pharmacists must focus on the broader issues of health, not the more narrow role defined by the treatment of disease with medications. Public health activities of health providers are part of the continuum of care.

The public-health–oriented pharmacist focuses on the key elements of health promotion and disease prevention (Box 19.1). Pharmacists practice in a manner that *promotes health* through proactive health activities, such as the encouragement of exercise, good nutrition, non-use of tobacco, minimization of alcohol intake, and the development of a healthy community. Second, pharmacists participate in *health protection* activities. These are actions that are intended to minimize disease and injury. For example, pharmacists are involved daily in drug safety issues. They often participate in encouraging public health issues that improve the environment, such as minimizing toxic automotive emissions. More common is the pharmacist's participation in *preventive health services*. These activities contribute to the minimization of chances for clinical health conditions such as cancer, health disease, and stroke. Preventive health services also include immunization activities, education, needle exchanges to diminish human immunodeficiency virus (HIV) infections, and other clinical services. Finally, and in many ways uniquely, pharmacists provide *surveillance, data collection,* and *data management* on drug usage. Pharmacists are well recognized, especially in complex health systems such as hospitals and managed care organizations, for their drug utilization review management systems.

Box 19.1   Public Health Objectives

Health promotion
Health protection
Preventive services
Surveillance, data collection, and data management

WHAT IS THE PHARMACIST'S ROLE?

The pharmacist has five basic roles (Box 19.2): information, screening, education, care, and referral/triage. Pharmacists must first be sources of information in their practices for their patients and colleagues. General health education messages can be distributed through brochures and booklets, presentations by pharmacists to providers and community groups, and "face-to-face" interactions with patients. Public health screening is another important pharmacist role. Pharmacists identify potential health concerns and refer patients to the appropriate health care providers. Pharmacists can screen for hypertension and many other early signs of illness and refer patients to appropriate sources.

Education is an important role. At the patient level, this is usually called counseling. However, pharmacists can participate in expanded education directed at the greater community in which they work and live. For example, immunization initiatives provide opportunities for pharmacists to provide care with a public health focus. Currently a somewhat controversial issue in the health care practice community, pharmacists can and do provide immunization screening and injections. Ultimately, because the pharmacist is in an accessible role as a provider and monitor of pharmacotherapy, referral is a natural and frequent disease prevention and health promotion activity.

Pharmacists must be competent in several areas to provide a public-health–oriented practice (Box 19.3). First, pharmacists must understand the basic elements of public

---

Box 19.2 Pharmacist Roles

Information	Brochures, booklets
Screening	Taking blood pressures
Education	Public lectures, counseling
Care	Immunizations, smoking cessation programs
Referral/triage	Connecting need with community resources

Box 19.3   Pharmacist Public Health Competencies

Understand the basic elements of public health

Know the pharmacist perspective on the major public
health issues

Know the relative importance of public health issues in
their practice communities

Be able to deliver relevant health screening and health
protection services

Know how to appropriate triage public health issues

health as they apply to the practice of pharmacy. It is imperative that the pharmacist be familiar with the health assessments of the population as a whole. Such a familiarity
might include the general nature of the immunization rates
of members of the community. Is the current rate in the
community sufficient to prevent an epidemic of influenza,
pneumonia in the elderly, or measles in children? Pharmacists must participate in the delivery of care that can assure
optimal health in the community. Continuing with the immunization example, pharmacists can establish clinics or
screening and referral services for at-risk patients or during
critical seasonal periods. Finally, pharmacists must participate in the formulation of public policy that creates a
healthy environment.

Pharmacists should know the public health conditions
and local issues in their practice community. These issues
include the rates of preventable or modifiable diseases, such
as cardiovascular illnesses, and the condition of the environment, such as water quality and sanitation programs.
Many pharmacists practice these public health activities as
members of community boards and councils. It is not unusual to find pharmacists as mayors of their communities
and chairpersons of community health panels.

Health screening and the delivery of health protection
services are important pharmacist activities. For decades,
pharmacists have provided screening for cardiovascular
diseases. Pharmacists are competent at taking blood pressures and do so with individual patients as the need presents
itself and in recurring, pharmacy-based screening programs. They are experts at taking medication histories, including immunization histories.

With their knowledge of the above issues, their grounding in science, and their centrality in their practice settings, pharmacists are in ideal positions to be able to appropriately refer patients and community public health concerns to the proper places. Individual patient public health referral is a relatively common part of the pharmacist's practice. Referral of community issues, such as the recognition that air pollution from selected sources has increased the number of patients with respiratory illnesses, brings the pharmacists' public health practice to a more complex and higher level.

CONTINUUM OF CARE

Health care providers link health promotion and disease prevention with the continuum of care. The basic premise is to teach the general population strategies to maintain good health and avoid illness. From this view, the continuum of care initiates with disease prevention (primary prevention), evolves to disease detection (secondary prevention), and ultimately leads to disease minimization (tertiary prevention) (Box 19.4).

Primary prevention encompasses health promotion, health protection, and preventive services. The goal is to prevent the emergence of a disease or injury. Examples of educational effort in primary prevention include strategies such as immunization, smoking cessation, education about rational use of alcohol, proper nutrition, and exercise.

Secondary prevention is central to preventive services and involves a focus of screening for early signs and symptoms of disease in an effort to provide cure or prevent disease progression. Examples of secondary prevention could

---

Box 19.4   Disease Prevention

DISEASE	PREVENTION
Primary	Prevent emergence of disease or injury
Secondary	Early detection of health problems
Tertiary	Disease minimization

include screening for cancer or hypertension and choles-terol monitoring to identify treatable risk factors for coro-nary diseases.

Tertiary prevention efforts generally involve preventive services for the patient with a chronic illness, for whom the goal is to prevent the progression of illness and improve functional status. Again, education plays a key role in this area. Guidelines for management of chronic illness are as-sembled to improve quality. Examples of tertiary preven-tion efforts include using evidence-based guidelines to as-sess the severity of asthma and provide appropriate therapy with the goal of decreasing symptoms and improving the quality of life for patients. From a public health or popula-tion perspective, ensuring access to the most current infor-mation about treatment should improve overall care to all persons with a chronic illness.

APPLICATION OF PUBLIC HEALTH TO PHARMACY

The United States' *Healthy People 2000* initiative focused on health promotion objectives. Many of these can be in-fluenced by pharmacists. These priorities are divided into three general categories: health promotion, health protec-tion, and preventive health services. Twenty-two priorities have been identified; not all priorities or objectives within priorities fit within the practice of pharmacists. The overar-ching activities that pharmacists can perform include com-munity level education, monitoring of pharmacotherapy, counseling, referral, and drug distribution and control. These recur from objective to objective.

➤ *Alcohol and Other "Drugs."* Drug distribution, the lim-ited access to hazardous substances, is a basic role of the pharmacist. Monitoring, managing, and counseling pa-tients on substance abuse is a routine role.

➤ *Clinical Preventive Services.* Pharmaceutical care ser-vices assess and assure the provision of public health care, a daily function of the pharmacist.

➤ *Communicable Diseases by Contact.* Pharmacists coun-sel and monitor the treatment of communicable dis-eases. In many communities, pharmacists assist in the distribution of needle exchange and condom distribution programs.

➤ *Community-Based Education.* Some pharmacists practice in facilities called pharmacies. These facilities, whether they are contained inside an institution or are free-standing in a community, become sources of health information. Pharmacists work within and outside these facilities to provide education programs to members of the "community" they serve.

➤ *Decrease Tobacco Use.* Pharmacists play an important role in assisting patients in decreasing and stopping their intake of nicotine through pharmacotherapy and support. Pharmacists can also assist such efforts by making the facility in which they practice "smoke-free," and by not selling tobacco products.

➤ *Drug Safety.* Pharmacists learn that their primary role is drug safety. The appropriate distribution, consumption, storage, and disposal of drugs are a major part of any practice.

➤ *Family Planning.* Patient counseling and appropriate referral of patients is an important role. Pharmacists counsel parents to assure that children have a healthy start, prenatally and postnatally.

➤ *Immunizations.* Pharmacists can refer, counsel, and in some communities provide immunizations to patients.

➤ *Improved Nutrition.* Pharmacists monitor patient health and distribute nutritional supplements in their practices. Nutrition support is a board certification area in pharmacy.

➤ *Infectious Disease Control.* Maintenance of appropriate pharmacotherapy can assist in the prevention of super-infections.

➤ *Maternal and Infant Health.* Because of their accessibility, pharmacists are key referral agents for maternal and infant health counseling.

➤ *Mental Health and Mental Disorders.* Pharmacists monitor the pharmacotherapy of patients with mental health disorders. It is often difficult for these patients to manage their medications, requiring pharmacists to work closely with health care providers and caregivers to assure optimal health outcomes and to minimize the misuse/abuse of medications.

➤ *Occupational Safety.* Knowledgeable about their community, pharmacists counsel on injury prevention in the workplace.

➤ *Physical Activity/Fitness*. Pharmacists provide community-level education on issues such as weight control and coronary health. At the individual level pharmacists monitor pharmacotherapy and counsel patients.

➤ *Prevention (Minimization) of Chronic Illness*. Pharmacotherapy management can minimize the progression or increased symptoms associated with chronic illness.

➤ *Surveillance and Data Systems*. Pharmacists participate in population-based medication management systems to monitor processes, predict outcomes, and optimize care.

➤ *Toxic Agent Control*. Medication safety, storage, and disposal, are pharmacist practice roles.

➤ *Unintentional Injuries*. Prevention of injuries related to medication use and specifically related to poisoning are important pharmacist roles.

➤ *Violence and Abusive Behavior*. In most states, pharmacists are mandatory reporters of abuse. Abuse of children, spouses, and elders can be reported when seen by pharmacists.

PUBLIC HEALTH SCREENING QUESTIONS

Public health screening questions are easy to ask. However, one must be prepared to deal with the answers one receives. Below are some screening questions for public health issues. Pharmacists must consider how they will choose to respond to the various answers they will receive.

Basic Screening Questions

These are questions that one can ask nearly every time one counsels a patient.

➤ Do you smoke or use smokeless tobacco products?
➤ Do you and your family members wear seatbelts and/or use car seats each time you are in the car?
➤ How do you use alcohol?
➤ Where do you currently store your medications and similar products?
➤ (If young children in the home) Do you have syrup of ipecac available in your home?
➤ (If young children in the home) Do you have the number of the poison center near your home telephone?

Age-Related Public Health Screening Areas

ALL AGES

Automobile safety: seatbelts, car seats.

Diet: proper, complete.

Home safety: smoke detectors, water heater thermostat, firearm storage.

Immunizations: asking age-appropriate questions about status of immunizations.

Personal safety: child, spouse, parent abuse.

Smoking: active, passive.

Alcohol use: consumption, driving.

PRENATAL

Prenatal health care visits.

Use of medications, over-the-counter (OTC) drugs, drugs of abuse, and alcohol.

YOUNG CHILDREN

Oral/dental health: fluorides.

Sport helmets.

Home safety: child proof; syrup of ipecac; stairs, gates, bed-rails, pool rails.

Storage of toxins: plants, cleaning fluids, medications.

ADULTS AND OLDER CHILDREN

Storage of toxins: drugs, especially abusable drugs.

Alcohol.

Other abusable drugs.

Sexual activity.

Routine health screening: Papanicolaou smears, cholesterol.

Skin protection.

Screening Questions for Selected Public Health Objectives

These questions are generally brought about by a clinical situation. If for example, a pharmacist is concerned about an individual's level of personal safety (abuse), questions on that issue can be asked.

➤ Alcohol and other "drugs."

- How do you use alcohol?
- How much alcohol do you drink each day? Week?
- Do you have any concerns about your alcohol intake?
- Do you use drugs recreationally, such as marijuana?
- Do you use drugs on a regular basis that are not for medical reasons?

➤ Communicable diseases by contact.

- Are you sexually active?
- Do you have more than one partner?
- Do you use condoms?
- Are you often exposed to colds?

➤ Decrease tobacco use.

- Do you smoke?
- How many packs per day?
- Do you chew tobacco or dip snuff?
- How often?
- May I offer you assistance to quit your tobacco use?

➤ Drug safety.

- Where do you keep your medicines in your home?
- Do you have any out-of-date medicines you can get rid of?

➤ Family planning.

- Are you sexually active?
- What are your practices and beliefs about family planning?
- Are you interested in discussing methods of preventing pregnancy?

➤ Immunizations.

- Are your (child's) immunizations up to date?
- (If appropriate) Did you get an immunization this year?

➤ Improved nutrition.

- Is your diet balanced in intake of fats, carbohydrates, proteins, and other nutrients?

➤ Infectious disease control.
- Do you take all of your antibiotics?
- Do you share antibiotics?
- Do you have any antibiotics left over that you can get rid of?

➤ Maternal and infant health.
- (For pregnancy and breast-feeding) What medications, including OTC medications, are you taking?
- (For pregnancy) Are you taking prenatal vitamins?
- (For pregnancy) Are you avoiding alcohol (fetal alcohol syndrome) and smoking (smaller birthweight babies)?
- (For infant) How is your baby feeling? Any concerns?
- (For infant) How often does your baby feed, need a diaper changed?

➤ Mental health and mental disorders
- Do you feel you are under a lot of stress?
- Do you have concerns about your moods?

➤ Occupational safety.
- Are you exposed to chemicals, toxins, or fumes in the workplace?
- Do you have a job where you need to do repetitive physical tasks?

➤ Physical activity/fitness.
- What do you do for exercise?
- How often do you exercise?
- What are your goals for your weight?

➤ Prevention (minimization) of chronic illness.
- Do you see your health care provider for preventive visits, e.g., a well-woman exam?
- Are you up to date on immunizations?

➤ Surveillance and data systems.
➤ Toxic agent control.
- Do you have the potential for toxic exposure in your workplace?
- Does your occupation require you to have poisonous substances in your home?
- Have you thought about the storage of pesticides, cleaners, and solvents?

➤ Unintentional injuries.

- Is your home child-proofed?
- Do you have a poison control telephone number by your telephone?
- Do you have plants in your home that can cause illness to your child?
- Do your young children use a car seat? Seatbelts?

➤ Violence and abusive behavior.

- Do you feel safe (at home)?

STRATEGIES FOR IMPLEMENTATION OF HEALTH PROMOTION/DISEASE PREVENTION ACTIVITIES BY PHARMACISTS

Although it may seem intuitive that pharmacists, particularly those with community-based practices, may be in an ideal situation to provide public health services, implementation of services may be difficult. Some of the challenges may involve lack of knowledge about models for providing such services and access to quality information. In the following sections, specific examples of pharmacy-based models of preventive care are discussed and examples of written and computer-based, on-line information are provided.

Primary Prevention

IMMUNIZATIONS

Immunization rates for preschool children in the United States were estimated to be 75% in April 1996. Although this represented an increase from a rate of 55% from 4 years earlier, it falls short of the goal of 90% immunization rates prescribed by the Public Health Service for 2000. The immunization record for the adult population is by comparison much lower, with estimated rates of death between 50,000 and 70,000 adults each year in the United States from diseases such as pneumococcal disease, influenza, and hepatitis B.

Pharmacists in virtually every type of practice have an opportunity to improve immunization rates. Community pharmacists can participate in activities such as public education, adding immunization records to profiles, and reminding patients of needs for immunizations. Some community pharmacies have served as sites for immunization programs. Hospital practitioners can include immunization histories in data collected on admission, screen patients at high risk because of certain diseases for appropriate immunizations intervention (e.g., patients with heart or pulmonary disease), advocate on pharmacy and therapeutics committees for immunization practices, and use computer databases to screen for disease conditions that can be controlled with appropriate immunizations. For example, patients older than 65 years of age could be screened for evidence of immunizations for influenza, pneumococcal disease, and diphtheria/tetanus.

The Centers for Disease Control and Prevention (CDC) has up-to-date information on practice guidelines for adult and childhood immunizations. These guidelines serve as a basis for evaluating current immunization status of both children and adults. To access the CDC's web page, enter http://www.cdc.gov/, where direct links to immunizations related to travel and a link to health information will be found. The health information link can be explored in a number of ways, but using the link option will provide access to immunization information. The immunization link can be explored to look at new information, publications, and services related to immunization programs.

ALCOHOL USE

Pharmacists commonly ask patients about alcohol use when taking medication histories. For pharmacists who take a proactive role in triage related to alcohol use and abuse, information contained in the National Institutes of Health's, National Institute on Alcohol Abuse and Alcoholism publication, "The Physician's Guide to Helping Patients with Alcohol Problems" may be particularly helpful. This document suggests a series of four steps for screening and brief intervention, including (1) asking about alcohol use, (2) assessing for alcohol-related problems, (3) advising appropriate action, and (4) monitoring patient progress. In

---

Box 19.5   Alcohol Use Assessment

REASONS TO MONITOR

Men: >14 drinks/week or 4 drinks/occasion
Women: >7 drinks/week or 3 drinks/occasion
Pregnancy
Medication use
History of dependency
Medical conditions
   Black-outs, chronic abdominal pain, depression,
    liver dysfunction, trauma, sleep disorders
Preoccupation with drinking
Unable to stop once started
Drinking to avoid withdrawal symptoms
Withdrawal symptoms
Increased alcohol tolerance
Positive response to CAGE format questions
   Cut down—feels they should
   Annoyed by criticism of drinking patterns
   Guilty feelings about drinking
   "Eye-opener" drink needed in the morning

*Source: National Institute on Alcohol Abuse and Alcoholism. The
Physician's Guide to Helping Patients with Alcohol Problems. 1995
NIH Publication No. 95-3769.*

---

particular, steps 1 and 2 will be helpful for pharmacists in
identifying patients at risk for alcohol-related concerns and
provide background foundation for referral to other
providers for more in-depth treatment. Box 19.5 outlines
indications for alcohol use assessment.

SMOKING CESSATION

Pharmacists are in a unique position to help patients stop
smoking. Increasingly, drug products such as nicotine
patches and gum are available in OTC forms, and pharmacists can help patients with efforts to stop smoking. A useful tool for pharmacists is a web-based publication by the
Agency for Health Care Policy and Research entitled,
"Helping Smokers Quit—A Guide for Primary Care Clini-

Box 19.6   Smoking Assessment and Support

Ask users about smoking habits regularly

Advise users to quit; use clinical knowledge of illnesses related to smoking

Inform users there are new, effective treatment therapies available

Refer and assist users who want to quit; these patients should be referred to pharmacists and other health care providers who are specialists in smoking cessation

Source: Agency for Health Care Policy and Research Guidelines of Smoking Cessation.

---

cians." Box 19.6 provides guidelines from the agency on smoking assessment and support. The overview provided on this web page gives practical advice to health care providers to enable them to help patients with smoking cessation. Links to the Clinical Practice Guidelines offer more in-depth information for providers organizing programs for their patients. Using the Table of Contents to explore General Strategies will provide more in-depth information in organizing programs. Although some pharmacists may not be in a position to offer intensive programs in smoking cessation, the initial intervention, follow-up, and referral to specialized programs when appropriate are important activities for the primary care pharmacist.

Box 19.7 provides additional information on internet-based sources of public health information.

Secondary Prevention

HYPERTENSION AND CHOLESTEROL SCREENING

Both hypertension and elevated cholesterol are risk factors for coronary disease. Early detection and treatment are important components of prevention of cardiac disease. Pharmacists in institutional settings and in community practices are involved with cholesterol screening programs. Likewise,

Box 19.7   Internet-Based Sources of Public Health
            Information

Centers for Disease Control and Prevention (Travel Immunizations and General Search)	http://www.cdc.gov
The Physician's Guide to Helping Patients with Alcohol Problems	http://silk.nih.gov/niaaa1/ publication/physicn.htm
Helping Smokers Quit—A Guide for Primary Care Clinicians	http://www.ahcpr.gov/ clinic/smokepcc.htm
National Institute's of Health—National Heart, Lung, and Blood Institute (Clinical Guidelines)	http://www.nhlbi.nih.gov/ index.htm
Sources of U.S. Government Documents Online	http://www.healthfinder. gov
Smoking Cessation	http://www. surgeongeneral. gov/tobacco/
Immunizations (Children)	http://www.cdc.gov/nip/ diseases/childvpd.htm
Immunizations (Adult)	http://www.cdc.gov/nip/ diseases/adultvpd.htm
Diet and Exercise	http://www.nhlbi.nih.gov/ health/public/heart/ obesity/lose_wt/ index.htm
Poison Prevention	http://www.aapcc.org/ preventi.htm

pharmacists can and should take an active role in screening, educating, and referring patients for hypertension. One source of information for providers related to both cholesterol and blood pressure screening is the National Institutes of Health's National Heart, Lung, and Blood Institute.

Table 19-1. Hypertension Risk Stratification

Blood Pressure (mm Hg)	Indicators	Therapy
130–139/85–89	None	Lifestyle modification
130–139/85–89	Target organ disease[a] Clinical cardiovascular disease Diabetes	Pharmacotherapy
140–159/90–99	None	Try lifestyle modification for 12 months, then pharmacotherapy
140–159/90–99	One risk factor[a]	Try lifestyle modification for 6 months, then pharmacotherapy
140–159/90–99	Target organ disease[a] Clinical cardiovascular disease Diabetes	Pharmacotherapy
>159/>99		Pharmacotherapy

[a] Target organ diseases are cardiovascular-related conditions. Risk Factors are smoking, dyslipidemia, diabetes mellitus, age older than 60 years, male gender, postmenopausal status (women), and family history of cardiovascular disease.

Source: National Institutes of Health, National Heart, Lung, and Blood Institute. The Sixth Report of the Joint National Committee on Prevention, Detection, Evaluation, and Treatment of High Blood Pressure. NIH publication no. 98-4080. Bethesda, MD: USGPO; 1997.

This agency publishes practice guidelines related to as-sessment, treatment, and follow-up for these and other conditions. As an example, the Sixth Report of the Joint National Committee on Prevention, Detection, Evaluation, and Treatment of High Blood Pressure was published in

1997. Table 19.1, adapted from this publication, is useful in providing guidelines for appropriate strategies for assessing and referring patients whose blood pressures are screened.

Tertiary Prevention

ASTHMA DISEASE MANAGEMENT

Pharmacists are important links in comanagement of chronic diseases with patients and other health care providers. One example of management of chronic disease is the care of patients with asthma. In the treatment of patients with asthma, pharmacists explain how medication works, clarify treatment goals, provide written materials, assess patient understanding, work with patients and their family to construct management plans, and look at potential barriers to appropriate treatment. The National Heart, Lung, and Blood Institute's 1997 Guidelines for the Diagnosis and Management of Asthma is a valuable resource for evidence-based information about the disease, assessment/diagnosis, treatment, patient education, and follow-up. Information provided in this publication is valuable for evidence-based information about the disease, assessment/diagnosis, treatment, patient education, and follow-up.

An exhaustive review of resources and materials is beyond the scope of this chapter. As pharmacists seek to become more involved with public health practice, searches of the primary literature should be beneficial in learning about models of practice established by other pharmacists. A useful computer link is http://www.healthfinder.gov/online. htm for looking at a broad array of government agency publications and information.

Suggested Readings

American Pharmaceutical Association. Pharmacists' Delivery of Primary Care. Washington, DC: American Pharmaceutical Association; 1994

Blenkinsopp A, Panton R. Health Promotion for Pharmacists. New York, NY: Oxford University Press; 1991.

Bush PJ, Johnson KW. Where is the public health pharmacist? Am J Pharm Educ. 1979;43:249–51.

Bush PJ, Johnson KW. Public health role of the pharmacist. In: Wertheimer AI, Smith MC, eds. Pharmacy Practice. Social and Behavioral Aspects. 3rd ed. Baltimore, MD: Williams & Wilkins; 1989:379–88.

Carter BL. Current recommendations of the joint national high blood pressure committee (commentary). Clin Pharm. 1993;12:53–7.

Eickhoff TC. Adult immunizations-how are we doing? Hosp Pract. 1996; 31(11) 107–108; 111–112; 115–117.

Ernst ME et al. Implementation of a community pharmacy-based influenza vaccination program. J Am Pharm Assoc. 1997;NS37:570–80.

Furmaga EM. Pharmacist management of a hyperlipidemia clinic. Am J Hosp Pharm. 1993;50:91–5.

Grabenstein JD. Pharmacists and immunizations: advocating preventive medicine. Am Pharm. 1988;NS28:25–33.

Hepler CD, Grainger-Rousseau TJ. Pharmaceutical care versus traditional drug treatment. Is there a difference? Drugs. 1995;49:1–10.

Hurd PD, Levin BL. Public Health and Prevention. In: McCarthy RL, ed. Introduction to Health Care Delivery. A Primer for Pharmacists. Gaithersburg, MD: Aspen Publishers; 1998:171–84.

Institute of Medicine. National Academy of Sciences. The Future of Public Health. Washington, DC: National Academy Press; 1988.

McKenney JM. An evaluation of cholesterol screening in community pharmacies. Am Pharm. 1993;NS33(7):34–40.

Munzenberger PJ. Improving adherence in patients with asthma. Am Pharm. 1993; NS33(8):32–7.

National Institutes of Health, National Heart, Lung, and Blood Institute. The Sixth Report of the Joint National Committee on Prevention, Detection, Evaluation, and Treatment of High Blood Pressure. NIH publication no. 98-4080. Bethesda, MD: USGPO; 1997.

Paluck EC, Stratton TP, Eni GO. Community pharmacists' participation in health education and disease prevention activities. Can J Public Health. 1994;85:389–92.

Turnock B. Public Health. What is It and How It Works. Gaithersburg, MD: Aspen Publishers; 1997.

U.S. Department of Health and Human Services Public Health

Service. Healthy People 2000-National Health Promotion and Disease Prevention Objectives. DHHS publication no. (PHS) 91-50213. Washington, DC: USGPO; 1990.

World Health Organization. The World Health Organization: A Report on the First Ten Years. Geneva, Switzerland: 1958.

Chapter 20

Approaches to Evaluating Drug-Related Problems

Timothy J. Hoon

A major responsibility of a pharmacist is the evaluation of drug therapy in an individual patient and the subsequent therapeutic recommendations based on the patient's specific clinical condition. In simple terms, there are four activities or responsibilities that are part of this process: (1) start a medication that is needed, (2) monitor current medication response to optimize efficacy, (3) vigilantly look for adverse effects, and (4) discontinue medications that are not needed, not effective, or producing adverse effects. This chapter provides the framework for the evaluation of drug-related problems that are typically defined as adverse effects. A discussion of the importance of differentiating drug-related versus disease-related problems is followed by an overview of the mechanistic causes of drug-related problems. This background information will support the problem-solving process of evaluating drug-related problems, including the collection of data necessary to reach appropriate conclusions. Lists of medications that have been associated with drug-induced problems are provided as a quick reference at the end of the chapter (Appendix 20.1). A more detailed discussion of drug-induced renal and hepatic dysfunction is found in the text.

DRUG VERSUS DISEASE ISSUES

From a pharmacist's perspective, a guiding philosophy in the identification of drug-related issues is the assumption that any new complaint or problem is drug-induced until proven otherwise. Other members of the health care team may focus on searching for pathophysiologic causes of new complaints while overlooking potential drug-induced causes. By looking first at a patient's medications, the pharmacist provides a valuable contribution by approaching the situation from a unique perspective. Likely drug-related causes of new problems should be sought first. Then, other potential causes should be investigated. Finally, the most likely cause of the new complaint or problem should be determined based on all available evidence.

It is important to understand that many drug-induced problems share a similar presentation to disease-related causes but have a unique feature that suggests that a particular drug is the causative agent. An example of this would be leukocytosis in patients receiving corticosteroids. An elevated white blood cell count is one indication that patients have an infection. Patients receiving corticosteroids are prone to infections due to the immunosuppressant effects of steroids. In addition to identifying the presence of a fever or other signs of infection, careful evaluation of the differential of the elevated white blood cell count can help determine whether the leukocytosis is infection-induced or drug-induced. If the elevated white blood cell count is due predominantly to mature neutrophils with few immature neutrophils (bands or stabs), leukocytosis is likely due to steroid-induced demargination of the mature cells from the endothelial surface of the vasculature. On the other hand, if there is an abundance of immature neutrophils (known as a left-shift) then infection is the likely cause of leukocytosis. It is evident from this example that a careful analysis of the situation is important to reach the correct clinical conclusion leading to an appropriate therapeutic recommendation.

PHARMACOLOGIC ISSUES

Drug-induced problems may result from an extension of the primary pharmacologic action of the drug. Examples of this situation are hypotension occurring from excessive lowering of blood pressure with an antihypertensive drug and hypoglycemia secondary to incorrect insulin dosing. In these cases, the problem is dose-related, and a search for excessive intake or reduced clearance often suggests a likely cause within agents known to produce the observed effect. It should also be kept in mind that duplication in therapy (e.g., multiple antihypertensive agents) may lead to excessive response and problems at doses of drugs within a regimen that, on an individual basis, do not seem excessively large.

IDIOSYNCRATIC REACTIONS

Problems unrelated to the primary mechanism of action of a drug can occur. These are typically termed idiosyncratic reactions if the problem cannot be predicted based on the expected pharmacologic effect. Toxicity unrelated to the primary pharmacologic mechanism may be due to cytotoxic reactions, immunologic reactions, or hereditary enzyme deficiencies. Cytotoxic reactions result from the covalent bonding of a reactive drug or metabolite species to tissue macromolecules resulting in local tissue injury. An example of a cytotoxic reaction is drug-induced hepatotoxicity. Another type of idiosyncratic reaction is an immunologic mediated reaction resulting from drug-induced antibody production which may lead to tissue damage by various mechanisms. Antibodies may attack a drug that is bound to tissue, resulting in damage to the tissue. Alternatively, drug or metabolite binding to tissue may render the host tissue antigenic and subject to attack from resulting autoantibodies. Also, various allergic reactions may occur, such as anaphylaxis, from antibodies reacting to drugs, metabolites, or inactive ingredients used in the production of the dosage form. These reactions are considered idiosyncratic because they are unpredictable in an individual patient and are not dose-related. However, it is known that certain drugs have more commonly been associated with these types of problems. This knowledge aids in the identification of a likely culprit.

GENETIC-BASED REACTIONS

Genetically determined deficiencies in certain metabolic enzymes also predispose patients to drug-induced problems. In these cases, the normal biochemical pathways of metabolism are altered or limited. Introduction of a drug to these patients may lead to an unexpected reaction due to the build up of metabolic precursors or other biochemical abnormalities that would not have resulted in a patient without a genetically altered metabolism. An example of this type of reaction is hemolytic anemia that may occur in patients with glucose-6-phosphate dehydrogenase (G6PD) deficiency who receive antimalarials, sulfonamide antibiotics, or other drugs known to cause this problem. In these cases, identification of the enzymatic deficiency can help predict a likely drug-induced problem with exposure to known offending agents. The risk of such reactions is often based on an index of suspicion based on a patient's ethnic background or family history. Metabolic markers can also be used to assess genetic predisposition to rates and pathways of metabolism; however, this is not routinely done in clinical practice. An adverse drug event sometimes provides the first clue to a genetic enzyme deficiency.

APPROACH TO EVALUATING DRUG-RELATED PROBLEMS

Based on the mechanisms listed above, there are four questions that should be addressed when evaluating a potential drug-induced problem.

➤ First, are the known pharmacologic effects of the medication plausible causes for the encountered problem?
➤ Second, was the time lag between medication initiation and problem presentation consistent with previous reports or the proposed mechanism of the adverse effect?
➤ Third, did the problem resolve or improve once the suspected drug was stopped?
➤ Fourth, did the problem recur with rechallenge of the suspected drug?

A solid case has been made for a drug-induced problem if the answers to all four of these questions are yes. This organized approach to analyzing drug-induced problems is very helpful but does have some limitations. An affirmative answer to the first question cannot be made in cases of idiosyncratic or allergic reactions to drugs. However, if there are reports of these types of problems with a particular drug, one could conclude that a potential link is plausible even if it does not involve the pharmacologic mechanism of action. Another obvious limitation is that many drug-induced problems are so severe that a rechallenge is out of the question. Conclusively determining a drug as a causative agent for a particular problem is not worth risking a potentially life-threatening reaction. Therefore, the questions above should be used to guide an investigation of possible links based on patient-specific information and literature reports.

When multiple potential causes for a new problem exist, how does one sort out the most likely causative agent? This necessitates exploring the details of the new problem including the characteristics of the presentation, speed of onset, and any other problem-specific data that may be useful in discriminating between etiologies. The timing of a new problem in relation to changes in a patient's medication regimen deserves further discussion.

A potentially drug-related problem often occurs that may be caused by more than one medication in a patient's regimen. To discern the most likely offending agent, a careful study of the details of the presenting problem should be made and compared to the characteristics of the adverse effects associated with all likely agents. All too often the last medication started is blamed for any new problem. Although one should seriously consider the latest alteration in a drug regimen, one should also consider the mechanistic cause of the problem. Does the adverse effect typically have an acute onset, such as anaphylaxis or other acute allergic reactions? Or does it typically require a prolonged exposure to a drug, such as amiodarone-induced pulmonary toxicity? By matching the clinical characteristics of the reaction with those reported from likely culprit medications, the pool of candidates is often limited. Careful inspection of the typical duration of exposure to the onset of the problem, relative to the timing of medication regimen changes, can often further narrow the list to one of two potential causes. Depending on the mechanism and severity of the reaction, it may be possible to eliminate drugs from the regimen one at a time to identify which drug was responsible for the problem. However, in many instances, more than one medication may be stopped, prohibiting the positive identification of a single causative agent.

DATA COLLECTION

In addition to obtaining a careful medication history that includes the drug name, dose, dosing interval, start date, indication, and compliance for all recent medications, the pharmacist should inquire about any use of over-the-counter products including nutritional supplements, vitamins, and herbals. The patient should also be asked about any recently discontinued medications and previous reactions to medications that led to discontinuation of use. The timing of initiation and termination of therapy is key when trying to determine the cause of a potentially drug-induced problem. If the patient is experiencing a dermatologic problem such as a rash, the pharmacist should also inquire about any change in body soaps, lotions, powders, or laundry products.

Data regarding the characteristics of the problem can come solely from a patient's complaint (e.g., nausea, dizziness) or may include physical examination and laboratory findings. Physical examination findings are particularly important in dermatologic reactions, because the appearance of the reaction may be the classic characteristic linking the problem to a drug. Nondermatologic problems may also manifest with physical examination findings that should be considered in evaluating the nature and severity of a new problem. Laboratory studies may support the presence of a new drug-induced problem or may be the only evidence that a problem exists in the early stages, such as in hyperglycemia or hyperkalemia.

SPECIFIC DRUG-RELATED PROBLEMS

Lists of medications that have been associated with various drug-induced problems are described in the following section and are organized by organ system. These lists should be consulted with two caveats in mind. First, just because a drug is not on the list does not mean that it cannot be the cause of a new problem. These lists are not all-inclusive. Further, new discoveries continue to link medications to adverse effects. There is a first time for every reported drug-induced problem. Second, just because a medication is listed does not mean that it is the cause of a new complaint or problem. Many of these problems can occur without a drug-induced etiology. Therefore, in a particular patient a medication may be mistakenly blamed for a condition that has arisen for other reasons. The pharmacist should search for all potential causes of a new complaint or problem and seek to determine the most likely cause in a particular patient before quickly casting blame on a drug. If a drug has been identified as the likely cause of a new problem, it is highly recommended that specialty texts, review papers, and even original reports are consulted to confirm that the clinical presentation matches previous reports. However, one must always use clinical judgment based on all available information.

Two organ systems are worthy of special mention, because they are often the targets of drug-induced problems and are also organs of drug elimination. Renal and hepatic injury can result from several etiologies. These are organ systems frequently monitored by pharmacists to assess not only potential drug toxicity, but also organ function as an indication of a patient's ability to clear a drug. Therefore, changes in organ function are often detected by laboratory assessments, leading to a search for the cause of injury that may be drug-induced.

In general, a rise in blood urea nitrogen (BUN) and serum creatinine concentrations are the first signs of a decline in renal function. There are three common causes of renal dysfunction: prerenal azotemia due to hypoperfusion, intrinsic renal damage, and postobstructive dysfunction. Postobstructive dysfunction involves a physical blockage of urine outflow downstream from the kidney. This is a physical abnormality, often due to renal stones or other anatomic abnormalities, that is typically not drug-induced. Relieving the obstruction usually restores kidney function.

Drug-induced prerenal azotemia, caused by a pharmacologic hypoperfusion of the kidneys, results in a drop in the glomerular filtration pressure and a decline in renal function. A rise in BUN and serum creatinine is noted with a BUN:creatinine ratio exceeding 20:1. This laboratory rule of thumb is helpful in assessing the reason for a decline in renal function. Drug-induced prerenal azotemia may result from excessive lowering of blood pressure with antihypertensive or antianginal agents, dehydration from excessive diuretic use, or alterations in the intrarenal hemodynamics from angiotensin-converting enzyme inhibitors, vasodilators, or agents that inhibit prostaglandin synthesis. Therefore, the first step in evaluating a decline in renal function is to evaluate not only the BUN and serum creatinine concentrations but also the ratio, in addition to other signs or risk factors for drug-induced renal hypoperfusion and dysfunction.

Intrinsic renal damage may also be the result of a drug-induced problem. Several problems producing direct injury to the kidneys can be associated with drugs as causative agents. These include interstitial nephritis, nephropathies, nephrotic syndrome, and tubular necrosis. Additionally, the kidneys' ability to excrete or preserve water and electrolytes may also be hampered by drugs, resulting in clinically relevant problems such as nephrogenic diabetes insipidus and renal tubular acidosis. In these cases of intrinsic renal damage, the BUN and serum creatinine both rise but typically with a ratio of less than 20:1.

Drug-induced hepatic dysfunction typically falls into three categories than can be classified by standard laboratory tests. A hepatocellular problem results from injury to the hepatocyte causing cell death. A cholestatic problem results from injury to bile ducts or canaliculi resulting in altered bile flow. A mixed problem may also result from a combination of cholestasis and hepatocyte necrosis. Allergic reactions may manifest as either hepatocellular or cholestatic problems. Liver function abnormalities range from asymptomatic cases, in which laboratory abnormalities or hepatomegaly observed on physical examination are the only evidence of a problem, to severe dysfunction evidenced by marked jaundice and encephalopathy. The time course of liver disorders may be described as acute, with symptoms and enzyme elevations lasting less than 3 months, or chronic, in which symptoms or enzyme elevations persist longer than 3 months. A fulminant course may occur in which acute liver injury progresses from normal function to severe dysfunction in a few days to weeks.

The characteristic hepatic enzyme elevation patterns associated with these disorders are summarized in Table 20.1. It is important to highlight that elevations in these enzymes are indicative of injury but may not reflect alterations in liver function. To assess alterations in metabolic function, an examination of the products of liver function needs to be made. Reductions in serum albumin or total protein may indicate liver dysfunction provided that the patient has been receiving adequate nutrition to build protein and has not undergone recent trauma or other severe stress

Table 20-1.   Hepatic Enzyme Elevation in Various Hepatic Disorders

Enzyme	Hepatocellular	Cholestatic	Chronic
Bilirubin (direct)	+	+++	+
Alkaline phosphatase (Alk Phos)	+	+++	+
γ-Glutamyltransferase (GGT)	+	+++	++
Aspartate aminotransferase (AST, SGOT)	+++	+	++
Alanine transferase (ALT, SGPT)	+++	+	++
Lactate dehydrogenase (LDH)	+++	+	+

Source: DiPiro JT et al., eds. Pharmacotherapy: A Pathophysiologic Approach. 4th ed. Stamford, CT: Appleton & Lange; 1999.

necessitating the catabolism of circulating proteins for energy. An elevation in the prothrombin time (PT) or international normalized ratio (INR) may also indicate liver dysfunction provided that the patient has not received anticoagulants that alter these coagulation test results. It should be borne in mind that patients with severe liver dysfunction may have altered coagulation, albumin, or total protein results but apparently "normal" liver enzymes if the damage occurred long ago and left the patient with a dysfunctional liver.

The impact of drug-induced renal and hepatic dysfunction carries two risks that must be handled. First, the causative agent needs to be identified and discontinued. Guidance has already been given on how to approach this challenge. Second, the impact of altered drug elimination must be evaluated to prevent the accumulation of other drugs to excessive amounts within the body, which may lead to additional toxicity.

A pharmacist should assume that any new problem is drug-induced until proven otherwise. A careful medication history, including the timing of therapy changes, is of prime importance in identifying likely causative agents. The lists provided in this chapter can support an investigation. However, confirmation using more detailed descriptions of these drug-induced problems is suggested. Additionally, a positive identification typically requires discontinuation and rechallenge with the suspected medication.

References

1. DiPiro JT et al., eds. Pharmacotherapy: A Pathophysiologic Approach. 4th ed. Stamford, CT: Appleton & Lange; 1999.
2. Young LY, Koda-Kimble MA, eds. Applied Therapeutics: The Clinical Use of Drugs. 6th ed. Vancouver: Applied Therapeutics, Inc.; 1995.
3. Wood AJJ. Adverse Reactions to Drugs. In: Fauci AS et al., eds. Harrison's Principles of Internal Medicine. 14th ed. New York, NY: McGraw-Hill; 1998.
4. Schrier RW. Renal and Electrolyte Disorders. 4th ed. Boston, MA: Little Brown & Co.; 1992.
5. Lipsky BA, Hirschmann JV. Drug fever. JAMA. 1981;245:851–4.
6. Mackowiak PA, LeMaistre CF. Drug fever: a critical appraisal of conventional concepts. Ann Intern Med. 1987;106:728–33.

Appendix 20.1:
Medications Associated With Medical Problems[1–6]

Multisystem Disorders

Drugs Associated with Anaphylaxis/Anaphylactoid Reactions

ACE Inhibitors

l-Asparaginase

Cephalosporins

Demeclocycline

Dextran

Immune globulin, intravenous

Insulin

Iodinated drugs/contrast media

Iron dextran

Lidocaine

Narcotic analgesics

Penicillins

Procaine

Psyllium

Streptomycin

Sulfonamides

Tetracyclines

Drugs Associated with Angioedema

ACE inhibitors

Penicillins

Drugs Associated with Lupus Erythematosus

Acebutolol

Asparaginase

Barbiturates

Bleomycin

Cephalosporins

Chlorpromazine

Hydralazine

Iodides

Isoniazid

Methyldopa

Penicillamine

Phenolphthalein

Phenytoin

Procainamide

Quinidine

Sulfonamides

Thiouracil

Drugs Associated with Vasculitis

Allopurinol

Cimetidine

Fluoxetine

Hydralazine

Ibuprofen

Indomethacin

Penicillins

Phenylbutazone

Phenytoin

Piroxicam

Procainamide

Propylthiouracil

Quinine

Sulfonamides

Thiazides

Warfarin

Drugs Associated with Serum Sickness

Antithymocyte globulin

Aspirin
Cephalosporins
Penicillins
Phenytoin
Propylthiouracil
Streptokinase
Streptomycin
Sulfonamides

Drugs Associated with Fever
Allopurinol
Aminosalicylic acid
Amphetamines
Amphotericin B
Antidopaminergics
Antihistamines
Asparaginase
Azathioprine
Barbiturates
Benztropine
Bleomycin
Carbamazepine
Cephalosporins
Chlorambucil
Chloramphenicol
Cimetidine
Clofibrate
Cocaine
Colistin
Cytarabine
Daunorubicin
Haloperidol
Hydralazine
Hydroxyurea
Immune globulin, intravenous

Interferons
Iodides
Iron Dextran
Isoniazid
Levamisole
Mebendazole
Mercaptopurine
Methyldopa
Metoclopramide
Neuroleptics
Nitrofurantoin
Nonsteroidal antiinflammatory agents
Pamidronate
Penicillins
Phenothiazines
Phenytoin
Procarbazine
Procainamide
Propylthiouracil
Prostaglandin E_2
Quinidine
Quinine
Rifampin
Ritodrine
Salicylates
Streptokinase
Streptomycin
Streptozocin
Sulfonamides
Sulindac
Tetracycline
Vancomycin

Dermatologic Disorders

Drugs Associated with Acne

Anabolic/androgenic steroids

Corticosteroids

Iodides

Isoniazid

Oral contraceptives

Drugs Associated with Alopecia

Busulfan

Carbamazepine

Clofibrate

Colchicine

Cyclophosphamide

Doxorubicin

Ethionamide

Etretinate

Fluconazole

Granulocyte colony-stimulating factor

Heparin

Hydroxyurea

Interferon alpha

Isotretinoin

Lithium

Methotrexate

Mitoxantrone

Oral contraceptive withdrawal

Phenytoin

Propranolol

Tricyclic antidepressants

Valproic acid

Vitamin A (high doses)

Warfarin

Drugs Associated with Photosensitivity

Amiodarone

Barbiturates

Captopril

Carbamazepine

Chlordiazepoxide

Doxorubicin

5-Fluorouracil

Furosemide

Griseofulvin

Ketoprofen

Mitomycin

Nalidixic acid

Naproxen

Oral contraceptives

Phenothiazines

Phenylbutazone

Piroxicam

Protriptyline

Quinidine

Simvastatin

Sulfonamides

Sulfonylureas

Sulindac

Tetracyclines (especially Demeclocycline)

Thiazides

Drugs Associated with Erythema Multiforme/Stevens-Johnson Syndrome

Acetaminophen

Allopurinol

Barbiturates

Carbamazepine

Cephalosporins

Chlorpropamide

Codeine

Ibuprofen

Imidazoles

Lamotrigine

Macrolides

Penicillins

Phenolphthalein

Phenylbutazone

Phenytoin

Piroxicam

Propranolol

Quinolones

Salicylates

Sulfadiazine

Sulfonamides

Sulfonylureas

Tetracyclines

Thiazides

Valproic acid

Drugs Associated with Toxic Epidermal Necrolysis

Allopurinol

Barbiturates

Carbamazepine

Chloramphenicol

Ibuprofen

Indomethacin

Iodides

Lamotrigine

Macrolides

Nalidixic acid

Penicillins

Phenolphthalein

Phenylbutazone

Quinine

Quinolones

Phenytoin

Sulfonamides

Sulindac

Tolmetin

Valproic acid

Drugs Associated with Skin Necrosis

Warfarin

Drugs Associated with Urticaria

Aspirin

Barbiturates

Captopril

Enalapril

Gold salts

Heparin

Ibuprofen

Immune globulin, intravenous

Indomethacin

Naproxen

Opiates

Penicillins

Radiocontrast media, iodinated

Sulfonamides

Sulindac

Tartrazine (FD&C Yellow Dye no. 5)

Tolmetin

*Drugs Associated with Fixed
   Drug Eruptions*
Barbiturates
Captopril
Carbamazepine
Dapsone
Digitalis
Diphenhydramine
Disulfiram
Erythromycin
Foscarnet
Gold salts
Griseofulvin
Hydralazine
Hydroxyurea
Ibuprofen
Metronidazole
Phenolphthalein
Phenothiazines
Phenylbutazone
Quinidine
Quinine
Salicylates
Sulfasalazine
Sulfonamides
Sulindac
Tetracycline
Trimethoprim

*Drugs Associated with
   Maculopapular Eruptions*
Allopurinol
Barbiturates
Benzodiazepines
Captopril
Carbamazepine

Chloramphenicol
Ciprofloxacin
Erythromycin
Enalapril
Ethionamide
Etoposide
Gold salts
Ibuprofen
Indapamide
Indomethacin
Isoniazid
Lamotrigine
Methyldopa
Nitrofurantoin
Ofloxacin
Penicillamine
Penicillins
Phenothiazines
Phenylbutazone
Phenytoin
Piroxicam
Rifampin
Streptomycin
Sulfonamides
Sulfonylureas
Sulindac
Tetracyclines
Thiazides
Tolmetin

*Drugs Associated with
   Purpura*
Aspirin
Clopidogrel
Corticosteroids

Drugs Associated with Altered Pigmentation

Amiodarone

Bleomycin

Busulfan

Chloroquine/antimalarials

Corticotropin

Cyclophosphamide

Doxorubicin

Gold salts

Hypervitaminosis A

Mechlorethamine

Oral contraceptives

Phenothiazines

Drugs Associated with Hypertrichosis

Cyclosporin

Minoxidil

Phenytoin

Pulmonary Disorders

Drugs Associated with Bronchospasm/Airway Obstruction

ACE inhibitors

Adenosine

Allergen extracts

l-Asparaginase

Aspirin

Benzalkonium chloride

Beta-adrenergic antagonists

Cephalosporins

Cholinergic drugs

Inhalational agents and aerosols

Iron dextran

Local anesthetics

Narcotic analgesics

Nonsteroidal antiinflammatory agents

Pancreatic extract

Penicillins

Pentazocine

Phenylbutazone

Psyllium

Radiocontrast media, iodinated

Smoke

Sulfites

Sulfonamides

Streptomycin

Tartrazine (FD&C Yellow Dye no. 5)

Tetracyclines

Drugs Associated with Cough

ACE Inhibitors

Drugs Associated with Nasal Congestion

Decongestants (topical overuse)

Guanethidine

Hydralazine

Isoproterenol

Methyldopa

Oral contraceptives

Prazosin

Reserpine

Drugs Associated with Pulmonary Edema

Heroin

Hydrochlorothiazide

Interleukin-2

Methadone

Morphine

Oxygen

Propoxyphene

Radiocontrast media

Drugs Associated with Pulmonary Infiltrates/Fibrosis

Acyclovir

Amiodarone

Azathioprine

Bleomycin

Bromocriptine

Busulfan

Carmustine

Chlorambucil

Cyclophosphamide

Gold salts

Mecamylamine

Melphalan

Methotrexate

Methysergide

Mitomycin

Oxygen

Nitrofurantoin

Paraquat

Procarbazine

Sulfonamides

Drugs Associated with Pulmonary Infiltrates with Eosinophilia (Loeffler's Syndrome)

p-Aminosalicylic acid

Imipramine

Methotrexate

Minocycline

Nitrofurantoin

Penicillins

Sulfonamides

Drugs Associated with Central Respiratory Depression

Alcohol

Barbiturates

Benzodiazepines

Narcotic analgesics

Sedative-hypnotics

Drugs Associated with Respiratory Muscle Myopathy/Dysfunction

Aminocaproic acid

Aminoglycosides

Clofibrate

Corticosteroids

Diuretics

d-Penicillamine

Polymyxins

Neuromuscular blockers

Cardiovascular Disorders

Drugs Associated with Arrhythmias

Antiarrhythmic drugs

Astemizole

Atropine

Anticholinesterase agents

Beta-adrenergic antagonists

Cocaine

Daunorubicin

Digitalis

Diltiazem

Doxorubicin

Emetine

Erythromycin

5-Fluorouracil

Guanethidine

Lithium

Papaverine

Pentamidine

Phenothiazines

Sympathomimetics

Theophylline

Thyroid replacement

Tricyclic antidepressants

Verapamil

Drugs Associated with Angina Exacerbation

Alpha-adrenergic antagonists

Beta-blocker withdrawal

Ergotamine

5-Fluorouracil

Hydralazine

Methysergide

Minoxidil

Nifedipine

Oxytocin

Sumatriptan

Thyroid replacement (excessive)

Vasopressin

Drugs Associated with Cardiomyopathy

Daunorubicin

Doxorubicin

Emetine

Lithium

Phenothiazines

Sulfonamides

Sympathomimetics

Drugs Associated with Heart Failure Exacerbation/Fluid Retention/Pulmonary Edema

Beta-adrenergic antagonists

Calcium channel blockers

Carbenoxolone

Corticosteroids

Estrogens

Indomethacin

Intravenous fluids

Mannitol

Methadone

Minoxidil

Morphine

Phenylbutazone

Radiocontrast media

Sodium salts of drugs

Verapamil

Drugs Associated with Hypotension

Amiodarone

Calcium channel blockers

Diuretics

Dopamine agonists

Interleukin-2

Levodopa

Morphine

Nitroglycerin

Phenothiazines

Phenytoin (parenteral)

Procainamide

Protamine

Quinidine

Drugs Associated with Hypertension

Clonidine withdrawal

Corticotropin

Cyclosporine

Corticosteroids

MAO inhibitors with sympathomimetics

Nonsteroidal antiinflammatory agents

Oral contraceptives

Sympathomimetics

Tricyclic antidepressants with sympathomimetics

Drugs Associated with Hyperlipidemia

Alcohol

Beta-adrenergic antagonists

Corticosteroids

Cyclosporin

Isotretinoin

Progestins

Protease inhibitors

Thiazides

Drugs Associated with Pericarditis

Emetine

Hydralazine

Methysergide

Procainamide

Drugs Associated with Pericardial Effusion

Minoxidil

Drugs Associated with Thromboembolism

Oral contraceptives

Tamoxifen

Gastrointestinal Disorders

Drugs Associated with Dry Mouth

Anticholinergics

Clonidine

Levodopa

Methyldopa

Tricyclic antidepressants

Drugs Associated with Gingival Hyperplasia

Calcium channel blockers

Cyclosporine

Phenytoin

Drugs Associated with Tooth Discoloration

Tetracycline

Drugs Associated with Taste Disturbances

Acetazolamide

Captopril

Clarithromycin

Griseofulvin

Lithium

Metronidazole

Penicillamine

Rifampin

Drugs Associated with Nausea or Vomiting

Anthracyclines

Cisplatin

Dacarbazine

Digitalis

Ergotamines

Estrogens

Ferrous sulfate

Levodopa

Mechlorethamine

Opiates

Potassium chloride

Tetracyclines

Theophylline

*Drugs Associated with Oral
    Ulceration*

Cytotoxic agents

Gold salts

Methotrexate

Penicillamine

*Drugs Associated with Peptic
    Ulceration or Hemorrhage*

Aspirin

Corticosteroids

Ethacrynic acid

Nonsteroidal antiinflammatory
agents

Reserpine

*Drugs Associated with
    Cholestatic Hepatitis*

ACE inhibitors

Acetohexamide

Anabolic steroids

Androgens

Azathioprine

Chlorpropamide

Clavulanic acid/amoxicillin

Cyclosporine

Erythromycin estolate

Fluoroquinolones

Gold salts

Haloperidol

Ketoconazole

Lovastatin

Methimazole

Nitrofurantoin

Nonsteroidal antiinflammatory
agents

Oral contraceptives

Oxacillin

Phenothiazines

Phenylbutazone

Propylthiouracil

Rifampin

Sulfonamides

Tricyclic antidepressants

*Drugs Associated with
    Hepatocellular
    Damage/Drug-Induced
    Hepatitis*

Acetaminophen

Acebutolol

Alcohol

Allopurinol

Aminosalicylic acid

Amiodarone

Carbamazepine

Carbenicillin

Carmustine

Chlorpropamide

Corticosteroids

Cyclophosphamide

Methyldopa

Misoprostol

Oral contraceptives

Reserpine

Ticlopidine

Drugs Associated with Biliary Obstruction

Ceftriaxone

Drugs Associated with Pancreatitis

Aminosalicylic acid

Ampicillin

l-Asparaginase

Azathioprine

Bumetanide

Cimetidine

Chlorthalidone

Cisplatin

Clozapine

Corticosteroids

Cytarabine

Didanosine

Enalapril

Estrogens

Ethacrynic acid

Furosemide

Ifosfamide

Lisinopril

Mercaptopurine

Methyldopa

Metronidazole

Opiates

Oral contraceptives

Pentamidine

Phenformin

Piroxicam

Procainamide

Salicylates

Sulfonamides

Sulindac

Tetracycline

Thiazides

Valproic acid

Zalcitabine

Renal Disorders

Drugs Associated with Bladder Dysfunction

Anticholinergics

Disopyramide

MAO inhibitors

Tricyclic antidepressants

Drugs Associated with Hemorrhagic Cystitis

Cyclophosphamide

Ifosfamide

Drugs Associated with Hemodynamic/Prerenal Azotemia

ACE inhibitors

Calcium channel blockers

Cyclosporin

Diuretics

Muromonab

Nonsteroidal antiinflammatory agents

Radiocontrast media

Tacrolimus

Dantrolene

Dapsone

Diclofenac

Erythromycin estolate

Ethionamide

Felbamate

Fluoroquinolones

Glyburide

Halothane/inhaled anesthetics

Isoniazid

Ketoconazole

Labetalol

Lovastatin

MAO inhibitors

Mercaptopurine

Methimazole

Methotrexate

Methoxyflurane

Methyldopa

Mithramycin

Niacin

Nifedipine

Nitrofurantoin

Nonsteroidal antiinflammatory
agents

Oxyphenacetin

Phenylbutazone

Phenytoin

Propoxyphene

Propylthiouracil

Quinidine

Retinoic acid and derivatives

Rifampin

Salicylates

Sulfonamides

Tacrine

Tetracyclines

Trazodone

Tricyclic antidepressants

Valproic acid

Verapamil

Vitamin A (high doses)

Zidovudine

*Drugs Associated with
    Constipation or Ileus*

Aluminum hydroxide

Barium sulfate

Calcium carbonate

Ferrous sulfate

Ganglionic blockers

Ion exchange resins

Opiates

Phenothiazines

Tricyclic antidepressants

Verapamil

Vincristine

*Drugs Associated with
    Diarrhea or Colitis*

Antibiotics (broad spectrum)

Clindamycin

Cisplatin

Colchicine

Digitalis

Guanethidine

Lactose

Lincomycin

Magnesium-containing
    antacids

*Drugs Associated with
    Postrenal Obstruction*

Ganglionic blocking agents

Sulfonamides

*Drugs Associated with
    Interstitial Nephritis*

Acetaminophen

Acetazolamide

Acyclovir

Allopurinol

Amiloride

Aminoglycosides

p-Aminosalicylic acid

Amphotericin B

Aspirin

Azathioprine

Aztreonam

Captopril

Carbamazepine

Cephalosporins

Chlorthalidone

Cimetidine

Ciprofloxacin

Clofibrate

Cyclosporine

Erythromycin

Ethambutol

Furosemide

Glyburide

Gold salts

Interferon-alpha

Lithium

Methyldopa

Nonsteroidal antiinflammatory
  agents

Penicillins, especially
    methicillin

Phenindione

Phenobarbital

Phenylpropanolamine

Phenytoin

Polymyxins

Propylthiouracil

Radiocontrast media

Ranitidine

Rifampin

Sulfinpyrazone

Sulfonamides

Tacrolimus

Tetracycline

Thiazides

Triamterene

Valproic acid

Vancomycin

Warfarin

*Drugs Associated with
    Nephrolithiasis/Calculi*

Acetazolamide

Magnesium antacids

Topiramate

Triamterene

Vitamin D

*Drugs Associated with
    Nephropathies*

Analgesics (phenacetin)

*Drugs Associated with
    Nephrotic Syndrome*

Captopril

Gold salts

Ketoprofen

Penicillamine

Phenindione

Probenecid

*Drugs Associated with
    Proteinuria*

Analgesic nephropathy

Aminoglycosides

Cyclosporin

See also interstitial nephritis

*Drugs Associated with Renal
    Tubular Acidosis*

Acetazolamide

Amphotericin B

Cyclosporin

Lithium

Spironolactone

*Drugs Associated with
    Tubular Necrosis*

Acetaminophen overdose

Aminoglycosides

Amoxapine

Amphotericin B

Carboplatin

Cephaloridine

Cisplatin

Colistin

Cyclosporine

Dextran, low molecular weight

Foscarnet

Ifosfamide

Immune globulin, intravenous

Mannitol

Methoxyflurane

Nonsteroidal antiinflammatory
    agents

Pentamidine

Polymyxins

Radiocontrast media

Sulfonamides

Tetracyclines

Endocrine Disorders

*Drugs Associated with
    Addisonian-Like Syndrome*

Busulfan

Etomidate

Ketoconazole

*Drugs Associated with
    Decreased
    Libido/Impotence*

Beta-adrenergic antagonists

Carbamazepine

Clonidine

Diuretics

Lithium

Major tranquilizers

Methyldopa

Oral contraceptives

Phenobarbital

Phenytoin

Primidone

Sedatives

*Drugs Associated with
    Impaired Ejaculation*

Bethanidine

Fluoxetine

Guanethidine

Thioridazine

*Drugs Associated with
    Priapism*

Trazodone

*Drugs Associated with
    Gynecomastia*

Calcium channel blockers

Clomiphene

Digitalis

Estrogens

Ethionamide

Griseofulvin

Isoniazid

Methyldopa

Phenytoin

Reserpine

Spironolactone

Testosterone

*Drugs Associated with
    Galactorrhea*

Domperidone

Methyldopa

Metoclopramide

Phenothiazines

Reserpine

Tricyclic antidepressants

*Drugs Associated with Altered
    Thyroid Function or Tests*

Acetazolamide

Amiodarone

Chlorpropamide

Clofibrate

Colestipol

Nicotinic acid

Dimercaprol

Gold salts

Iodides

Lithium

Oral contraceptives

Phenindione

Phenothiazines

Phenylbutazone

Phenytoin

Sulfonamides

Tolbutamide

Metabolic Disorders

*Drugs Associated with
    Hypercalcemia*

Antacids with absorbable
  alkali

Calcium supplements

Lithium

Thiazides

Vitamin A

Vitamin D

*Drugs Associated with
    Hypocalcemia*

Barbiturates

Calcitonin

Cisplatin

Furosemide

Oral phosphorus supplements

Mithramycin

Phenytoin

*Drugs Associated with
    Hyperglycemia*

l-Asparaginase

Chlorthalidone

Corticosteroids

Diazoxide

Ethacrynic acid

Furosemide

Growth hormone

Niacin

Oral contraceptives

Pentamidine

Phenytoin

Thiazides

Drugs Associated with Hypoglycemia

Insulin

Octreotide

Oral hypoglycemics

Pentamidine

Quinine

Drugs Associated with Hyperkalemia

ACE inhibitors

Alpha-adrenergic agonists

Amiloride

Beta-adrenergic agonists

Cyclosporin

Cytotoxics

Heparin

Lithium

Nonsteroidal antiinflammatory agents

Pentamidine

Potassium supplements/salt substitutes

Potassium salts of drugs

Spironolactone

Succinylcholine

Triamterene

Trimethoprim

Drugs Associated with Hypokalemia

Amphotericin B

Carbenicillin

Carbenoxolone

Cisplatin

Corticosteroids

Diuretics

Drug-induced alkalosis

Gentamicin

Insulin

Laxative abuse

Mineralocorticoids

Osmotic diuretics

Sympathomimetics

Theophylline

Vitamin B_{12}

Drugs Associated with Hypernatremia

Acetohexamide

Alcohol

Amphotericin B

Cisplatin

Colchicine

Demeclocycline

Foscarnet

Glyburide

Lithium

Loop diuretics

Methoxyflurane

Norepinephrine

Osmotic diuretics

Phenytoin

Radiocontrast media

Tolazamide

Vinblastine

Vitamin D

Drugs Associated with Hyponatremia

Acetaminophen

Amitriptyline

Antipsychotics

Carbamazepine

Chlorpropamide

Clofibrate

Cyclophosphamide

Desmopressin

Diuretics

Enemas

Immune globulin, intravenous

Mannitol

Narcotic analgesics

Nicotine

Nonsteroidal antiinflammatory
  agents

Octreotide

Vincristine

*Drugs Associated with
  Hypomagnesemia*

Alcohol

Aminoglycosides

Amphotericin B

Cisplatin

Cyclosporin

Diuretics

Sodium loads

*Drugs Associated with
  Hypermagnesemia*

Lithium

Magnesium-containing
  antacids

*Drugs Associated with
  Hypophosphatemia*

Androgens

Antacids

Calcium salts

Corticosteroids

Diuretics

Glucose

Epinephrine

Fructose

Glucagon

Insulin

Lactate

Salicylates

Sucralfate

*Drugs Associated with
  Hyperuricemia*

Aspirin

Chlorthalidone

Cyclosporine

Cytotoxics

Ethacrynic acid

Furosemide

Hyperalimentation

Pyrazinamide

Thiazides

*Drugs Associated with
  Metabolic Acidosis*

Acetazolamide/carbonic
  anhydrase inhibitors

Ethylene glycol ingestion

Metformin

Methanol ingestion

Salicylates

Spironolactone

*Drugs Associated with
  Metabolic Alkalosis*

Antacids in renal failure

Carbenicillin, high doses

Diuretics

Milk-alkali syndrome ($CaCO_3$, $NaHCO_3$)

Penicillin, high doses

Hematologic Disorders

Drugs Associated with Agranulocytosis

Acetaminophen

Acetazolamide

Allopurinol

p-Aminosalicylic acid

Benzodiazepines

Beta-lactam antibiotics

Brompheniramine

Captopril

Carbamazepine

Carbimazole

Cefotaxime

Ceftriaxone

Chloramphenicol

Chlorpropamide

Cimetidine

Clindamycin

Clomipramine

Clozapine

Colchicine

Cotrimoxazole

Cytotoxics

Dapsone

Desipramine

Doxycycline

Ethacrynic acid

Ethosuximide

Flucytosine

Fosphenytoin

Furosemide

Ganciclovir

Gentamicin

Gold salts

Griseofulvin

Hydralazine

Hydroxychloroquine

Ibuprofen

Imipenem-cilastatin

Imipramine

Indomethacin

Isoniazid

Levodopa

Meprobamate

Methazolamide

Methimazole

Methyldopa

Metronidazole

Nitrofurantoin

Nonsteroidal antiinflammatory agents

Oxyphenbutazone

Penicillamine

Pentazocine

Phenothiazines

Phenylbutazone

Phenytoin

Primidone

Procainamide

Propranolol

Propylthiouracil

Pyrimethamine

Quinine

Rifampin

Streptomycin

Sulfonamides

Sulfonylureas

Thiazides

Ticlopidine

Tocainide

Tolbutamide

Tricyclic antidepressants

Vancomycin

Zidovudine

*Drugs Associated with
    Hemolytic Anemia*

Acetaminophen

p-Aminosalicylic acid

Cephalosporins

Chlorpromazine

Chlorpropamide

Dapsone

Hydralazine

Hydrochlorothiazide

Imipenem-cilastatin

Interferon alpha

Insulin

Isoniazid

Levodopa

Mefenamic acid

Melphalan

Methadone

Methyldopa

Methysergide

Nomifensine

Nonsteroidal antiinflammatory
    agents

Omeprazole

Penicillins

Phenacetin

Probenecid

Procainamide

Quinidine

Quinine

Rifampin

Streptomycin

Sulfonamides

Tacrolimus

Tetracycline

Tolbutamide

Triamterene

*Drugs Associated with
    Hemolytic Anemia in G6PD
    Deficiency*

p-Aminosalicylic acid

Aspirin

Chloramphenicol

Cotrimoxazole

Dapsone

Methylene Blue

Nalidixic acid

Nitrofurantoin

Phenacetin

Phenazopyridine

Primaquine/antimalarials

Probenecid

Procainamide

Quinidine

Sulfonamides

Vitamin C

Vitamin K

*Drugs Associated with
    Megaloblastic Anemia*
p-Aminosalicylic acid
Azathioprine
Chloramphenicol
Colchicine
Cyclophosphamide
Cytarabine
5-Fluorouracil
Folate antagonists
Hydroxyurea
Mercaptopurine
Methotrexate
Neomycin
Nitrofurantoin
Oral contraceptives
Phenobarbital
Phenytoin
Primidone
Pyrimethamine
Sulfasalazine
Triamterene
Trimethoprim
Vinblastine

*Drugs Associated with
    Aplastic Anemia*
Acetazolamide
Antihistamines
Carbamazepine
Carbimazole
Chloramphenicol
Chloroquine
Chlorothiazide
Cytotoxics

Felbamate
Furosemide
Gold salts
Indomethacin
Interferon-alpha
Mepacrine
Mephenytoin
Methimazole
Oxyphenbutazone
Penicillamine
Pentoxifylline
Phenobarbital
Phenothiazines
Phenylbutazone
Phenytoin
Potassium perchlorate
Propylthiouracil
Quinacrine
Quinidine
Sulfonamides
Sulfonylureas
Ticlopidine
Thiouracils
Trimethadione
Zidovudine

*Drugs Associated with
    Thrombocytopenia*
Abciximab
Acetazolamide
Allopurinol
Aminosalicylic acid
Amphotericin B
Amrinone
Aspirin

Carbamazepine
Carbenicillin
Chlorothiazide
Chlorpropamide
Chlorthalidone
Cimetidine
Colchicine
Co-trimoxazole
Desipramine
Diazepam
Didanosine
Digitoxin
Disopyramide
Fluconazole
Furosemide
Ganciclovir
Gold salts
Heparin
Hydrochlorothiazide
Hydroxychloroquine
Imipenem-cilastatin
Indomethacin
Interferon
Isoniazid
Meclofenamate
Methyldopa
Milrinone
Morphine
Moxalactam
Nonsteroidal antiinflammatory
  agents
Novobiocin
Oxyphenbutazone
Penicillin

Phenylbutazone
Phenytoin
Procainamide
Quinidine
Quinine
Rifabutin
Rifampin
Sulfisoxazole
Sulfonylureas
Thiazides
Ticarcillin
Ticlopidine
Trimethoprim
Valproic acid
Vancomycin

*Drugs Associated with Pure
  Red Cell Aplasia*

Azathioprine
Chlorpropamide
Isoniazid
Phenytoin

*Drugs Associated with
  Leucocytosis*

Corticosteroids
Lithium

*Drugs Associated with
  Eosinophilia*

p-Aminosalicylic acid
Chlorpropamide
Drug allergy
Erythromycin estolate
Imipramine
l-Tryptophan
Methotrexate

Nitrofurantoin

Procarbazine

Sulfonamides

Ocular Disorders

*Drugs Associated with Blurred
    Vision/Decreased Acuity*

Amantadine

Amiodarone

Carbamazepine

Chloroquine/hydroxychloroqu
    ine

Clomiphene

Cyclophosphamide

Cyclosporine

Digitalis

Fludarabine

Ibuprofen

Lithium

Mexiletine

Nalidixic acid

Nifedipine

Phenylbutazone

Piroxicam

Quinidine

Retinoids

Trimethadione

Vigabatrin

*Drugs Associated with Color
    Vision Disturbances*

Barbiturates

Digitalis

Ethambutol

Nalidixic acid

Sulfonamides

Thiazides

Trimethadione

*Drugs Associated with
    Glaucoma*

Corticosteroids

Ipratropium bromide

Mydriatics

Sympathomimetics

*Drugs Associated with
    Cataracts*

Allopurinol

Amiodarone

Busulfan

Carbamazepine

Chlorambucil

Corticosteroids

Deferoxamine

Gold salts

Phenothiazines

Phenytoin

*Drugs Associated with Optic
    Neuritis*

Aminosalicylic acid

Amiodarone

Chloramphenicol

Cisplatin

Clioquinol

Ethambutol

5-Fluorouracil

Ibuprofen

Isoniazid

Metronidazole

Minoxidil

Nalidixic acid

Penicillamine

Phenothiazines

Phenylbutazone

Quinine

Streptomycin

*Drugs Associated with
Retinopathy*

Chloroquine

Corticosteroids

Didanosine

Interferons

Leuprolide

Phenothiazines

Otic Disorders

*Drugs Associated with
Hearing Loss*

Aminoglycosides

Ampicillin

Aspirin

Bleomycin

Capreomycin

Carboplatin

Chloramphenicol

Chloroquine

Cisplatin

Colistin

Cotrimoxazole

Cytarabine

Dactinomycin

Deferoxamine

Erythromycin

Ethacrynic acid

Interferons

Loop diuretics

Mechlorethamine

Nonsteroidal antiinflammatory
agents

Nortriptyline

Oral contraceptives

Paromomycin

Polymixin B

Propoxyphene

Propylthiouracil

Quinidine

Quinine

Rifampin

Tricyclic antidepressants

Vincristine

*Drugs Associated with
Tinnitus*

Aminoglycosides

Aminophylline

Antihistamine

Antimalarials

Aspirin

Bleomycin

Caffeine

Capreomycin

Carbamazepine

Carboplatin

Clindamycin

Cytarabine

Dactinomycin

Deferoxamine

Doxycycline

Erythromycin

Ethacrynic acid

Haloperidol

Hydroxychloroquine

Levodopa

Lidocaine

Loop diuretics

MAO inhibitors

Mechlorethamine

Metaproterenol

Methotrexate

Metronidazole

Molindone

Morphine

Nonsteroidal antiinflammatory agents

Penicillamine

Pentazocine

Primaquine

Propoxyphene

Propranolol

Propylthiouracil

Quinidine

Quinine

Salicylates

Sulfonamides

Tetracycline

Thiabendazole

Tricyclic antidepressants

Vincristine

Drugs Associated with Vestibular Disturbances

Aminoglycosides

Chloroquine

Cisplatin

Cytarabine

Erythromycin

Ethacrynic acid

5-Fluorouracil

Indomethacin

Loop diuretics

Minocycline

Paromomycin

Quinidine

Quinine

Neurologic Disorders

Drugs Associated with Extrapyramidal Effects

Haloperidol

Levodopa

Methyldopa

Metoclopramide

Oral contraceptives

Phenothiazines

Reserpine

Tricyclic antidepressants

Drugs Associated with Peripheral Neuropathy

Amiodarone

Chloramphenicol

Chloroquine

Chlorpropamide

Cisplatin

Clioquinol

Clofibrate

Demeclocycline

Disopyramide

Ethambutol

Ethionamide

Glutethimide

Hydralazine

Isoniazid

Methysergide

Metronidazole

Nalidixic acid

Nitrofurantoin

Perhexiline

Phenelzine

Phenytoin

Polymyxin

Procarbazine

Streptomycin

Tolbutamide

Tricyclic antidepressants

Vinblastine

Vincristine

Drugs Associated with Seizures

Amphetamines

Analeptics

Antiepileptics

Bupropion

Imipenem

Isoniazid

Lidocaine

Lithium

Maprotiline

Meperidine

Nalidixic acid

Penicillins

Phenothiazines

Physostigmine

Theophylline

Tricyclic antidepressants

Vincristine

Drugs Associated with Tremor

Beta-adrenergic agonists

Valproic acid

Drugs Associated with Myasthenia Gravis Exacerbation

Aminoglycosides

Penicillamine

Musculoskeletal Disorders

Drugs Associated with Myopathy, Myalgia, Rhabdomyolysis

Amphotericin B

Carbenoxolone

Chloroquine

Cimetidine

Clofibrate

Corticosteroids

Gemfibrozil

Lovastatin

Oral contraceptives

Zidovudine

Drugs Associated with Osteomalacia

Aluminum hydroxide

Anticonvulsants

Glutethimide

Drugs Associated with Osteoporosis

Aluminum antacids

Anticonvulsants

Corticosteroids

Cyclosporin

Heparin

Lithium

Phenothiazines

Tetracycline

Psychiatric Disorders

*Drugs Associated with
Delirium, Confusion, or
Hallucinations*

Amantadine

Aminophylline

Anticholinergics

Antidepressants

Beta-adrenergic antagonists

Bromides

Cimetidine

Corticosteroids

Digitalis

Isoniazid

Levodopa

Meperidine

Methyldopa

Narcotic analgesics

Penicillins

Pentazocine

Phenothiazines

Ranitidine

Sedatives/hypnotics

Topiramate

Tricyclic antidepressants

Vigabatrin

*Drugs Associated with
Drowsiness*

Antiepileptics

Antihistamines

Anxiolytic drugs

Clonidine

Haloperidol

Methyldopa

Narcotic analgesics

Phenothiazines

Reserpine

Tricyclic antidepressants

*Drugs Associated with
Insomnia*

Amphetamines

Anorexiants

Corticosteroids (high dose,
oral)

Levodopa

Felbamate

SSRIs

Sympathomimetics

Theophylline

*Drugs Associated with
Depression*

Amphetamine withdrawal

Beta-adrenergic antagonists

Clonidine

Corticosteroids

Levodopa

Methyldopa

Reserpine

*Drugs Associated with Mania
or Excitation*

Corticosteroids

Levodopa

MAO inhibitors

Sympathomimetics

Tricyclic antidepressants

Drugs Associated with Schizophrenic/Paranoia Reactions

Amphetamines

Bromides

Corticosteroids

Levodopa

MAO inhibitors

Tricyclic antidepressants

Appendix I:
Medical Abbreviations, Terms, and Notations

A

$\bar{a}$ before

A₂   aortic second sound

AA   amino acid

AAA   abdominal aortic aneurysm

AAF   African American female

AAOC   antacid of choice

Abd   abdomen; abductor

ABE   acute bacterial endocarditis

ABG   arterial blood gases

ABO   blood group system (A, AB, B, and O)

ABW   actual body weight

ABX   antibiotics

AC   before meals

ACE   angiotensin-converting enzyme

ACLS   advanced cardiac life support

ACMV   assist-controlled mechanical ventilation

ACS   acute coronary syndrome

ACT   activated clotting time

ACTH   corticotropin (adrenocorticotrophic hormone)

ADD   attention deficit disorder

ADH   antidiuretic hormone

ADHD   attention deficit hyperactivity disorder

ADL   activities of daily living

ad lib   as desired; at liberty

ADM   admission

ADR   adverse drug reaction

AF   acid-fast; atrial fibrillation

AFB   acid-fast bacilli

AFEB   afebrile

A Fib   atrial fibrillation

Afl   atrial flutter

AFP   alpha-fetoprotein

AFVSS   afebrile, vital signs stable

AG   aminoglycoside; anion gap

A/G   albumin to globulin ratio

AGN   acute glomerulonephritis

AHCPR   Agency for Health Care, Policy, Research

AHF   antihemophilic factor

AHFS   American Hospital Formulary Service

AI   accidentally incurred; aortic insufficiency; artificial insemination

AICD   automatic implantable cardioverter/defibrillator

AIDS   acquired immunodeficiency syndrome

AIHA autoimmune hemolytic anemia

AIMS Abnormal Involuntary Movement Scale; Arthritis Impact Measurement Scales

AKA above-knee amputation

Alb albumin

ALG antilymphocyte globulin

ALL acute lymphoblastic leukemia; acute lymphocytic leukemia

ALS amyotrophic lateral sclerosis (Lou Gehrig Disease)

Al(OH)³ aluminum hydroxide

ALT alanine transaminase (SGPT)

AM adult male; morning (a.m.)

AMA against medical advice; American Medical Association

AMI acute myocardial infarction

AML acute myelogenous leukemia

AMP ampicillin; amputation

m-AMSA acridinyl anisidide

ANA antinuclear antibody

ANC absolute neutrophil count

ANF atrial natriuretic factor

ANLL acute nonlymphoblastic leukemia

ANT anterior

ante before

A & O alert and oriented

A&O × 3 awake and oriented to person, place, and time

AOC antacid of choice

AODA alcohol and other drug abuse

AODM adult onset diabetes mellitus

AOM acute otitis media

AP alkaline phosphatase; apical pulse

A&P anterior and posterior; assessment and plans; auscultation and percussion

A₂>P₂ second aortic sound greater than second pulmonic sound

APACHE Acute Physiology and Chronic Health Evaluation

APAP acetaminophen

APC aspirin, phenacetin, and caffeine; atrial premature contraction

appr. approximate

appt. appointment

APPY appendectomy

aPTT activated partial thromboplastin time

ARA-A vidarabine

ARA-C cytarabine

ARC AIDS related complex

ARDS adult respiratory distress syndrome

ARF acute renal failure; acute respiratory failure; acute rheumatic fever;

AS aortic stenosis

ASA aspirin (acetylsalicylic acid)

AS/AI aortic stenosis/aortic insufficiency

ASAP as soon as possible

ASCVD arteriosclerotic cardiovascular disease

ASD atrial septal defect

ASHD arteriosclerotic heart disease

ASO antistreptolysin-0 titer

AST aspartate transaminase (SGOT)

ATB antibiotic

ATC around the clock

At Fib atrial fibrillation

ATG antithymocyte globulin

ATN acute tubular necrosis

ATPase adenosine triphosphatase

AU both ears

AUC area under the curve

AVF arteriovenous fistula

AVM arteriovenous malformation

AVN arteriovenous nicking; atrioventricular node; avascular necrosis

AVR aortic valve replacement

AVSS all vital signs stable; afebrile, vital signs stable

AWI anterior wall infarct

AWOL absent without leave

ax axillary

AZA azathioprine

AZT zidovudine (azidothymidine)

B

B_1 thiamine HCl

B_2 riboflavin

B_2M beta 2 microglobulin

B_6 pyridoxine HCl

B_7 biotin

B_8 adenosine phosphate

B_{12} cyanocobalamin

BACOP bleomycin, adriamycin, cyclophosphamide, vincristine, and prednisone

BAD bipolar affective disorder

BaE barium enema

BAERs brain stem auditory evoked responses

BAL bronchoalveolar lavage

BAND band neutrophil (stab)

BBB bundle branch block

B Bx bone biopsy; breast biopsy

BC birth control; blood culture

BC/BS Blue Cross/Blue Shield

BCC basal cell carcinoma

BCCa basal cell carcinoma

B cell large lymphocyte

BCG bacillus Calmette-Guérin vaccine

BCNU carmustine

BCP birth control pills; carmustine, cyclophosphamide, and prednisone

BE barium enema; base excess

BEP bleomycin, etoposide, and cisplatin

BF black female

B. frag *Bacillus fragilis*

BIA bioimpedance assay

Bicarb bicarbonate

BID twice daily

BIL bilateral

Bili bilirubin

BKA below knee amputation

bl cult blood culture

BLEO bleomycin sulfate

BM black male; bone marrow; bowel movement

BMR basal metabolic rate

BMT bone marrow transplant

BO body odor

B & O belladonna and opium (suppositories)

BOM bilateral otitis media

BP bathroom privileges; blood pressure

BPD bronchopulmonary dysplasia

BPH benign prostatic hypertrophy

BPM beats per minute; breaths per minute

BPR blood per rectum

BRBPR bright red blood per rectum

BS blood sugar; bowel sounds; breath sounds

BSA body surface area

BSN Bachelor of Science in Nursing

BSO bilateral salpingo-oophorectomy

BUN blood urea nitrogen

Bx biopsy

C

C ascorbic acid; Celsius; Centigrade; hundred

ε with

CD$_4$ T-lymphocyte (helper)

C$_1$ . . . C$_7$ cervical nerve 1 through 7; cervical vertebra 1 through 7

CII controlled substance, class 2

CA carcinoma; cardiac arrest; carotid artery

Ca calcium

CAA crystalline amino acids

CABG coronary artery bypass graft

CaCO$_3$ calcium carbonate

CAD coronary artery disease

CAF cyclophosphamide, doxorubicin, and fluorouracil

CAH chronic active hepatitis

CAO chronic airway (airflow) obstruction

CAP capsule; community acquired pneumonia

Ca/P calcium to phosphorus ratio

CAPD chronic ambulatory peritoneal dialysis; continuous auto peril dialysis

CAT computed axial tomography

cath. catheter; catheterization

CBC complete blood count

CBD common bile duct

CBI continuous bladder irrigation

CBRF community-based residential facility

CBZ carbamazepine

CC chief complaint; cubic centimeter (cc), (mL)

CCE clubbing, cyanosis, and edema

CCNU lomustine

CCPD continuous cycling (cyclical) peritoneal dialysis

C$_{cr}$ creatinine clearance

CCU coronary care unit; critical care unit

CDB cough and deep breath

CDC Centers for Disease Control

CEA carcinoembryonic antigen; carotid endarterectomy

CEV cyclophosphamide, etoposide, and vincristine

CF cystic fibrosis

CFNS chills, fever, and night sweats

CHAD cyclophosphamide, adriamycin, cisplatin, and hexamethylmelamine

CHB complete heart block

CHD congenital heart disease

CHF congestive heart failure

CHOP cyclophosphamide, doxorubicin, vincristine, prednisone

CI cardiac index

CIG cigarettes

Cis-DDP cisplatin

CK creatine kinase

Cl chloride

CL/CP cleft lip and cleft palate

CLL chronic lymphocytic leukemia

Cl liq clear liquid

CM Caucasian male; centimeter (cm)

cm^3 cubic centimeter

CMC carpal metacarpal (joint)

CMF cyclophosphamide, methotrexate, and fluorouracil

CMG cystometrogram

CMI cell-mediated immunity

CML chronic myelogenous leukemia

CMML chronic myelomonocytic leukemia

CMV cytomegalovirus

CN cranial nerve

CN II–XII cranial nerves 2 through 12

CNS central nervous system; Clinical Nurse Specialist

CO carbon monoxide; cardiac output

C/O complained of

CO_2 carbon dioxide

COAD chronic obstructive airway disease

COPD chronic obstructive pulmonary disease

CP cerebral palsy chest pain

CPAP continuous positive airway pressure

CPB cardiopulmonary bypass

CPK creatinine phosphokinase (BB, MB, MM are isoenzymes)

CPmax peak serum concentration

CPmin trough serum concentration

CPP cerebral perfusion pressure

CPPB continuous positive pressure breathing

CPR cardiopulmonary resuscitation

CPT chest physiotherapy

CR controlled release

CR_1 first cranial nerve

CrCl creatinine clearance

CREST calcinosis, Raynaud's, esophageal dysmotility, sclerodactylia, and telangiectasia

CRF chronic renal failure

CRIT hematocrit

C&S culture and sensitivity

C/S culture and sensitivity

CsA or CSA cyclosporin

CSF cerebrospinal fluid; colony-stimulating factors

CT chest tube; computed tomography

CTA clear to auscultation

CT & DB cough, turn, and deep breath

CTX cyclophosphamide (Cytoxan®)

CTZ chemoreceptor trigger zone

Cu copper

CUP carcinoma of unknown primary (site)

CV cardiovascular

CVA cerebrovascular accident; costovertebral angle

CVAT costovertebral angle tenderness

CVP central venous pressure

CVS cardiovascular surgery

Cx cervix; culture

CXR chest x-ray

CYSTO cystoscopy

D

D day; diarrhea

D4T stavudine

D50 50% dextrose injection

DA dopamine; drug addict

DAT daunorubicin, cytarabine, (ARA-C), and thioguanine

DAW dispense as written

DB date of birth

DBP diastolic blood pressure

d/c, DC decrease; discharge; discontinue

DDAVP® desmopressin acetate

DDC zalcitabine

DEA# Drug Enforcement Administration number

DDI didanosine

Decub decubitus

DES diethylstilbestrol

DFO deferoxamine

DHPG ganciclovir

DI diabetes insipidus; drug interactions; drug information

D&I dry and intact

DIC disseminated intravascular coagulation

DIFF differential blood count

DIG digoxin

DIP distal interphalangeal (joint)

DJD degenerative joint disease

DKA diabetic ketoacidosis

D_L maximal diffusing capacity

D5LR dextrose 5% in lactated Ringer's solution

DM dermatomyositis; Dextromethorphan; diabetes mellitus

DMARD disease modifying antirheumatic drug

DME durable medical equipment

D_5 1/2NS dextrose 5% in 0.45% sodium chloride solution

DNI do not intubate

DNR do not resuscitate

D_5NSS 5% dextrose in normal saline solution

DO Doctor of Osteopathy

DOA date of admission; dead on arrival

DOB date of birth

DOC drug of choice

DOE dyspnea on exertion

DOSS docusate sodium (dioctyl sodium sulfosuccinate)

DP diastolic pressure; dorsalis pedis (pulse)

DPH phenytoin (diphenylhydantoin)

DPT diphtheria, pertussis, and tetanus (immunization)

DPUD duodenal peptic ulcer disease

Dr. doctor

DRG diagnosis-related groups

DS double strength

DSA digital subtraction angiography

DSMIII Diagnostic & Statistical Manual, 3rd Edition

DSMIV Diagnostic & Statistical Manual, 4th Edition

DSS docusate sodium

DST dexamethasone suppression test

DT delirium tremens; diphtheria tetanus; diphtheria toxoid

DTIC dacarbazine

DTR deep tendon reflexes

DTs delirium tremens

DUE drug use evaluation

DUI driving under the influence

DUR drug use review; duration

DVI atrioventricular sequential pacing; digital vascular imaging

DVM Doctor of Veterinary Medicine

DVT deep vein thrombosis

D$_5$W 5% dextrose in water solution

DWI driving while intoxicated

Dx diagnosis

E

EC enteric coated

ECG electrocardiogram

ECHO echocardiogram

ECM erythema chronicum migrans

ECMO extracorporeal membrane oxygenation (oxygenator)

ECOG Eastern Cooperative Oncology Group

ECT electroconvulsive therapy

ED emergency department

EDTA edetic acid (ethylenediamine tetraacetic acid)

EEG electroencephalogram

EENT eyes, ears, nose, and throat

EES® erythromycin ethylsuccinate

EF ejection fraction

EFAD essential fatty acid deficiency

e.g. for example

EKG electrocardiogram

ELISA enzyme-linked immunosorbent assay

Elix elixir

EMD electromechanical dissociation

EMG electromyelogram; electromyograph

EMIT enzyme multiplied immunoassay technique

EMS emergency medical services; eosinophilia myalgia syndrome

EMT emergency medical technician

ENDO endoscopy

ENT   ears, nose, throat

EOC   enema of choice

EOM   external otitis media; extraocular movement

EOMI   extraocular muscles intact

EOS   eosinophil

EPI   epinephrine

EPO   erythropoietin

EPS   electrophysiologic study; extrapyramidal syndrome (symptom)

EPSE   extrapyramidal side effect

EPT®   early pregnancy test

ER   emergency room

ER+   estrogen receptor-positive

ERCP   endoscopic retrograde cholangiopancreatography

ESR   erythrocyte sedimentation rate

ESRD   end-stage renal disease

ET   endotracheal

et   and

et al   and others

ETC   and so forth; estimated time of conception

ETCO$_2$ end tidal carbon dioxide

ETOH   alcohol

ETT   endotracheal tube; exercise tolerance test; exercise thallium test

Exp. Lap.   exploratory laparotomy

EXT   extension; extremity

F

F   Fahrenheit; female

F II   factor II (two)

F VIII   factor VIII (8)

FA   folic acid

FAB   digoxin immune Fab (Digibind®)

FABER   flexion, abduction, and external rotation

FAS   fetal alcohol syndrome

FB   fasting blood (sugar); foreign body

FBRCM   fingerbreadth below right costal margin

FBS   fasting blood sugar

5-FC   flucytosine

FC   fever, chills

F & D   fixed and dilated

FDA   Food and Drug Administration

FDP   fibrin-degradation products

FDS   first day surgery; for duration of stay

Fe   iron

FEM   femoral

Fem-Pop   femoral popliteal (bypass)

FeSO$_4$ ferrous sulfate

FEV$_1$ forced expiratory volume in one second

FFP   fresh frozen plasma

FH   family history

FiCO$_2$ fraction of inspired carbon dioxide

FiO$_2$ fraction of inspired oxygen

FMH family medical history

F+N fever and neutropenia

FSH follicle stimulating hormone

FSP fibrin split products

FT foot (ft)

FT$_3$ free triiodothyronine

FT$_4$ free thyroxine

F/U follow-up

5-FU fluorouracil

FUO fever of undetermined (unknown) origin

FVC forced vital capacity

Fx fracture

FXN function

FYI for your information

G

G gram (g); gravida

G+ Gram-positive

G− Gram-negative

Ga gallium

GABA gamma-aminobutyric acid

Ga scan gallium scan

GC *gonococci* (gonorrhea)

GCSF granulocyte colony-stimulating factor

GE gastroesophageal

GENT gentamicin

GERD gastroesophageal reflux disease

GFR glomerular filtration rate

GGT gamma-glutamyl transpeptidase

GH growth hormone

GI gastrointestinal

GM+ Gram-positive

GM− Gram-negative

gm% grams per 100 milliliters

GMC general medical clinic

GIMC general internal medicine clinic

GM-CSF granulocyte macrophage colony stimulating factor

GN glomerulonephritis

GNB Gram-negative bacilli

GNR Gram-negative rods

GP general practitioner

G/P gravida/para

GpIIa/IIIb glycoprotein 2b/3a inhibitor

G$_3$P$_3$ 3 pregnancies (gravida), 3 went to term

GPC Gram-positive cocci

GRD gastroesophageal reflux disease

Gr$_2$P$_1$AB$_1$ two pregnancies, one birth, and one abortion

GSW gunshot wound

GT gastrostomy tube

GTT drop; glucose tolerance test

GU genitourinary

GVHD graft-versus-host disease

H

H heart; hydrogen

HA headache; hemolytic anemia; hyperalimentation

HAT hepatic artery thrombosis

HAV hepatitis A vaccine

HbA$_{1c}$ glycosylated hemoglobin

HB$_e$ AB hepatitis B$_e$ antibody

HB$_c$Ag hepatitis B$_c$ antigen

HB$_e$ AG hepatitis B$_e$ antigen

HBIG hepatitis B immune globulin

HbS sickle cell hemoglobin

HbsAg hepatitis B surface antigen

HbSC sickle cell hemoglobin C

HAART highly active antiretroviral therapy

HBV hepatitis B vaccine; hepatitis B virus

HC hydrocortisone

HCG human chorionic gonadotropin

HCO$_3$ bicarbonate

HCT hematocrit

HCTZ hydrochlorothiazide

HD hemodialysis; Hodgkin's disease

HDL high-density lipoprotein

HEENT head, eyes, ears, nose, and throat

HEPA high efficiency particular air

H flu *Hemophilius influenzae*

HG hemoglobin

Hgb hemoglobin

HH hiatal hernia

H&H hematocrit and hemoglobin

HHC home health care

HI head injury

Hi-cal high caloric

HIV human immunodeficiency virus

HIV-RNA viral load

HJR hepato-jugular reflex

HLA (−) heart, lungs, and abdomen negative

HLA human lymphocyte antigen

HMO Health Maintenance Organization

H&N head and neck

HO house officer

H/O history of

H$_2$O water

H$_2$O$_2$ hydrogen peroxide

HOB head of bed

H&P history and physical

HPI history of present illness

HPLC high-pressure (performance) liquid chromatography

HR   heart rate; hour

HS   bedtime; herpes simplex

HSC   human subjects committee

HSV   herpes simplex virus

HSVI   herpes simplex virus type 1

HSVII   herpes simplex virus type II

HT   height; hypertension

HTN   hypertension

HUC   health unit coordinator

Hx   history

HZV   herpes zoster virus

I

IABP   intra-aortic balloon pump

IBD   inflammatory bowel disease

IBS   irritable bowel syndrome

IBW   ideal body weight

ICF   intermediate care facility

ICP   intracranial pressure

ID   identification; infectious disease (physician or department); intradermal

IDS   Investigational Drug Service

I&D   incision and drainage

IDDM   insulin-dependent diabetes mellitus

i.e.   that is

IF   interferon; internal fixation

IFN   interferon

IFOS   ifosfamide

IgA   immunoglobulin A

IgD   immunoglobulin D

IGDM   infant of gestational diabetic mother

IgE   immunoglobulin E

IgG   immunoglobulin G

IGIV   immune globulin intravenous

IgM   immunoglobulin M

IHSS   idiopathic hypertrophic subaortic stenosis

IJ   internal jugular

IL$_{( )}$ interleukin (1, 2, etc.)

IM   intramuscular

IMC   intermediate care intermediate care unit

IMI   inferior myocardial infarction

IMP   impression

In   inches

Inc Spir, IS   incentive spirometer

IND   Investigational New Drug

ING   inguinal

✓ing   checking

INH   isoniazid

INR   international normalization ratio

Inj   injection; injury

Inpt   inpatient

INR   international normalized ratio

Intol   intolerance

Intub   intubation

I&O intake and output

IO intraocular pressure

IOF intraocular fluid

IOP intraocular pressure

IP intraperitoneal

IPG impedance plethysmography

IPN intern's progress note

IPP inflatable penile prosthesis

IPPB intermittent positive pressure breathing

IQ intelligence quotient

IRB institutional review board

IRR irrigate

Irreg irregular

IT intrathecal

ITP idiopathic thrombocytopenia purpura

IU international unit

IV four; intravenous (i.v.); symbol for class 4 controlled substances

IVC inferior vena caval filter

IVF intravenous fluid(s)

IVH intraventricular hemorrhage

IVIG intravenous immunoglobulin

IVP intravenous push; intravenous pyelogram

IVPB intravenous piggyback

J

Jnt joint

JODM juvenile onset diabetes mellitus

JP Jackson-Pratt (drain)

JRA juvenile rheumatoid arthritis

JT jejunostomy tube joint

J-Tube jejunostomy tube

Juv. juvenile

JVD jugular venous distention

JVP jugular venous pressure; jugular venous pulse

K

K potassium; thousand; vitamin K

K/PTx kidney/pancreas transplant

K₁ phytonadione

KA ketoacidosis

kcal kilocalorie

KCl potassium chloride

KD Kawasaki's disease

KDA known drug allergies

kg kilogram

KI potassium iodide

kilo kilogram

KISS saturated solution of potassium iodide

Kleb Klebsiella

KMnO₄ potassium permanganate

KO keep open

KOH potassium hydroxide

KTx kidney transplant

KUB   kidney, ureter, and bladder

KVO   keep vein open

KW   Keith-Wagener (ophthalmoscopic finding, graded I-IV)

L

L   fifty; left; lente (insulin); liter

L̲   left

L₁–L₅   lumbar nerve 1 through 5; lumbar vertebra 1 through 5

LA   left atrial; left atrium; local anesthesia

L+A   light and accommodation

LAD   left anterior descending

LAK   lymphokine-activated killer

LAM   laminectomy

LAP   laparoscopy; laparotomy

L-ASP   asparaginase

LAT   lateral

LB   low back; pound

LBP   low back pain

LBW   lean body weight

LCD   coal tar solution (*liquor carbonis detergens*)

LCFA   long-chain fatty acid

LCM   left costal margin

LD   lactic dehydrogenase (formerly LDH); learning disability; lethal dose; living donor; loading dose

LDH   lactic dehydrogenase (see LD)

LDL   low-density lipoprotein

L-dopa   levodopa

LE   left ear; left eye; lower extremities; lupus erythematous

LES   lower esophageal sphincter

LF   left foot

LFT(s)   liver function test(s)

LG   large

LH   left hand; luteinizing hormone

LHF   left heart failure

Li   lithium

LICM   left intercostal margin

Li₂CO₃   lithium carbonate

Lido   lidocaine

LIG   ligament

LIH   left inguinal hernia

LIQ   liquid

LIS   left intercostal space; low intermittent suction

LK   left kidney

LKS   liver, kidneys, spleen

LL   left leg; left lower; left lung; lower lid; lower lobe; lymphocytic leukemia

LLE   left lower extremity

LLL   left lower lid; left lower lobe (lung)

LLQ   left lower quadrant (abdomen exam)

LMD   local medical doctor; low molecular weight dextran

L/min   liters per minute

LMP   last menstrual period

LMWD   low molecular weight dextran

LMWH   low molecular weight heparin

LOA   leave of absence

LOC   laxative of choice; loss of consciousness

LOM   left otitis media; loss of motion

LOS   length of stay

LOZ   lozenge

LP   lumbar puncture

LPA   left pulmonary artery

LPN   Licensed Practical Nurse

LR   lactated Ringer's (solution)

L→R   left to right

LRD   living related donor

LS   left side; liver spleen; lumbosacral

L-Spar   Elspar (asparaginase)

LT   left; light

LTB   laryngotracheo-bronchitis

LTC   long-term care

LTCF   long-term care facility

LUL   left upper lobe (lung)

LV   left ventricle

LVDP   left ventricular diastolic pressure

LVEDP   left ventricular end diastolic pressure

LVEDV   left ventricular end diastolic volume

LVEF   left ventricular ejection fraction

LVF   left ventricular failure

LVFP   left ventricular filling pressure

LVG   living

LVH   left ventricular hypertrophy

LVP   large volume parenteral; left ventricular pressure

Lymphs   lymphocytes

Lytes   electrolytes (Na, K, Cl, CO_2)

M

M   male; meter (m); molar; Monday; thousand

MA   medical assistance

MAB   monoclonal antibody

MABP   mean arterial blood pressure

Mag Cit   magnesium citrate

Mag Sulf   magnesium sulfate

Malig   malignant

m-AMSA   amsacrine

MAOI   monoamine oxidase inhibitor

MAP   mean airway pressure; mean arterial pressure

MAR   medication administration record

MAST   mastectomy

Max   maximal

MBC   minimal bacteriocidal concentration

MBD minimal brain dysfunction

MCA motorcycle accident

mcg microgram (μg)

mcg/kg/min microgram per kilogram per minute

MCH mean corpuscular hemoglobin

MCHC mean corpuscular hemoglobin concentration

MCT medium chain triglyceride

MD manic depression; medical doctor; multi-dose

MDE major depressive episode

MDI metered dose inhaler

MDR minimum daily requirement

MEC meconium

MED medial; medication; medicine medium

mEq milliequivalent

mEq/24 H milliequivalents per 24 hours

mEq/L milliequivalents per liter

MET medical emergency treatment; metastasis

METS metastasis

MG milligram (mg)

Mg magnesium

mg% milligrams per 100 milliliters

mg/dL milligrams per 100 milliliters

MGF maternal grandfather

mg/kg milligram per kilogram

mg/kg/hr milligram per kilogram per hour

MGM maternal grandmother

MGN membranous glomerulonephritis

MgO magnesium oxide

MgSO₄ magnesium sulfate (Epsom salt)

MI mitral insufficiency; myocardial infarction

MIC minimum inhibitory concentration

MIN minimum; minute (min)

MIP metacarpo-interphalangeal (joint)

MISC miscellaneous

mL milliliter

MLC mixed lymphocyte culture

MLNS mucocutaneous lymph node syndrome

MM malignant melanoma; millimeter (mm); mucous membrane

mM. millimole

M&M morbidity and mortality

mmHg millimeters of mercury

mmol millimole

MMP multiple medical problems

MMPI Minnesota Multiphasic Personality Inventory

MMR measles, mumps, and rubella

MMWR Morbidity & Mortality Weekly Report

MN midnight

Mn manganese

MO month (mo); months old

MOA mechanism of action

MoAb monoclonal antibody

MOM milk of magnesia

mono. infectious mononucleosis

MOPP mechlorethamine vincristine procarbazine prednisone

mOsm milliosmole

mOsmol milliosmole

6-MP mercaptopurine

MPGN membranoproliferative glomerulonephritis

MPSS methylprednisolone sodium succinate

MR magnetic resonance; may repeat; mental retardation; mitral regurgitation

MR × 1 may repeat times one (once)

MRI magnetic resonance imaging

MRM modified radial mastectomy

MRSA methicillin-resistant *Staphylococcus aureus*

MRSE methicillin-resistant *staphylococcus epidermitis*

MS mental status; mitral stenosis; morphine sulfate; multiple sclerosis; muscle strength

MSE Mental Status Examination

MSH melanocyte-stimulating hormone

MSIR® morphine sulfate immediate release tablets

MSL midsternal line

MSPN medical student progress notes

MSW Master of Social Work

MT metatarsal

MTX methotrexate

MU million units

mU milliunits

MUE medication usage evaluation

MUGA multiple gated acquisition

MV millivolts; mitral valve; multiple vitamin (po)

MVA motor vehicle accident

M-VAC methotrexate, vinblastine, doxorubicin, and cisplatin

MVAC methotrexate, vinblastine, doxorubicin, and cisplatin

MVI multiple vitamin injection

MVI® trade name for parenteral multi-vitamins

MVI 12® trade name for parenteral multivitamins

MVO₂ myocardial oxygen consumption

MVR mitral valve regurgitation; mitral valve replacement

Myelo myelocytes

N

N negative; Negro; nerve; normal; NPH insulin; size of sample

N₂ nitrogen

Na sodium

NA Native American; not applicable; not available; nursing assistant

NaCl sodium chloride (salt)

NAD no acute distress; no apparent distress

NaF sodium fluoride

NAF nafcillin

NaHCO₃ sodium bicarbonate

NaI sodium iodide

NAPA N-acetyl procainamide

Na Pent Pentothal Sodium®

NARC narcotic(s)

NAS no added salt

NB note well

NC nasal cannula; no change

NCI National Cancer Institute

NDA New Drug Application

NE norepinephrine

NEC necrotizing enterocolitis

NEG negative

NF Negro female

NG nanogram; nasogastric

NGB neurogenic bladder

NGR nasogastric replacement

NGU nongonococcal urethritis

NGT nasogastric tube

NH nursing home

NH₃ ammonia

NH₄Cl ammonium chloride

NHL non-Hodgkin's lymphomas

NICU neonatal intensive care unit

NIDD non–insulin-dependent diabetes

NIDDM non–insulin-dependent diabetes mellitus

NIH National Institutes of Health

Nitro nitroglycerin

NJ nasojejunal

NKA no known allergies

NKDA no known drug allergies

NKMA no known medication allergies

NL normal

NLT not later than; not less than

NM neuromuscular

nmol nanomole

NMP normal menstrual period

NMR nuclear magnetic resonance (same as magnetic resonance imaging)

NMS neuroleptic malignant syndrome

NMT not more than

NN neonatal

NO nitrous oxide

N_2O nitrous oxide

$N_2O:O_2$ nitrous oxide to oxygen ratio

Noc. night

Noct nocturnal

NOR-EPI norepinephrine

Norm normal

NP nasal prongs; nurse practitioner

NPH Isophane insulin

NPO nothing by mouth

NPR normal per rectum

NPT nocturnal penile tumescence

NQWM1 non–Q-wave myocardial infarction

NR no refills; no response

NRC Nuclear Regulatory Commission

NREM nonrapid eye movement

NREMS nonrapid eye movement sleep

NS normal saline solution (0.9% sodium chloride solution); not significant

NSA normal serum albumin

NSAIA nonsteroidal anti-inflammatory agent

NSAID nonsteroidal anti-inflammatory drug

NSC no significant change

NSG nursing

NSR normal sinus rhythm

1/2 NSS sodium chloride 0.45% (or 1/2 normal saline solution)

NSVD normal spontaneous vaginal delivery

NSY nursery

NT nasotracheal

NTI nortriptyline

N&T nose and throat

NTE not to exceed

NTG nitroglycerin

NTP Nitropaste® (nitroglycerin ointment); sodium nitroprusside

NTT nasotracheal tube

Nullip nullipara

NV nausea and vomiting

N&V nausea and vomiting

NVD nausea, vomiting, and diarrhea; neck vein distention

NYHA New York Heart Association (classification for heart disease)

O

O eye; objective findings; oral; oxygen; zero

O_2 oxygen

OA osteoarthritis

OB obstetrics

OBG obstetrics and gynecology

Ob-Gyn obstetrics and gynecology

Obj objective

Obl oblique

OC on call; oral contraceptive

Occl occlusion

Occup Rx occupational therapy

OCD obsessive-compulsive disorder

OCP ova, cysts, parasites; oral contraceptive pills

OD Doctor of Optometry; overdose; right eye

OI opportunistic infections

OJ orange juice

OK all right

OKT$_3$ muromonab

OLT orthotopic liver transplantation

OM otitis media

ON Ortho-Novum®

ONC oncology

OOB out of bed

OOC out of control

OP outpatient

O&P ova and parasites

op cit in the work cited

OPP opposite; outpatient pharmacy

OPS operations; outpatient surgery

OPV oral polio vaccine

OR operating room; open reduction

ORCH orchiectomy

ORIF open reduction internal fixation

ORN operating room nurse

OR × 1 oriented to time

OR × 2 oriented to time and place

OR × 3 oriented to time, place, and person

OS left eye; ophthalmic suspension; ophthalmic solution

OSHA Occupational Safety & Health Administration

OSN off service note

OSS osseous

OT occupational therapy

OTC over the counter

OTD out the door

OTH other

OTO otology

OT/RT occupational therapy/recreational therapy

OU both eyes

oz ounce

P

P para; peripheral; phosphorus; pint; plan; protein

p̄ after

P450 cytochrome oxidase metabolic enzymes

PA physician assistant; posterior-anterior; pulmonary artery

P&A percussion and auscultation

PAB premature atrial beat

PAC premature atrial contraction

PaCO$_2$ partial arterial carbon dioxide tension

PACU post anesthesia care unit

PAE postantibiotic effect

PAF paroxysmal atrial fibrillation

PAH pulmonary arterial hypertension

Pa Line pulmonary artery line

PALN para-aortic lymph node

PALS pediatric advanced life support

2-PAM pralidoxime

PAN polyarteritis nodosa

PAO$_2$ partial arterial oxygen tension

PAP prostatic acid phosphatase; pulmonary artery pressure

Pap smear Papanicolaou smear

PAR postanesthetic recovery

PARA number of pregnancies

para paraplegic

PAS pulmonary artery stenosis

PAT paroxysmal atrial tachycardia

Path. pathology

PAWP pulmonary artery wedge pressure

PB phenobarbital

Pb lead; phenobarbital

PBI protein-bound iodine

PBN polymyxin B sulfate, bacitracin, and neomycin

PBS phosphate-buffered saline

PBZ phenoxybenzamine; phenylbutazone

ΦBZ phenylbutazone

PC after meals; packed cells

PCA patient controlled analgesia

PCBs polychlorinated biphenyls

PCE® erythromycin particles in tablets

PC&HS after meals and at bedtime

PCKD polycystic kidney disease

PCI percutaneous coronary intervention

PCM protein-calorie malnutrition

PCN penicillin

PCO$_2$ carbon dioxide pressure (or tension)

PCP phencyclidine; *Pneumocystis carinii* pneumonia

PCV packed cell volume

PCWP pulmonary capillary wedge pressure

PD peritoneal dialysis

PDA patent ductus arteriosus

PDE paroxysmal dyspnea on exertion

PDN prednisone

PDR Physician's Desk Reference

PE physical examination; physical exercise; pulmonary edema; pulmonary embolism

P_1E_1® epinephrine 1%, pilocarpine 1% ophthalmic solution

PEARLA pupils equal and react to light and accommodation

PEB cisplatin, etoposide, and bleomycin

Peds pediatrics

PEEP positive end-expiratory pressure

PEG percutaneous endoscopic; gastrostomy; polyethylene glycol

PEN penicillin

PERC percutaneous

Perf. perforation

PeriCare perineum care

PERL pupils equal, reactive to light

per os by mouth

PERRLA pupils, equal, round, reactive to light and accommodation

PERRRLA pupils equal, round, regular, react to light and accommodation

PET position-emission tomography

PETN pentaerythritol tetranitrate

PEx physical examination

PF preservative free

PFC persistent fetal circulation

PFT pulmonary function test

PG pregnant

PGE posterior gastroenterostomy prostaglandin E

PGE2 prostaglandin E2

PG-1 post-graduate year one

PG-2 post-graduate year two

PG-3 post-graduate year three

PH past history

PHA pharmacist assistant

Pharm Pharmacy

PharmD Doctor of Pharmacy

PICC peripherally inserted central catheter

PID pelvic inflammatory disease

Pit Pitocin®

PIV peripheral intravenous

PKU phenylketonuria

PLS plastic surgery

PLT platelet

plts platelets

PM afternoon; pacemaker; petit mal; polymyositis

PMD private medical doctor

PMH past medical history

PMI past medical illness; point of maximal impulse

PMN polymorphonuclear leukocyte

PMP previous menstrual period

PMS premenstrual syndrome

PNB percutaneous needle biopsy; pulseless nonbreather

PNC penicillin

PND paroxysmal nocturnal dyspnea

PNET- primitive neuroectodermal tumors-MB medulloblastoma

PO by mouth (*per os*)

PO$_2$ partial pressure of oxygen

PO$_4$ phosphate

POD 1 postoperative day one

POMP prednisone, vincristine, methotrexate, and mercaptopurine

poplit popliteal

POS positive

"POST" post mortem examination (autopsy)

Post op postoperative

P&P policy and procedure

PPB positive pressure breathing

PPD packs per day; purified protein derivative (tuberculin skin test)

PPI patient package insert

PPM parts per million

PPNG Penicillinase producing *Neisseria gonorrhoeae*

PPO preferred provider organization

PR patient relations; per rectum

PRBC packed red blood cells

PRC packed red cells

Pred prednisone

Pre-op before surgery

Prep prepare for surgery

PRN as occasion requires

PRO protein; prothrombin

PROM passive range of motion

PSA prostate-specific antigen

PSF posterior spinal fusion

PSGN post streptococcal glomerulonephritis

PSI pounds per square inch

PSVT paroxysmal supraventricular tachycardia

PT paroxysmal tachycardia; patient physical therapy or therapist; pint; prothrombin time

P&T Pharmacy and Therapeutics; peak and trough

PTA percutaneous transluminal angioplasty; prior to admission

PTCA percutaneous transluminal coronary angioplasty

PTH parathyroid hormone

PTLD post-transplant lymphoproliferative disorder

PTSD post-traumatic stress disorder

PTT partial thromboplastin time

PTU propylthiouracil

PU peptic ulcer

PUD peptic ulcer disease

PUFA polyunsaturated fatty acids

pul. pulmonary

PUVA psoralen-ultraviolet-light (treatment)

PV per vagina

PVB premature ventricular beat

PVC polyvinyl chloride; premature ventricular contraction

PVD peripheral vascular disease

PVK penicillin V potassium

PVR peripheral vascular resistance; postvoiding residual; pulse-volume recording

PVT private

PWB partial weight bearing

PWP pulmonary wedge pressure

Px physical exam; pneumothorax; prognosis

PZI protamine zinc insulin

Q

q every

QA quality assurance

QAM every morning

QC quality control

qd every day

q2h every two hours

qh every hour

qhs every night

qid four times daily

qod every other day

qpm every evening

qt quart

qwk once a week

R

R rectum; regular; respiration; right

R̲ right

RA rheumatoid arthritis; right atrium; room air

RAA renin-angiotensin-aldosterone

RAD ionizing radiation unit; reactive airway disease

RAN resident's admission notes

RAS renal artery stenosis

RBBB right bundle branch block

RCA right coronary artery

RCC renal cell carcinoma

RCM right costal margin

R.D. Registered Dietitian

RDA recommended daily allowance

RDS respiratory distress syndrome

RDW red (cell) distribution width

RE reticuloendothelial; right ear

RE ✓ recheck

REC recommend

REE resting energy expenditure

Regurg regurgitation

Rehab rehabilitation

REM rapid eye movement

REMS rapid eye movement sleep

REP repeat

RES resident; reticuloendothelial system

Resp. respirations

Retic reticulocyte

REV review

RF rheumatic fever; rheumatoid factor

Rh Rhesus factor in blood

RHD rheumatic heart disease

rHmEPO recombinant human erythropoietin

RIA radioimmunoassay

R→L right to left

RL Ringer's lactate

RLD related living donor

RLE right lower extremity

RLL right lower lobe

RLQ right lower quadrant

RM room

RMSF Rocky Mountain spotted fever

RN Registered Nurse

RO routine order

R/O rule out

ROM range of motion; right otitis media; rupture of membranes

RoRx radiation therapy

ROS review of systems

R.Ph. Registered Pharmacist

RPT Registered Physical Therapist

RQ respiratory quotient

RR recovery room

R/R rales-rhonchi

R&R rate and rhythm

RS renal scan

RSR regular sinus rhythm

RSV respiratory syncytial virus

RT radiographic tech; respiratory therapist; right

RTA renal tubular acidosis

RTC return to clinic

rtPA recombinant tissue plasminogen activator

RTx radiation therapy; renal transplant

RU routine urinalysis

RUA routine urine analysis

RUL   right upper lobe

RUQ   right upper quadrant

RV   right ventricle

RVH   right ventricular hypertrophy

S

S   second(s); subjective findings; suction; sulfur

s̄   without

S₁   first heart sound

S₂   second heart sound

S₃   third heart sound (ventricular gallop)

S₄   fourth heart sound (atrial gallop)

S₁–S₅   sacral vertebra 1 through 5

SA   salicylic acid; sinoatrial; surface area; sustained action

SAD   seasonal affective disorder

SAH   subarachnoid hemorrhage

Sang   sanguinous

SAT   saturated; saturation; Saturday

SB   sinus bradycardia; small bowel; spina bifida

SBA   serum bactericidal activity

SBFT   small bowel follow through

SBO   small bowel obstruction

SBP   systolic blood pressure

SC   subcutaneous

SCC   squamous cell carcinoma

SCCa   squamous cell carcinoma

SCI   spinal cord injury

SCID   severe combined immunodeficiency disorders

SCIO   severe combined immunodeficiency syndrome

SCr   serum creatinine

SD   septal defect

SDH   subdural hematoma

SE   side effect

Se   selenium

Sec   second

SED   sedimentation

SEG   segment

SF   spinal fluid; sugar free

SG   serum glucose; specific gravity; Swan-Ganz

SGA   small for gestational age

SGOT   serum glutamic oxaloacetic transaminase (see AST)

SGPT   serum glutamic pyruvic transaminase (see ALT)

SH   social history

SI   International System of Units

SIADH   syndrome of inappropriate antidiuretic hormone secretion

SIDS   sudden infant death syndrome

Sig. let it be marked

SIM Similac®

SL sublingual

SLE systemic lupus erythematosus

Sl. tr. slight trace

SLUD salivation, lacrimation, urination, and defecation

SM small

SMA sequential multiple analyzer; simultaneous multichannel auto-analyzer

SMZ sulfamethoxazole SUZ/TMP

SNP sodium nitroprusside

SOAP subjective, objective, assessment, and plan

SOB shortness of breath

SOM serous otitis media

S/P status post

SPA albumin human (formerly known as salt-poor albumin)

SPF split products of fibrin; sun protective factor

SQ subcutaneous

SR sinus rhythm; sustained release

SROM spontaneous rupture of membrane

SRT sustained release theophylline

SS half; sliding scale

S&S signs and symptoms

SSKI saturated solution of potassium iodide

SSS sick sinus syndrome

S/SX signs/symptoms

ST sinus tachycardia; skin test

stab. polymorphonuclear leukocytes

staph *Staphylococcus aureus*

STAT immediately

STD sexually transmitted diseases

STD TF standard tube feeding

STG split thickness graft

STI soft tissue injury

Strep *streptococcus*

STSG split thickness skin graft

SUBL sublingual

Subcu subcutaneous

sub q subcutaneous

SUP superior

supp suppository

SVPB supraventricular premature beat

SVPC supraventricular premature contraction

SVR supraventricular rhythm systemic vascular resistance

SVT supraventricular tachycardia

SWOG Southwest Oncology Group

Sx signs; symptoms

syr syrup

SYS BP systolic blood pressure

SZ seizure

T

3TC lamivudine

T tablespoon (15 mL); tender

T$_{1/2}$ half-life

T3 Tylenol® with codeine 30 mg

T$_3$ triiodothyronine

T$_4$ levothyroxine

T&A tonsillectomy and adenoidectomy

TAB tablet

TAC tetracaine, adrenalin, and cocaine

TAH total abdominal hysterectomy

TAHBSO total abdominal hysterectomy, bilateral salpingo-oophorectomy

TAO troleandomycin

TB tuberculosis

TBA to be added; to be admitted; total body (surface) area

TBG thyroxine-binding globulin

T bili total bilirubin

tbl. tablespoon (15 mL)

TBR total bed rest

Tbsp tablespoon (15 mL)

TBW total body water

TC throat culture; tissue culture

T&C type and crossmatch

T&C#3 Tylenol® with 30 mg codeine

TCA tricyclic antidepressant

T cell T-lymphocyte

TCN tetracycline

TD tardive dyskinesia; tetanus-diphtheria toxoid (pediatric use)

Td tetanus-diphtheria toxoid (adult type)

TDD thoracic duct drainage

TDM therapeutic drug monitoring

TDNTG transdermal nitroglycerin

TE trace elements; tracheoesophageal

TEDS® Anti-embolism Stockings

TEE transesophageal echocardiography

TEN® Total Enteral Nutrition

TENS transcutaneous electrical nerve stimulation (stimulator)

TERB terbutaline

TF tube feeding

TFTs thyroid function tests

TG triglycerides

6-TG thioguanine

TGA transposition of the great arteries

TH total hysterectomy

THAM® tromethamine

THC tetrahydrocannabinol (dronabinol)

TH CULT throat culture

THR total hip replacement

TI tricuspid insufficiency

TIA transient ischemic attack

TIBC total iron-binding capacity

TID three times a day

TIG tetanus immune globulin

tinct tincture

+tive positive

TIW three times a week

TKA total knee arthroplasty

TKO to keep open

TKR total knee replacement

TKVO to keep vein open

TLC tender loving care; total lung capacity; total lymphocyte count; triple lumen catheter

TM Thayer Martin (culture); tympanic membrane

TMJ temporomandibular joint

TMP trimethoprim

TMP/SMX trimethoprim sulfamethoxazole

TNA total nutrient admixture

TNF tumor necrosis factor

TNG nitroglycerin

TO telephone order

TOA tubo-ovarian abscess

TOF tetralogy of Fallot

TOGV transposition of the great vessels

Tomo tomography

TOPV trivalent oral polio vaccine

TORCH toxoplasmosis, other (syphilis, hepatitis, Zoster), rubella, cytomegalovirus, and herpes simplex (maternal infections)

TOTBILI total bilirubin

TP total protein

tPA alteplase, recombinant (tissue plasminogen activator); total parenteral alimentation

TPN total parenteral nutrition

TP & P time, place, and person

TPR temperature, pulse, and respiration

T PROT total protein

TR trace

TRA to run at

trach. tracheal

TRH protirelin (thyrotropin-releasing hormone)

TSF triceps skin fold

TSH thyroid-stimulating hormone

TSP teaspoon; total serum protein

TT tetanus toxoid; thrombin time

TTE transthoracic echocardiograph

TTP thrombotic thrombocytopenic purpura

TU tuberculin units

TUN total urinary nitrogen

TURBT transurethral resection bladder tumor

TURP transurethral resection of prostate

TV television; tidal volume

TVH total vaginal hysterectomy

TW tap water

TWE tap water enema

Tx therapy; transfer; transfuse; transplant; treatment

T & X type and crossmatch

Tyl Tylenol®

U

U ultralente insulin; units

UA umbilical artery; uric acid; urinalysis

UAC umbilical artery catheter

UC ulcerative colitis; urine culture

UCHD usual childhood diseases

UCX urine culture

UD as directed

UE upper extremity

UES upper esophageal sphincter

UFH unfractionated heparin

UGDP University Group Diabetes Project

UGI upper gastrointestinal series

UGISBFT upper gastrointestinal small bowel follow through

UK unknown

ULQ upper left quadrant

ULYTES electrolytes, urine

umb ven umbilical vein

UNa urine sodium

ung ointment

UNK unknown

UO urinary output

Uosm urinary osmolality

✓ up check up

U/P ratio urine to plasma ratio

UR utilization review

Urol urology

URTI upper respiratory tract infection

US ultrasonography

USN ultrasonic nebulizer

USP United States Pharmacopeia

USPHS United States Public Health Service

ut dict as directed

UTI urinary tract infection

UV ultraviolet

UVA ultraviolet A light

UVB ultraviolet B light

V

V five

x Ventilation (L/min)

VA valproic acid; Veterans Administration

vag. vagina

VAG HYST vaginal hysterectomy

VAH Veterans Administration Hospital

VATER vertebral, anal, tracheal, esophageal, and renal anomalies

VBG venous blood gas; vertical banded gastroplasty

VBL vinblastine

VC vena cava; vital capacity

VCR vincristine sulfate

VCU voiding cystourethrogram

VD venereal disease

Vd volume of distribution

V&D vomiting and diarrhea

Vdg voiding

VDRL Venereal Disease Research Laboratory (syphilis test)

VENT ventilation; ventilator

VF ventricular fibrillation

V. Fib ventricular fibrillation

VG very good

VI six

vib vibration

VIP etopside, ifosfamide, and cisplatin; vasoactive intestinal peptide

VIT vitamin

vit. cap. vital capacity

VLDL very low density lipoprotein

VM26 teniposide

VMA vanillylmandelic acid

VO verbal order

VOCAB vocabulary

VOL volume

VP etoposide

VP-16 etoposide

VPC ventricular premature contractions

VQ ventilation perfusion

VRI viral respiratory infection

VS versus; vital signs

VT; v. tach. ventricular tachycardia

VWD von Willebrand's disease

VWF von Willebrand's factor

VZ varicella zoster

VZIG varicella zoster immune globulin

VZV varicella zoster virus

W

w week; weight

WA while awake

WB weight bearing

WBC white blood cell (count)

WBE whole blood electrolytes

W Bld whole blood

WBN wellborn nursery

WC ward clerk; white count; whooping cough

WD well developed

W→D   wet to dry

WDM   white divorced male

WDWN-BF   well-developed, well-nourished black female

WDWN-BM   well-developed, well-nourished black male

WDWN-WF   well-developed, well-nourished white female

WDWN-WM   well-developed, well-nourished white male

WE   weekend

WF   white female

wgt   weight

W/I   within

wk   week

WK   week

WM   white male

WMF   white married female

WMM   white married male

WN   well nourished

WND   wound

W/O   water in oil; without

WPW   Wolff-Parkinson-White

WT   weight (wt)

W/U   workup

W/V   weight to volume ratio

X

X   cross; crossmatch; times

$\overline{x}$ except

X3   orientation as to time, place, and person

X-ed   crossed

XKO   not knocked out

XR   x-ray

XRT   radiation therapy

XV   fifteen

Z

Z-E   Zollinger-Ellison (syndrome)

ZIG   zoster serum immune globulin

ZnO   zinc oxide

Other Notations

$\pm$ either positive or negative; plus or minus

$>$ greater than

$\geq$ greater than or equal to

$<$ caused by; less than

$\uparrow$ elevated; increase

$\downarrow$ decrease; falling

$\rightarrow$ causes to; results in

$\leftarrow$ resulted from

$\downarrow\downarrow$ flexor; testes descended

$\uparrow\uparrow$ extensor; positive Babinski; testes undescended

$\checkmark$ check

\#   number; pound

$\therefore$ therefore

+ plus; positive; present

− absent; minus; negative

/ slash mark signifying per, and, or, with

? questionable

∅ no; not

@ at

1° first degree; primary

2° second degree

3° third degree

♂ male

♀ female

■ deceased male

● deceased female

□ living male

○ living female; standing position; recumbent position; sitting position

M μ micro; mu

′ feet; minutes (as in 30′)

″ inches; seconds

2 × 2 gauze dressing folded 2″ × 2″

4 × 4 gauze dressing folded 4″ × 4″

Note: There are many individual variations as to how these are arranged. By knowing normal values, most of these variations can be readily identified.

140	100	20			NA	Cl	BUN	
3.8	28	105			K	CO₂	CR	*glucose*

Na = 140, Cl = 100, BUN = 20, K = 3.8, CO₂ = 28, glucose = 105

$$\frac{sodium}{potassium} \quad \frac{chloride}{bicarbonate} \quad \frac{BUN}{creatinine} \quad glucose$$

$$\frac{calcium}{phosphorus} \quad \frac{protein}{albumin} \quad \frac{AST}{ALT} \quad \frac{LDH}{Alkalinephos} \quad bilirubin$$

segmented neutrophils	lymphocytes	eosinophils
banded neutrophils	monocytes	basophils

hemoglobin	WBC
hematocrit	platelets

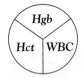

REFERENCES

1. Chabner DE. Medical Technology: A Short Course. Philadelphia, PA: W.B. Saunders Co; 1991:156–220.

2. Steves N, Adler J. Introduction to Medical Terminology. Spring-house, PA: Springhouse; 1992:252–260.

3. Austrin MG, Austrin HR. Learning Medical Terminology. St. Louis, MO: Mosby Year Book; 1991:456–461.

4. Bergman HD. Medical Terminology. US Pharm; 1980;1:42–48.

5. Davis NM. Medical Abbreviations: 7000 Conveniences at the Expense of Communication & Safety. Huntington Valley, PA: Davis Associates; 1991.

Appendix II:
Common Anatomic Terms

Anatomic Planes

Frontal (Coronal Plane). An imaginary line that divides an organ or the body into front and back portions or anterior and posterior portions.

Median (Midsagittal, Midline) Plane. An imaginary plane that passes from the front to the back through the center of the body and divides the body into right and left equal portions.

Sagittal Plane. An imaginary line that divides an organ or the body into a right and left portion.

Transverse Plane. An imaginary line that divides an organ or the body into upper (cranial) and lower (caudal) portions.

Anatomic Positions

Erect. Standing position.

Knee-Chest (Genupectoral). Kneeling with chest resting on same surface.

Lateral Recumbent (Sim's). Lying on left side with thigh and knee drawn up.

Prone. Lying face down.

Reverse Trendelenburg. Lying supine with the *head tilted upward* 45° or less.

Supine (Dorsal). Lying on the back.

Trendelenburg Position. Lying supine with the *head tilted downward* 45° or less.

Regions of the Body
Chest and Abdomen

Axillary. Axillary (ampit) and its borders.

Clavicular. Region on either side of the sternum (breastbone), extending the length of the clavicles (collarbones).

Epigastric. Upper mid area of the abdomen.

Hypochondrium. Right and left areas of the epigastric region.

Hypogastric. Middle region of the lower portion of the abdomen.

Infraclavicular. Region below the clavicles.

Infraspinous. Located below a spinous process.

Infrasternal. Located below the sternum.

Inguinal (Iliac). On either side of the hypogastric region, triangular in shape, also known as the groin area.

Lateral Abdominal. Lying on either side of the umbilical region.

Mammary. Area relating to the breasts.

Pubic. Area near the pubic bone.

Sternal. Region over the front of the sternum.

Subclavian. Region beneath the clavicle.

Subdiaphragmatic (Subphrenic). Located below the diaphragm.

Sublingual. Just below the inguinal region.

Supraclavicular. Area above the clavicles.

Suprapubic. Region above the pubic area.

Umbilicus. Umbilical area of the abdomen.

Head

Auricular. Located around the ears.

Buccal. Region pertaining to the cheeks.

Infraorbital. Located immediately beneath or in the floor of the eye.

Mental. Region of the chin.

Occipital. Area relating to the lower back of the head.

Orbital. Region around the orbit or eyes.

Sublingual. Region located beneath the tongue.

Submandibular. Region below the lower jaw.

Submaxillary. Region below the upper jaw.

Submental. Region below the chin.

Supraorbital. Region above the eyebrows.

Posterior Trunk

Coxal. Area just below the lumbar regions in the back and lateral abdominal regions on either side, they are bordered by gluteal regions (area over the buttocks).

Infrascapular. Area below scapulae (shoulder blades), extending down to the last ribs.

Loin. Part and sides of the body between the ribs and pelvis.

Lumbar. Region immediately below the infrascapular region, extending down to the crest of the ilium.

Medial Region of Back. Central zone of the back, extending from the neck as far down as the base of the sacrum.

Nuchal. Area located at the back of the neck.

Sacroiliac. Area over the sacrum at the base of the median region.

Scapular. Areas on either side covering the scapula.

Suprascapular Region. Region above or in the upper part of the scapula.

Terms for Determining Directions

Abduction. Movement away from the body midline.

Adduction. Movement toward the midline or beyond the body midline.

Anterior. At or near the ventral (front) surface of the body.

Caudal. Towards the lower end of the body (cauda means tail).

Cavity. A hollow part or space in a structure.

Central. Toward the center of the body.

Cranial (Cephalic). Toward the head.

Distal. Away from the point of origin or away from the body.

Eversion. A turning outward.

Extension. The straightening of a limb.

External. Outside.

Flexion. The bending of a limb so that the proximal and distal parts are brought together.

Inferior. Below or beneath some part of a structure.

Internal. Inside.

Inversion. A turning inward.

Lateral. Farther from the midline or to the side of the body.

Medial. Near to or toward the midline.

Palmer. Involving the palm of the hand.

Peripheral. Away from the center of the body.

Posterior. At or near the dorsal (back) surface of the body.

Proximal. Nearest to the point of attachment or to the point of origin.

Superior. Above or over some part of a structure.

Supination. Turning the palmar side upward.

Index

Note: Page numbers in *italics* denote figures; those followed by t denote tables; and those followed by b denote boxed material.